SOCIAL
ADMINISTRATION

THE MANAGEMENT OF THE SOCIAL SERVICES

SOCIAL
ADMINISTRATION

THE MANAGEMENT OF
THE SOCIAL SERVICES

7607

EDITED BY

SIMON SLAVIN

Published jointly by

THE HAWORTH PRESS

NEW YORK

and

COUNCIL ON SOCIAL WORK EDUCATION

NEW YORK

The opinions expressed in this publication are solely those of the contributors and do not necessarily reflect the policy or position of the Council on Social Work Education. No official endorsement of the views presented should be inferred unless it is so indicated.

HV
41
.S6 18

© 1978 by The Haworth Press. All rights reserved. No part of this book may be reproduced in any form or by any means without permission in writing from the publisher.
The Haworth Press, 149 Fifth Avenue, New York, New York 10010
Council on Social Work Education, 345 East 46th Street,
New York, New York 10017
ISBN 0-917724-01-1 *Cloth*
ISBN 0-917724-02-X *Paper*
Library of Congress Catalog Card Number 77-88090
Printed in the United States of America

To Jean
    Rayna
    Vicky
    Johanna

CONTENTS

PART III

SOME ORGANIZATIONAL PERSPECTIVES

PART IV

THE STRUCTURE AND USES OF AUTHORITY

A. THE GOVERNING BOARDS

B. EXECUTIVE AUTHORITY

C. BOARD–EXECUTIVE RELATIONSHIPS

PART V

RESOURCES—ALLOCATION, CONTROL, AND ACCOUNTABILITY

A. BUDGETING

B. PROGRAM BUDGETING AND COST ANALYSIS

C. MANAGEMENT BY OBJECTIVES

D. ZERO-BASE BUDGETING

E. ACCOUNTABILITY

F. SYSTEMS ANALYSIS

PART VI

ADMINISTERING SOCIAL SERVICE PERSONNEL

A. SOCIAL SERVICE MANPOWER

PART VII

SOCIAL SERVICE INFORMATION SYSTEMS

THE AUTHORS

ELIZABETH ANGELL, Regional Business Administrator, East St. Louis Region, State of Illinois, Department of Children and Family Services, Chicago, Illinois, at the time this paper was written.

ALOYSIUS J. BECKER, M.S.W., ACSW, Regional Social Service Administrator, East St. Louis Region, State of Illinois, Department of Children and Family Services, Chicago, Illinois, at the time this paper was written.

CHERYL BLACKBURN, Director of Emergency Services, Dede Wallace Center, Nashville, Tennessee, at the time this paper was written.

GEORGE BRAGER, PH.D., Professor, School of Social Work, Columbia University, New York, New York.

THOMAS L. BRIGGS, M.S.S., Professor and Director of the Division of Continuing Education and Manpower Development, School of Social Work, Syracuse University, Syracuse, New York.

SHIRLEY M. BUTTRICK, D.S.W., Dean, Jane Addams College of Social Work, University of Illinois at Chicago Circle, Chicago, Illinois.

H. R. CATHERWOOD, Principal, Kansas-Denver Associates, Denver, Colorado.

STEPHEN R. CHITWOOD, M.P.A., PH.D., J.D., Associate Professor of Public Administration, School of Government and Business Administration, George Washington University, Washington, D.C.

JUDITH CINGOLANI, M.S.W., Regional Social Service Specialist, East St. Louis Region, State of Illinois, Department of Children and Family Services, Chicago, Illinois, at the time this paper was written.

JACK M. DONAHUE, M.S.W., ACSW, Assistant Deputy Director, Program Operations, Cook County, State of Illinois, Department of Children and Family Services, Chicago, Illinois.

KENNETH P. FALLON, JR., M.S.W., Psychotherapist, Langdon Clinic, Anchorage, Alaska.

MALVERN J. GROSS, C.P.A., Partner, Price Waterhouse & Co., Washington, D.C.

MURRAY GRUBER, D.S.W., Associate Professor, School of Social Work, University of Michigan, Ann Arbor, Michigan.

BURTON GUMMER, PH.D., Associate Professor, School of Social Welfare, State University of New York at Albany, Albany, New York.

ARCHIE HANLAN, Associate Professor, Department of Social Work, University of Pennsylvania, Philadelphia, Pennsylvania, at the time this paper was written.

MARY S. HANLAN, ACSW, Director of Consultation and Education, West Philadelphia Community Mental Health Consortium, Inc., Philadelphia, Pennsylvania.

ADAM W. HERBERT, PH.D., Director of Research, Joint Center for Political Studies, Washington, D.C.

GEORGE HOSHINO, D.S.W., Professor, School of Social Work, University of Minnesota, Minneapolis, Minnesota.

HOWARD HUSH, Executive Director, Family Service of Detroit and Wayne Counties, Detroit, Michigan (ret.).

JOSEPH H. KAHLE, M.S.W., Executive Director, Family and Child Service of Metropolitan Seattle, Seattle, Washington.

JOEL KOTIN, M.D., Assistant Adjunct Professor, Department of Psychiatry and Human Behavior, University of California at Irvine, Irvine, California, and in the private practice of psychiatry in Orange, California.

ABRAHAM S. LEVINE, PH.D., Division of Intramural Research, Office of Research and Demonstrations, Social and Rehabilitation Service, United States Department of Health, Education and Welfare, Washington, D.C.

HAROLD LEWIS, D.S.W., ACSW, Dean, School of Social Work, Hunter College, City University of New York, New York.

CATHERINE LOVELL, PH.D., Assistant Professor, Graduate School of Administration, University of California, Riverside, California.

THOMAS MC DONALD, M.S.W., Research Associate, School of Social Work, University of Wisconsin-Madison, Madison, Wisconsin.

RODERICK K. MACLEOD, Partner, Coopers & Lybrand, San Francisco, California.

DARYL G. MITTON, B.CH.E., M.B.A., PH.D., Professor of Management, San Diego State University, San Diego, California.

SCOTT MULLIS, PH.D., Director, Office of Technical Services Support, Bureau of Police, Portland, Oregon.

MARILYN NELSON, M.S.W., Regional Social Service Specialist, East St. Louis Region, State of Illinois, Department of Children and Family Services, Chicago, Illinois, at the time this paper was written.

BERNARD NEUGEBOREN, Chairman, Administration Sequence, Graduate School of Social Work, Rutgers—The State University, New Brunswick, New Jersey.

EDWARD NEWMAN, PH.D., Professor, School of Social Administration, Temple University, Philadelphia, Pennsylvania.

EDWARD J. O'DONNELL, Consultant, United States Department of Health, Education and Welfare, at the time this paper was written.

JOSEPH A. OLMSTEAD, PH.D., Director, Columbus, Georgia Research Office, Human Resources Research Organization, Columbus, Georgia.

RINO J. PATTI, D.S.W., Professor, School of Social Work, University of Washington, Seattle, Washington.

FELICE PERLMUTTER, PH.D., Professor, School of Social Administration, Temple University, Philadelphia, Pennsylvania.

IRVING PILIAVIN, D.S.W., Professor, School of Social Work, University of Wisconsin-Madison, Madison, Wisconsin.

MELVYN C. RAIDER, PH.D., Associate Professor and Assistant to the Dean, School of Social Work, Wayne State University, Detroit, Michigan.

OTTO M. REID, PH.D., Chief, Division of Health Services Research and Demonstrations, Health Care Financing Administration, Washington, D.C.

ARTHUR J. ROBINS, PH.D., Professor, Department of Psychiatry, University of Missouri-Columbia, Columbia, Missouri.

GEORGE E. ROSS, PH.D., Salem Area Administrator, State of Illinois, Department of Children and Family Services, Chicago, Illinois.

MYRON R. SHARAF, PH.D., Research Psychologist, Boston State Hospital, and Assistant Professor of Psychiatry, Tufts University School of Medicine, Boston, Massachusetts.

LAWRENCE C. SHULMAN, M.S.W., Divisional Director, Department of Social Work Services, Long Island Jewish-Hillside Medical Center, New Hyde Park, New York.

SIMON SLAVIN, ED.D., Dean, School of Social Administration, Temple University, Philadelphia, Pennsylvania.

IRVING A. SPERGEL, D.S.W., Professor, School of Social Service Administration, The University of Chicago, Chicago, Illinois.

HERMAN D. STEIN, D.S.W., University Professor, Case Western Reserve University, Cleveland, Ohio.

MILTON TAMBOR, M.S.W., Institute of Labor and Industrial Relations, Wayne State University, Detroit, Michigan, and Union President, Local 1640, American Federation of State, County, and Municipal Employees, Council 77, AFL-CIO, Detroit, Michigan, at the time this paper was written.

JERRY TUREM, PH.D., Project Director, Social Services Research Program, The Urban Institute, Washington, D.C., at the time this paper was written.

MARGO L. VIGNOLA, Senior Policy Analyst, American Public Welfare Association, Washington, D.C.

COLIN WHITTINGTON, M.A., Lecturer in Social Work Studies, Department of Sociology and Psychology, Chelsea College, University of London, London, England.

VERNON R. WIEHE, PH.D., Associate Dean, College of Social Professions, University of Kentucky, Lexington, Kentucky.

DAVID W. YOUNG, D.B.A., Assistant Professor, School of Public Health, Harvard University, Cambridge, Massachusetts.

ACKNOWLEDGMENTS

PART I

Lewis, H. Management in the Nonprofit Social Service Organization.
Reprinted with permission of the author and the Child Welfare League of America, Inc. from Child Welfare, Vol. LIV, No. 9, November 1975, pp. 615–623.

Gummer, B. Social Planning and Social Administration: Implications for Curriculum Development.
Reprinted with permission of the author and the Council on Social Work Education from Journal of Education for Social Work, Vol. 11, No. 1, Winter 1975, pp. 63–73.

Spergel, I. A. Social Development and Social Work.
Reprinted with permission of the author from Administration in Social Work, Vol. 1, No. 3, Fall 1977, in press.

PART II

Mullis, S. Management Applications to the Welfare System.
Reprinted with permission of the author and the American Public Welfare Association from Public Welfare, Vol. 33, No. 4, Fall 1975, pp. 31–34.

Hanlan, A. From Social Work to Social Administration.
Reprinted with permission of the publishers from Social Work Practice, 1970. Copyright © 1970 by National Conference on Social Welfare. New York: Columbia University Press, 1970, pp. 41–53.

Neugeboren, B. Developing Specialized Programs in Social Work Administration in the Master's Degree Program: Field Practice Component.
Reprinted with permission of the author and the Council on Social Work Education from Journal of Education for Social Work, Vol. 7, No. 3, Fall 1971, pp. 35–48.

PART III

Whittington, C. Organizational Research and Social Work: Issues in Application Illustrated from the Case of Organic and Mechanistic Systems of Management.
Reprinted with permission of the author and the British Association of Social Workers from British Journal of Social Work, Vol. 5, No. 1, Spring 1975, pp. 59–73.

Olmstead, J. A. Organizational Factors in the Performance of Social Welfare and Rehabilitation Workers.
Reprinted with permission of the author from Working Papers No. 1: National Study
of Social Welfare and Rehabilitation Workers, Work and Organizational Contexts.
Washington, D.C.: U.S. Department of Health, Education and Welfare, 1971, pp.
89–103; 126–130.

PART IV

Mitton, D. G. Utilizing the Board of Trustees: A Unique Structural Design.
Reprinted with permission of the author and the Child Welfare League of America, Inc.
from Child Welfare, Vol. LIII, No. 6, June 1974, pp. 345–351.

Robins, A. J., and Blackburn, C. Governing Boards in Mental Health: Roles and Train-
ing Needs.
Reprinted with permission of the senior author from Administration in Public Health,
Summer 1974, pp. 37–45.

O'Donnell, E. J., and Reid, O. M. Citizen Participation on Public Welfare Boards and
Committees.
Reprinted with permission of the second author from Welfare in Review, Vol. 9, No. 5,
September/October 1971, pp. 1–9.

Kotin, J., and Sharaf, M. R. Management Succession and Administrative Style.
Copyright © 1967 by the William Alanson White Psychiatric Foundation, Inc. Reprinted with permission of the senior author and by special permission of the copyright holder, The William Alanson White Psychiatric Foundation, Inc. from Psychiatry, Vol. 30, 1967, pp. 237–248.

Fallon, K. P., Jr. Participatory Management: An Alternative in Human Service Delivery
Systems.
Reprinted with permission of the author and the Child Welfare League of America,
Inc. from Child Welfare, Vol. LIII, No. 9, November 1974, pp. 555–562.

Kahle, J. H. Assessing Executive Performance.
Reprinted with permission of the author and the Family Service Association of America
from Social Casework, Vol. 52, No. 2, February 1971, pp. 79–85.

Herbert, A. W. The Minority Administrator: Problems, Prospects, and Challenges.
Reprinted with permission of the author and the American Society of Public Administration from Public Administration Review, November/December 1974, pp. 556–563.

Hanlan, M. S. Women in Social Work Administration: Current Role Strains.
Reprinted with permission of the author from Administration in Social Work, Vol. 1,
No. 3, Fall 1977, in press.

Stein, H. D. Board, Executive, and Staff.
Reprinted with permission of the author and the publishers from The Social Welfare
Forum, 1962. Copyright © 1962 by National Conference on Social Welfare. New
York: Columbia University Press, 1962, pp. 215–230.

Perlmutter, F. Citizen Participation and Professionalism: A Developmental Relationship.
Reprinted with permission of the author and the American Public Welfare Association
from Public Welfare, Vol. 31, No. 3, Summer 1973, pp. 25–28.

PART V

Gross, M. J. The Importance of Budgeting.
Reprinted with permission of the author and The Ronald Press Company from Financial and Accounting Guide for Nonprofit Organizations, Second Edition, pp. 293–308. Copyright © 1974, The Ronald Press Company, New York.

Macleod, R. K. Program Budgeting Works in Nonprofit Institutions.
Reprinted with permission of the author and the copyright holder from Harvard Business Review, September/October 1971, pp. 46–56. Copyright © 1971 by the President and Fellows of Harvard College; all rights reserved.

Levine, A. S. Cost-Benefit Analysis and Social Welfare Program Evaluation.
Reprinted with permission of the author and the copyright holder from Social Service Review, Vol. 12, No. 2, June 1968, pp. 173–183. Copyright © 1968 by The University of Chicago Press.

Wiehe, V. R. Management by Objectives in a Family Service Agency.
Reprinted with permission of the author and the Family Service Association of America from Social Casework, Vol. 54, No. 3, March 1973, pp. 142–146.

Raider, M. C. Installing Management by Objectives in Social Agencies.
Reprinted with permission of the author from Administration in Social Work, Vol. 1, No. 3, Fall 1977, in press.

Vignola, M. L. The Latest in Federal Spending Control: Zero-Base Budgeting.
Reprinted with permission of the editor from Washington Report, Vol. 11, No. 8, September 1976, p. 1–4. Washington, D.C.: American Public Welfare Association.

Hoshino, G. Social Services: The Problem of Accountability.
Reprinted with permission of the author and the copyright holder from Social Service Review, Vol. 47, No. 3, September 1973, pp. 373–383. Copyright © 1973 by The University of Chicago Press.

Newman, E., and Turem, J. The Crisis of Accountability.
Reprinted with permission of the National Association of Social Workers from Social Work, Vol. 19, No. 1, January 1974, pp. 5–16.

Chitwood, S. R. Social Equity and Social Service Productivity.
Reprinted with permission of the author and the American Society for Public Administration from Public Administration Review, January/February 1974, pp. 29–35.

Piliavin, I., and McDonald, T. On the Fruits of Evaluative Research for the Social Services.
Reprinted with permission of the senior author from Administration in Social Work, Vol. 1, No. 1, Spring 1977, pp. 63–70.

Patti, R. The New Scientific Management: Systems Management for Social Welfare.
Reprinted with permission of the author and the American Public Welfare Association from Public Welfare, Vol. 33, No. 2, Spring 1975, pp. 23–31.

Gruber, M. Total Administration.
Reprinted with permission of the author and the National Association of Social Workers from Social Work, Vol. 19, No. 5, September 1974, pp. 625–636.

PART VI

National Association of Social Workers. Standards for Social Service Manpower.
   Reprinted with permission of the National Association of Social Workers from Standards for Social Service Manpower. Washington, D.C.: National Association of Social Workers, 1973, pp. 4–19.

Briggs, T. L. A Critique of the NASW Manpower Statement.
   Reprinted with permission of the author and the Council on Social Work Education from Journal of Education for Social Work, Vol. 11, No. 1, Winter 1975, pp. 9–15.

Slavin, S., and Perlmutter, F. Perspectives for Education and Training.
   Reprinted with permission of the authors and Columbia University Press from A Design for Social Work Practice. New York: Columbia University Press, 1974, pp. 243–265.

National Association of Social Workers. NASW Standards for Social Work Personnel Practices.
   Reprinted with permission of the National Association of Social Workers from NASW Standards for Social Work Personnel Practices. Washington, D.C.: National Association of Social Workers, 1971, pp. 9–10; 23–32.

Buttrick, S. M. Affirmative Action and Job Security: Policy Dilemmas.
   Reprinted with permission of the author and the publisher from The Social Welfare Forum, 1976, copyright © 1977 National Conference on Social Welfare. New York: Columbia University Press, 1977, pp. 116–125.

Lovell, C. Three Key Issues in Affirmative Action.
   Reprinted with permission of the author and the American Society for Public Administration from Public Administration Review, Vol. 34, No. 3, May/June 1974, pp. 235–237.

Tambor, M. Unions and Voluntary Agencies.
   Reprinted with permission of the National Association of Social Workers from Social Work, Vol. 18, No. 4, July 1973, pp. 41–47.

Shulman, L. C. Unionization and the Professional Employee: The Social Service Directors View.
   Reprinted with permission of the author from a paper presented at a meeting for Directors of Social Service Departments, Carnegie Endowment Center, New York, New York, March 11, 1970.

Hush, H. Collective Bargaining in Voluntary Agencies.
   Reprinted with permission of the author and the Family Service Association of America from Social Casework, Vol. 50, No. 4, April 1969, pp. 210–213.

PART VII

Donahue, J. M., Angell, E., Becker, A. J., Cingolani, J., Nelson, M., and Ross, G. E. The Social Service Information System.
   Reprinted with permission of the senior author and the Child Welfare League of America, Inc. from Child Welfare, Vol. LIII, No. 4, Spring 1974, pp. 243–255.

Catherwood, H. R. A Management Information System for Social Services.
Reprinted with permission of the author and the American Public Welfare Association
from Public Welfare, Vol. 32, No. 3, Summer 1974, pp. 54–61.

Young, D. W. Management Information Systems in Child Care: An Agency Experience.
Reprinted with permission of the author and the Child Welfare League of America,
Inc. from Child Welfare, Vol. LIII, No. 2, February 1974, pp. 102–111.

PART VIII

Slavin, S. Concepts of Social Conflict: Use in Social Work Curriculum.
Reprinted with permission of the Council on Social Work Education from Journal of
Education for Social Work, Vol. 5, No. 2, Fall 1969, pp. 47–60.

Patti, R. J. Organizational Resistance and Change: The View from Below.
Reprinted with permission of the author and the copyright holder from Social Service
Review, Vol. 8, No. 3, September 1974, pp. 367–383. Copyright © 1974 by The
University of Chicago Press.

Brager, G. Helping vs. Influencing: Some Political Elements of Organizational Change.
Reprinted with permission of the author from a paper presented at the National Conference on Social Welfare, San Francisco, California, May 1975.

PREFACE

The past few years were witness to an escalation of interest in the administration of the social services. The enormous expansion of these services in the last decade, and the pressure from unsympathetic administrations to contain the public expenditures they called forth, led to a call for more efficient management and more clearly delineated accountability. Federal grants were made to several schools of social work and to the Council on Social Work Education for the purpose of furthering the study and development of curricula in administration and management, with special encouragement to engage in cooperative activity with schools of business administration and departments of public administration.

The growth in programs and enrollment in social administration, the development of joint degrees between graduate schools of social work and business and public administration, and the appearance of a new professional journal devoted to the management of the social services all attest to this new focus on an old subject. After all, administration may be the oldest of the practices in social work—the first social agency surely had to be administered.

For all its importance to the social services, the literature on its administration is relatively scanty and sporadic. Full treatment of the subject in the United States is contained in a mere handful of books that appeared during the past four decades. Works by Atwater (1940), Trecker (1946), and Street (1947) were published in the forties. In 1950, Trecker revised and enlarged his slim volume, and in 1959, Spencer prepared the Council on Social Work Education's Curriculum Study volume on administration. Nothing seems to have appeared during the next decade on this subject. The sixties seemed preoccupied with community action and organization following upon the national effort to deal with delinquency and poverty.

In 1970, the Council on Social Work Education published two volumes edited by Schatz, a reader and casebook. One year later, Trecker (1971) recast his former work and produced the only conventional text now available. More recently, Ehlers, Austin, and Prothero (1976) published a programmed text.

The periodical literature on administration of the social services, however, has grown noticeably during the past ten years. In looking for recent material to include in courses on administration, the thought occurred to the editor to compile the most notable writings that have appeared during the past decade reflecting the preoccupation of administrators and educators with current processes and practices in social service management. New subject matter appeared on the scene, i.e., affirmative action and zero-base budgeting; and older content took on new meaning, i.e., collective bargaining in public social agencies and management information processes. There appeared to be a significant enough corpus of material prepared by, for, and about practitioners in the human services in the context of the social service system to warrant the appearance of a new volume.*

The material that follows is intended to reflect the "state of the art" in the administration and management of the social services. It is necessary, then, to set forth the boundaries of the field to which it is addressed, and indicate the concept of administrative practice that ties together the many ideas found in these selections. Implicit in this effort is the idea that social administration is a definable and distinctive field, comparable to such kindred enterprises as educational administration and health administration. In spite of elements of overlap in all fields of administration, particularly those dealing in some way with human services, there is a demonstrable sense in which social service administration deals with central problems of only peripheral or no interest to other pursuits. In other words, programmatically viewed, a book about social administration should in major ways look different from its cognate disciplines. A casual comparison of texts in the several administrative fields demonstrates this difference, though many common organizational and administrative concepts find their way into each.

Defining the field encompassed by the social services is at best a difficult task. Boundaries in human affairs tend to be arbitrary. Disciplines compete with one another in establishing their respective domains, and newly emerging patterns challenge time-honored jurisdictional claims. Perhaps the most complete and thorough treatment to date of the social services in the United States is that of Kamerman and Kahn (1976). They identify for analysis "those public—and private—sector benefits, services, entitlements, and policies which are informed by other than market concerns" (p. 7), and which are not included in the other basic social program fields—income maintenance, health, education, housing, and employment. These are "helping, access and socialization—development services" made available to clients of social agencies. The main service fields covered in their comprehensive study are:
- Child Welfare Programs
- Child Care and Related Programs

* Editor's note: As is the usual practice in a book of readings, all selections are faithfully reproduced from the original, and thus the appearance of certain currently objectionable terminology—especially certain uses of the personal pronoun, "he"—was unavoidable.

- Social Services for the Aged
- Social Services for Families
- Homemakers, Home Help, Home Health Aides
- Veterans Programs
- Correctional and Penal Services
- Community Centers, Settlements, Group Programs
- Access Services, i.e., Information, Referral, Advice, Case Advocacy, Liaison
- Special Programs for Refugees, Native Americans, Migrant Workers
- Components of Community Mental Health, Retardation Programs, Community Development

Social services provided in schools, in hospitals and health care, in housing and in manpower programs should also be seen as part of the social service system. Additionally, one might include activity in social planning, and policy development programs in both private agencies and the public welfare system.

Social administration is concerned with that aspect of professional practice in the social agency which organizes the means to make a service possible (Reynolds, 1942, p. 41). According to Reynolds, "Skill in administration consists not only in building organizational machinery which is adapted to the work to be done, but also in so dealing with the human parts of the machine that they will work at their individual and collective best" (pp. 35–36). If administration is "organization to get something done" (p. 207), then that "something" in social administration is the delivery of a social service. The processes that organize and monitor the social service delivery in an agency do so in the light of an explicit or implicit social policy which provides direction and purpose for the service system. However, "neither the process nor the organization of administration can be understood in isolation from each other: they are two different ways of describing the same phenomena" (Donnison & Chapman, 1965, p. 36).

The social administrator's task is to link the three universal elements that are engaged in the service experience: clients (consumers), practitioners (providers), and the organization (agency) which brings them together. Each of these elements is imbedded in a social network within the organization, and develops distinctive relationships one to the other. The primary constituencies of the administrator consist of the staff, the clients, and the board of trustees, which is the legal embodiment of the agency. Much of the administrator's energy and time is devoted to managing their respective activities in the light of the organization's philosophy, objectives, and policies, and their interactive relationships.

None of these relationships, however, develops in an institutional vacuum, for each of the primary constituencies has its own constituencies who are ready to intercede in the ongoing activities of the agency, sometimes implicitly, at other times openly and forcefully. The primary staff group reflects the norms and standards of the profession to which it belongs and to which it refers when questions of professional practice are raised. Similarly, trade union organizations representing the staff constituency actively participate in establishing conditions of work.

In like manner, clients frequently belong to consumer organizations, or parent associations, or tenant groups that reflect client interests and often become part of the process of establishing conditions affecting client service. In some instances, such associations become part of decision-making bodies, thus reflecting formal recognition of this essential interest in the organization's activities and purposes.

The service-giving agency also has its direct relationship with other bodies in the institutional environment. Of primary interest here are service networks of which they are a part, such as sectarian and nonsectarian local service systems, and citywide, statewide, or national networks. Funding sources, either voluntary or public, similarly represent immediate organizational relationships that affect the ability of social agencies to provide services. Each of these primary and secondary constituencies is a part of the organizational life space of the social administrator.

There is, finally, a third tier that is part of this organizational reality, one that affects each of the elements in common ways. Located here are the general public whose sanction is the ultimate source of organizational legitimacy, the media in both press and T.V., legislative bodies, regulatory agencies, and the like. Each of these has its occasions for making its influence felt on the service-giving function, sometimes to the ultimate detriment of the service, sometimes to its flowering. This hierarchy of constituencies is pictured in Table 1. This delineation suggests the vast complexity of the administrative enterprise and points to the many forces in the institutional environment with which the administrator must perforce be concerned.*

The practice detailed in the body of this book is a professional pursuit, calling upon skills, knowledge, values, and philosophical orientation that provide a creative dimension to organizational development. It has its technical and scientific aspects, but it is also in part an art, enlightened by practice wisdom, disciplined role performance, and balanced judgment.

A basic assumption underlies the organization and content of all that follows, namely, that social administration is an identifiable field of practice, more or less bounded and distinct from other administrative pursuits and rooted in the organization of the social services. While aspects of its work find parallels elsewhere, as a constellation of skills, knowledge, and values, it is sufficiently unique to warrant special study, application, and training. Although interdisciplinary in many ways, it relies heavily on the

---

* For a somewhat comparable depiction, see Negandhi (1975), "successive environment organization boundaries: (a) organizational environment; (b) task environment; and (c) societal environment."

TABLE 1
Organizational Life Space of Social Administration:
The Constituencies of the Social Administrator

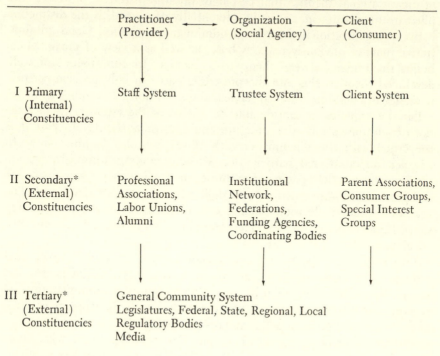

	Practitioner (Provider)	Organization (Social Agency)	Client (Consumer)
I Primary (Internal) Constituencies	Staff System	Trustee System	Client System
II Secondary* (External) Constituencies	Professional Associations, Labor Unions, Alumni	Institutional Network, Federations, Funding Agencies, Coordinating Bodies	Parent Associations, Consumer Groups, Special Interest Groups
III Tertiary* (External) Constituencies	General Community System Legislatures, Federal, State, Regional, Local Regulatory Bodies Media		

* These are illustrative and not intended to be comprehensive.

accumulated and recorded experience over many decades of the core profession in the social services, social work.

THE PLAN OF THE BOOK

Part I provides an overview of the administration of the social services. It introduces the reader to considerations concerning the nature of the administrative enterprise and to the vexing questions about boundaries, and conceptual overlaps with cognate disciplines and between processes and methods internal to social practice.

Part II examines some theoretical issues explored in the literature. It provides perspectives for looking at social administration, and indicates some multidisciplinary contributions that can be readily incorporated into theory building. Some distinctive philosophical and technical characteristics are indicated and suggestions made for the integration of practice and theory in educational programs.

Part III reviews selected organizational research relevant to an understanding of social work practice in the social services and looks at a range of organizational theories that cast light on administrative processes. Implicit in this discussion, and only inferentially developed, is the distinction between organizational theory and administrative theory. Good administrative practice obviously requires both, as well as a view of praxis which builds the bridge between theory and practice. In the absence of well-developed theories, this and the preceding part can only provide perspectives. Theory building in social service administration has a long way to go.

Part IV explores in considerable detail one of the essential characteristics of administration—the structure and uses of authority. In part it is concerned with the dilemma recently posed by John Gardner—how to advance organizational participation without eroding administrative authority. The parallel systems of authority in social agency governance—lay and professional—are described and their internal processes developed. The roles of trustees in decision-making, and of executives in providing professional leadership, are stressed. The essential relationships between the two are elaborated.

Two neglected aspects of social agency (as well as other institutional systems) administration are reviewed—the special problems of racism and sexism. The issues confronted by minority and feminine administrators are set forth, as is the need to understand and deal with the existent patterns of discrimination on both policy and operational levels.

The recent preoccupation with managerial techniques in a wide range of service organizations is the subject of Part V. It explores the relatively scanty literature on the allocation and control of social service resources, and gives special attention to conventional and program budgeting, cost analysis, management by objectives, and zero-base budgeting. A relevant literature on the last has not yet appeared. The final chapters analyze issues and problems of accountability in both its formal requisites and its equity considerations, and indicate some provocative aspects of contemporary systems analysis when applied to the social welfare system.

Part VI includes material on personnel administration of special relevance to the social services and points to the ways in which affirmative action and labor relations affect manpower considerations. Documents from the professional association on personnel practices and manpower classification are included.

Part VII provides some guidelines for the development of modern information management and includes illustrations of actual agency experience in their application. The importance of sophisticated approaches to data handling in the interest of coordinated client service is highlighted.

Finally, the perennial issues and problems of organizational conflict and change are presented in Part VIII. Concepts and strategies in their management are identified, and the inevitable difficulties and constraints encountered by practitioners located variously in the organizational hierarchy are elaborated.

This book is intended for use in schools of social work and other educational enterprises that deal with human services management. It can be used in undergraduate courses on administration as an introduction to the field, and in graduate courses both as overview and as the beginning of a sequence of courses geared to the preparation of social administrators.

Administrators of social agencies will also find the combination of theoretical and practical material relevant to their preoccupation with day-to-day managerial concerns.

The material included in the volume reflects significant developments which took place in the past decade, during which most of the selections were written. I am indebted to my students in graduate classes in administration at the School of Social Administration, Temple University, who tested and evaluated these readings. I owe much to their comments and suggestions.

SIMON SLAVIN

REFERENCES

Atwater, Pierce. *Problems of Administration in Social Work*. Minneapolis: The University of Minnesota Press, 1940.

Donnison, D. V., Chapman, Valerie, and others. *Social Policy and Administration*. London: George Allen and Unwin Ltd., 1965.

Ehlers, Walter H., Austin, Michael J., and Prothero, Jon C. *Administration for the Human Services: An Introductory Programmed Text*. New York: Harper and Row, 1976.

Kamerman, Sheila B., and Kahn, Alfred J. *Social Services in the United States: Policies and Programs*. Philadelphia: Temple University Press, 1976.

Negandhi, Anant R. "Comparative Management and Organization Theory: A Marriage Needed." *Academy of Management Journal* 18, no. 2 (June, 1975).

Reynolds, Bertha C. *Learning and Teaching in the Practice of Social Work*. New York: Rinehart and Co., 1942.

Schatz, Harry A. *Social Work Administration*. New York: Council on Social Work Education, 1970.

———. *A Casebook for Social Work Administration*. New York: Council on Social Work Education, 1970.

Spencer, Sue. *The Administration Method in Social Work Education*. New York: Council on Social Work Education, 1959.

Street, Elwood. *A Handbook for Social Agency Administration*. New York: Harper and Bros., 1947.

Trecker, Harleigh B. *Group Process in Administration*. New York: The Woman's Press, 1946; Revised and Enlarged Edition, 1950.

———. *Social Work Administration*. New York: Association Press, 1971.

INTRODUCTION

This book provides an urgently needed addition to the social work literature responsive to the current burgeoning interest in social work administration. Recent estimates indicate that a substantial number of all social work practitioners report administration as their primary job function. In the past ten years the number of schools of social work offering concentrations in administration or management has more than tripled. Growth in the education and practice of social administration has been paralleled by increasing concern over the need to improve competence in the administration and management of the expanding social welfare enterprise. What are the sources of this widespread concern?

A primary emphasis in the first schools of social work was the preparation of students for employment in the charity organization societies, which saw as their mission increasing efficiency in the use of resources to improve the condition of the poor. Paradoxically, however, in the first three decades of this century little emphasis was given in social work education to the teaching of administration per se, perhaps due to the relatively undeveloped state of relevant theory. From approximately 1930 through the late 1950s social work focused on the sociopsychological interaction of individual caseworkers and group workers with clients and their families. It seems fair to say that, despite rare exceptions, during this period, most schools of social work did not adequately exploit the emerging body of administrative knowledge which was rapidly developing in other fields and disciplines. Although the worker-client relationship was perceived as paramount then as now, the fact remains that most social workers practice in complex organizational settings where the level of administrative competence can often make the difference between effective or ineffective service delivery outcomes.

The rapid growth of public expenditures for health, education, and welfare services in the 1960s brought widespread demands for program evaluation and accountability. Concommitantly, the social welfare enterprise began to witness the proliferation of new programs, new fields of practice, ever-changing rules and procedures, new organizational structures, and complex and frequently fragmented service delivery systems. With these changes came new expectations by the general public, funding sources, and clients. The increasing democratization of social institutions during the period modified agency-consumer and agency-staff roles. Today, these developments have focused responsibility on the social welfare administrator as the central figure in orchestrating the above forces so that program processes and outcomes satisfy very different internal and external professional and lay audiences. Thus there is a demand for the development and dissemination of materials which will enable current and prospective social welfare administrators to improve their administrative and managerial competence and to keep abreast of the latest developments in administrative theory and technology.

Successfully managing any enterprise requires a profound knowledge of the technology it employs. The primary technology and dominant profession in social welfare is social work. Social welfare administrators need a firm grounding in social work not only to understand and share the values which underly the above concerns, but also to execute most effectively organizational policies associated with those concerns. Knowledge of social work will enhance the administrator's performance in such key roles as recruiting and developing staff, identifying and translating agency priorities, and determining acceptable standards for service delivery. Perhaps more importantly, administrators must have a profound knowledge of the stance of service consumers toward the organization delivering the service. For example, as business managers need to understand how retail customers differ from wholesale customers in their ways of relating to business organizations, social welfare administrators need to understand how the stance of social welfare consumers will be affected by whether the services are purchased, utilized voluntarily or involuntarily, and so on. Hence, there is a need for social workers to manage the social welfare enterprise. Yet, being a social worker does not guarantee administrative competence. While there is general agreement that many social work administrators need to gain greater mastery of management principles, there also is a need for social welfare administrators from other disciplines to gain more understanding of social work. For better or worse, it has long been observed that styles of top administrators tend to permeate organizations. Therefore, it is not merely sentimental or self-serving to claim that the achievement of social welfare objectives is enhanced by employing administrators who can blend social work concerns with management principles. Both elements in this blending are essential. As social welfare administrators become increasingly attuned to the importance of management principles, they need to be wary of the cult of management which sees management as an end unto itself. As new converts to a management ideology, they need to understand that the danger in inflating the importance of accountability and cost-benefit analysis above client service and primary organizational mission is equal to the danger of ignoring them.

All of these issues are well treated in this volume, which achieves a balanced approach to social administration. In so doing it is a valuable resource for social work administrators seeking to learn more about management, as well as other social welfare personnel seeking to improve their application of management principles to the social welfare enterprise. This volume contains 45 articles in eight parts which cover key areas of concern to practitioners, educators, and students of social administration. Its content ranges from diverse theoretical perspectives and their application to a broad spectrum of practice-based wisdom. The articles cover most major concerns of social welfare administrators, including boards and executive authority, various forms of budgeting and accountability, administering personnel, management information systems, and organizational conflict and change. What sets this book apart is its treatment of all of these areas with a keen articulation of their unique applications to social welfare organizations with their common and distinctive elements.

This book also makes a much-needed contribution to social work education. Administration has had a shorter history than other methods in social work education programs and therefore has fewer reading materials related specifically to social work. Not only does this volume reduce this shortage, but it contains material which directly addresses social work curricula in administration, describes essential content, and develops implications for patterning this content.

The issues regarding administration curricula in social work education are many. Do students who are not administration majors need to learn about administration in order to accept or affect organizational procedures? If so, what do they need to learn? What kinds of field placements can be used to ensure that administration majors will be assigned meaningful administrative responsibilities? (It is well known that many field agencies are reluctant to assign administrative responsibilities to beginners, but are willing to turn over crucial life decisions of clients to them.) What is the optimal interdisciplinary thrust for teaching administration to social work students? How can education in schools of business, management, and others be affected by exposure to social work, just as schools of social work are affected by them? Where shall schools of social work place administration in their curricula? As a separate method concentration by itself? Or as an integrated whole with policy and planning? These are but a few of the timely educational issues illuminated by the authors.

Therefore, the Council on Social Work Education views with great pleasure the opportunity to co-publish this volume. The Council has long been concerned about the need, by practitioners and educators alike, for more reading material in social welfare administration. We commend Simon Slavin and the many contributors for this outstanding addition to the literature.

RICHARD LODGE, D.S.W.
EXECUTIVE DIRECTOR
COUNCIL ON SOCIAL WORK EDUCATION

Part I

INTRODUCTION—
MAPPING THE TERRITORY

EDITOR'S INTRODUCTION

Although administration is among the oldest of the methods of social practice—the first social agency had to be administered—there remain a series of unresolved issues in determining its conceptual and practical territory. The delineation of the social services given in the Preface suggests their functional boundaries, but leaves unanswered questions concerning the relationship between the several systems of administration. The historical connection between social administration and the development and evaluation of the social services suggests that there is a core professional discipline that organizes the essential skill, technique, knowledge, values, and objectives required for effective service delivery. In like manner, medicine remains the core discipline that organizes health and hospital administration, and education is the profession that directs the public schools.

Yet, these disciplines, with their distinctive traditions and areas of expertise, are not fully bounded or discrete. There are aspects of each that draw on the same research and that utilize similar procedures. Such overlap of interest often includes structural considerations. Thus social administration of governmental services is part of public administration, social service departments in hospitals are part of health administration, school social work and counseling part of educational administration. As social administrators deal with planning, allocation and control of financial resources, institutional maintenance functions, personnel management, and the like, it is difficult to distinguish some of these organizational behaviors from those of business administration and management.

Thus, there are common and overlapping aspects that inhere in any administered system, at the same time that each system has its own set of preoccupations—of values, techniques, goals, policy dimensions, consumer targets, intervention modes, and knowledge constellations. Both general (G) and specific (S) elements require explication for an adequate understanding of each of the respective administrative disciplines. Social and behavioral research informs all administrative action, and organizational theory and perspectives provide especially significant insight into administrative behavior.

Paralleling these external conceptual and organizational relationships of social administration are somewhat similar considerations respecting social policy and social planning, processes internal to social work practice. The literature and practice both support the observation that administration incorporates at its core the development and implementation of policy, and that planning processes are integral to its operation. Here, too, we see both common (G) and distinctive (S) features. The development of policy, if it is not to be moribund, implies implementation (administration is essentially the implementation of policy), while administration defines its operations in the light of either explicit or implicit policy.

A look at models of practice of administrators and policy developers suggests that at the extremes there is an essential differentiation. Perhaps the critical variable is the closeness of such practitioners to the actual delivery of client services. The administrator of a family service agency or an institution for the retarded spends a significant part of his or her time dealing with problems that are quite different from those of, say, a regional official in a state department of welfare or a policy analyst in a consultant firm. One is in close touch with clients, providers of service, and supervisors; the other with developing, monitoring, and evaluating programs, grant proposals, and transmission of guidelines.

Schools of social work divide in their teaching of administration between those that organize their curricula to differentiate social policy-planning from administration in both classroom instruction and in field work placements, and those that have a single, integrated concentration (Kazmerski & Macarov, 1976). More experience and study is required before one can confidently declare the superiority of one pattern over the other. One possible pathway to resolve these differences is to plan curricula that reflect both overlap and distinctive elements in theory and in practice. Some experimentation along these lines is currently under way.*

The selections in this section deal, in part, with some of the issues suggested above. Lewis reviews some of the distinctive characteristics of social service organizations and discusses the cultural differences between them and business organizations. Special stress is placed on the meaning of nonmarket mechanisms for service evaluation. He analyzes such common managerial concepts as accountability, efficiency, and effectiveness, and suggests the importance of considering political and economic factors that bear upon managerial decision-making. Balancing considerations of unit costs with client satisfaction, effect with effectiveness, and, especially, knowledge and value, is seen as an important aspect of professional managerial practice.

The case for viewing social planning, social policy, and social administration as one "seamless web" of activity is persuasively argued by Gummer.

---

* The School of Social Administration at Temple University bases its administrative concentration on this assumption.

He sees this unitary character as a continuum of ends and means, of goals and operations. Curriculum implications for this view are explicated, and contrasts to other approaches indicated.

Spergel looks at macro practice—he calls it social development—and analyzes its constituent parts: social policy, planning, community organization, and administration. He then explores their relation to traditional and characteristic social treatment concerned with individual or group change rather than organizational or institutional development.

The demand by social agency boards for trained service-providing administrators will likely continue at an accelerated pace in the years ahead. The same will, in all likelihood, be true of policy analysts, program developers, and program evaluators, particularly in the public welfare system and among national, standard-setting organizations. The selections in this section are intended to bring to professional awareness some issues that call for further probing.

REFERENCE

Kazmerski, Kenneth J., and Macarov, David. *Administration in the Social Work Curriculum*. New York: Council on Social Work Education, 1976.

1/MANAGEMENT IN THE NONPROFIT SOCIAL SERVICE ORGANIZATION

HAROLD LEWIS

The late 1950s and early 1960s in social service organizations were bullish years for innovators. The mid-1960s to the end of the decade saw "problem solvers" come into their own. Today, as resources contract and demand expands, the call is out for managers. Is it only by chance that this cycle, often repeated in social welfare history, appears to coincide with periods of major social unrest, liberalization and reaction? Coincidence or not, the fact is that managers now enter center stage, as economic distress and political reaction threaten social services in all fields. In the eyes of professionals who must deliver the service, talk of budget cuts, personnel freezes, program retrenchment, and organizational rigidity linked to demands for accountability, is managerial talk. Managers in such trying circumstances find themselves speaking of efficiency, when the professionals—in daily practice—speak of insufficiency. Managers had best be strong and wise people, for theirs is an unenviable lot.

The need for intelligent and concerned management of nonprofit social service organizations has never been greater. There are more of these organizations, they are involved in increasingly complex and costly operations, they now influence the lives and livelihoods of millions. But greater need does not necessarily attract better or greater resources. Administrators have always been there, minding the store in social service agencies. But apparently in the eyes of managers who can judge, these administrators are not very good managers.

Among social service administrators, there are many who accept this evaluation, readily expressing their own feelings of inadequacy. The upsurge in management courses and concentrations in schools of social work, the experiments in joint programs with schools of business administration and public administration, and seminars on management, all testify to a degree of agreement between the outside evaluators and those evaluated. On the assumptions that such agreement exists and that it is the social work managers who seek to learn more about management from the business school managers, and not the other way around, this discussion takes the perspective of a client seeking the service of managerial specialists.

DIFFERENT CULTURES

It is important to clarify the situation of social service administrators; what it is we want help with, and what factors in our circumstances condition the use we can make of help that may be provided. We come from a culture very different from that of the business manager. We operate nonprofit organizations and can, with little effort, spend for good purposes more than we have, thereby incurring a deficit, but no loss in profit. When our consumers no longer need our services, an optimistic interpretation is that success has been achieved; this is hardly the case in business when customers stop buying a firm's product. In the social service organization concern for fairness often takes precedence over efficiency. The service ethic considers unequal advantage justified only if it raises the expectations of the least advantaged. Since the most disadvantaged are also more likely to experience difficulty in making appropriate use of opportunities, special and costly effort may be required to reach out to them. This, despite the fact that other claimants who do not need this special effort are sufficient in number to absorb totally the available resources. What business would spend resources to attract the most difficult to serve and usually most deprived customer when there are more than enough cooperative and affluent customers prepared to buy all it has to sell?

In business, when competition doesn't bring efficiency, adversity will. In social service, rarely does competition compel efficiency, and adversity is not likely to be the result of a client taking his business elsewhere. Given our lack of resources, selective inefficiency may be a necessity for organizational survival. In one city I know well, if the society to protect children from neglect and abuse systematically and efficiently reached out and informed the total community of its charge and the services it was expected to provide, not only would it be overwhelmed with needy cases, but its overload would swamp the courts, public assistance agencies, and children's institutions. In our field, where need—our definition of demand—far exceeds allocated resources, a certain amount of selected inefficiency appears essential for survival. Organizational cultures differ in important respects from that of business, and unless we understand these differences, it may be difficult to play an appropriate service role.

DIFFICULT DAYS AHEAD

The clamor for our services that will increase with rising unemployment and inflation is not, of course, evidence of a healthy demand. Success measured in terms of basic human needs met and social problems overcome is increasingly unlikely in these difficult times. We have more than once experienced times when our clients increased in number as the means for meeting their needs declined. We on the firing line know our consumers are restless. They take seriously the promise of justice and fairness. They will not accept an efficient operation that leaves their needs unattended. We may be devoted to our tasks, but we are also human. Managerial help, to be useful, should provide supplements to our courage and convictions, to prepare us to suffer the anger and distrust that will be heaped on our heads not for our failings, though they be many, but for the failings of our profit-oriented political and economic institutions.

An important characteristic of social service organizations is their monopoly over the type of resource they offer their clientele. Usually, as noted earlier, there are no competitive services that offer the consumer options. Moreover, since the cost is rarely carried by consumer payments, the threat of nonpayment or withdrawal by individual recipients may be irritating, but rarely fatal. Unlike the private monopoly that public policies regulate to protect the consumer from exploitation and profiteering, the nonprofit social service organization can hardly be accused of exercising these negative options for its own gain. The critic of these organizations must look elsewhere to find fault, and this leads to the traditional charges that have always hounded the managers of social service programs: laxity, antiquated methods, ineffective and inefficient operations. What ill serves the consumer, our critics assume, must be because of mismanagement, since motives seem to be absent. How the agency offers service, the service offered and the lack of responsiveness of the program to changing conditions are the key targets.

Another characteristic of social service organizations is the use of unit service cost, in the absence of profit, as a measure of efficiency. When goals are displaced as functions, this also serves as one measure of success. Those who recall the Ormsby-Hill Family Agency cost studies and their followups will remember how cost measures were used in these ways. Thus, while the nonprofit organization and the profit organization both want to maximize client-consumer satisfaction and minimize client-consumer ill will, the former would achieve this purpose at the minimum cost per unit service, while the latter would achieve it without threatening maximum profits. That the social service organization can incur deficits without a loss of profit suggests the role of service costs as an equivalent to profit as an indicator of managerial achievement.

PROMOTING TRUST

Client satisfaction in the nonprofit social service agency is in part dependent on the quality of service and in part on the quality of the processes and procedures through which the service is provided. Since much of the service entails intimate human contact between the worker and client, these two elements—what is being provided and how it is being provided—

are not readily separable. For close helping relationships to serve successfully as vehicles for service, mutual trust is crucial. Trust is evident in the
ability, willingness and opportunity to share one's self with another. A
client seeking social service help more often than not chooses an agency,
not a particular worker. Thus, trusting the agency is a major requisite for
instilling trust in the worker-client relationship. Good management should,
therefore, embody in the agency's organization work those elements that
promote trust. Developing trust must have a high priority in any procedure
instituted to assure accountability.

Returning to the unit cost and satisfaction functions, it is apparent that
good management should seek an appropriate mix of both, normally somewhere between the minimum of the former and the maximum of the latter.
An effective manager would provide guidance in approaching this ideal
blend. An unwise manager would focus on one element to the exclusion of
the other. What social service managers need help with is the body of
established principles of practice in approaching this blend.

Costs per unit in the condition of excessive demand and fixed income
that typically confronts the social service organization can be altered by
changing worker productivity, operational efficiency, quality of service and
characteristics of clients. The options to increase the price and extend the
market are not usually available. Managers, then, face limited internal
choices in seeking to lower unit costs without courting client ill will. They
can hire less costly staff, require more productivity of staff, limit waste, give
less to each client, choose only the clients who need less. If none of these
options works, the manager can control intake in order to manage with
available resources, but this would not necessarily control unit costs.

PRIVACY AND ANONYMITY

A third characteristic of the social service organization is that it must respect the privacy of the client, while distinguishing privacy from anonymity. To develop trust, opportunity must be provided to demonstrate its
presence. Both the client and worker must have something they are free
to share with the other. Where there is no privacy, there can be no free
choice to share, and trust is hardly likely to infuse the relationship. Privacy,
therefore, requires sufficient personal contact to permit recognition of differences and idiosyncratic attributes. It requires a feeling and knowing
human interface between client and agency. Anonymity masks client differences and seeks to assure uniform treatment. It minimizes worker judgments. The destructive result of failure to appreciate the difference between
privacy and anonymity has been amply demonstrated in the New York
City experience with the separation of income maintenance and service in

the Department of Social Services. The clientele of this agency lost trust in the agency's program.

EFFECT AND EFFECTIVENESS

Two popular terms in the language of managers, "effect" and "effectiveness," should not be confused with issues of efficiency and accountability. Effectiveness measures are based on criterion variables intended to judge achievement of goals associated with terminal values. Effect, on the other hand, is measured in relation to criteria derived from purposes associated with instrumental values. The former helps in judging a program's success; the latter provides the basis for judging the achievements of a practice. Those who base managerial decisions solely on effect measures risk the tyranny of small decisions. On the other hand, those who base managerial decisions solely on effectiveness measures risk remaining in doubt as to what, in fact, did or did not help. An appropriate mix of both types of outcome measures provides a basis for choices to be informed by functional and goal achievements. For example, at the functional level it is important in a child neglect situation to determine if the help given did provide supervision previously absent. This is a measure of effect. On the other hand, it is important to know that as a result of such improved supervision, the child attended school regularly, experienced less interruption in expected routines because of illness, imprisonment, etc. The latter measure shows whether the social purpose of the program was achieved. With the foregoing discussion as background, it is possible to address specific issues of efficiency and accountability, areas in which those who manage nonprofit social service organizations need most assistance.

EFFICIENCY

Consider the following not uncommon experience in social service agency personnel management. The agency proposes to upgrade the educational preparation of its staff to improve the quality and efficiency of its services. In addition to setting up an inservice training program, it proposes to underwrite, by released time or scholarship, the costs of employees attending graduate programs in areas useful to the agency. It selects the best candidates available on its staff; they attend the program, return after graduation for an obligated period, and leave the agency.

The worker who received the education has increased his economic options. The new competence brings a wider range of job choices, and greater maneuverability. The worker seeks out the best agency, not necessarily the one that invested in the worker. But the agency may still want to pursue this policy. It can be rationalized as preparing personnel for the profession, thus assuring the presence of competent practitioners in other programs to which this agency often must turn for help with its clients. Theoretically, if all agencies followed the same route, the general level of practice would improve, and the market would ultimately distribute appropriately the various talents needed. There may, however, be another reason for maintaining this policy.

Suppose the agency, as much as the talented worker, recognizes the low level of its practice, but has a locked-in senior staff, with little likelihood of turnover. Also assume the agency has a relative monopoly on employment opportunities for a particular skill. In these circumstances staff at the lower level in the agency program have no place to go, in the agency or elsewhere. Discontent is inevitable, and the politics of organizational practice can be brutal. The more talented, frustrated employees may use their ability to highlight, for client and community alike, the limitations of the quality of service, and may organize the staff to "Fanshen" (to turn over)—as the Chinese say. Faced with this possibility, the organization's leadership can opt for education as an effective tool to defuse the powderkeg, decapitating the potential leadership through a process that provides the more able with the options to go elsewhere.

This hypothetical case points up the need to examine both the political and economic factors that influence managerial decisions. Failures to do so may be the major inefficiency in social service organizations. Discussions of technology, of rational decision mechanisms based on up-to-date information retrieval, of sound management of fiscal resources, of control and planning systems, of quality control, of organizational statemanship, of personnel administration, of goal-directed practice—all make for interesting and useful dialogues, but still one encounters the cases of the Pennsylvania Railroad, Lockheed, the Pan Am syndrome. In social service organizations with access to the more sophisticated technological hardware and software—such as large public welfare departments—the same syndrome is evident. Obviously, help is needed in formulating principles of managerial practice to guide political and economic judgments. Such principles will at least promote a principled practice, using the best available technologies to achieve goals and purposes.

ACCOUNTABILITY

The issue most in need of attention in relation to accountability is posed by the question: Accountability to whom? Lacking the choice to go elsewhere, social service consumers form a natural base for a political pressure group with considerable sustaining energies.

But there is also accountability to the funding source, to the community, to the profession, to one's superior and, last but not least, to oneself. Which of all these accountabilities deserves the highest priority? Mechanisms and techniques for assuring accountability differ in accordance with the interests of those for whom the results are intended. Obviously, groups that can exercise the major influence will demand and get the major attention. If the funding source threatens to cut off payment, its interest will be attended to, and soon. In a review of the clout likely to be available to the different populations to whom one can be accountable, the weakest group may well be the least organized. A unionized staff or an organized profession can make a more telling demand than individual persons. A board, a single or major funding source, or collaborating funding sources can speak in a more commanding voice when united than when disagreements produce no clear message. Weakest of all is the unorganized client whose problems bring him to the agency, and whose personal inability to manage seriously limits his energies and other resources needed to command accountability. The major help social service managers need with the problem of accountability is a set of guiding principles to inform the use of technologies in a manner that would assure a just and fair, not merely a convenient, response to requests for accountability. This may require, at times, that we assist in organizing future trouble makers. In the short run, it is unlikely that managers will promote a source of power that can be used to restrict their choices. In the long run, failure to do so may not only restrict choices, but eliminate choice entirely.

THE PRACTICE SCIENCE OF MANAGEMENT

I agree with those management experts who recognize a distinction between theoretical science and practice science. Although we need the former to tell us where to look and what to look for, the latter provides us with the "how." Practice science is formulated in terms of principles and rules, not laws. And since practice sciences intend consequences, they are never value-free. This paper was intended to emphasize the linkage of knowledge and value in professional managerial practice.

SUMMARY

I have noted the following areas where assistance would serve both our immediate and long-term concerns. We need to know principles of management that:

1) will communicate in the organizational work of the agency those elements that promote trust and concurrently respect privacy;

2) will help us approach an appropriate mix of unit-cost and client satisfaction functions;

3) can provide a basis of choosing an appropriate mix of effect and effectiveness measures to inform managerial decisions;

4) will guide us in making appropriate political and economic judgments affecting organizational efficiency; and

5) will inform our use of technologies in a manner that will assist us in assuring a just and fair, not merely a convenient, response to requests for accountability.

This paper was presented at the Seminar on Education for Management of Social Sciences, at the University of Pennsylvania, January 5, 1975. The seminar was made possible by a grant from the U.S. Department of Health, Education and Welfare.

The writer is indebted to Albert O. Hirschman, author of *Exit, Voice and Loyalty: Responses to Decline in Firms, Organizations and States* (Cambridge, Mass.: Harvard University Press, 1970), for a number of analogs used in this paper.

2/SOCIAL PLANNING AND SOCIAL ADMINISTRATION: IMPLICATIONS FOR CURRICULUM DEVELOPMENT

BURTON GUMMER

An important problem facing social work educators is clarification of the conceptual and operational issues contained in the relationship between social planning and social administration. Increased understanding of these areas will lead to more coherent and rational curriculum planning and, ultimately, to more effective social work practitioners. The present paper will identify some of the major conceptual issues involved, and discuss implications for the development of curriculum at the master's degree level.

The first problem encountered is a definitional one due to the fact that both social planning and social administration are not unitary concepts but umbrella terms that subsume a variety of activities. Gurin, for instance, notes that the term "social planning" is sometimes used synonymously with community organization; this is further complicated by the various meanings attributed to community organization, ranging from community development through interorganizational relations to social action.[1]

For the purposes of this paper the definition of social planning used is the one developed by Kahn, who views planning as "policy formulation and realization through choices and rationalization. . . . It includes elements of: (1) research (including fact-finding, projection, and inventory-taking); (2) value analysis and facilitation of expression of value positions, sometimes through political mechanisms; (3) policy formulation; (4) administrative structuring (programming); and (5) measurement and feedback."[2]

The field of social administration seems to be free of the definitional and conceptual confusion that has plagued social planning, since it can be taken to refer exclusively to the management of social welfare organizations. Closer inspection, however, quickly reveals at least two distinct activities under the name of administration: first, the identification of the goals of an organization and the development of appropriate structures for implementing those goals. Selznick refers to this as "institutional leadership," the defining characteristic of which is "the definition of institutional mission and role."[3] The second, and more commonly accepted notion of what is meant by administration, refers to the coordination and integration of organizational subsystems into coherent mechanisms for the attainment of organizational goals—usually referred to as "management."[4]

The literature on social administration clearly identifies this dual nature of administration.[5] Moreover, there is agreement that effective administration involves both activities. The following position taken by Spencer is representative of current thinking:

the administrative process is not limited to the intraagency management of resources, nor to the fulfillment of an assignment made to the agency by an outside body. . . . There is general agreement that administration is the conscious direction of the internal relationships and activities of the enterprise toward the achievement of goals. . . . Administration is also the conscious intervention in the interacting forces operating between the agency and the larger community.[6]

TWO AREAS OF OVERLAP

Given these definitions of planning and administration, there are at least two areas of activities in which these fields overlap: the first is the identification and explication of program goals (i.e., the social purpose of organizational activities), and the second is the planning and development of appropriate structures for the implementation of goals. In general this overlap is not viewed as problematic, but merely reflective of the multifaceted nature of this kind of activity. Thus Kahn notes that "planners, community organizers, and administrators are . . . in closely interrelated and interacting roles. . . . Each is readily found functioning in the domain of the other and defining it as his own."[7]

Although there is a lack of clear boundaries between planners and administrators this does not necessarily pose major conceptual problems. But it can become problematic in practice. Frequently an activity is not specifically assigned to anyone and it then is not performed. This situation is conducive to "buck passing." If the assumption is that *everyone* has responsibility for some activity, then it becomes easier for *any one* individual to forego work in a specific area since there is an assumption that *someone* will do it.

Thus while the theory of social administration posits a holistic approach—one that unites the goal-setting and management aspects of the administrative process—administrators honor this concept more often in the breach than in practice. There is a preoccupation by top-level administrators with the internal management and stability of their organizations, which often involves a disregard of the stated goals. This leads to "goal displacement" whereby "an instrumental value becomes a terminal value."[8] This phenomenon has been empirically documented in the areas of employment counseling,[9] medical care,[10] family counseling,[11] and public welfare.[12] Social planners, on the other hand, are frequently accused of a preoccupation with developing highly-refined statements of purpose with little consideration for the structural and administrative arrangements necessary to achieve them.[13]

This tendency by planners and administrators to disregard some activities and emphasize others is a result of their respective roles in the organizational structure. The administrator, as the chief line officer, has the ultimate responsibility for the ongoing operation of the organization. Moreover, as Selznick points out:

Once an organization becomes a "going concern," with many forces working to keep it alive, the people who run it can readily escape the task of defining its purposes. . . . In part . . . there is the wish to avoid conflicts with those in and out of the organization who would be threatened by a sharp definition of purpose, with its attendant claims and responsibilities.[14]

The planner, on the other hand, is frequently assigned a staff function outside the main line operation. This is generally seen as beneficial since "by getting out of the firehouse environment of day-to-day administration, policy analysis seeks knowledge and opportunities for coping with an uncertain future."[15] The planner's role can, however, have negative consequences if it produces an inclination to deemphasize or lose sight of administrative requirements for program implementation.

The implications of this analysis for social work education are many and pose a challenge to the educator to develop a curriculum that will increase the capacities of both planners and administrators to deal with the situations described above. The rest of this paper will be concerned with culling from the foregoing analysis of planners and administrators, guidelines for the development of curriculum.

GENERAL OBSERVATIONS
ON CURRICULUM DEVELOPMENT

Before moving to specific concerns about curriculum for planning and administration, some general observations about approaches to curriculum development for professional education are needed. An educational curriculum can, in some ways, be seen as analogous to a theoretical model. The process of model formation has been described as:

conceptually marking off a perceptual complex. It involves . . . replacing part or parts of a perceptual complex by some representation, or symbol. . . . Each model stipulates . . . some correspondence with reality, some relevance of items in the model to the reality, and some verifiability between model and reality.[16]

The process of modelling can be seen as one of abstracting from any phenomenon those elements seen as crucial to an understanding of the dynamics involved in its operation, and subjecting those elements to intensive examination. One way to classify models, then, is the degree to which they recapitulate reality; that is, some models will be overly-simplistic in their representation of a phenomenon while other, more complex ones, will represent the phenomenon in its actual form.

Pursuing the analogy, an educational curriculum aimed at the preparation of practitioners can be seen as heuristically marking off some complex of activities. Curriculum development involves taking an area of activity such as planning and administration, identifying essential elements in the operation of that activity, and then structuring some form of educational mechanism (e.g., courses, modules, field-experiences) that will teach students how to perform it. To complete the analogy, curricula can also be classified in terms of the degree to which they accurately recapitulate the complexity of the activity for which they are preparing students.

CURRICULUM DEVELOPMENT IN SOCIAL WORK

Turning now to curriculum development in social work, there are at least two factors determining the degree to which a curriculum accurately models the activity for which it is preparing students. The first is the initial definition of what that activity is. This can range from a narrow definition (e.g., casework as consisting exclusively of interviewing and other counselling skills), to a much broader one (e.g., the foregoing discussion of planning, administration, and community organization as one "seamless web" of activity). The second factor is the nature of the administrative arrangements for "packaging" content areas.

The definition of the problem does not seem critical for curriculum development in planning and administration. As noted in the first part of this paper, one can observe a consensus in the various conceptual approaches in this area around the theme that planning and administration are broad-based activities involving several interrelated and interacting components, and attempts to define whether a specific activity should be administration or planning is not a productive approach. The second factor, however, seems to be the more critical; moreover, the nature of its impact is not a straightforward one and requires some elaboration.

As noted earlier, one of the problems in the field of social welfare is a tendency on the part of planners and administrators to develop vested interests in certain aspects of their overall responsibilities to the exclusion of others; this is generally seen in terms of a preoccupation with either means or ends. If social work education is to have a corrective impact on this tendency it is essential that curriculum be designed to accomplish two major objectives: to enable the student to acquire a firm grasp of the essentially unitary nature of the policy-planning-administation process; and to enable the student to acquire in-depth training of the overall process.

What is meant by a unitary nature is that there seems to be a natural continuum that underpins the policy-planning-administration process and has the identification of goals at one end and the development of means at the other. Figure 1 presents a typology of activities based on this continuum. It ranges from a primary emphasis on the nature of the goals to be pursued (policy) to a primary emphasis on the operation of organizational structures aimed at achieving these goals (management). Moreover, this

ENDS		MEANS
Policy–Planning	Planning–Administration	Administration–Management
Social-philosophical analyses of normative approaches to social welfare	Conceptual and operational identification of program goals	Securing and maintaining a resource base for organizational operations
Analyses of long-range trends; analyses of anticipated and unanticipated consequences of current and prospective programs	Articulating program purposes with social welfare values	Coordination and integration of organizational subunits
	Design of appropriate structures for program implementation	Design of organizational structures to improve program effectiveness
Development of new models for program analysis and program development	Monitoring-evaluation of program activities	Inducing participation in appropriate organizational activities
Improving the base of social data	Developing coherent and rational systems of service	

FIGURE 1.   Sphere of Activities Covered by the Concept of Social Administration

entire range of activities is what the present writer understands to be the operationalization of the concept of "social administration," particularly as this concept has been developed by Titmuss and his colleagues.[17]

Within this range of activities there seems to be at least three natural groupings: policy-planning, planning-administration, and administration-management. Moreover, as with most phenomena that are conceptualized in terms of continua, their essential nature is usually found somewhere in the middle-range. This is due to the fact that the ends of the continuum are more appropriately seen as the *boundaries to some system of activities*. There is a tendency for these activities to lose some of the characteristics of the system of which they are a part and take on those of the external systems with which they are in contact.

This phenomenon can be seen quite clearly in social welfare where polar activities are frequently seen as blurring into other fields. Thus there has been a continual debate as to whether social policy analysis is really a social welfare activity or in fact belongs to the more generic sphere of public policy analysis.[18] Likewise, the literature on social agency administration continues to address the question of whether this area should more appropriately come under the purview of management science.[19] This debate can only be resolved by an empirical investigation of each case. But it is first necessary to clarify the primary character of social administration so that there will be criteria for evaluating how far away any particular activity is from the core.

SOCIAL ADMINISTRATION

The point of view that will be developed here is that social administration is most appropriately viewed as that middle range of activities where social purposes are wedded to social structures.[20] The primary task for social administration is "to choose key values and to create a social structure that embodies them."[21] The first responsibility of the social administrator is to be evermindful of the highly normative nature of all social welfare activities. Social welfare is infused with value judgments since all welfare activities ultimately are informed by one or another view of what social justice is.[22]

Moreover, there is generally little consensus among these various conceptions of what *should be*, for, as Donnison points out, "there is no generally understood state of 'social health' toward which all people strive; our disagreements on this question form the subject matter of politics the world over."[23] The social administrator, then, must first have an explicitly and systematically developed point of view about the purposes of social welfare; he should be an "expert in the promotion and protection of values."[24]

While a clear and strong normative orientation is necessary for social administration, it is not sufficient; it must be combined with substantive knowledge about institutional dynamics so that the structure developed to carry out the purpose of a program will be consonant with the nature of the purpose. Social welfare takes place almost exclusively within an organizational context. Therefore the social administrator must possess sufficient technical knowledge about the nature of institutional and organizational behavior to be able to make informed judgments and decisions in the area of goal-implementation.

This analysis points to an activity that only has meaning if it is able to maintain a middle-range position between two polar attractions. On the one hand, the policy end of the continuum offers the allure of normative and conceptual purity. On the other hand, the management end offers an equally compelling attraction in the form of perfecting operational arrangements. Maintaining the middle position is precarious, but to move in either direction would be to abandon the social administration function.

What this means for curriculum planning is that the educator is faced with the difficult problem of designing a program that will enable students to develop a base of knowledge and skill sufficient for the performance of the social administrator role while at the same time building in safeguards against distortion by overspecialization in some aspect of the activities associated with the role. The word "sufficient" is used advisedly, since the critical question is not *what* should be taught but *how much*.

Some guidelines for dealing with this situation are suggested in Etzioni's discussion of the related problem of the appropriate background for an administrator of any professional organization.[25] The organizational dilemmas encountered in that situation are analagous to the dilemmas inherent in the role of the social administrator:

On the one hand the role should be in the hand of an expert in order to ensure that the orientation of the head of the authority structure will mean that expert activity is recognized as the major goal activity and that the needs of professionals will be more likely to receive understanding attention. On the other hand organizations have functional requisites that are unrelated to their specific goal activity. Organizations have to obtain funds to finance their activities, recruit personnel to staff the various functions, and allocate the funds and personnel. . . . Organizational heads must know how to keep the system integrated. . . . An expert may endanger the integration of the professional organization by overemphasizing the major goal activity.[26]

One solution is to have professional organizations headed by a semi-expert—"a person who combines an expert background and education with a managerial personality and role."[27] In a similar sense, the social administrator can be viewed as a semiexpert, but one who combines a background in the normative, analytical, and programming skills of social policy and social planning, with the ability to operate effectively in an administrative capacity. This notion has important implications both for curriculum development and the nature of this function as a professional role in the social welfare field.

INTEGRATION OF POLICY, PLANNING, AND ADMINISTRATION

The first recommendation that comes out of the above analysis is that a curriculum for social administration should strive for as much integration as possible among the areas of social policy, social planning, and administration. This integration has to be of two kinds—conceptual and administrative. It is hoped that this paper will add to conceptual clarity in this area; work of this sort should be seen as a priority item on one's research agenda. The next task is to examine alternate patterns for structuring curriculum in this area in order to determine which patterns maximize integration.

In a recent survey by the Council on Social Work Education it was found that 46 percent of the 85 graduate schools of social work contacted listed some offering in administration during the academic year 1972–73.[28] On the basis of the descriptive material reported in this survey one can identify three approaches to structuring curriculum in this area: (1) administration as a distinct two-year concentration; (2) administration as a subspecialty within a combined policy, planning, and administration concentration; and (3) administration as a second-year concentration following specialization in either service delivery or social planning and community organization.

The conceptual approach to social administration developed in this paper seems to find its fullest expression in the second approach. Neugeboren, in presenting the rationale for this approach, argues that:

administration of direct service agencies is one specialized area of practice of organizing and planning in social work. Therefore, we view the knowledge and skill required for direct service administration as having common elements with planning and administration in other areas of practice as social work in planning and allocating agencies.[29]

Sarri, on the other hand, concedes the interrelated nature of policy, planning, and administration, but argues for the first approach on pedagogical grounds:

Although the two specializations in administration and policy were closely linked, a distinctive curriculum was designed for each. This was done deliberately to stimulate and challenge the faculty and students to identify elements which were distinctive to each other.[30]

Finally, the argument generally put forth in support of the third approach is that the administrator should have substantive knowledge about, and practice skills in, the services being administered.

TENTATIVE OBSERVATIONS

Since most of these programs are in their beginning stages it is too early to tell which of the three patterns will prove most effective, or even if different patterns will have to be developed. However, some tentative observations can be made on the basis of the experiences thus far. The major concern for the educator is to structure curriculum in such a way that the student develops a firm grasp of the dual requirements of effective social administration (i.e., creating structural arrangements that allow for the attainment of socially-valued goals).

This consideration suggests that a program in social administration should concentrate primarily on the areas of policy analysis, planning, and organizational and managerial dynamics. This is not to say that the student should not receive information *about* the nature of the services that social agencies offer, but that he should not be expected to develop skill in the actual delivery of those services. One possible exception to this generalization is the case of the administrator of a highly-clinical service, for example, individual or family counseling. In this situation a strong case can be made for an educational program that gives the student substantive experience in the delivery of social services, as well as skills in the area of administration.

With the one exception noted it seems that the second curriculum pattern—a combined program of administration and planning—offers the greatest possibility for the education of effective social administrators. The strongest alternative to this seems to be the first pattern—a separate concentration in administration—for the reasons noted by Sarri. The ultimate test for any of these approaches, however, will have to await more extensive experiences with them on the part of students, faculties, and agencies.

NOTES

1. Arnold Gurin, "Social Planning and Community Organization," in *Encyclopedia of Social Work*, Vol. II (New York: National Association of Social Workers, 1971), p. 1324. Also see Jack Rothman, "Three Models of Community Organization Practice," *Social Work Practice, 1968* (New York: Columbia University Press, 1968).
2. Alfred J. Kahn, *Theory and Practice of Social Planning* (New York: Russell Sage Foundation, 1969), pp. 17–18.
3. Philip Selznick, *Leadership in Administration: A Sociological Interpretation* (New York: Harper & Row, 1957), p. 61.
4. See Parsons' distinction among the technical, managerial, and institutional levels of an organization. Talcott Parsons, *Structure and Process in Modern Societies* (Glencoe, Ill.: The Free Press, 1969), pp. 60–69.
5. For a good overview of current approaches to social administration see Harleigh B. Trecker, *Social Work Administration: Principles and Practices* (New York: Association Press, 1971), pp. 22–28. Also see Ralph M. Kramer, "Community Organiza-

tion and Administration: Integration or Separate but Equal?" *Journal of Education for Social Work,* Vol. 2, No. 2 (Fall 1966), pp. 48–56; John C. Kidneigh, "Administration and Community Organization in Social Work," *International Social Work,* Vol. 11 (July 1968), pp. 17–22; Rosemary C. Sarri, "Administration in Social Welfare," in *Encyclopedia of Social Work,* Vol. I (New York: National Association of Social Workers, 1971); and Bernard Neugeboren, "Developing Specialized Programs in Social Work Administration in the Master's Degree Program: Field Practice Component," *Journal of Education for Social Work,* Vol. 7, No. 3 (Fall 1971), pp. 35–47.

6. Sue W. Spencer, "The Administrative Process in a Social Welfare Agency," in *Social Work Administration: A Resource Book,* ed. Harry A. Schatz (New York: Council on Social Work Education, 1970), pp. 135–136.

7. Kahn, *op. cit.,* p. 23. Also see Sue Spencer, *The Administration Method in Social Work Education,* Vol. III, Social Work Curriculum Study (New York: Council on Social Work Education, 1959), pp. 35–36.

8. Robert K. Merton, *Social Theory and Social Structure,* 3rd rev. ed. (New York: The Free Press, 1968), p. 253.

9. Peter M. Blau, *The Dynamics of Bureaucracy* (Chicago: University of Chicago Press, 1963).

10. Charles Perrow, "Organizational Prestige: Some Functions and Dysfunctions," *American Journal of Sociology,* Vol. 66 (January 1961), pp. 335–341.

11. Richard A. Cloward and Irwin Epstein, "Private Social Welfare's Disengagement from the Poor: The Case of Family Adjustment Agencies," in *Community Action Against Poverty,* ed. George A. Brager and Francis P. Purcell (New Haven: College and University Press, 1967).

12. Burton Gummer, "The Effects of Patterns of Interorganizational Relations on the Delivery of Social Services" (Ph.D. diss., Bryn Mawr College, 1973), pp. 174–183.

13. Rein, for instance, argues that "the study of social policy involves the interaction between values, operating principles, and outcomes. If any of these is lost sight of, the analysis tends to be nonproductive." Martin Rein, "Social Policy Analysis as the Interpretation of Beliefs," *Journal of the American Institute of Planners,* Vol. 37 (September 1971), p. 298. Community mental health centers offer a good example of lack of articulation between goals and structures. See Felice Perlmutter and Herbert A. Silverman, "CMHC: A Structural Anachronism," *Social Work,* Vol. 17, No. 2 (March 1972), pp. 78–84.

14. Selznick, *op. cit.,* p. 25.

15. Aaron Wildavsky, "Rescuing Policy Analysis from PPBS," in *Public Expenditures and Policy Analysis,* ed. Robert H. Haveman and Julius Margolis (Chicago: Markham Publishing Co., 1970), p. 462.

16. Paul Meadows, "Models, Systems and Science," *American Sociological Review,* Vol. 22 (February 1957), p. 4.

17. See Richard M. Titmuss, "The Subject of Social Administration," in *Commitment to Welfare* (New York: Pantheon Books, 1968), pp. 13–24; and David V. Donnison, "The Evolution of Social Administration," *New Society* (October 20, 1966), and *The Development of Social Administration* (London: Bell, 1962).

18. See Kenneth E. Boulding, "The Boundaries of Social Policy," *Social Work,* Vol. 12, No. 1 (January 1967), pp. 3–11; Martin Rein, *Social Policy: Issues of Choice and Change* (New York: Random House, 1970)), pp. 3–20; and Yehezkel Dror, "Policy Analysts: A New Professional Role in Government Service," *Public Administration Review,* Vol. 27 (September 1967), pp. 197–203.

19. See Edward E. Schwartz, "Some Views of the Study of Social Welfare Administration," in *Research in Social Welfare Administration: Its Contributions and Problems,* ed. David Fanshel (New York: National Association of Social Workers,

1962), pp. 33–43; Trecker, *op. cit.*, pp. 17–30; and Edward H. Litchfield, "Notes on a General Theory of Administration," *Administrative Science Quarterly*, Vol. 1 (1956), pp. 1–29.

20. The following discussion owes much to the writings of Philip Selznick. See especially his *Leadership in Administration, op. cit.*, and *TVA and the Grass Roots: A Study in the Sociology of Formal Organizations* (New York: Harper Torchbooks, 1966).

21. Selznick, *Leadership, op. cit.*, p. 60.

22. See Charles Frankel, "The Moral Framework of the Idea of Welfare," in *Welfare and Wisdom*, ed. John S. Morgan (Toronto: University of Toronto Press, 1966), pp. 147–164.

23. David V. Donnison, "Observations on University Training for Social Workers in Great Britain and North America," *Social Service Review*, Vol. 29 (December 1955), p. 350.

24. Selznick, *Leadership, op. cit.*, p. 28.

25. Amitai Etzioni, "Authority Structure and Organizational Effectiveness," *Administrative Science Quarterly*, Vol. 4 (1959), pp. 43–67.

26. *Ibid.*, pp. 53–55.

27. *Ibid.*

28. "Concentration and Special Learning Opportunities in the Master of Social Work Curricula of Graduate Schools of Social Work: 1972–1973," mimeographed (New York: Council on Social Work Education, November 1972).

29. Neugeboren, *op. cit.*, p. 38.

30. Rosemary C. Sarri, "Education for Social Welfare Administration—Today and Tomorrow" (Paper presented at the 17th Annual Program Meeting of the Council on Social Work Education, Cleveland, Ohio, January 23, 1969), p. 11.

3/SOCIAL DEVELOPMENT

AND SOCIAL WORK

IRVING A. SPERGEL

Social development is a relatively new term which may be used to describe "macro-structural" practice. It may be regarded as a basic perspective of social work, cognate with social treatment. Its end like that of social treatment is individual welfare, personal and social improvement, but the route is less direct. Social development practice focuses on the institutions of community and society and their social impact on the individual. Social treatment focuses on the social relationships of the individual to other individuals and groups in various situations—family, school, work, neighborhood, corrections, health care, recreation, etc.

Social work addresses social welfare problems. In particular the functions of social work are to change individuals and institutions.[1] The extent to which social work carries out these functions and the nature of their interactions have been a source of long-term debate and discussion. More recently the effectiveness of these efforts has been brought into question.[2]

There is little question that social work practice has become increasingly complex, diverse, and specialized in recent years, especially since the era of "Great Society" programs. While there have been efforts to describe these new and changing areas of individual or institutional practice, there has been possibly less interest in how the practice pieces fit together, either within the two major practice sectors—social treatment and institutional practice—or across them.

Integrative or synthetic conceptions of practice are periodically needed to provide a sense of general mission and to make explicit the parameters of a field of professional intervention. These conceptions become a basis for the improvement of professional practice and role preparation. Often they signal or recognize significant change in professional practice already occurring. Occasionally they may precede or generate practice innovations.

The purpose of this essay is to address partially the task of conceptual integration, mainly of certain elements of social development practice—community organizing, social policy formation and analysis, social planning, and administration. Much of the thinking about social development in the sense used here began at the School of Social Service Administration of the University of Chicago in 1972 with a concern over curriculum fragmentation, especially duplicated courses.* A more effective educational pattern on the "macro" side of the master's curriculum was sought.

An assumption of the discussion by some of the faculty was that social work was carried out, not only in social welfare organizations, but in other types of organizations or systems of society. Policies and actions in certain national, state, and urban arenas or domains, e.g., taxation, education, urban transportation, civil rights, had clear and sometimes immediate consequences for the social welfare of individuals. The distintions as to whether one area had more or less impact for the social welfare of individuals seemed unclear. It was possible that social workers were or should be practicing social work, at least at the institutional change or development level, in each of these areas. Furthermore, the boundaries of the social develop-

---

* Involved in these discussions, still ongoing, have been Jack Meltzer, Mary Davidson, Earl Durham, Harold Richman, Lynn Vogel, Sheldon Tobin, Frank Breul, Pastora Cafferty, Laurence Hall, Arnita Boswell, and others. Jack Meltzer is chairman of the Social Development Program at the master's level.

ment modalities—policy administration, community organization, and planning—to deal with these issues and problems of individuals at a structural level were blurred. It therefore appeared important in a practice profession to look at the specifics of method—at least "macro" methods—within a consistent frame of values, and to identify some underlying concepts.

THE VALUE BASE OF SOCIAL DEVELOPMENT

The goal of social work is the fulfillment of human potential and the prevention of social problems. The general objective of social development is the creation of effective institutional structures to meet human social needs. On the one hand, social development may call for institutional development or reform, especially when institutional arrangements fail to meet existing social needs. On the other hand it may be extremely important to sustain, protect, and enhance already effective social institutions when they clearly contribute to personal development and social adjustment.

The concept of social development indicates not only the creation of effective institutions of social provision, social protection, social control, social rehabilitation, and social problem prevention. It also suggests a *weltanschauung* or general view about society and the role of all institutions in contributing to social betterment of individuals. In Wilensky and Lebeaux's terms, it is an "institutional" rather than a "residual" view:

As the residual conception becomes weaker . . . and the institutional conception increasingly dominant, it seems likely that distinctions between welfare and other types of social institutions will become more blurred. Under continuing industrialization all institutions will be oriented toward and evaluated in terms of social welfare aims. The "welfare state" will become the welfare society, and both will be more reality than epithet.[3]

A moral imperative underlies the social development approach. It implies an unfolding historical process. Society is evolving a set of social concerns or stages of social reform. Myrdal suggests:

Social reform policies may be conceived as passing through three stages. A paternalistic conservative era, when curing the worst ills was enough; a liberal era when safeguarding against inequalities through pooling the risks is enough; and a social democratic era, when preventing the social ills is attempted. The first was the period of curative social policy through private charity and public poor relief; the second was the period of social insurance, broad in scope but still merely symptomatic; and the third may be called a period of protective and cooperative social policy. . . .[4]

Finally, we should note that, in practice, social development and social treatment may represent overlapping areas of activity. Both are concerned with prevention and cure, with individuals and institutions. A social worker may simultaneously, interactively or sequentially emphasize social development and social treatment in his practice. Nevertheless, in social treatment there is a tradition of emphasis on diagnosis and modification of personal and interpersonal problems within existing institutional frameworks. In social development the emphasis has been probably more on the prevention of problems, especially the modification rather than simply the support of institutional arrangements which seem to create or aggravate individual disorders. Both orientations, nevertheless, need to emphasize even more the positive rather than the remedial aspects of human development and realization of individual social potentials.

The idea of social development in terms of substantive strategies has generally been absent from public and professional group discussions. This is not quite the case in European countries, particularly in planned economies, where social development policies have been extensively debated, formulated, and applied in economic, manpower, and social welfare areas. Nevertheless, there is some beginning attention to the idea of social development in the United States, for example, in relation to "reallocative public policy" which seeks to redistribute substantial resources from high-income individuals and corporations to the lower and middle classes. The formulation and testing of models of income policies and service delivery systems have begun, and relevant policy critiques have been initiated.

SOCIAL DEVELOPMENT MODALITIES

Furthermore, it may be that the means or modalities, as well as the strategies and objectives to achieve social development, are not so coherent after all. It is obvious that the means to institutional change lie in the principles and technologies developed in such disciplines as policy analysis, administration, planning, and community organization rather than in casework or group work. However, we are still not clear what the scope and character of these "macro" methodologies are, to what extent they overlap, and how they may be integrated. Indeed, an examination of the practice of the policy analyst, the planner, the community organizer, or administrator may reveal large areas of similarity, if not equivalence. A specification of these relevant practice areas may therefore be a first step in examining where we are, what constitutes social development practice, and of viewing it in a somewhat integrative manner. Some clarity also about the complementarity and sequence of these modalities is essential to a rational approach to role behavior in social development practice.

Social Policy
The term refers to legislative, political, organizational decision-making mainly at national or state levels in such arenas as aging, mental health,

taxation, transportation, welfare, community development, housing, and employment—usually in relation to specific issues—although it is also relevant to decision-making in nonpublic sectors at small community and agency levels. Social policy is also a result as well as a decision-making process. It suggests some general consequence or wide ramification of action for the welfare of a broad segment of people. Methodologically, it has been regarded as the "principles and general procedures guiding a course of actions dealing with aggregate social relationships in a society."[5] It has been suggested that social policy is the "development of strategic moves that direct an organization or a set of the organization's critical resources toward perceived opportunities in a changing environment."[6]

Policy thus may suggest not only a social mandate or explicit prescription for action but an ongoing process. It is largely an intellectual activity involving perception, conceptualization, analysis, and choice. It deals mainly with social, political, and legal process, and finally the formulation of organizational structure, program measurement, budget allocation, evaluation, and sanctions in some particular problem area or social arena. While policy may indicate what should be done, and to some extent how to do it, it usually does not do so clearly or in detail. Furthermore, a policy statement may not provide sufficient rationale for a particular course of action. Most important, it may not explicate who will get what benefits and who will suffer what losses as a result of a given course. Policy in this sense is, at best, a useful framework for planning, administration, and the delivery of services.

The role of the social work policy analyst also may be quite different from that of the actual policy-maker or decision-maker, e.g., the politician, legislator, or administrator. His major activities may be mainly research and evaluation, budget analysis in relation to particular legislative issues and agency programs, and their differential social consequences. However, depending on the reputation and power of his organization, his own position, skill, and experience, he may utilize not only his cognitive and analytic skills, but organizational, interorganizational, and political influence as well as expertise. The line between policy analysis and decision-making is thus not clear.

Planning

Planning is a term often used interchangeably with policy development or analysis. It may also signify a set of tasks, within an organizational, interorganizational, social problem or social service arena, involving community organizing and administration as well. In the urban planning tradition, it has historically signified a rational, detailed, and program-related process. Kahn says that planning is "policy choice and programming in the light of facts, projections, and the application of values." The planner's key contribution is the formulation or definition of the planning task. This for-

mulation is a result of a continual playback between assessment of the
relevant aspects of social reality and the preferences of the relevant community, whether geographic, interest, or problem based.[7] A recent United Nations document stated that planning was a "marriage between perspective
and detail."[8]

The social consequences of values and priorities are much clearer at the
level of planning than policy. Thus it is more likely that ideological, political, community, and professional debates and conflicts would break out at
the planning stage of a program. For example, the concept of decentralization may be entirely acceptable to various groups during general policy
discussion but stir a great deal of debate and conflict over particular community plans, program strategies, and specific budget allocations.

The idea of social planning has also been associated with large-scale
institutional change or development at community, national, and international levels. In this sense, social planning may be viewed as a major source
of social change, rather than a response to it. Planning in the former sense
is not characteristic in the United States. Social planning in centralized
and a large-scale version is more common in other societies. Thus, planning
in the American context, to be realistic, must take into consideration highly
pluralistic, decentralized, or varied interest group contexts and pressures.

Kahn suggests that planning probably achieves more when it focuses on
particular programs than when it deals more generally with changing institutions. The variety of sophisticated planning tasks which presently exist—
cost benefit analysis, PPBS, priorities planning, PERT, MBO, etc.—may
be more useful in relation to program development tasks than for purposes
of institution creation or institutional problem elimination, where politics
and a variety of contingent factors may play predominant roles.

While the planner "backs" into the policy analysis or policy-maker roles,
he also treads the community organizer's "turf." He may organize public
and agency interest in the recognition of a problem or issue or stimulate a
coalition of agencies to accept a particular planning approach. He may also
negotiate community sanction for a set of plans and programs, lobby for a
financial or legislative support, and even engage in the actual implementation or administration of a service system or program.

Community Organization

Community organization or development—we shall use the terms interchangeably—refers to a point of view different from policy analysis, social
planning, and administration. As we move to a community organization
emphasis within the larger social development perspective, we may shift
from complex political, bureaucratic, professional, and program decision-
making to citizen involvement. In a critical sense the shift may be from a
top-down to a bottom-up, client decision-making perspective. A larger requirement for citizen or client involvement and leadership development

may exist at the community organization level than the other social development levels of intervention.[9]

In the past decades, community organization practice appears to have focused on coordination of social welfare agencies and on attempts to balance available community resources with existing needs of local people as efficiently as possible. In recent years community organization has changed emphasis somewhat to problem-solving, resource and economic development, and grass-roots participation. More community groups and workers appear to be active than ever before, and employing a greater variety of tactics—cooperative, advocacy, and conflictual—to achieve their objectives. At the same time, policy analysis, planning, and program administration may be part and parcel of the organizer's role. Nevertheless, if we focus on distinctive kinds of role behavior, the *organizer* tends to be more activist or political, especially at the local community level, but also likely to engage in the development or administration of services.

Furthermore, community organization or community development and social treatment practices may overlap, especially at the neighborhood or grass-roots level. The organizer may need not only to help community people to express their concerns, interests in organization change and program development, but to obtain certain high-priority or emergency services as quickly as possible. His provision of advocate or brokerage services in effect may be a significant bridging, referral, brief counseling, or crisis-intervention service in itself. Furthermore, citizen leadership is not necessarily facilitated without considerable support, training, and even ongoing "counseling" by the community organizer or developer. These efforts clearly require interpersonal sensitivity and interviewing skills. Institutional and individual change may be simultaneous, if not interdependent, considerations in the course of a relationship which the community organizer may have with a committee member or community leader.

Administration

Ideally we should define social welfare administration as a process of efficient and effective implementation of social policy and plans within a framework of community values and support. However, it is not clear that social welfare administration theory and practice distinctively exist. While the notion of social administration or development administration may have meaning in other countries, the terms are not ordinarily employed in the United States, and social welfare administration here means simply administration in the context of a social welfare agency.

General organizational and management theory, research, and usually social welfare experience are the traditional guides to administrative practice. Stein describes administration as a "process of defining and attaining the objectives of an organization through a system of coordinated and cooperative effort."[10] Sarri's definition is more sophisticated: "administration is a method concerned with 1) translation of societal mandates into operational policies and goals to guide organizational behavior; 2) design of organizational structures and processes through which the goals can be achieved; 3) securing of resources in the form of materials, staff, clients, and societal legitimation necessary for goal attainment and organizational survival; 4) selection and engineering of the necessary technologies; 5) optimizing organizational behavior directed toward increased effectiveness and efficiency; and 6) evaluation of organizational performance to facilitate systematic and continual problem solving."[11]

While these definitions emphasize the rational or explicit purposes of administration and bureaucracy, there are other definitions which center on informal structures, system relations, human relations, and appropriate decision-making procedures.

Administration has also been viewed at three levels of activity and function, each overlapping or interacting—executive or institutional, managerial, and technical. At the institutional level, the administrator needs to translate and implement certain social, community, or legal mandates into action. A key activity is the determination of organizational boundaries, i.e., the scope of the particular organization's relations to its environment. This includes the pattern of resource acquisition needed in relation to the kind of social product delivered. The executive function determines the nature of exchange relations with other agencies—cooperative, competing, conflictual (or nonrelationship)—to be developed.

At the managerial level, major activities are mediation between consumers and the technical subunits of the organization. The role behaviors of this level of administrator are directed toward procurement and allocation of services, structural design, interunit coordination, staff direction and development, including recruitment, selection, training, and supervision of staff. At the technical level, which includes such subroles as consultation, case managing, teaching, evaluation, referral, monitoring, and even the direct delivery of a client service, emphasis is on such matters as standardization, routinization, periodic assessment, and evaluation.

As with the policy analyst or policy-maker, community organizer, or social planner, so too with the administrator—it is difficult if not impossible to set firm boundaries on what is expected of a particular social development role. Each role interacts with or overlaps another in some fashion. There may be a set of core concepts required for performance of each of these roles which includes—in addition to intelligence and imagination—social commitment, use of social relationship, information, communication, and decision-making, sanction and control, politics, problem analysis and problem-solving, program evaluation, resource acquisition and allocation, consensus and conflict, and citizen participation. While these ideas, and the skills they entail, may be building blocks of the general social development role, knowledge of them is still mainly located within traditional discipline boundaries of policy analysis, community organization, planning, and administration. Nevertheless, they would appear to be the key elements or clusters of elements needed by the worker to deal with the creation, growth, and change of social welfare programs and institutions.

CONSISTENCY WITH THE SOCIAL WORK PARADIGM

There is no necessary dissonance between the social development and social work paradigms. Social development is consistent with social work's historic reform mission and practice character. We have approached the analysis of social development modalities as an elaboration of the social growth and specialization of practice activities. We have centered attention, however, on institutional factors and the means to influence them, in relation to individual human problems and needs.

However, we may need to compare social development with social work, mainly as it has traditionally emphasized social treatment, particularly in its application. The comparison should be in terms of such professional categories or considerations as ideology, worker qualification, use of "relationship," influence, scientific method, and resource complexity and constraint. The similarities and differences between the two paradigms are implicit in the discussion already, but we shall try to make them a little clearer, particularly from the view of role performance.

Ideology
Both social development and social treatment workers are preeminently concerned with respect for the individual person, his right to self-determination and maintenance of his personal dignity. Emphasis by both kinds of workers is on meeting social needs and doing this through social relationships, whether the impact on personal need and welfare is direct or indirect. However, these moral imperatives for the social development worker mean that he must operate with a focus on institutional and program structure rather than individual personality. There is greater concern with structural inequities rather than with personal disorders. The social development worker acts more directly on the assumption that the inequities of wealth, income, race, and status, as well as social services, are responsible for the problems which people have. Social workers, as treatment or clinical workers, do not or cannot structurally or functionally act as readily on these beliefs. Nor can the social development worker, on his part, deal in any extensive or detailed fashion with a particular individual's social dysfunction. This does not mean there may not be great variation, including radical or conservative approaches to practice within and across these perspectives. These terms, however, have different meaning in social treatment than in social

development. Indeed, the political use of these terms has far more relevance to social development than to social treatment practice.

Worker Qualification

Both social development and social workers are qualified for their roles by virtue of special education and training and also by special social sensitivities, emotional and social maturity, and a capacity to empathize with people in special need—the poor, the mentally, physically, and socially handicapped. The social development worker may require also an extra modicum of aggressiveness, resourcefulness, and ability to operate not only inside but outside existing agency structures. Since laws, policies, social service systems, and programs are sometimes viewed as contributing to the problems of people, the social development worker needs critically to question present social and organizational realities and operate in some quasi-independent, yet professionally and organizationally relevant, fashion.

"Use of Relationship"

Both social development and social treatment workers are unique in their concern for the quality of social relationships. They are concerned with the use of socially helpful and disciplined relationships. The social development worker must be able to create these special relationships not only directly, but structurally or indirectly as well. Both types of workers, as professionals, must be aware of their own personality strengths and weaknesses, and use "professional self" to facilitate patterns of social relationships which are helpful to clients or constituents. A considerably larger proportion of time, however, must be spent by the social development worker in dealing with organizational and interorganizational, intellectual, and political issues. The social development worker must therefore deal with a task environment which is not only more complex, but his disciplined use of "self" must extend to a different type of relationship as well. Facilitation of positive or helpful relationships with a particular agency may have quite different meaning and ramifications than the development of a helping relationship with a client in need. The social development worker may consequently encounter greater difficulty in the creation of a balance of objectivity and involvement or "partisanship" on behalf of both agencies and clients in need.

Influence

In effect, the social development worker may differ from the social treatment worker mainly in respect to his use of organizational, community, and political influence. He is more concerned with the importance of modifying policies and procedures than with directly changing client relationships. He uses staff, data, laws, plans, facilities, resources, et al., politically and organizationally, on behalf of people in need. He is more interested in the organizational and political uses of people as institutional representatives than in directly helping people as clients. In general, he is more concerned with the exercise of influence than in the use of relationship, particularly in relation to clients. Power and pressure, both collective and individual, direct and indirect, are tools he employs. It should be noted that principles of influence are not articulated in the traditional social work paradigm. They are clearly ignored in the clinical social work role. A basic criterion of effective practice, rarely raised by the clinical social worker, is who benefits and who loses from a particular social problem, program or service delivery system. The social treatment worker is probably less likely than the social development worker to raise questions about the value of a given program effort. The social development worker has to think in community, system, and organizational change and development terms. These, then, become the primary objects of his influence efforts.

Scientific Method

Both types of worker are committed to rationality and reality testing. Both rely heavily on inductive and intuitive procedures. Differences are mainly in relation to the kind of data collection and analysis used as a basis for decision. The social development worker finds survey and quantitative technologies more congenial than case approaches to the demands of his job. A more formal approach to hypothesis testing and to the acquisition of data may be required. The social development worker probably needs to develop greater mastery of research and evaluative procedures than does the social treatment worker. Both kinds of worker, however, are likely to emphasize output rather than outcome or long-term effectiveness.

Resource Complexity and Constraint

While both the social development and social worker are confronted with complexity, variability, and constraints in their efforts to help people, the problems may be greater for the social development worker. He may have to contend not simply with more practice variables, but he has relatively less direct control over the means to achieve his objectives. The time frame in which program, organizational, and community change occur may be much longer than that for individual or family change to occur.

It is possible, therefore, that the social development role is more vulnerable to dysfunction than the typical social work role, in its classic treatment emphasis. The social development worker thus may be subject to greater frustration, ritualistic behavior, i.e., "bureaucratic" activity, opportunism, and corruption, than the social treatment worker. The lack of immediacy and insufficient interpersonal interaction with clients also may dull the social sensitivities of the social development worker over time. In other words, the social development worker appears to be faced with greater complexity and constraint on the performance of his role. As a result he may be less likely than the social treatment worker to achieve his objectives.

CONCLUSION

Social development is a principal perspective of social helping inherent in the tradition of social work, basically compatible with social treatment. It is possible, however, that institutional and individual practice emphases can be drawn so sharply that the links between the two are lost. To the extent that this occurs, these professional subsectors become culturally and politically isolated from each other. The profession may decompose, for example, into groups of therapists or clinicians and managers. While the vitality of the profession depends on the one hand on continued specialization and the existence of creative tension between practice components, on the other its durability may depend on the ability of theorists and practitioners to implement and conceptualize common interests and ideals on a continuing basis.

NOTES

1. See Porter R. Lee, *Social Work As Cause and Function, and Other Papers* (New York: Columbia University Press, 1937); Mary E. Richmond, *Social Diagnosis* (New York: Russell Sage Foundation, 1917).
2. See, for example, Joel Fisher, *The Effectiveness of Social Casework* (Springfield, Ill: Charles C Thomas, 1976); Henry Meyer, Edgar F. Borgatta, and Wyatt C. Jones, *Girls at Vocational High* (New York: Russell Sage Foundation, 1965).
3. Harold L. Wilensky and Charles H. Lebeaux, *Industrial Society and Social Welfare* (New York: Free Press, 1965), p. 147; see also John M. Romanyshyn, *Social Welfare* (New York: Random House, 1971).
4. Alva Myrdal, *Nation and Family* (New York: Harper and Bros., 1941), p. 152.
5. Alvin L. Schorr and Edward C. Baumheer, "Social Policy," *Encyclopedia of Social Work* (New York: National Association of Social Workers, 1971), 2:1361–76.
6. Raymond A. Bauer and Kenneth J. Gergen, eds., *The Study of Policy Foundation* (New York: Free Press, 1968).
7. Alfred Kahn, *Theory and Practice of Social Planning* (New York: Russell Sage Foundation, 1969).
8. United Nations, Economic Commission For Asia and the Far East, *Social Development in Asia—Restrospect and Prospect* (New York: United Nations, 1971), p. 53.
9. Irving A. Spergel, "Social Planning and Community Organization: Community Development," *Encyclopedia of Social Work*, vol. 2 (New York: National Association of Social Workers, forthcoming).
10. Herman A. Stein, "Social Work Administration," in *Social Work Administration: A Resource Book*, ed. Harry A. Schwartz (New York: Council on Social Work Education, 1970), pp. 7–11.
11. Rosemary C. Sarri, "Administration in Social Welfare," *Encyclopedia of Social Work*, 1971, 1:42–43.

Appreciation is especially expressed to Sheldon Tobin for comments and suggestions.

Part II

SOME
THEORETICAL PERSPECTIVES
ON SOCIAL ADMINISTRATION

EDITOR'S INTRODUCTION

The literature on social administration is noticeably devoid of material of theoretical interest. A growing list of empirical studies parallels writing devoted to elaborations of practice wisdom. The best that one can find are certain perspectives that help identify the material to be studied and organized.

There are several theoretical streams in the general literature on administration that are potentially useful for the social services. Viewing the social agency as an open system directs attention to the external organizational environment and to the host of interorganizational relationships with which it must inevitably interact. In this day of extensive governmental support and regulation, the social agency is increasingly dependent on other organizations for its stability and growth. Few can be self-generating and self-directing.

Furthermore, service-giving organizations are imbedded in a network of constituencies that help define their objectives, policies, and ongoing operations. Each of their universal elements—providers, consumers, and the organization that brings them together—has its essential internal and external constituencies. Practitioners look to unions, staff organizations, and professional societies to help secure their standards and interests. Clients frequently establish parent associations, alumni groups (i.e., ex-offenders), client organizations (i.e., The Welfare Rights Organization). Organizations and their trustees are closely tied to coordinating bodies, funding sources, and, often, accrediting agencies.

Each of the networks in turn, and in common, directs attention to broad, general constituencies that affect public acceptance and legitimacy—the media, legislative bodies, administrative areas of government, and the like. Public relations and social action inevitably become important aspects of administrative action, both individually and collectively. Agencies in special fields band together for the purpose not only of setting standards and advancing levels of adequacy in delivering services, but also to enhance the public awareness of social need and to assure governmental assumption of responsibility where this seems indicated. Thus, open system perspectives help define the broader parameters of administrative behavior, and add important insight to the traditional concern for internal dynamics and management.

Another influential stream of thought comes quite naturally to social administration—human relations theory and research. Much that developed since the early Hawthorne research on the effect of social and cultural variables on work organizations parallels similar work on the social and psychological foundations of social work practice. The nature of social system attributes and their effect on social administration provide important clues for administrative practitioners. The significance of value systems, social norms, power constellations, sentiments, reward patterns, goals, and tension management are generally recognized by astute managers as they deal with problems of organizational stability, conflict, and change. Much work remains to be done before the literature of social administration will reflect more of the practice wisdom that grows out of day-to-day experience with organizational encounters.

A recent emphasis in management thought, contingency theory, has hardly begun to influence social administration thinking, yet can potentially provide useful perspectives. Less a theory than a point of view, contingency suggests that few general propositions in administration hold under all circumstances, that it is necessary to specify the unique conditions under which one or another principle is likely to obtain. Such an approach directs attention to the importance of organizational diagnosis, of identifying variables in the organization that condition its ability to achieve its objectives, of highlighting the factors (contingencies) affecting decision-making and courses of action that meet the requirements of the organization and the needs and interests of its several constituencies (Morse & Lorsh, 1970).

These perspectives are drawn from the general management literature. It is appropriate to suggest some specific orientations which come from the vantage point of the administration of the social services. One such derives from a view of the often competing interests of the essential elements that constitute the social agency. While client, practitioner, and organization come together to achieve common goals, in practice their requirements and preferences often diverge. Because of their differing interests, internal contradictions abound. Client demands for service availability often conflict with staff convenience. Agency pressures for containing cost run into staff demands for salary increments. Client requirements for comprehensive service compete with agency focus on specialized offerings. Professional dominance, client urgings, and bureaucratic procedures frequently engage with one another in a struggle for control of the service encounter (Freidson, 1970). An essential task of the administrator is to bring these divergent needs, interests, and pressures into some form of balance, moving from one steady state to another in the process of program development.

Where the administrator stands in relation to this force field is crucial with respect to charting administrative strategy. Because of the necessarily interdependent relationships of the several constituencies in the organization, a prime focus on one element directs energy to engender compliance on the part of the others. When agency needs are seen as primary, client and practitioner must conform, often to the ascendancy of organizational maintenance requirements and to the detriment of service adequacy. Such is frequently the circumstance in large bureaucracies. Where practitioner needs are seen as primary, service requirements are often ignored. Thus, medical personnel in hospitals eschew research and treatment of common and widespread illness in favor of "exotic" conditions, such as open-heart surgery.

Finally, when the administrator assumes a client perspective, and client need and service integrity become the primary orientation for administrative action, agency and staff are moved to compliance in furtherance of those objectives. Client service requirements become the constant, and organization and practitioner are encouraged to adapt.

There are two important consequences of such a view. Primacy of orientation to the client and to the integrity of client service leads naturally to a posture of administrative advocacy. While it is true that administrators are formally accountable to their employer—the legal entity that represents the organization—they implicitly assume accountability to the client for the quality of the service. Internal and external constraints on that quality become fundamental targets of administrative action. This may well have the consequence of bringing the administrator into conflict with agency trustees, supporting organizations, and funding sources, as well as members of the staff. The true ethic of professional behavior, however, lies in concern for the clients and their needs. Professional skill is concerned precisely with the ways in which the administrator balances and orchestrates the interests of divergent constituencies, but from a client perspective as an organizing principle.

Finally, the issue of compliance referred to above moves administrators to an interest in organizational change, taking their clue from the shifting environment of social practice and the response of current and prospective clients to the social and psychological pressures that attend such social changes. Organizations rarely remain static, but move from one equilibrium to another, absorbing and adapting to the requirements of both internal and external pressures and circumstances. These processes are akin to Piaget's concepts of assimilation and accommodation (Piaget, 1968), the give and take between the organism and its environment. The process of equilibration, which balances the intrusions of the social and physical environment with the organism's need to conserve its structural systems, describes quite precisely the administrative function. When internal dislocation or external turbulence seem to disturb the existing state of affairs, administrative leadership serves the equilibrating requisites. The ethical guide to this function derives from administrative identification with client service requirements.

The selections in this section deal with a variety of theoretical perspectives for social agency administration. Mullis reviews several schools of thought in management and organizational theory, without making a distinction between the two, and stresses recent emphasis on contingency approaches and systems concepts. The context of his analysis is public welfare, from which he draws several examples of the application of management thinking.

Hanlan presents three models of administration which are relevant to the education and practice of social work. They represent an overlapping continuum of theories, knowledge, and skills, and are based on differing assumptions, goals, and interventions. Social work administration flows from a synthesis of social work methods and stresses clinical skills; social welfare administration relies on social science knowledge and directs its application to social welfare policy and program evaluation; social administration encompasses a view of the societal context of service delivery systems represented by other political, social, and economic institutions, and focuses attention on advocacy and social action. Hanlan's brief is to move beyond narrow professional concerns, beyond clinical, managerial, or organizationally defined activist approaches, to a concern for dealing with broad social problems and issues with a view of helping achieve the requisite resources for which they call. His is a plea for social responsibility of the administrator and the profession.

Neugeboren identifies the essential skill areas of social welfare administration—analytical, interactional, and technical—and describes how one school of social work based its training program on these aspects of practice. In presenting patterns of field work, he indicates some issues raised in orienting students to both organizational maintenance and system change activities.

REFERENCES

Friedson, Eliot. *Professional Dominance: The Social Structure of Medical Care*. New York: Atherton Press, 1970.

Morse, John J., and Lorsch, Jay W. "Beyond Theory Y." *Harvard Business Review*, May-June, 1970, pp. 37–44.

Piaget, Jean. *Six Psychological Studies*. New York: Vintage Books, 1968, pp. 100–114.

4/MANAGEMENT APPLICATIONS
TO THE WELFARE SYSTEM

SCOTT MULLIS

In relating management and organization concepts to welfare programs two clear problems emerge. The first is the degree to which welfare professionals are able to understand principles of management and organization. The second problem, while perhaps more subtle, is the converse of the first. Professional managers have tremendous difficulty understanding welfare.

The purpose of this article is to close some of the differences between management and welfare thinking. It is beyond its scope to resolve most questions, and in particular it is impossible to determine if welfare can, indeed, be managed. Attempted here are two things: (1) an update to management and organizational concepts and (2) an application of some recent trends in organizational thought to welfare.

In the absence of ongoing education, many middle- and top-level managers today are not generally cognizant of changes in the scope and direction of management and organization theory. Similarly, welfare professionals, often with early training in sociology and political science, are handicapped by their extensive exposure to bureaucracy as *the* form of organization. While we are not about to observe the "death of bureaucracy,"[1] other organizational models are available and an understanding of situations where these contingent forms apply is essential.

An important current trend in management and organization theory is movement away from set, "universal" principles toward a contingency view.[2] This means roughly that the correct organizational structure and management plan is dependent on the situation. Much of the current empirical work in management and organization is directed toward isolating situational variables and developing scenarios where certain principles work consistently. This focus can be exemplified by work in the area of leadership.[3] It was once generally agreed that group participation and concern for subordinates were uniformly good. More recent analysis indicates that in some situations performance requires an autocratic, production-oriented leadership.[4]

So, too, use of the bureaucratic model (and its principles of organization) is increasingly recognized as only one possible form. Longitudinal empirical evidence is scant, but at least three other forms are appearing in organizations. These are project, matrix, and free-form typologies. All of these violate in some way the classical bureaucratic model.[5] They are, however, effective in some situations and for certain kinds of tasks.

The significant generalization seems to be that when an organization is faced with a fairly stable environment, and when tasks are repetitive, a strict bureaucratic structure can work efficiently. However, when goals and objectives are more general, and when the relevant environment can generate great variety, then a more open, less structured, and consequently more responsive organization seems to work well.[6]

MANAGEMENT AND ORGANIZATIONAL THEORY

Management and organizational theory can be traced through four schools of thought: process, behavioral, quantitative, and systems. The currently emerging school described as contingent or situational has potential for uniting these highly divergent approaches.[7]

Process

The process school, as the name implies, sees management as a series of activities. The original thinking in this view goes back to the early twentieth century with Fayol's plan—organize, command, coordinate, and control.[8] Though Fayol's work was published in Europe early in this century, translation into English did not become generally available until the late 1940s. While there has been much elaboration on Fayol's theme, there has been little development in this school beyond the original.

Organizational precepts associated with the process school are bureaucratic. The "universal" prescriptions for efficiency included increasing division of labor or specialization, hierarchy, a set of formal abstract rules, and impersonal relations.

Behavioral

The extreme mechanistic view implicit in the process approach, as well as its failure to provide "universal" answers to organizational problems, led many to seek alternative approaches.

Psychological factors received increasing attention and with the Hawthorne Studies at Western Electric, a behavioral approach was born. The first attempts were primarily a reaction to the mechanics of the bureaucratic model and, in their own way, were severely constrained. Most of the discussion involved looking at psychological factors within the bureaucratic prescription with little attention to other structural forms. The net result was the "happiness equation" of the human relations movement. According to this school, productivity was a function of morale. This simplistic explanation fell rapidly into disrepute as practitioners and students alike increasingly recognized the complexity of the organization-human interaction.

More recently the behavioral approach can be characterized as an assemblage of concepts drawn from all behavioral sciences unified in the conceptual framework of the organization-human interaction as mutually dependent systems. This view is partially the result of influence from the systems approach to management.

Systems

The systems view of management has its roots in developments during and after World War II. The great promise of general systems theory is the idea of tying together many approaches into a unified whole—and therein lies the problem. As a general science of just about everything, it explains just about nothing. As one of its founders points out, there is great difficulty in moving from interesting analogy to a productive model.[9]

This is not to say that general systems theory is without value. As will be developed below, some concepts have great power to assist through "explanation in principle."[10] But the promise is not fulfilled. General systems theory will require years of work and new approaches to mathematics to become the all powerful science of sciences.

Quantitative

The quantitative approach to management, which also developed during and immediately following World War II, is properly viewed as a lineal descendant of scientific management of Frederick W. Taylor (circa 1910). The reason that this merits rating as a major school of management is a function of two factors.

First, in an industrial society there is great impetus to quantify and measure. Often this holds even if it can't be shown that the proper variables are being measured. This emphasis on quantification and measurement is the nemesis of the quantitative school as well as its forte. Too often so much is abstracted from problems in order to force a situation into a given model that any hope of realistic application is lost.

The second factor which brings the quantitative school to the status of a major school of management is the development of the computer. Without the computer many of the techniques and models would never have been developed, much less implemented. As the computer becomes ever faster and more capable in storage and retrieval, quantitative approaches become more viable. The problem of abstraction and consequent oversimplification is ameliorated as the computers become capable of handling models in increasing variety and complexity.

In summary then, students and practitioners of management and organization theory are divided in their approach. This situation has recently changed with the development of a contingency approach. The contingency frame of reference starts with the assumption that universal prescriptions (like universal truths!) are difficult to find.

This approach is not eclipsing the other schools. Contingent analysis has contributed to further development of principles in the four major schools. The behavioralists have for some time now looked to situational contin-

gencies to explain effective leadership. The quantitative approach applies
different models to different situations although the methodology remains
the same. More important, one of the principles of general systems theory
is that of equifinality.[11] This means that given an open system there is more
than one way to accomplish an end. This is the contingency approach in a
most abstract form. The following section takes two selected concepts, one
drawn from the systems school and the other from the behavioral school,
and applies contingent analysis to the welfare system.

CONTINGENCIES IN ORGANIZATION OF THE
WELFARE FUNCTION

The Systems Model
The systems school views an organization as having inputs, transformation
processes, and outputs which are measured on certain variables. The results
of the measurements are then fed back as part of the inputs to the next cycle. Figure 1 depicts this conceptual framework.

This framework points directly to three groups of questions extremely
important to organizational analysis. The first set of questions involves the
outputs. What is the organization supposed to accomplish? Further, how
is this accomplishment to be measured? The second set involves the inputs.
What exactly is available to the organization in terms of resources? Also,
what is the nature of the environment? What factors beyond the direct
control of the organization impinge upon the operations? Finally, the last

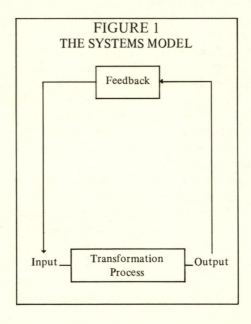

FIGURE 1
THE SYSTEMS MODEL

Feedback

Input — Transformation Process — Output

set of questions looks at the transformation processes. These include: What are the steps that lead to a given end? Can certain steps be bypassed? Can the process be accelerated? Can it be slowed?

These are not surprising questions. An experienced manager would ask these questions and many others if asked to analyze this organization. What this framework does provide is an organized whole—a checklist of areas of possible improvement. Thus, such a framework can at least be used to unify diverse areas of concern.

Beyond such analysis, however, is the possibility of using such a framework to actually structure an organization. It is clear that the kind of analysis alluded to above will not automatically flow from a standard organization chart. Why not use such a systems framework in lieu of the normal bureaucratic organizational chart, thus organizing in terms of process instead of physical entities connected by lines of authority? Much credit must be given F. H. Allport for his view of structure as a cycle of events.[12]

In looking at a welfare organization such a structure might develop along the following lines:

Output

A welfare department has responsibility for acting on social and economic problems of certain individuals. The desired output then is defined in terms of the proper social and economic variables. The objective in a given case may be a degree of improvement, prevention of a further negative trend, or a deceleration of a negative trend. This definition of output must meet the test of "operationality" to allow measurement. Once the proper output and measurement is determined, the next task is to analyze the inputs to understand the necessary and available transformation tasks.

Inputs

Inputs to the system include physical and human resources, plans, and mandates. The most important input is the people who are to be served. The people that enter the welfare system enter because of some need or set of needs. The input function is charged with defining that set of needs for which the organization can provide. This is done through the eligibility process. Once eligibility is established, the client enters into the transformation process, where transformation includes slowing or stabilizing a regressive situation, as well as improvement.

Transformation Process

In a welfare program the transformation process would be identified as the programs providing aid and services, which generally include income maintenance, and medical and social services. These programs all converge at the individual client level to define a major portion of his life. To artificially separate income maintenance from services at the organizational level as presently mandated really misses the point.

One of the principal reasons for separation of services is to divorce the client-oriented services aspect from the eligibility-oriented income maintenance function.[13] This follows from the idea that the eligibility process is degrading and has highly negative connotations with respect to clients. It should have been apparent that care is required in eligibility determination because a welfare office must be responsible to taxpayers as well as clients (who may also pay taxes). Whenever resources are scarce, and they always are, criteria must be set up. Eligibility is a problem in social services as well as income maintenance.

What follows from this kind of longitudinal analysis of the client as he moves through the system is that the organization could be designed around that flow. Specific recommendations would include the separation of all aspects of the transformation process from the input. Instead of a separation by programs we would implement a separation by flow. When clients entered the system, they would go through the eligibility process once, not twice or more. Out of this screening the client would receive a checklist of all services and other benefits which can be provided by the agency.

Figure 2 depicts this kind of systems framework applied to welfare.

CENTRALIZATION-DECENTRALIZATION:
A CONTINGENCY APPROACH

The second example of analysis of welfare organization in the context of management and organization theory involves the classic question of whether an organization is more effective when closely controlled at the

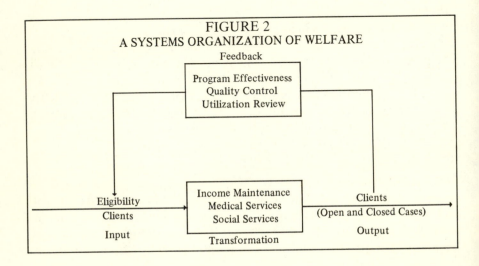

FIGURE 2
A SYSTEMS ORGANIZATION OF WELFARE

Feedback

Program Effectiveness
Quality Control
Utilization Review

Eligibility
Clients

Input

Income Maintenance
Medical Services
Social Services

Transformation

Clients
(Open and Closed Cases)

Output

top through centralization or when lower-level members are given more responsibility and authority for decision making. Most schools of management address this question, and all agree that advantages of decentralization generally outweigh advantages of centralization. The process school sees decentralization as necessary because of the excessive time lag between a developing situation and remote decision making. The behavioral school points to more satisfaction at lower levels when participants have more input and control on their jobs. The systems school would look not only at increased speed of response but also to the ability of the organization to be more diverse and flexible in its response to nonroutine matters.

Decentralization, for all its popularity, is not uniformly accepted. Many organizations try decentralization but move back to a more centralized form. Decentralization, it is found, is not a universal principle. Rather decentralization is a matter of degree, and the proper degree is dependent on the situation.

This contingency approach to the centralization-decentralization question is generally discussed in terms of the whole organization. The welfare organization indicates centralization of some functions and decentralization of others.[14]

As indicated above, the degree of decentralization involves a trade off of close uniform control against more rapid flexible decision making. The proper degree of decentralization, then, depends on the relative importance of uniformity and flexibility, as well as elements in the specific situation affecting these variables. In the welfare organization, income maintenance and medical and social services each present a different situation; therefore, differing degrees of centralization are appropriate.

Income maintenance involves money, and money is a scarce resource with uniform acceptance by and predictable benefits to the recipient. Equity and uniform treatment of clients dictate a closely controlled centralized operation with minimal variance in policy decisions on an individual basis. The client should know what to expect, and should not be able to "work the system." On the supply side, taxpayers demand accountability and protection from fraud whether perpetrated by client or employee. All of these considerations dictate a highly centralized closely audited payments function.

Client needs, however, are not uniform, nor can they be adequately evaluated in a centralized situation. Provision of social services can, to some extent, pick up the slack. However, it is very likely that local discretionary decisions about money will be required at the local level. Such local discretion should be exercised with a local funds matching scheme and should be centrally monitored for both excessive and insufficient use. The ratio of such discretionary funds to the total aid bill should be low.

Medical, too, should be closely monitored and centralized for services payments. The situation is different from income maintenance, but the result is the same. Medical services are locally provided, but payments for services are centralized.

The problem in medical is to avoid fraudulent claims. It is also necessary to assure adequate client care and to avoid experimental treatments. Accomplishing these goals requires a highly integrated utilization-review procedure based on statistical analysis. Centralization of payments provides the opportunity for such close control. The negative aspect of such centralization is turnaround time or the delay of payments. In many states the first requirement is to clean up the medical claims processing; only then can any kind of control become feasible.

Social services provide an interesting variant to the above analysis. Both income maintenance and medical assistance present clear-cut problems when compared with social services. In both cases there are generally accepted, available units of measurement with relatively predictable results in the provision of funds or services. Also, for the most part, in both payments and medical the objective of maintenance is predominant. Social services also involves an implicit mandate to bring about change and prevent deterioration.

Social services do not lend themselves to generally accepted, available units of measurement. This is, of course, because there is little generally accepted operational theory or body of knowledge behind services. This area is emerging as a science and depends to a large degree on an eclectic approach which includes many minor theories, often inconsistent and contradictory, and a smattering of empirical evidence in the form of case histories and poorly controlled experiments and surveys. As a result, there is a great deal of question as to the value of social services in general.

This situation calls for carefully centralized monitoring of services provided, and recording of precedent and subsequent conditions to allow evaluation. But decisions as to which service to provide and the method of provision are most properly made at the local level by truly professional staff. Local decision making provides the variety and the rapid response necessary to cope with the very individual approach required. This is so because the need for service varies significantly between individuals; there is great variety in delivery method as well as availability of service; and, finally, local conditions will affect the proper prescription of service. Most services cannot be standardized at this time.

CONCLUSION

This short paper attempts a review of some of the most recent developments in the field of management as applied to the context of public welfare. Application of systems concepts in organizing around client flow and the contingency analysis of relative decentralization of three major functions provide practical examples of how management thinking can contribute to welfare. Purposely avoided are the problems related to federal mandates and matching formulas, which are beyond the scope of this article. It is hoped that some questions have been raised for the practitioner.

NOTES

1. Warren Bennis, "The Death of Bureaucracy," in David C. Cleland and William R. King, eds., *Systems, Organizations, Analysis, Management: A Book of Readings* (New York: McGraw-Hill Book Co., 1969), pp. 11–17.
2. Fred Luthans, "The Contingency Theory of Management," *Business Horizons,* June 1973, pp. 57–72.
3. Fred E. Fiedler, *A Theory of Leadership Effectiveness* (New York: McGraw-Hill Book Co., 1967).
4. Ibid., pp. 142–48.
5. It is beyond the scope of this article to elaborate on these forms. Further development can be found in Fred Luthans, *Organizational Behavior* (New York: McGraw-Hill Book Co., 1973), pp. 168–79.
6. Y. K. Shetty and Howard M. Carlisle, "A Contingency Model of Organizational Design," *California Management Review* 15 (Fall 1972): 40.
7. Luthans, "The Contingency Theory of Management," pp. 57–72.
8. Henri Fayol, "Administration Indústrielle et Générale," *Bulletin de la Société de l'Industrie Minérale,* 5th series, vol. 10, pt. 3 (1916), pp. 1–162.
9. Ludwig Von Bertalanffy, *General Systems Theory,* rev. ed. (New York: George Braziller, Inc., 1969), pp. 33–36.
10. Ibid., p. 33.
11. Ibid., p. 46.
12. Floyd H. Allport, "The Structuring of Events: Outline of a General Theory with Application to Psychology," *Psychological Review* 61, no. 5 (September 1954): 281–303; and Floyd H. Allport, "A Structuronomic Conception of Behavior, Individual and Collective. I. Structural Theory and the Master Problem of Social Psychology," *Journal of Abnormal and Social Psychology* 64 (1962): 3–30.
13. U.S., Department of Health, Education, and Welfare, Social and Rehabilitative Service, Community Services Administration, *The Separation of Services from Assistance Payments,* HEW pubn. no. (SRS) 73–23015 (Washington, D.C.: Government Printing Office, 1972), pp. 5–8.
14. We are talking now on the state level. The centralization of payments at the federal level in the adult categories was unnecessary and has resulted in untold human misery as a highly efficient centralized bureaucracy, the Social Security Administration, operating in a very stable environment, learned that it is not capable of handling the higher variety and more pressing need of the welfare population. The people and their characteristics did not change by act of Congress. As a result state and county welfare administrators are forced to pick up the slack. The goal of more equitable treatment under federalization should have been accomplished with more leadership from the Department of Health, Education, and Welfare.

5/FROM SOCIAL WORK TO
SOCIAL ADMINISTRATION

ARCHIE HANLAN

"Activism" is a term that has enjoyed popular usage since, a few years ago, California college students wore necklaces of mutilated IBM cards and protested an administration that they regarded as unresponsive, alienating, and sometimes even brutal. These students were the advance guard of a new militancy, an activist orientation on the part of some college students and young professionals. In recent years they have been joined by such diverse groups as organized tenants, welfare recipients, and welfare workers who consider computerized welfare budgets and welfare directors to be symbols of the steel-hearted administrators who do the dirty work of our society.[1]

The increasing protest and demonstration against the administration of our social welfare agencies are only part of a larger debate in this country. Administrators of all the agencies and organizations of society have been characterized as members of an elite class in a class-torn system. They are portrayed as symbols of authority who are implacable in the face of our pervasive social needs and problems. In one of the more flamboyant descriptions of twentieth-century man, he is described as psychologically and economically split asunder by the "Omnipotent Administrators" who rule over the "Supermasculine Menials."[2] Thus, the rhetoric on administration is a curious mixture of psychological, economic, and sociological arguments. In social welfare and elsewhere, we can no longer wish away or dismiss the arguments simply because they are rhetorical.

These emotionally charged views of administration make it difficult to discuss the subject, and even in the profession of social work, "administration" has become an obscene fourteen-letter word. It is argued that the executive constrains the development of the autonomous practitioner. He is the captive of elitist power groups in the community. He is punitive, self-interested, and, worse yet, an anal-compulsive personality who imposes his will on a powerless clientele. The ghosts of Freud, Marx, and Weber are invoked: we are confronted by unresolvable Oedipal conflicts, inevitable class struggles, and uncontrollable bureaucracies.[3]

Yet all of these dialectical dilemmas obscure crucial administrative goals and interventions for achieving the needed social changes in our society. We will not humanize our social agencies and institutions by bromides or by random, irrational behavior. It is only through some reasoned and rational explication of social change, by debureaucratizing our organizations, and by demonstrably effective strategies for achieving the desired changes, that we may lead ourselves to something other than an apocalyptic end to our recurring social crises.

An initial step for social work, then, is to strain toward some conceptual clarity when ambiguity and distortion exist. Our literature and research suggest that there are at least three models of administration in the education and practice of social workers. These models are not separate and mutually exclusive entities; rather, they represent an overlapping continuum of theories, knowledge, and skills. Yet some important distinctions can be made among them in terms of their differing emphases on assumptions, goals, and interventions. And these distinctions are significantly related to the way in which we perceive the social work profession in relation to the larger society.

This continuum of administration in social work will be divided into three segments: (1) social work administration; (2) social welfare administration; and (3) social administration. These three represent a broad spectrum of perspectives and activities within the profession which range from micro- to macro-emphases on the human being and his environment. The three models will be explicated in terms of their assumptions, goals, and interventions.

SOCIAL WORK ADMINISTRATION

Perhaps the largest percentage of social workers employ the social work administration model. For example, a recent survey of members of the National Association of Social Workers (NASW) was concerned with the primary job functions of social workers. Almost half of the respondents (49.7 percent) reported that administration is their primary job function.[4] Only one third (33.4 percent) reported casework as their primary job function; 2 percent, community organization; and one percent, group work. Given the method focus of our practice, and the NASW's exclusion of administration from that practice,[5] what is the knowledge and skill base for this large body of social workers whose major function is administration?

Presumably, the answer lies in the term "social work administration," which most frequently has referred to the method approach.[6] That is, it has generally referred to a combination of the knowledge and skills of one or more of the three methods, applied by the social work administrator. Rather than articulating new knowledge and skills, the emphasis is upon some synthesis of methods in the interventions employed by social workers in administrative positions.

This model of administration is logically related to the career patterns of many social work executives. In other words, the directors of many casework agencies have moved from caseworker to supervisor to administrator. Group work agencies are most frequently administered by group workers, and this small group of practitioners has produced a large portion of the social work texts on administration.[7] Health and welfare councils and planning agencies tend to draw their executives from social workers who have had community organization training, and some recent social work literature links administration with community organization.[8]

Basic assumptions for social work administration derive, then, from the assumptions inherent in our three methods. Each method has implied a distinct social work body of knowledge and skills, and this assumption logically holds for social work administration. Thus, the knowledge base for social work administration is to be found primarily in the substantive areas of social work, not in other disciplines.

Interventions generated by social work administration follow the methods approach. There is particular emphasis on use of clinical skills in individual and group interpersonal relations among employees. These skills are compatible with the human relations approach in management literature, with growing interest in administrative use of sensitivity training, and with an emphasis on leadership styles and behavior.[9] Given a dominance of the casework method in social work, it is reasonable to expect reliance on clinical skills as the social worker moves into administration.

The assumptions underlying our practice are closely intertwined with the major goals of the profession, and the goals for social work administration are clearly within the broad social work goal of enhancement of social functioning.[10] Drawing upon more specific goals suggested by Rosen and Connaway, social work administration is clearly compatible with these purposes of the profession: providing and distributing societal resources and helping persons to use maximally the social resources available to them.[11] With emphasis upon existing goods and services, existing programs and agencies, these purposes are essentially residual social welfare functions.[12] Within this context, this model of social work administration is well within the mainstream of social work practice.

SOCIAL WELFARE ADMINISTRATION

Social welfare administration is distinguished from social work administration in terms of the degree of emphasis rather than in absolute differences. The term has been used to stress the relevance of social science knowledge in the management of human service organizations.[13] While this point of view does not necessarily deny the knowledge and skills base of the three social work methods, it does place those methods in a broader context of knowledge which social workers need for the administration of social welfare programs and agencies.[14] On the continuum, this model may be seen as moving away from a central concern with indigenous social work knowledge and away from a major focus on individual and group behavior. Instead, it moves toward a critical and differential extrapolation of existing and developing social science knowledge in the areas of social welfare policy and administration.

The assumptions which pertain here derive from more than an internal perspective of social work. Rather than accepting some prior definitions of methods and practice in social work, this model assumes that it is the interface between social work and social science knowledge which is important, and a central task is to apply the social science knowledge to goals and tasks of the profession. The model does not require clinical skills.

Interventions generated by social welfare administration are related more to social science-management tasks than to any one of the social work methods. Thus, components of the decision-making process become a series of interrelated activities and interventions for the administrator.[15] Priority is given to means for constantly assessing and analyzing the current operations of an agency; and these devices serve as important sources of information for the social welfare administrator when he engages in his decision-making activities.

A major goal of social welfare administration is the enhancement of social functioning. More specifically, in regard to the goal of distribution of resources, this model encompasses the major monitoring and implementing positions in the field of social welfare. Social workers who administer the social welfare goods and services of our society from this perspective are the key group in the profession's attainment of this goal.

SOCIAL ADMINISTRATION

Social administration, although not widely known in American social work, represents a model which has been in existence in Western Europe for several decades.[16] In terms of the continuum here, social administration moves further away from American social work's emphasis on residual functions and the concomitant stress on a model of individual achievement-failure.[17] Social administration moves toward the opinion that knowledge and skills of the profession are interrelated not only with the social sciences but also with the values, priorities, and resources of the larger social institutions. Thus, social administration focuses on the policies, planning, and administration of social welfare goods and services in relation to the political, social, and economic institutions and to the determinants of the distribution of national resources to social welfare needs.

The related term "national development" refers to the broad social and economic resources, and to the establishment of priorities which crucially determine the goals and functions of the social work profession in a given society.[18] In this context, social administration is directly linked to the social work profession, but from the broader vantage point of social welfare and from the perspective of other social and economic institutional influences on national social welfare development. Compared with the other two models, this approach may be seen as less in the mainstream of American social work. At the same time, it provides a comparative analysis which may indicate new directions and alternatives for the profession, especially as American national priorities and social welfare planning change the distribution of social welfare resources. And we have a questionable illustration of such change in the family assistance program now before Congress.

The major assumptions stem from a macro-view of the social work profession as a subsystem of social welfare which, in turn, is a subsystem of the larger social, political, and economic institutions of society.[19] Thus, while social administration does not deny that social work may initiate, from within its own profession, a definition of its boundaries, practices, and resources, this viewpoint does assume that the perimeters of the profession's initiative are constantly bounded and determined by events in the larger system. Social administration, then, assumes a systems approach within which such social work and social welfare issues as autonomy, interventions, clientele, programs, and agencies are constantly being redetermined by the larger societal context.

Interventions generated by social administration derive from this basis. Thus, interventions are carried out less in terms of isolated administrative decisions than in terms of decisions related to other parts of the system, with special emphasis on a highly differentiated use of manpower resources. In some respects, the social administrator may be regarded as a catalyst upon other individuals and groups in the system, so that they can intervene with alternatives and resources not previously considered. The interventions of the social administrator are constantly determined by the needs, especially the unmet needs, of client-consumer groups of the social welfare agency. His interventions might be described as those of a middleman between the upper reaches of policy-making and the firsthand implementation of policy.

Goals for social administration include those of the other two models. On the continuum proposed here, this model distinctly concerns itself with the creation of new societal resources for distribution. Social administration, in contrast with the other two models, focuses upon the creation of new social welfare goods and services, upon an institutional function of social welfare.[20]

Social administration, then, is concerned with the redistribution of priorities and resources in the social welfare field. It is concerned with new delivery systems, with the extension of existing social welfare goods and services, and with the creation of new goods and services. Importantly, it claims a legitimate role in the establishment and monitoring of social welfare indicators as a rational base for the redistribution and creation of these goods and services.[21]

To recapitulate, these three models of administration generate differing assumptions, goals, and interventions in regard to social work practice, the profession, and the relationships of these factors to the larger society. At the same time that these models provide an important comparative analysis of administration in social work, they may not reveal some commonalities that cut across the three models. Some of the social work literature on advocacy and social action suggests a range of strategies that may be employed by all social workers, including those in administrative positions.[22] Thus, the conceptualization of the social worker as an administrative activist borrows heavily from some of our advocacy and social action literature, and it suggests some general strategies that may be applicable to all the models on the continuum.

ADMINISTRATIVE ACTIVIST

The term "activist" has been used to indicate direct action in both leftist and rightist political matters.[23] Here the term "administrative activist" is used not to imply a specific political ideology but rather to indicate direct administrative action, initiative, and leadership by social work executives.[24] Thus, this perspective counters the stereotyped view of the administrator as a passive pawn of the status quo.

In a general context, an activist orientation tends to be associated with conflict strategies and interventions and with an emphasis on system change. By contrast, consensus strategies tend to be associated with a more conservative orientation and with emphasis upon maintenance of the system. The limited research and literature regarding executives with the master's degree in social work (MSW) suggests that they are in the latter category and that they employ consensus-type strategies and emphasize maintenance of the social welfare administrative system.[25] A recent survey suggests that this is only partially correct. Initial analysis of data collected from a small sample of social work executives finds that they are much more activist-oriented than our literature has so far indicated.

The survey reported here borrows from Epstein's continuum of consensus and conflict type strategies in social work.[26] Through a partial replication of Epstein's study, data were collected from eighteen executives in the St. Louis area (median age fifty-two years) and from seventy-one social workers who graduated from the George Warren Brown School of Social Work in 1968 and 1969 (median age twenty-nine years). Popular opinion in social work holds that recent social work graduates are more activist-oriented than social work executives, but the survey findings suggest that such a generalization requires important qualifications. While conflict strategies are approved slightly more by the recent graduates than by the executives with the MSW degree, the same strategies are actually used by these executives more frequently than by recent graduates. Thus, on these dimensions, the differences between our executives and recent graduates do not appear to be significant.

Additional interview data from other social work executives suggest that they are, in fact, employing conflict strategies within their own agencies and among their own staff. Basic changes in the system are not necessarily the goals, but, more likely, better service delivery within the system. Thus, some executives may employ conflict strategies to counter staff resistances to change, to increase service productivity, and to create administrative structures which will lead to more effective services delivery.[27]

These conflict strategies are illustrated by an executive of a large staff of social workers in a psychiatric hospital. He has developed his own typology of strategies which include: (1) stimulating change among staff by introducing his own ideas and personal persuasion in staff meetings, conferences, etc.; (2) exposing staff to new ways for delivering social work services by assigning them tasks to explore or developing new delivery systems within or outside the hospital; (3) making explicit use of his own clinical skills in encounter groups with staff, encouraging group discussion of interpersonal conflicts and tensions in work relationships, with the goal that the staff will engage in new treatment modalities and new organizational arrangements for services.[28] This same executive is developing agency structures which foster collegial rather than traditional hierarchical relations among staff. Similar explorations are under way in a number of social agencies.[29]

The administrative activist, then, performs important functions which may cut across all three models of administration. These functions apply regardless of the method employed by the social worker as an administrator. Thus, the administrative activist represents important interventions toward achieving better distribution and use of social welfare programs and services. Yet, in themselves, these strategies do not lead to a focus on the goal of, and the interventions for achieving, new and desperately needed social welfare resources. For these, we must move beyond the administrative activist.

TOWARD NEW SOCIAL WELFARE RESOURCES

An essential step if social work is to deal substantively with the third major goal of social work is to assign some priority and support to the education for, and practice of, the social administration model. Leadership in the NASW has resulted in statements that favor some sort of guaranteed income, document the need for a family allowance system, explicate the arguments for resident control of neighborhood facilities and for effective, grass-roots political participation. Yet the rhetoric of our professional association does not match the reality.

Social workers have had minimal influence because we have had minimal knowledge. We have had minimal knowledge because only a small portion of our educational and practice resources has been deployed to anything more than a residual model of social work knowledge and practice; and this model has dominated our practice as administrators. In our preoccupation with narrower professional concerns, too many of us have defaulted on knowledge leadership which might lead toward the beginning of some institutional functions in American social welfare.

This is not to deny the value of residual social welfare services and programs. Nor is it to suggest that social work's attention to a social administration model will provide a panacea. Yet it will be a beginning by allocating some of our own resources to counterbalance the forces in our society which make it possible for American social welfare still to be characterized by nineteenth-century laissez-faire economics and Social Darwinism. Too much of social work practice can still be subsumed under these characteristics.

We must move, then, beyond only clinical or managerial or activist approaches in social work to a model of social administration which will meet the urban-racial realities of the twentieth-century United States. It must address itself to the diverse interests of our peoples, affirming a nonpathological view of social and personal conflict.[30] It will require that we be less concerned with the autonomy and protection of the social work profession and agencies than with a firm integration of both our values and the facts regarding the disadvantaged and high-risk people who continue to suffer from the benign neglect that results from our current national priorities and our social welfare policies. It will require that we venture beyond the province of our profession to the knowledge and activities in other disciplines and in other arenas of power that can influence the field of social welfare.

NOTES

1. For accounts of the organization of welfare recipients and workers, see Joseph E. Paull, "Recipients Aroused: the New Welfare Rights Movement," *Social Work*, XII, No. 2 (1967), 101–6; Lee Rainwater, "The Revolt of the Dirty-Workers," *Transaction*, V, No. 1 (1967), 2, 64. For a broader view of recent protest movements, see Jerome H. Skolnick, *The Politics of Protest* (New York: Ballantine Books, 1969).

2. Eldridge Cleaver, *Soul on Ice* (New York: Dell Publishing Co., 1968), pp. 179–80.

3. These dialectical conflicts are embraced in the writings of Marcuse and discussed by George Kateb, "The Political Thought of Herbert Marcuse," *Commentary*, XLIX, No. 1 (1970), 48–63. For an incisive comment on social work's misuse of the theories of Marx and Weber, see S. K. Khinduka, "Community Development: Potentials and Limitations," in *Social Work Practice, 1969* (New York: Columbia University Press, 1969), p. 18.

4. Alfred M. Stamm, "NASW Membership: Characteristics, Deployment, and Salaries," *Personnel Information*, NASW, XII, No. 3 (1969), 39.

5. For the working definition of social work, see Harriett M. Bartlett, "Toward Clarification and Improvement of Social Work Practice," *Social Work*, III, No. 2 (1958), 3–8.

6. Although the working definition of social work practice excludes administration

from practice, other social workers have strained to define social work administration as a full partner in professional practice. For example, see E. Elizabeth Glover, "Social Welfare Administration: a Social Work Method," *Child Welfare*, XLIV (1965), 431–39. Heffernan suggests that many of the professional issues are far from resolved: W. Joseph Heffernan, Jr., "Some Dysfunctions in the Teaching of Administration in Schools of Social Work," in Heffernan and Sue Spencer, eds., *Education of the Welfare Administrator* (Nashville, Tenn.: University of Tennessee School of Social Work, 1967; mimeographed), pp. 14–20.

7. For example, Harleigh B. Trecker, *Group Process in Administration* (New York: Woman's Press, 1950); Arthur L. Swift, Jr., *Make Your Agency More Effective* (New York: Association Press, 1941). For administration as a combination of casework, group work, and "the emerging principles of administration," see Ray Johns, *Executive Responsibility* (New York: Association Press, 1954), p. 26.

8. See Arnold Gurin, "The Community Organization Curriculum Development Project: a Preliminary Report," *Social Service Review*, XLII (1968), 421–34. For an overlapping of administration with community organization, see the "social planning model" in Jack Rothman, "Three Models of Community Organization Practice," in *Social Work Practice, 1968* (New York: Columbia University Press, 1968), pp. 16–47.

9. The human relations approach is summarized in Daniel Katz and Robert L. Kahn, *The Social Psychology of Organizations* (New York: John Wiley & Sons, Inc., 1966), pp. 396–425.

10. Werner W. Boehm, "The Nature of Social Work," *Social Work*, III, No. 2 (1958), 10–18.

11. Aaron Rosen and Ronda S. Connaway, "Public Welfare, Social Work, and Social Work Education," *Social Work*, XIV, No. 2 (1969), 91–92.

12. In a similar context, it has been noted that the residual aspects of social work generate a "preoccupation with process and with personality that keeps community development from becoming an effective instrument for large-scale institutional change" (Khinduka, *op. cit.*, p. 25). The distinctions between residual and institutional functions are drawn in Harold L. Wilensky and Charles N. Lebeaux, *Industrial Society and Social Welfare* (New York: Free Press, 1965), pp. 138–40.

13. Sarri contrasts social welfare administration with some dysfunctions in the social work method approach to administration. See Rosemary Sarri, "Education for Social Welfare Administration: Today and Tomorrow," Council on Social Work Education Annual Program Meeting, 1969 (mimeographed), pp. 4–5. For an interesting "intermediate" model outside social work, see Daniel J. Levinson and Gerald L. Klerman, "The Clinician-Executive," *Psychiatry*, XXX (1969), 3–15.

14. A NASW committee report outlines some of the behavioral and social science knowledge relevant to social work administration, without reference to the methods issues which have been raised in the past. See *Social Work Administration* (New York: National Association of Social Workers, 1968).

15. See Katz and Kahn, *op cit.*, pp. 259–99.

16. See Barbara N. Rodgers, John Greve, and John S. Morgan, *Comparative Social Administration* (New York: Atherton Press, 1968); David Vernon Donnison and Valerie Chapman, *Social Policy and Administration* (London: George Allen & Unwin, Ltd., 1965); Kathleen M. Slack, *Social Administration and the Citizen* (London: Michael Josephs, 1966). For the impact of cybernetics on policy and administration in American social welfare, see Allen Shick, "The Cybernetic State," *Trans-action*, LXX, No. 4 (1970), 15–26.

17. These features of American social work are described in David M. Austin, "Social Work's Relation to National Development in Developing Nations," *Social Work*, XV, No. 1 (1970), 97–106.

18. From this perspective, "Social work will champion a planned and comprehensive overhaul of moribund institutions while searching constantly for substitute structures for those which are unjust or unworkable. Emphasis on the macro and intermediate levels of professional intervention will, of necessity, entail a corresponding turning away from such approaches of social work that are geared primarily to enhancing individual adjustment." S. K. Khinduka, "Social Work and the Third World" (1970; mimeographed), p. 20.

19. This systems view is illustrated in W. J. M. Mackenzie, *Politics and Social Science* (Baltimore: Penguin Books, 1967). Shick (*op. cit.*, p. 23) predicts that the major analytic constructs for the policy sciences will be "systems and communication nets."

20. Wilensky and Lebeaux, *op. cit.*

21. For a description of the importance of these functions, see U.S. Department of Health, Education, and Welfare, *Toward a Social Report* (Washington, D.C.: U.S. Government Printing Office, 1969). For a critique of this report see Michael Springer, "Social Indicators, Reports, and Accounts: toward the Management of Society," *Annals*, Vol 388 (1970), 1–13.

22. For a description of some of the new roles and strategies, see Gerald M. Shattuck and John M. Martin, "New Professional Work Roles and Their Integration into a Social Structure," *Social Work*, XIV, No. 3 (1969), 13–20.

23. Seymour Lipset, "Students and Politics in Comparative Perspective," *Daedalus*, XCVII, No. 1 (1968), 1–20.

24. The term "administrative activism" has been applied to Daniel Moynihan's writings and criticized on the grounds that it "underestimates the persistence of old-fashioned power relationships and conflicts." Michael Harrington, "The New Elite," book review, *Commentary*, XLIX, No. 2 (1970), 84. Rothman, responding to some social work objections to activism, states: "An activist, social-change orientation is seen as compatible with democratic process and *not* contrary to the achievement of functional capacity goals." Jack Rothman, "An Analysis of Goals and Roles in Community Organization Practice," *Social Work*, IX, No. 2 (1964), 30.

25. For example, see W. Joseph Heffernan, Jr., "Political Activity and Social Work Executives," *Social Work*, IX, No. 2 (1964), 18–23; Paul Weinberger, "Executive Inertia and the Absence of Program Modification," in Weinberger, *Perspectives on Social Welfare* (New York: MacMillan, 1969), pp. 387–94.

26. Irwin Epstein, "Social Workers and Social Action: Attitudes toward Social Action Strategies," *Social Work*, XV, No. 2 (1968), 101–8. Students at the George Warren Brown School of Social Work, in *Social Work 585*, collected and tabulated these data in the fall of 1969.

27. These statements are drawn from students' written summaries of their tutorials with executives in the St. Louis area. These executives may be similar to those "whose referent is the professional staff of his agency as much as his board, the administrator for whom professional reputation may provide the basis for present or future success, [and who] will not totally ignore the norms of the field in favor of powerful community forces." George A. Brager, "Institutional Change: Perimeters of the Possible," *Social Work*, XII, No. 1 (1967), 65.

28. Excerpted from paper by William Hunt, George Warren Brown School of Social Work, January, 1970.

29. See Joseph H. Kahle, "Structuring and Administering a Modern Voluntary Agency," *Social Work*, XIV, No. 1 (1969), 21–28.

30. For the conceptualization of conflict as a normal social process, see Mary Parker Follett, *Creative Experience* (London: Longmans, Green, and Co., 1924).

6/DEVELOPING SPECIALIZED PROGRAMS IN SOCIAL WORK ADMINISTRATION IN THE MASTER'S DEGREE PROGRAM: FIELD PRACTICE COMPONENT

BERNARD NEUGEBOREN

Social welfare administration as an area for professional practice for social workers has become especially relevant in these days when critics question the value of existing social welfare programs. As the results of evaluative research raise the issue of the effectiveness of existing social service efforts and clients and staff are more militant in their demands for change, attention is focused on the need for more pertinent training for those who design and direct these social welfare programs.[1] A consequence is that goals for professional education in social work are being examined with attention given to training for leadership roles and functions. The question posed is what kind of education is required to prepare administrators of social welfare organizations to fulfill their responsibilities for maintaining and changing these agencies more adequately in order to serve human needs more efficiently and effectively.

This question of education for professional practice in social welfare administration is discussed here through a description and analysis of a program of training for administration of direct service agencies at the Rutgers University Graduate School of Social Work. This program description will focus on the field practice training component including educational objectives, the kinds of learning experiences students have received and the methods of instruction used. Issues will be raised as to constraints and opportunities for conducting training in social work administration.

RATIONALE AND STRUCTURE OF RUTGERS ADMINISTRATION PROGRAM

The general rationale for the administration training program at Rutgers is based on the assumption that administration of direct service agencies is one specialized area of practice of organizing and planning in social work. Therefore, we view the knowledge and skill required for direct service administration as having common elements with planning and administration in other such arenas of practice as social work in planning and allocating agencies. Thus, at Rutgers we have developed a Social Planning Track including common and specific knowledge and skill for students concentrating in organizing and planning in direct service agencies as well as in planning and allocating agencies and agencies concerned with social policy analysis and planning.[2]

The class and field curriculum is designed around a four-term 16-month program with class learning concentrated in the earlier terms and field learning in later terms. The class curriculum and field experiences provide learning of analytic, action, and technical skills for maintaining and changing direct service organizations. Foundation knowledge of structure and functions of complex organizations is provided the first term as a basis for later learnings in class and field. Field placements are in a single agency and cover three terms—two days in the field the first term, three days in each of the last two terms. Students are placed as administrative aide trainees to executives of such large, complex public direct service agencies as institutions for the retarded, correctional institutions, general hospitals, public welfare departments, mental health agencies, and central offices of state divisions and departments. These are selected as field placement settings in line with the program stress on training for administration of public social welfare programs in which many of the students had previous experience and expect to return to after graduation. Thus, the program emphasizes career goals in the public sector of social welfare where we feel there is the greatest need for trained administrators. In this regard it is of interest to note here that about 75 percent of the students who graduated from the Michigan program obtained jobs in public agencies after graduation.[3]

Field placements in administration also provide learning experience directed toward development of analytic, interactional, and technical management skills. Tasks assigned to students range from problem analysis utilizing methods for collecting and analyzing data to problem solution involving program implementation and change.[4] Opportunities are also available for students to learn specific technical skills such as research, staff development and budgeting. Particular students can select a concentration in program analysis which trains students for administrative positions requiring research skills.[5] This concentration includes additional courses in research as well as placements in settings that provide supervised experience in program analysis. The importance of research skills for administration is also recognized through a required course in administrative research designed around each student systematically studying an administration problem selected from his field placement agency. Therefore, field experiences provide opportunities for students to develop a range of administrative skills with particular attention given to preparing some students for program analysis roles.

The course in administrative research is an illustration of our effort to integrate field practice with classroom instruction. This objective is also facilitated by close liaison with agency executive field instructors through regular visits of faculty and periodic meetings and seminars at the school. Efforts are made to assist students in the integration of their learnings through a continuous seminar over the last three terms. This seminar, together with our system of advising and field liaison, provides for individualization of students by giving these responsibilities (seminar instructor, advisor, field liaison) for about ten students to one faculty member. This is based on the assumption that the faculty member, because of his involvement in class teaching, as well as field liaison, can better help the student integrate foundation analytic knowledge with skill learning in field in relation to his individual abilities, interests and career goals. The rationale and structure of the Rutgers program has the objective of training for administrative positions particularly in large complex direct service public social welfare organizations. Stress is on integration of academic and field instruction in a structure that facilitates meeting students' individual educational needs.

This analysis is based on data obtained from the verbal and written reports of fifteen field instructors and detailed reporting on daily logs by thirty students of their activities in the field. Additional information was obtained from student papers and conferences. This report covers two classes of students—one graduated in December 1969 and the second graduated in December 1970. Although this analysis essentially uses qualitative data, we are also in the process of developing a system for measuring quantitatively the kinds of field activities in which students are engaged.

Objectives of Field Practice Component
The basic objective of the field practice component of the Rutgers program is for students to learn to integrate and apply general principles to organization theory and decision-making to specific tasks assigned to them in their field placement situation. The goal is the development of analytic, interactional, and technical administrative skills that can be used to enhance as well as to change existing social welfare programs to serve client needs more efficiently and effectively. These general principles include a variety of theoretical approaches to understanding organizational behavior and leadership roles and functions. These skills, both cognitive and affective, are viewed as basic dimensions of administrative leadership and are assumed to facilitate the goals of maintaining and modifying social agency programs. The definitions of analytic and interactional leadership skill will be presented first, followed by a discussion of technical skills.

Analytic skill is defined as the application of principles of organizational function, structure, and process in gaining an understanding of intra- and inter-organizational problems. It is the ability to view the organization as a totality so that administrative problems can be accurately diagnosed and solved with an awareness of the consequences in the choice of different alternative solutions. This requires the application of knowledge of organizational performance within a systematic method of decision-making. Analytic administrative skill permits the student to understand organizational problems so that they can be successfully solved by taking into account the constraints and opportunities present in the system. Understanding these factors necessitates various strategies and leadership abilities appropriate for solution of particular problems and within specific organizational context. This skill is viewed primarily as cognitive in nature, particularly requiring conceptual abilities.

In contrast, *interactional* administrative skill depends upon the ability of the student to work with and through people by applying knowledge of principles of human behavior, interpersonal relations, and human motivation. This interactional skill depends more on affective abilities required to influence others in the implementing of solutions to problems in contrast to the cognitive problem analysis skills. It necessitates the application of various interpersonal methods on individual and group levels to achieve individual and group integration and consensus. It promotes individual need satisfaction so that personal and organizational goals are made complementary. It provides support through individual relationships as well as by facilitating group interaction and cohesiveness.

The leadership literature has reported on skills analogous to these two dimensions of analytic and interactional skill. Although there is some similarity between analytic and interactional skills and such dualities of leadership skills as "initiating structure" and "consideration,"[6] administrative, and human relations skills,[7] and instrumental and expressive leadership,[8] the former attempts to make a sharper differentiation between cognitive and affective skills. This is similar to that made by Katz and Kahn in their discussion of the relationship between various cognitive and affective leadership skills and abilities and organizational locus of leadership influencing different kinds of organizational change.[9] Their model hypothesizes that *both* cognitive and affective leadership abilities and skills are required to achieve change in organizations but that the level of administrative position and the nature of the change will require different combinations of cognitive and affective skills. We shall return to this formulation later when we discuss its implications for designing leadership training programs.

Analytic and interactional skills, in their most basic meaning, refer to such polarities as the thinker and the doer plus the ability to use logic and reason in contrast to the ability to take action through interpersonal transactions. The objective of the field training component is therefore the development in the students of both kinds of skills which are assumed to be required for managerial effectiveness of social welfare organizations. This objective is achieved by providing students with specific administrative tasks which give them the opportunity to have experience from which they can learn both skills.

In contrast to these general administrative skills, specific *technical* skills are also needed to perform particular organizational tasks.[10] Technical administrative skills are associated with routine organizational functions such as personnel management, budgeting, service delivery, program evaluation, public relations, etc. It requires fairly specific and distinctive knowledge and skills associated with the particular task area. As technical skills often may be associated with certain organizational positions such as supervisor of direct service workers, budget analyst, personnel director, etc., these skills are usually related to particular career goals.

Therefore, in addition to the general analytic and interactional skills, the program is concerned with helping the student prepare for particular career goals by helping him develop the specific technical skills needed to perform in the specific management positions. Training to meet individual students' needs is also required because of different interests, abilities, and previous work experience of students. Therefore, the objectives of the program are concerned not only with generic management skills but also with developing special competencies related to the student's particular career goals, interests, and abilities.

Although it is difficult to foresee the career goals of students accurately, it can be assumed that they will assume various administrative roles on different organizational levels depending on such factors as job opportunities as well as individual abilities, interests, and experience.

Data from the survey of Michigan graduates does indicate variation in types of administrative positions taken in the early period after graduation.[11] Thus, it can be expected that students will enter line positions such as supervisor of direct service workers, middle level administrator, as well as sub-executive and executive level positions. In contrast, other positions may require staff specialist roles such as administrative aide to executives involving such activities as program design, development and evaluation. Since at this time it appears that there are job opportunities in all areas of administration, the decision as to what kind of career goals to train for may be influenced primarily by the particular interests, experience and abilities of students.

Content of Field Practice Component
Observation of the performance of the students in the Rutgers Program reveals variation in their potential for developing analytic and interactional skills. In general, we find that analytic and interactional abilities tend to be *inversely* related. That is, students with very good analytic skills as measured by class performance do not generally perform well in field tasks requiring them to work with and through people. The reverse also appears to be true in that those students who are considered good performers in

action situations do not do well in class. It is evident that the "interactional" students seem to be able to capitalize on their intuitive abilities to understand what is expected of them and, more important, they tend to be somewhat more outgoing in dealing with people and situations. Their action abilities are in contrast to the analytic students, who are more cautious in making decisions even though, once they analyze a problem, they usually arrive at excellent understanding and solutions. The field instructors' evaluations reflect this in that the analytic students' abilities are recognized later in the year in contrast to those students with better interactional skills who receive positive evaluation throughout the year.

The possibility that analytical and interactional skills may be inversely related in most people has been discussed in the social science literature. Bales[12] has indicated that instrumental and expressive roles and functions in a group are not usually performed by the same individual. Research on leadership skills has also found that these two types of skills are usually independent in most persons[13] as well as possibly inversely associated.[14]

The observation that students' analytic and interactional abilities are related to performance in class and field suggests that perhaps student selection for administration training could be guided by this knowledge. Our experience at Rutgers, however, has led us to avoid screening students for our administration training program because we have been unable to measure those characteristics which predict student performance in class and field work. Thus, correlations of such factors as college grades, scores on the Concept Mastery Test, and amount of previous work experience were not found to relate significantly to either class or field grades. This has led us to the policy of providing the student with complete information on what is involved in our program and then letting the student make the decision as to whether he wants to enroll and with what kind of agency he would like to be placed. This is possible because the students do not make a final decision on their area of concentration until the middle of the first term at school. Giving students freedom of choice is stressed throughout the program both in terms of their initial decision and subsequently in the selection of elective courses. In general, we have found that placing responsibility on students to make their own decisions in shaping their educational experiences has resulted in a high degree of motivation and involvement in the learning process, with the result of very adequate performance by all students. However, as indicated, there is variation between students in that some show more potential for analytic leadership roles while others are more competent in the interactional areas of management.

This variation has implications for the design of the field training component in administration which in turn can affect career patterns. If analytic and interactional abilities are inversely related, then how much emphasis should be put into building on a student's strengths and abilities in contrast to compensating for weaknesses? Should we expect that all students should have a minimum of all leadership skills and what mixture of these proficiencies are required for various future administrative positions? Should there be two tracks within administration training programs —one for the analytic type and the other stressing interactional skills? Which skill is most relevant for system maintenance and system change goals and for staff and line roles? How can practice training aid in the learning of these skills?

Mann, in his studies of the three leadership skills (administrative, human relations, and technical), suggests that the combination of these will vary by organizational level so that what is effective on one level may not be on another level.[15] He suggests that the technical and human relations skills would be more important at the lower levels while administrative skills are more pertinent on the upper levels. This is based on the rationale that lower-level supervisory staff have the critical task of dealing with the motivational problems of the lower-level employee's integration of personal and organizational goals. As congruence between the personal and organizational goals of upper-level employees is greater, there is less need for managers on this level to have human relations skills. This suggests that we may be able to individualize our educational program in terms of specific career goals of students as well as in relation to individual abilities.

Information on the kinds of tasks performed by our students in their practice training sheds some additional light on these questions, particularly in relation to the kinds of opportunities and limits placed on their learning experiences in the field placement agencies. In general, we find that our students perform primarily staff "trouble shooting" types of roles rather than tasks having line responsibilities. These learning opportunities therefore stress use of analytic skills required for problem analysis with a minimum of tasks requiring interactional and technical line administration skills. Student assignments also stress system maintenance goals with there being little involvement in activities directed toward agency structural change.

There are several explanations why the students are not provided more opportunities for line administrative responsibility. Agency executives may be reluctant to risk giving authority to students. It is possible they do not think it appropriate since the student not being an employee cannot be held fully accountable. A related concern may be their uncertainty as to whether a student would be capable of successfully assuming responsibility.

The finding that most of the student's activities are involved in system maintenance rather than change activities is not surprising as it is unusual for any organization to be involved in major organizational change efforts. This has implications for the achievement of one of the major objectives of our program—for students to develop skills that will aid them in modifying social welfare programs in order to make them more responsive to client needs. If it is true that most administrative activity is concerned primarily with system maintenance, then how can students learn to develop the skills required to change these programs? Even if we were able to structure our training so that students could learn these skills, what opportunity would they have to use these skills after they entered practice?

A possible answer to this dilemma lies in how we define system maintenance and change. If we view organizational change as a continuum which involves using, bending, and changing agency structure, then we can design our training accordingly. The literature in social work has tended to be somewhat global in the discussion of the need for and our ability to accomplish "social change." It seems important for those developing programs for training "inside" change agent administrators to be more specific as to change goals so that we can know more precisely the kinds of learning experiences necessary for students to fulfill expectations in a more realistic manner after they graduate.

As indicated previously, an answer to the question posed as to whether programs in social work administration should specialize according to students' analytic and interactional abilities may be found in Katz and Kahn's model referred to above. It will be recalled that this model suggests that various cognitive and affective leadership skills are associated with the organizational position of the individual as well as the level of change goals. *Major structural change* is considered to be possible if top level staff are involved who have the cognitive skill of an internal and external systemic perspective as well as a charismatic affective ability.

Bending (or interpolation) of structure is most appropriate for middle level administrative staff who need to have a cognitive sub-system perspective and two-way orientation as well as the affective human relations skill to achieve integration of primary and secondary relations. *Better use* of existing structure (the usual definition of administration) is appropriate for lower administrative levels with cognitive technical knowledge of the system of rules and the affective skill in being concerned with equity in use of rewards and sanctions.

The purpose of presenting the above summary of the Katz and Kahn model is not to discuss its application here to social work administration in its specifics but rather to suggest that different administrative skills can be associated with career lines related to positions on different organizational levels. Thus, a student with good interactional (i.e., human relations) abilities might be encouraged to pursue a career in middle management while those students who have superior analytic abilities (i.e., system perspective) may be encouraged to seek positions close to the top level in the agency. Finally, those students who appear to be most able to deal with existing structure and are interested and able to develop specific technical skill may be encouraged to assume lower level positions.

The obvious problem with this formulation is that it does not take into account mobility up the hierarchy. Perhaps this would be dealt with by there being two career ladders, one stressing cognitive and the other affective abilities and skills. The above is obviously speculative at this time. It is presented here for purposes of developing a rationale for structuring our programs for training in administration. It is also proposed in the hope that it will stimulate some systematic study of leadership roles in social work to test out some of the hypotheses included in these formulations.

In summary, questions have been raised as to the constraints and opportunities for providing learning experiences in the practice field training in social work administration.

The issue was raised of educating students to learn *both* analytic and action skills when there is the tendency for students to favor one *or* the other ability. Opportunities for practice field training also may limit the kinds of training possible to analytic and system maintenance kinds of tasks. The implications of these issues are that it may not be possible to educate students as "generalists" in that they are expected to be able to perform in *all* kinds of administrative roles. It may be more strategic to capitalize on individual students' abilities, interests, and career goals and to develop flexibility in our training programs that would enable the individual to develop his particular abilities and talents. This stress on individualization of the students' education should not preclude the teaching and learning of the more general principles of administration to avoid a narrow, specialized vocational training of students.[16]

NOTES

1. Henry J. Meyer, Edgar F. Borgatta and Wyatt C. Jones. *Girls at Vocational High*, New York, Russell Sage, 1965. Gordon Brown, ed. *The Multi-Problem Dilemma*, The Scarecrow Press, 1968. (Ludwig Geismar, "The Rutgers Family Life Improvement Project and Other Outcome Studies: Some Findings and Their Implications for Social Policy and Practice," paper presented at 97th National Conference on Social Welfare, June, 1970.)
2. *Curriculum for Social Welfare Planning Track*, mimeo, Rutgers Graduate School of Social Work, 1969.
3. R. Sarri, *op. cit.* A complicating factor is the influence of public-voluntary auspice on an organization's ability to perform a training function. Thus it was found in the psychiatric clinic field that public auspice was positively associated with training. Bernard, Neugeboren, *Psychiatric Clinic—A Typology of Service Patterns* (Metuchen, New Jersey, Scarecrow Press, 1970). It appears most placement agencies used by schools of social work may be under voluntary auspice (personal communication from staff member of C.S.W.E.). This raises the issue of whether administrative skills developed through training in agencies under voluntary auspice is transferable to careers in public service administration.
4. Bernard Neugeboren, "Evaluation of Learning Experiences of Students in Administration Field Placements During 1969," mimeo; Ina Sullivan, "Summary Term II, Field Placement," May, 1970, mimeo; and "Typical Task Assignments in Administration Field Placements, 1970," October, 1970, mimeo, Rutgers Graduate School of Social Work.

5. Bernard Neugeboren, "Rationale for Field Training in Program Analysis at Rutgers Graduate School of Social Work," December, 1969, mimeo, Rutgers Graduate School of Social Work.

6. R. M. Stogdill, and A. E. Coons (eds.), *Leader Behavior: Its Description and Measurement* (Research Monograph No. 88, Ohio, Bureau of Business Research, The Ohio State University, 1957), pp. 6–38.

7. F. C. Mann, "Toward an Understanding of the Leadership Role in Formal Organizations," in R. Dubin, G. Homans, F. C. Mann and D. C. Miller, *Leadership and Productivity* (San Francisco: Chandler Publishing Company, 1965), pp. 68–103.

8. R. F. Bales, "Task Roles and Social Roles in Problem-Solving Groups," in Eleanor J. Maccoby, T. M. Newcomb, and E. L. Hartley (eds.), *Readings in Social Psychology*, 3rd edition (New York: Holt, Rinehart and Winston), pp. 437–447. Amitai Etzioni, "Dual Leadership in Complex Organizations," *American Sociological Review*, Vol. 30, No. 5, pp. 688–698.

9. Daniel Katz and Robert Kahn, *Social Psychology of Organizations* (New York: John Wiley & Sons, Inc. 1967), p. 312.

10. F. C. Mann, "Toward an Understanding of the Leadership Role in Formal Organizations," in R. Dubin, G. Homans, F. C. Mann, and D. C. Miller, *Leadership and Productivity* (San Francisco: Chandler Publishing Company, 1965), p. 73.

11. R. Sarri, *op. cit.*

12. Bales, *op. cit.*

13. E. A. Fleischman and D. A. Peters, "Interpersonal Values, Leadership Attitudes and Managerial Success," *Personal Psychology* (1962), Vol. 15, pp. 127–143.

14. Aaron Lorwin et al., "Consideration and Initiating Structure: An Experimental Investigation of Leadership Traits," *Administrative Science Quarterly*, Vol. 14, No. 2, (June 1969), pp. 238–253. Amitai Etzioni, *op. cit.*

15. Mann, *op. cit.*, p. 76.

16. Individualization in educational programs for students is also emphasized in the C.O. Development Projects recommendations: "Because of the diversity of practice for which the program is designed to prepare students, the wide range of subject matter to be covered, and the differences among students entering the programs," Gurin, Arnold, *op. cit.*, p. 178.

This paper was originally prepared for a workshop held at the 18th annual program meeting of the Council on Social Work Education, Seattle, Washington, January 1971.

The author is indebted to Dr. Bernard P. Indik, Rutgers Graduate School of Social Work, for his assistance in the preparation of this paper and in the development of the Administration Program at the Rutgers Graduate School of Social Work.

Part III

SOME ORGANIZATIONAL
PERSPECTIVES

EDITOR'S INTRODUCTION

Social services are provided by complex organizations for the most part, often in large-scale bureaucracies. In popular usage, bureaucracy has taken on invidious meaning, and "bureaucrat" is frequently used as an epithet. In its technical meaning, bureaucracy refers to a particular set of organizational characteristics originally identified by Max Weber. The theory of bureaucracy arose in response to the need for rational patterns or organization of the newly developing industrial mechanisms of the nineteenth century if they were to be efficient and to withstand the competition inherent in a free enterprise, capitalist economy. Rationality and efficiency were to substitute for nepotism and political convenience as the road to organizational stability in business, government, and voluntary associations.

The essential feature of the "ideal" form of bureaucratic organization was based, in Weber's concept, on the following six principles (Mansfield, 1973):

1. There are fixed and official jurisdictional areas which are generally ordered by rules.

2. Organizations have a strict hierarchical system of authority.

3. Administration is based on written documents.

4. Management presupposes thorough and expert training.

5. Bureaucratic activity is a full-time occupation.

6. The management of the bureaucracy follows general rules which are more or less stable, more or less exhaustive, and which can be learned.

In Weber's view, these principles would tend to make it possible for organizations to achieve their results in the most efficient manner. In actuality, bureaucracies have often been plagued with unintended consequences that seemed to subvert the very virtues they proclaimed. The dysfunctional features of bureaucracy are well known: ritualism, red tape, overconformity, rigidity, impersonality, and consequent nonresponsiveness to individual need (Stein, 1961). The literature has tended to focus on these negative aspects.

There is, however, another side to the argument (Whatcott, 1974). Some inherent strengths of bureaucracies, when their most rational principles are fully applied, can lead to productive and effective organizational functioning. Impersonality and objectivity avoid nepotism and special privilege—all applicants for service are equally treated. Objective criteria for standards of personnel performance promote competence, avoid nepotism, and provide motivation for career planning. Specification and predictability of roles avoids role invasion and conflict. In general, bureaucratic organization can lead to stability, order, and permanence. The very fact that there are positive and negative potentials provides an agenda for administrative action—how to accentuate the one and delimit the other (Pruger, 1973).

In his review of selected organizational research and social work in England, Whittington contrasts two forms of organization, mechanistic and organic, the former essentially bureaucratic, the latter replacing hierarchy of office with a network of shared authority. He elaborates the implications of both forms of organization, pointing to the importance of studying the conditions under which one or the other is relevant to the social tasks undertaken. The specific context of this discussion is the reorganization of the social services in Britain. The work of important English researchers in industrial organizations—Burns and Stalker, Woodward, Pugh and Jacques —is reviewed, and consideration given to some of their possible implications for social work.

Olmstead identifies and analyzes several different ways of looking at organizations, and suggests their significance for understanding organizational behavior. The several organizational approaches are grouped as follows: structural theories, group theories, individual theories, decision theories, and systems theories. While some of this review covers ground previously included by Mullis—the one dealing with management theory the other with organizational theory—it should be apparent that there are fundamental differences in purpose and context between these two modes of analysis. The former is essentially descriptive, the other prescriptive. One undertakes to explain and understand, the other to provide courses of action. The contrast is between an intellectual pursuit and a professional practice. The fact that there is an intimate relation between the two, is, of course, obvious, and administrators require profound insight into this essential relationship.

REFERENCES

Mansfield, Roger. "Bureaucracy and Centralization: An Examination of Organizational Structure." *Administrative Science Quarterly* 18, no. 4 (December, 1973): 477.
Pruger, Robert. "The Good Bureaucrat." *Social Work* 18, no. 4 (July, 1973).
Stein, Herman. "Administrative Implications of Bureaucratic Theory." *Social Work* 6, no. 3 (July, 1961).
Whatcott, Weston E. "Bureaucratic Focus and Service Delivery." *Social Work* 19, Vol. 4 (July, 1974).

7/ORGANIZATIONAL RESEARCH AND SOCIAL WORK: ISSUES IN APPLICATION ILLUSTRATED FROM THE CASE OF ORGANIC AND MECHANISTIC SYSTEMS OF MANAGEMENT

COLIN WHITTINGTON

In the period which followed the report of the Seebohm Committee,[1] there was an upsurge in attention to managerial and organizational matters in social work. The Committee's conclusion that improvements in the personal social services should be sought through major organizational change emphasized, as never before, the significance of the organizational context of social work. Consistent with this the Report recommended the study of administrative structures during professional training (para. 557), and management training at the post-professional training level (para. 548). Moreover, paragraph 620 stated that

The objective should be to secure that most of the heads of the social service departments are people qualified in social work . . . who have received training in management and administration . . . or administrators with qualifications in social work.

Thus the scene was set for the study of organizations and of management to take their place on the list of 'highly recommended' subjects for social workers. These two subjects, however, though related, pose distinctive problems. In the case of the former there is the problem of selecting material. The literature on organizations in general is vast, while the material on social work organizations in particular is probably inadequate. In the case of the study of management, which is how to organize, the problem of a voluminous general literature is overshadowed by the question of whether we are yet in a position to prescribe for the problems and objectives of the diversely populated and perceived arena that is a social services organization.

Despite these difficulties, however, some writers, anticipating or responding to the Social Services Act 1970, ventured to suggest what shape social services departments should and should not take. Among them were those who were prepared to give a lead as to the kind of material from organizational research that was relevant. There was general agreement that a special kind of organizational structure was required (Barter,[2] Hopkins,[3] Rea Price,[4] Heal,[5] Phillips and Birchall,[6] Algie[7]). This should not be 'bureaucratic', and in particular a tall hierarchy should be avoided.[3,4,6] The structure should also be flexible,[6,7] offering adaptability to changing conditions;[2,7] minimize internal conflict;[5] and promote both co-operative effort among members,[2,5] and open and free communications.[2,4] No doubt these kinds of proposals could expect a sympathetic reception among those committed in principle to the rejection of bureaucratic structures and their widely discussed dysfunctions. More widespread support would be likely to follow the provision of an empirical rationale for such recommendations.

Taking three of the works referred to above, Barter,[2] Rea Price,[4] and Heal,[5] we find that the same empirically derived concept, that of the 'organic' (also known as 'organismic') organization, developed by the researchers Burns and Stalker,[8] crops up in each. The attempts by the three authors to prescribe, in varying degrees of specificity, this particular organizational form for social services departments are of interest here for two reasons (note 1). First, they stimulate us to consider some of the possible implications for social work of Burns and Stalker's influential industrial study and, in particular, of the organic organizational form which has become well known and canvassed in some social work circles. Secondly, they help us to illustrate, through a critical approach of the three authors' proposals, the kinds of problems that may await the increasing number of social workers wishing to apply material from organizational research to social work organization. These two themes will be pursued concurrently in this paper through a discussion of the following areas which appear to be central to any attempt to apply Burns and Stalker's mechanistic and organic concepts to social services organizations:

1. The prevailing organizational pattern of social services departments.
2. Environment and change.
3. Status and power.
4. Boundaries and the individual worker.
5. Managers, commitment, and consensus.

The discussion will make most use of illustrations from the articles by Barter and Rea Price. Reference to Heal, like his to Burns and Stalker, will be fairly brief. No critique of Burns and Stalker's approach will be attempted, for this has been conducted elsewhere (Silverman).[9] We will be concerned with issues in the application of their material and it is not within our scope to deal with the important but different question of the tenability of their underlying theoretical assumptions.

Since, however, none of the articles referred to provides an outline of

Burns and Stalker's findings, the main part of the paper will be prefaced by a brief outline of it.

MECHANISTIC AND ORGANIC SYSTEMS OF MANAGEMENT

In their study of firms in the electronics industry, Burns and Stalker arrived at the view that management systems could be polarized into two ideal types, 'mechanistic' and 'organic' (pp. 119–25).[8] The mechanistic form closely resembles Weber's bureaucracy,[10] being characterized by a clear hierarchy of offices involving functionally specific roles, a tendency to vertical communication, and dependence on the 'top' to relate each person's specialism to organizational goals. In contrast, the organic type has a 'network structure of control, authority, and communication' replacing the hierarchy, and involves the 'adjustment and continual redefinition of individual tasks through interaction with others' (p. 121).[8] The co-ordination of functions takes place through regular meetings between managers, and communications are lateral rather than primarily vertical. Communication between people of different rank resembles consultation rather than command, and the content consists of advice and information, as opposed to instructions and decisions. The head of the concern is no longer considered omniscient. Rather, there is shared responsibility for relating individual tasks to the current requirements of the organization.

Burns and Stalker suggest that 'the two management systems . . . represent . . . the two polar extremes of the forms which systems can take when they are adapted to a specific rate of technical and commercial change' (p. 119).[8] They conclude that a mechanistic type is appropriate for concerns like the rayon firm, which was studied as a preliminary to the main study, using an unchanging technology under relatively stable market conditions (pp. 1–2).[8] 'The organic system is appropriate to changing conditions, which give rise constantly to fresh problems and unforeseen requirements for action which cannot be broken down or distributed automatically' via functionally specific roles in a hierarchical structure (p. 119).[8] Such was the position in the electronics industry itself.

Burns and Stalker consider that the extent to which any particular organization approximates a mechanistic or organic form is determined by the operation of three variables. The first, already mentioned, is the rate of technical and market change. The second concerns the strength of commitment of individual members to the defence or enhancement of status or power. Members may have commitments to power or prestige, promotion or privilege, as well as to the organization. The outcome of status or political manoeuvrings may be the retention or imposition of a mechanistic system in conditions where an organic form would be appropriate, or vice versa. The third variable involves the capacity of the top management to interpret the requirements of the technical and market situation, that is of the 'environment', and to lead the organization to the appropriate structural form. More will be said of these variables later.

The organizations in the Burns and Stalker study had, for the most part, been equipped at their inception with systems of a mechanistic type. In the face of changing conditions, many failed to make use of the organic form which, Burns and Stalker say, would have assisted their performance: 'In these concerns the effort to make the orthodox bureaucratic system work . . . produced dysfunctional forms of the mechanistic system' (p. ix).[8]

Burns and Stalker's findings are striking, and seem to provide the foundations for a potent critique of organizations which we may hold to be bureaucratic, and which we may wish to alter. It is as well to bear in mind, therefore, one of the most important conclusions which they reach: that there is no one most efficient organizational form which is appropriate to all conditions. Different situations demand different structures, some requiring a bureaucratic form, and others a more fluid one. Thus, despite the emphasis by writers such as Rea Price[4] on the dysfunctions of mechanistic systems and their hierarchies, an approach consistent with Burns and Stalker's findings will acknowledge that such systems are no less 'functional' under certain conditions than are organic ones.

Attempts by social workers to make use of the Burns and Stalker study may, however, give rise to objections concerning the application of findings from industrial studies to the organization of social services departments. The latter, it may be argued, are 'service' organizations whereas those in the Burns and Stalker study were 'business' concerns. A crucial difference between the types, according to Blau and Scott, is that only the service organizations are faced with the problems of 'establishing social relations with the objects of their endeavours and of having to motivate them in various ways.'[11] To adapt their example, the success of the social worker may depend on the solution of these problems; that of the electronics engineer does not.

This immediately raises questions about an assertion made by Barter. He writes that 'Joan Woodward (1965) has shown empirically that there is a recognizable link between the technology employed by a given manufacturing concern and its organizational structure. It is likely that this holds good for service organizations such as the proposed social service departments . . .' (p. 1221).[2] No evidence is given by Barter to support his assertion, nor are any possible constraints upon extrapolation discussed by him. In particular, we might have expected reference to the question of the transferability of the concept of technology from the sphere of industrial to that of service organizations.

On the other hand, there are limitations to an approach which classifies organizations according to common manifest functions like 'business' and 'service'. Charles Perrow, for example, claims that such models neglect important structural variations within categories, and overlook similarities among differently classified organizations.[12] According to this argument, some social services departments may in fact be run like factories, while the structures of some factories may resemble those of therapeutic communities. Furthermore, Goffman has shown in his concept of the 'total' institution, that organizations like mental hospitals, concentration camps, and monasteries which possess what might be thought important differences, also share certain central, structural characteristics.[13] There are grounds for the view, therefore, that imaginative extrapolation from one area of study to another may be extremely fruitful, although the process seems to call for more reflectiveness than Barter displays. With these points in mind, we can move on to the issues raised by the Burns and Stalker study, and by the recommendations of Barter, Rea Price and Heal.

THE PREVAILING ORGANIZATIONAL PATTERN OF SOCIAL SERVICES DEPARTMENTS

The question of evidence, raised above, arises again in the discussions of the prevailing pattern of social service organization. In positing the need for a change to organic systems the prevalence of a mechanistic pattern is asserted by Barter and Rea Price. Thus, Barter writes, 'The organizational structures so far devised for local authority personal social services are seldom more than what Burns has called inorganic bureaucracies' (p. 1221).[2] Similarly, Rea Price refers to 'an inappropriate bureaucratization' of social service developments since 1948 (p. 2315).[4]

Prevalence of the mechanistic type is taken by both Barter and Rea Price as axiomatic, and the need for empirical support for their assertions is not acknowledged. This observation may seem niggardly since it is 'well known' that local authority social services are, and have long been, mechanistically organized. The problem, however, is that this sort of assumption fails, as do Barter and Rea Price, to raise questions about the *degree* of bureaucratization. Rea Price's reference on the one hand to 'bureaucratization' and 'extended hierarchies', and on the other to the 'few' social work departments which have 'opted for an organic management structure', seems to suggest a dichotomy of organizational form (pp. 2315/6).[4] But as Burns and Stalker point out, 'the two forms represent a polarity, not a dichotomy; there are . . . intermediate stages between the extremities . . .' (p. 122).[8] Furthermore, 'A concern may (and frequently does) operate with a management system which includes both types' (p. 122).[8]

According to this we might expect to find some variation between social services departments in their approximation to a mechanistic or organic form. Similarly, differences may be found among and between the functional divisions, area offices, or teams in the same department. This might also be said of the former health, welfare and children's departments, suggesting a possibly fruitful but neglected perspective on the problems encountered during and after amalgamation into social services departments. More recently, the perspective may be directed to issues arising from the reorganization of local government and of the health services. One consideration is the possible impact upon members when two units of differing organizational form, say a hospital social work department and an area office of a social services department, are expected to coalesce.

In the absence of evidence on the form taken by social service departments, the possibility of variations within and between them should be kept in mind. Let us now consider the subject of the environment of these agencies and its rate of change.

ENVIRONMENT AND CHANGE

Mechanistic structures, Barter writes, 'militate against effective social work practice' (p. 1221).[2] Correspondingly, we are told by Rea Price that 'The most successful social work departments have been the few . . . that have consciously opted for an organic management structure . . .' (p. 2316).[4] The mechanistic and organic forms, as we have said, are held by Burns and Stalker to be appropriate for conditions, respectively, of relative stability and relatively rapid change. According to their model, then, these assertions by Barter and Rea Price require demonstration of the presence of a relatively high rate of change in the environment of social work.

Before pursuing this idea, however, a brief comment is necessary concerning effectiveness and success in social work, although only a full article on these subjects could begin to do them justice. Barter and Rea Price do not specify what is meant by their use of the terms, or how effectiveness or success might be measured. Many and competing perceptions of effectiveness and success may intersect in the social services, and it is necessary, therefore, to state clearly the standards by which these characteristics are being judged. Success for the manager may not be success for the client!

To continue, a first step in establishing the rate of environmental change in Burns and Stalker's term, is to specify both the technology and market of a social services department. A precise definition of social work or industrial technology is not to be found in the works under review. Barter refers only to the social worker's 'technology of enablement' (p. 1220),[2] while Burns and Stalker go no farther than to mention scientific discoveries and technical inventions (p. 96).[8] A general definition, embracing people-processing and changing organizations like social services departments, as well as other kinds of organizations, is suggested by Perrow. Technology, he says, 'is the action that an individual performs upon an object, with or without the aid of tools or mechanical devices, in order to make some change in that object'.[14] People are included in the meaning of 'object'. This definition is sufficiently general to allow us to describe the casework, groupwork, community work and associated techniques of field and residential workers in a social services department as their technology. Concealed within this description, however, are enormous complexities which will confront attempts to analyse the technologies of social workers. Whatever approach is adopted to this problem, it will not be possible to speak of the technology of a social services department without extending analysis beyond the activities of social workers to include the work of personnel like home helps, occupational therapists, and day centre staff.

The other facet of the environmental variable is the market situation. The concept of 'market', with its connotations of exchange is, however, central to the distinction which some writers would make between the spheres of business and the social services. For example, Titmuss writes: 'The grant, or gift or unilateral transfer is the distinguishing mark of the social (in policy and administration) just as exchange or bilateral transfer is a mark of the economic.'[15] This view adds a further dimension to the earlier discussion of extrapolation from one field to another, and appears to rule out a definition of market which is applicable across the fields of business and the social services. Titmuss, however, does tentatively suggest the concept of the 'social market' which he distinguishes from the 'economic market'.[15] With this in mind, we might define the 'market' of a social agency, briefly, as embracing existing and potential clients, the community which it serves, other agencies, local and national social, political, and economic conditions, and new legislation, government regulations and circulars.

The elements of the environment identified by Burns and Stalker are, therefore, amenable to definition in the social services as well as the industrial sphere. The inadequacy of these definitions, however, will be seen as we go on to consider the issue of change. This is held by Burns and Stalker to be the crucial factor in determining the appropriate organizational form. Rea Price cites Algie who argues for a non-mechanistic social service structure to respond to today's conditions of complexity and social change (p. 2316).[4] Similarly, Barter refers to the 'constantly evolving' tasks of social work organizations (p. 1221).[2] He also notes the development of 'new or refined technologies', 'increasing expertise', 'uncertainty', 'unstable conditions', and social change (p. 1221).[2] In neither case, however, are we given evidence of the change and unpredictability in the environment. Yet, in so far as the Burns and Stalker model is concerned, this evidence is necessary to justify arguments for an organic system.

One possible reason for the juxtaposition of a mechanistic pattern and a constantly changing environment, Burns and Stalker tell us, is the inability of the top management to recognize and adapt the organization to the requirements of the technical and market situation. If the intention is that social work managers should acquire this ability, then what is held to constitute change and stability in the environment must surely be specified. An important consideration, however, is that different units within the organization, for example, a day centre for physically handicapped clients, and an area office, may vary in the degree of change experienced in their environment. This raises questions about the boundaries of a particular unit, and what is held to constitute its environment of which the rate of change is to be measured. It is evident, as suggested above, that more work will be necessary on defining 'environments'.

One of the problems for managers in operationalizing Burns and Stalker's findings is the latters' own limited specification of the concept of change. This refers to the appearance of novelties either in the form of new techniques, or requirements for products not previously available to or demanded by the market (p. 96).[8] What remains to be worked out, however, is when the element of change can be said to have reached the point at which the label 'relative change' should replace that of 'relative stability', and vice versa. Furthermore, how might different types on the mechanistic–organic continuum be matched with 'appropriate' points on the stability–change continuum? It is difficult to see how Burns and Stalker's organizational concepts could be introduced with confidence by managers without further work on these questions (note 2).

STATUS AND POWER

A second possible cause of an 'incongruent' environment–structure relationship, (and it has yet to be demonstrated that one exists in social services departments), concerns, we are told, distortions arising from members' commitments to the improvement or defence of status or power. The operation, on one level, of these kinds of commitments is illustrated in Rea Price's discussion which suggests that 'the growing [hierarchical] pyramid beneath him has seemed one way in which the chief officer could rise to parity of esteem and influence within the local authority. . . . Hierarchies have also developed from the need to create career opportunities for social workers, assuring status for the department . . .' (p. 2315).[4]

It is interesting that Burns and Stalker found that no firm was without some serious political conflict and division (p. 204).[8] This existed between and, in some cases, across departments and functional divisions, suggesting possible parallels with, say, field and residential services, on the one hand, or field-work services at team and divisional or central level on the other. Some managers in the Burns and Stalker study, feeling their authority threatened, arranged for communications difficulties and restricted interaction between staff and line. Other tactics to advance or protect status included avoidance and withholding information. In the latter case, 'information required for the proper functioning of the organization is not passed from person to person in accordance with the needs issuing from the tasks to be performed, but is used . . . to demonstrate superior worth or status' (p. 152).[8] Also of interest is the recurrent link which Burns and Stalker found between the political conflicts in the organizations studied and 'the appearance of a new group, or the rapidly enhanced importance of an existing group' (p. 205).[8] This description corresponds with the view which some hold of field social workers, and which others hold of their managers. Burns and Stalker note that distortions to the working organization consequent upon power and status conflicts are not restricted to the continuation or emergence of inappropriate mechanistic systems. An inappropriate organic form may arise in a situation of stability. The discussion of power and status interests suggest the significance of individuals' definitions of situations in the development of management systems. Let us now consider one important distinction for the individual between work in the different systems.

BOUNDARIES AND THE INDIVIDUAL WORKER

Burns and Stalker point out that one of the major distinctions between the two management systems is that the mechanistic system defines the members' functions, tasks and powers, with the result that boundaries of responsibility are set. It is common to read of the inhibiting effect on individual creativity of the working arrangements in which these boundaries arise (p. 2315).[4] In organic systems, however, 'the boundaries of feasible demands on the individual disappear' (p. viii).[8] Thus Heal, after Burns and Stalker, writes that 'any individual employed by an "organismic" social service department must regard himself as "fully implicated in the discharge of any task appearing over his horizon" . . .' (p. 21).[5] He adds that 'roles and responsibilities [will] be redefined continuously as new tasks emerge . . .' (p. 21).[5] This dissolution of boundaries is further emphasized by Barter, who writes that the type of organization which best contains social work practice is one which lacks functional and hierarchical differentiation, and in which tasks are perpetually redefined by interaction (p. 1221).[2] Similarly, Rea Price, quoting Burns and Stalker, notes that

the less definition can be given to status, roles and modes of communication, the more do the activities of each member of the organization become determined by the real tasks of the firm as he sees them than by instruction and routine. The individual's job ceases to be self-contained; the only way in which 'his' job can be done is by participating continually with others in the solution of problems which are real to the firm and put in a language of requirements and activities meaningful to them all (p. 2316).[4]

What Rea Price omits, however, is the succeeding and possibly crucial sentence in the passage which states that: 'Such methods of working put much heavier demands on the individual' (p. 125),[8] although at another point he does refer to the painful consequences among the upper hierarchies (p. 2316).[4] Heal also points out that work in such a department would be 'uncomfortable', but some members may find that this understates the experience of work in an organic structure (p. 21).[5] Social work, as both Rea Price and Barter emphasize, can be a stressful and anxiety-provoking activity and, it may be added, these effects are not necessarily confined to the level of field worker. One characteristic found in mechanistic organizations which may help to limit stress is the setting of boundaries of responsibility. It can be very consoling to be able to pass a problem on to someone with 'the responsibility' for dealing with it. Even where boundaries exist for reasons quite independent of a member's possible psychological needs, their removal, if they have been effective in reducing stress, may not be welcomed by him. Indeed, Burns and Stalker found that whilst the absence of clarity, definition and boundaries significantly increased the effectiveness of the management in conditions of unpredictability and change, this happened 'at the cost of personal satisfactions and adjustment . . .' (p. 135).[8] Moreover, as Pugh and his associates point out, Elliot Jaques's Glacier investigations found that: 'Where there is some confusion of role boundaries, or where multiple roles occupied by the same person are not sufficiently distinguished, insecurity and frustration result.'[16]

MANAGERS, COMMITMENT AND CONSENSUS

Willingness to tolerate the observed additional stresses of work in the organic organization is facilitated, it seems, by the individual's commitment to the organization and its goals. Furthermore, Burns and Stalker tell us that

the emptying out of significance from the hierarchic command system, by which co-operation is ensured and which serves to monitor the working organization under a mechanistic system, is countered by the development of shared beliefs about the values and goals of the concern. The growth and accretion of institutionalized values, beliefs, and conduct, in the form of commitments, ideology, and manners, around an image of the concern in its . . . setting make good the loss of formal structure (p. 122).[8]

The key members in establishing these shared commitments, we are told, are the top managers, especially the managing director. One of the functions of 'direction' is to define 'the demands of the working organization for commitment, effort and self-involvement which the individual should regard as feasible, and should attempt to meet' (p. 102).[8] Burns and Stalker emphasize the importance of the manager's aptitude and skills for motivating commitments to the working organization and its tasks (p. 232).[8]

Thus Barter tells us that 'social work management requires . . . the establishment of a common system of values shared freely by all the members of the organization. The achieving of goals then becomes the accepted responsibility of all its members' (p. 1220).[2] His ultimate objective is a unified social organization. In a similar vein Rea Price argues that: 'A primary task of the manager both at headquarters and at local level is to motivate the organization as a whole, and establish the commitment of the staff to the ends it is committed to meet' (p. 2374).[4]

What is not explained, however, is precisely how social work managers should achieve this aim. Burns and Stalker are of little help here, for they give us no way of telling how members come to define objectives, and themselves provide no clear indication of how managers may induce the kinds of commitment which characterize the organic organization. One suggestion, from Rea Price, is that a 'charismatic style of leadership' may be helpful (p. 2374).[4] Ironically, however, in view of Rea Price's opposition to hierarchic management structures, Burns and Stalker observe that the existence of charismatic leadership has often been regarded as a 'substantial justification for organization according to hierarchic forms and the concentration of power in the person at the top' (p. 215).[8] It is also the case that the operation of charismatic leadership depends upon the perceptions of those being led. It is not clear how the necessary perceptions of the leader may be induced in social workers. Another possible answer involves the provision of open discussion between managers and others of feelings and psychological difficulties. This is mentioned briefly by Burns and Stalker (p. 258),[8] and by Rea Price who emphasizes the special qualities which professionally trained social workers have to offer such managerial functions (p. 2374).[4] Barter also stresses these considerations in the appointment of senior managers and chief executives, making this a central theme of his paper.

The detailed procedures of these psychological techniques are not made clear in the works under review, but they appear to range from sympathetic discussion to what might best be termed 'therapeutic management'. They also carry certain risks whch ought parenthetically to be mentioned. First, managerial definitions in social work may be assumed to be 'right' or 'healthy,' and be used as a basis for judging the health or pathology of workers' attitudes and activities. This has been observed by Scott in the relationship between supervisor and social worker and discussed under the heading of 'therapeutic supervision'.[17] Secondly, the use of psychological 'enabling' and conflict-managing techniques by managers (p. 1220),[2] may be no less concerned with control than more overt methods, but this may go unrecognized. Thirdly, an emphasis on psychological perspectives may deflect attention from structural factors. For example, Barter suggests that conflicts in social work 'are more usually expressed within the organization than in the field of practice where they usually originate' (p. 1220).[2] The interaction of worker and client, he argues, revives elements of their parent–child relationships producing complex feelings and ambivalence. Professional restraint prevents the worker from expressing his antagonisms and these are fed back into the organization where they 'characterize its internal relationship unless recognized and dealt with' (p. 1220).[2] Adopted alone, this approach to conflict renders unnecessary the consideration of structural factors within the organization, such as unequal power among groups in the allocation of resources, or different objectives associated with different roles or statuses, and justifies its treatment in the worker by trained managerial therapists who aim to reduce it to 'non-destructive' proportions (p. 1220).[2]

To continue with the issue of commitment, Heal asserts that the person employed by an 'organismic' social services department 'must commit himself to the goals of the department . . .', but he also provides no guidance on managerial procedures for inducing this commitment (p. 21).[5] The worker's main incentive to adopt the orientations and commitments which characterize the organic system seems to be belief in Heal's assertion that these are required for the performance of the function placed upon the department by wider society. Failure to perform this function (which is not defined), may result in withdrawal of resources by the 'social environment', and the worker will be out of a job (pp. 19 and 21).[5] This argument alone is unlikely to convince organization members with a knowledge of Burns and Stalker's study, who will know that the researchers, apparently unlike Heal, do not hold the organic system to be functional for all conditions. Even with the environmental conditions fulfilled, however, social workers may remain unconvinced by Heal's argument. That is to say, if Rea Price and Barter are correct, a majority work in organizations which have long been mechanistically organized, but despite this employment opportunities appear to have increased overall, rather than declined (note 3).

It would also be helpful to know how members are to reach and sustain a consensus upon goals, themselves recognized by Heal as problematic, when these have been shown to be variously, multiple, conflicting, differently perceived and subject to change (Smith).[18] The same may be asked of Rea Price and Barter. Furthermore, although the latter conceives of two sub-cultures, social work and management, which await unification, this probably oversimplifies a situation in which, to take the example of a recent study of social workers' ideologies, it may not be solely the perspectives of different status groups which require reconciliation, but also differences among members of the *same* group (Smith and Harris).[19]

Heal is aware of the potential for conflict between different hierarchical levels in social services departments. Indeed, it is this which moves him to recommend the organismic organization in the first place. His suggestion that conflict in social services departments may be solved by setting up an organic system is no doubt fostered by the image contained in the ideal type of shared values, goals and commitments among members, and its attractions to managers are obvious. It would be a mistake, however, to slip into the assumption that this system or organization can be brought into operation in abstraction from the membership. A revised organizational form may exist in the minds and intentions of those with a mandate to organize, but in so far as organic organization describes the nature and pattern of relationships and orientations of the members, to gain the necessary commitment and action for the functioning of this organizational form is likely to require more than a decree that it shall be so. In any event, Burns and Stalker do not offer the organic system as a solution for organizational conflict. According to their view, the introduction of an organic form as Heal suggests, without reference to the rate of environmental change, may result in an organization 'inappropriately' adjusted to its environment.

The final point concerning commitment to the organization relates to the clients. Assuming that the type and degree of involvement advocated among members are feasible, we have to ask: would this state of affairs be in the interests of clients? One possibility is that it would not; that the desired level of commitment would diminish criticism by members to the ultimate disadvantage of the clients. For example, Barter states that: 'The primary task of the management of a social service department is to convert the aspirations of people in distress into programmes of action' (p. 1221).[2] Problems are raised, however, for those clients whose aspirations are not held to be legitimate by 'the management', and who have lost representation among social workers because the management have successfully established a common system of values shared 'by all the members of the organization' (p. 1221).[2]

CONCLUSION

Barter, Rea Price and Heal propose, in varying degrees of specificity, the introduction of an organic organizational form in social services departments. The critique of their proposals should not be taken as opposition *per se* to the introduction of such organizational forms. Rather, at certain points, and in terms of the findings which gave rise to the concept, the adequacy of their grounds for advocating the introduction of an organic form have been challenged. At other points, difficulties which attempts to establish this type might hold for managers, social workers, or clients have been identified. There are, undoubtedly, aspects of the organic style which are consistent with the values of some social workers. It offers, for example, an organizational form providing for individualization and flexibility in confronting social problems. It also proposes wide participation in decision-making, and stratification based on expertise rather than administrative position. Indeed, there seems to be some equation between, on the one hand, the organic approach to mobilizing special knowledge and experience to the common task and, on the other, the principle of a generic, team-based service in the integrated personal social services. Despite their possible attractions for social workers, however, organic systems like mechanistic ones have their limitations.

Some of the implications of Burns and Stalker's findings for social services departments have been suggested, together with certain constraints on a direct prescriptive use of their material. Illustrations from the articles utilized have also enabled us to identify some more general issues arising from the study of organizations and their management.

While the discussion has focused upon 'problems' rather than 'opportunities', this has in no way been designed generally to discourage the application of material from organizational research to social work organizations. Instead, the intention has been to draw attention to the complexities which may be involved. One hazard facing social workers engaged in this task, especially those confronted daily with organizational problems, is that a sense of urgency in identifying the implications of a piece of research may result in over-simplification of the findings. Another is that they may fail to evaluate critically the study itself. Short of ignoring research material completely, however, social workers may feel that avoiding these dangers is too time-consuming. For some the solution will be to turn to more intendedly prescriptive literature on management, although such a move will not obviate the need for a critical approach. Peter Leonard has observed that 'social work has sometimes swallowed too easily the knowledge methods and theories which have come from outside social work . . .'.[20] If this trap is to be avoided in the sphere of social work management it is essential that the expectation of ready-made solutions to organizational problems be resisted. This article has therefore favoured an approach which treats concepts arising in the study of organizations as problematic and not as given.

NOTES

1. The articles also raise other matters which are not the subject of discussion in this paper.
2. The development of more precise specifications of variables, however, would not meet all objections to attempts to use such research material prescriptively. See the discussion of this and related issues in Paul Filmer et al. (1972), *New Directions in Sociological Theory*, Collier-Macmillan, London.
3. To what extent this employment situation will be altered by the economic problems reported by central and local government during 1974 remains to be seen.

REFERENCES

1. *Report of the Committee on Local Authority and Allied Personal Social Services* (1968), Cmnd. 3703, H.M.S.O.

2. Barter, John (1969) 'Management in Social Service,' *Brit. Hosp. J. and Soc. Serv. Rev.*, Vol. 79, No. 4132, pp. 1220–1.
3. Hopkins, Jeff (1969) 'Social Work Organizations—New Models for Old', *Case Conference*, Vol. 16, No. 8, pp. 306-11.
4. Rea Price, John (1971), 'Hierarchy and Management Style' (Parts 1 and 2), *Brit. Hosp. J. and Soc. Serv. Rev.*, Vol. 81, 6 Nov., pp. 2315–6 (Part 1), and 13 Nov., pp. 2373–4 (Part 2).
5. Heal, Kevin (1971) 'Conflict and the Social Service Department', *Social Work Today*, Vol. 1, No. 11, pp. 19–22.
6. Phillips, Maurice and Birchall, Elizabeth (1971) 'Structuring an Area Office to Meet Client Need', *Social Work Today*, Vol. 1, No. 10, pp. 5–11.
7. Algie, J. (1970) 'Management and Organization in the Social Services', *Brit. Hosp. J. and Soc. Serv. Rev.*, Vol. 80, June, pp. 1245–8.
8. Burns, Tom and Stalker, G. M. (1966) *The Management of Innovation*, 2nd edn. Tavistock, London.
9. Silverman, David (1970) *The Theory of Organizations*. Heinemann, London.
10. Weber, Max (1947) *The Theory of Social and Economic Organization*. Free Press, New York.
11. Blau, Peter M. and Scott, W. Richard (1963) *Formal Organizations*. Routledge & Kegan Paul, London. p. 41.
12. Perrow, Charles (1970) *Organizational Analysis: A Sociological View*. Tavistock, London, p. 28.
13. Goffman, Erving (1968) *Asylums*. Penguin, Harmondsworth.
14. Perrow, Charles (1967) 'A Framework for the Comparative Analysis of Organizations', *Amer. Sociological Rev.*, Vol. 32, No. 2, p. 195.
15. Titmuss, Richard M. (1968) *Commitment to Welfare*. George Allen & Unwin, London, p. 22.
16. Pugh, D. S., Hickson, D. J. and Hinings, C. R. (1971) *Writers on Organizations*, 2nd edn., Penguin, Harmondsworth, p. 132.
17. Scott, W. Richard (1969) 'Professional Employees in a Bureaucratic Structure: Social Work', in A. Etzioni (ed.), *The Semi-Professions and their Organizations*. Free Press, New York, pp. 102–10.
18. Smith, Gilbert (1970) *Social Work and the Sociology of Organizations*. Routledge & Kegan Paul, London, pp. 5–8.
19. Smith, Gilbert and Harris, Robert (1972) 'Ideologies of Need and the Organization of Social Work Departments', *Brit. J. of Social Work*, Vol. 2, No. 1, pp. 27–45.
20. Leonard, Peter (1970) 'Experiments in Post-Professional Education', *Social Work Today*, Vol. 1, No. 4, p. 5.

I would like to thank Paul Bellaby and Joyce Warham of Keele University, and Brian Whittington of Bradford University for their helpful comments on an earlier draft of this article. I also wish to acknowledge my award under the Fellowship Scheme for Advanced Studies administered by the Central Council for Education and Training in Social Work, which has made possible the ongoing work from which this article arises. Responsibility for the views expressed, of course, remains my own.

8/ORGANIZATIONAL FACTORS IN THE PERFORMANCE OF SOCIAL WELFARE AND REHABILITATION WORKERS

JOSEPH A. OLMSTEAD

THEORIES OF ORGANIZATION

The organizational literature is characterized by numerous points of view, each of which seems to possess a certain degree of legitimacy. The problem is that the one phenomenon, an organization, can be validly approached from a number of different standpoints. Thus the systems developed by business theorists, social scientists, behavioral scientists, and operations researchers usually consist of widely different concepts and variables. Stogdill (1966) lists 18 separate ways of conceptualizing organizations and groups and says that this is not an exhaustive list. Yet each approach has a certain relevance, and each contributes to better understanding of organizations.

One major contributor to the proliferation of approaches is a certain duality which has existed throughout much recent history of the field. The division ultimately reduces to the old question of organizational requirements vs. needs of the individual. Although Barnard (1938) early recognized the necessity for balance between the two elements, the work of most writers has reflected one emphasis or the other but rarely both. Some writers, such as Argyris (1957) and McGregor (1967), have even made the conflict keystones of their systems. Only in the past several years have a few theorists, such as Bennis (1966), attempted to reconcile the differing viewpoints in an integrated position.

Recognition of these approaches and of the attempts to reconcile them is essential to understanding the point at which organizational research has arrived. Accordingly the major positions will be summarized, and a few landmarks will be reviewed.

STRUCTURAL THEORIES

The problem of structure is a recurring theme in organizational theory. All organizations have to provide for the meshing of members' activities. Thus tasks must be allocated, authority (the right to make decisions) must be assigned, and functions must be coordinated. These requirements lead to development of a hierarchical framework which is called the "structure" of the organization.

The putative father of structural theory is Max Weber, the German sociologist, who developed his concept of bureaucracy around the formal structure of organizations. Weber (1947) noted that, in an organization, authority is vested in positions rather than individuals and is exercised through a formal system of rules and procedures. The positions are arranged in a hierarchy with each position exercising authority over all of those below it. According to Weber, the formalism characteristic of bureaucracies minimizes variability in problem solutions and maintains high standards of internal efficiency. From this viewpoint, "an organization is a social device for efficiently accomplishing through group means some stated purpose; it is the equivalent of the blueprint for the design of the machine which is to be created for some practical purpose" (Katz and Kahn, 1966, p. 16).

Weber wrote on bureaucracy around the turn of the century. Until recently, most structural theorists followed him in stressing the rational aspects of organizations. Most concerned themselves with deriving more and more ideal structures and with analyzing how such factors as objectives, size, geographical dispersion, and techniques of operation influence the shapes of hierarchical frameworks. Because a scientist does not often get an opportunity to manipulate the structures of existing organizations, much of this work was descriptive.

Most of the earlier theorists were concerned with increasing effectiveness through improved structural designs. However, in recent years, more attention has been given to the attitudes, values, and goals of subordinate units and to the ways in which these unintended consequences can actually modify an organization's structure. This development began with Merton (1940) and continued with Dubin (1949) and Selznick (1957). As one example, Selznick demonstrated in a study of the Tennessee Valley Authority that Weber's description of a formal bureaucracy left out the problems that occur when organizational leaders delegate some of their authority, which inevitably they must. Delegation increases unit specialization and thus emphasizes conflicts of interest between units and between a unit and the organization as a whole. Such conflicts hamper the effectiveness anticipated when ideal structures are designed.

These recent developments have expanded the perspectives of structural theorists. Although there is still a vigorous concern with organizational design (Thompson, 1966) and with linkages, levels, and bonds of organizations (Haire, 1959; Marschak, 1959), most present-day theorists (Selznick, 1957; Dubin, 1959; Rapoport, 1959) attempt to bring internal processes into their systems. Primary emphasis remains upon structure, but there is now recognition that disregard of the human variable may have serious disrupting effects upon an ideally designed organization.

Structural theory has numerous critics. In particular, the older theories of bureaucracy have been attacked from many sides. According to Bennis, "Almost everybody, including many students of organizational behavior, approaches bureaucracy with a chip on his shoulder. It has been criticized for its theoretical confusion and contradictions, for moral and ethical reasons, on practical grounds such as its inefficiency, for its methodological weaknesses, and for containing too many implicit values or for containing too few" (1966, p. 5).

Some criticisms appear to be more valid than others. However, several limitations of structural theory are readily apparent and have particular relevance for this discussion. The first major limitation is that structural theories usually focus upon the anatomy of organizations rather than their behavior. A knowledge of anatomy is important for understanding any organism; however, it is only a small part of the story. Viewing an organization solely from the standpoint of structure is like looking at an iceberg. The greater portion of it is never seen.

This limitation would not seem so critical if theoretical understanding were the only consideration. The trouble is that structural theories held predominance for so long and they offer such easy answers that many practitioners—administrators, managers, military commanders, etc.—look to organizational design as the solution to problems whose sources often lie elsewhere. When difficulties arise within an organization, the most obvious solution is to redesign a job, change the authority structure, or modify the span of control, when in fact these aspects may be only tangentially relevant to the real problems.

A second limitation is that structural theories most frequently are concerned with derivation of ideal structures rather than with the design of real-life organizations. While ideal structures can contribute to thinking about real organizations, many of the discussions are simply irrelevant to practical situations.

A final limitation is that most structural theories ignore the effects that the personalities of members may exert upon the shape of an organization. A strong leader or team of leaders may exercise dramatic modifications upon the allocation of responsibility and authority. In a similar way, single positions or entire structures are sometimes changed to fit the competencies or limitations of incumbents. Structural theories rarely take such factors into account.

Despite these limitations, structural theories make valuable contributions to knowledge of organizational behavior. For example, an understanding of the ways in which such factors as missions, objectives, size, and techniques of operation determine optimum structure is critical for efficient functioning. Furthermore, the question of structure, of the linkage between positions, is closely associated with problems of information processing and decision making. The number of links in a system and the concomitant allocations of authority may have serious consequences for communication load and vulnerability to information loss. It seems clear that structural concepts, when viewed in the proper perspective, have an important place in any systematic theory of organizational functioning.

GROUP THEORIES

Weber himself eventually got around to expressing fear that the bureaucratic way of life tends to smother individual potentialities. He was the forerunner of a large number of writers who have sounded the alarm against practicing bureaucracy. Indeed, Bennis, in a discussion of "the decline of bureaucracy," states:

. . . it would be fair to say that a great deal of the work on organizational behavior over the past two decades has been a footnote to the bureaucratic "backlash" which aroused Weber's passion: saving mankind's soul "from the supreme mastery of the bureaucratic way of life." At least, very few of us have been indifferent to the fact that the bureaucratic mechanism is a social instrument in the service of repression; that it treats man's ego and social needs as a constant, or as nonexistent or inert; that these confined and constricted needs insinuate themselves into the social processes of organizations in strange, unintended ways; and that those very matters which Weber claimed escaped calculation—love, power, hate—not only are calculable and powerful in their effects but must be reckoned with (1966, p. 7).

Bennis probably overstates the case when he envisions concerted movement to save "mankind's soul from the supreme mastery of a bureaucratic way of life." Certainly, there has been a recent flurry of writings concerned with the inhibiting effects of organizational life. These will be discussed in the section on individual theories. However, the earliest, and still continuing, attack came not so much from a concern for the repressive effects of organizations as from discovery of a basic fallacy in classical structural theory. The fallacy was that structural theory fails to recognize the effects of informal groups upon motivation, behavior, and performance in organizations.

Group theories of organization stem from two unrelated sources. The first was the work begun by Mayo (1933) at the Hawthorne plant of Western Electric and continued by Roethlisberger and Dickson (1939). These writers "discovered" the influence of the face-to-face informal group upon motivation and behavior in a work situation. However, for them, there was no essential conflict between man and the organization. Rather, satisfying the workers' social and psychological needs was seen as congruent with the organization's goals of effectiveness and productivity.

Directly descending from Mayo are Whyte (1959, 1961), Homans (1950), and Zaleznik (1964). Working with data drawn from business organizations (usually obtained by intensive case study of a single firm), these theorists developed such findings as the following: the output of a worker is determined as much by his social relations as by his abilities and skills; noneconomic rewards are extremely important in the motivation and satisfaction of personnel; group-held norms and attitudes play a major role in an individual's evaluation of his work situation; and informal leaders can develop who may possess more actual power than appointed supervisors.

The second source of group theories was the work of Kurt Lewin (1947) who stressed the importance of group decision making and participation in motivating people. Following Lewin, there has appeared a long series, of which the most notable for this paper are the leadership studies of Lewin, Lippitt, and White (1939), the participation studies of Coch and French (1948), and the work on morale and productivity by Katz and Kahn (1952). Although not yet finished, the work of Lewin's successors reached a landmark with the publications of Likert's *New Patterns of Management* (1961). In this book, Likert proposes a "modified" theory of management in which he stresses the importance of group forces in worker motivation, the necessity for managers and supervisors to serve as "linking pins" between the various groups and levels within an organization, and the essentiality but relative independence of both productivity and morale. Likert has further elaborated on his theory in a more recent book, *The Human Organization* (1967).

Although the lineal descendents of Mayo and Lewin have remained apart in their general approaches, many common elements can be identified. In both approaches, the principal emphasis was changed from Weber's rational bureaucracy to an organizational model which takes account of unanticipated consequences, such as feelings, attitudes, norms, sentiments, and perceptions. The behavior of an organization is seen as less mechanistic but also more unpredictable.

The acceptance of social relationships as a major determinant of organizational behavior was a significant development in the theory of organizations. The strong reaction of group theorists to the older rational models was highly valuable in calling attention to a hitherto ignored facet in organizational functioning. On the other hand, the aversion of group theorists, especially the Lewinians, to anything resembling a hierarchy in organization has been something of a limitation. So far, there have been few attempts to relate group behavior to organizational functioning in any systematic way. Likert comes closest, but his concepts become rather pallid when he moves into discussion of groups in relation to hierarchical levels.

Many group theorists have been reluctant to give full weight to formal authority relationships. In fact, this reluctance has been so pronounced that Cartwright, one of the more eminent group theorists, has accused group psychology of being "soft on power" (1959). Especially for groups within hierarchical organizations, power is a critical variable. Because organizations are structured on the basis of authority relationships, groups within organizations are different from those outside. This fact can never be ignored.

INDIVIDUAL THEORIES

The rubric "Individual Theories" embraces two approaches that are only remotely related. On the one hand, a rather large group of researchers and a smaller number of theorists are concerned with psychological factors that affect the performance of individuals within organizations. On the other hand, a small but increasing number of writers, in violent reaction against rational structural theories and the practices based upon them, have emphasized the conflict between organizational requirements and the needs of the individual. Both approaches are concerned with the performance of individuals. However, the first addresses itself to improving performance through better selection, training, leadership, etc. The second approach starts with the notion of a basic incompatibility between organization and individual and then attempts to modify organizations and their practices in ways intended to permit greater opportunities for need satisfaction by personnel.

The first approach centers around those activities commonly considered to be within the purview of traditional "industrial psychology." Stemming from a long and respectable history of applied work, there has developed a considerable body of studies concerned with such concrete problems as selection, training, conditions of work, methods of payment, human engineering, etc. In these areas, a genuine contribution has been made in fitting the man to the job. Until recently, this contribution has been mainly in terms of methods. Most work has relied on analyses of single problems in unique situations rather than systematic studies of generalized phenomena.

This limitation has subjected individual theorists to criticism by a number of writers who desire a more systematic understanding of the problems studied. For example, Pugh (1966) contends that all of the studies on industrial selection have "contributed little more to the understanding of human behavior than a series of (usually modest) validity coefficients." Pugh credits the individual theorists for being the only ones who have tackled the problem of the validity of data, but he also contends that their emphasis upon a "factorial-statistical" approach has usually resulted in a theoretically arid formulation.

Another limitation of the traditional individual approach is that many attempts to improve performance of individuals do not take the organizational context into full account. Personnel selection again provides an illustration. Selection procedures are desired so that an organization can be composed of the most adequate individuals. Yet one can conceive of a highly adequate person in an organizational setting where his own adequacy is relatively independent of organizational effectiveness. Conversely, a highly effective organization could conceivably be composed of only average persons. Although the adequacy of each individual is important, the operational processes characteristic of the particular organization and the ways in which members' activities are integrated and coordinated can be equally critical.

At present, this traditional approach to individual effectiveness appears to be embarking on a new stage of development. Over the past decade, there has developed a growing body of data concerned with motivation and its more complex relationships with performance. Motivation has, of course, been recognized in industrial psychology for a long time. However, it is only recently that psychologists have produced genuinely sophisticated studies and theories concerned specifically with the composition of those motives most relevant to performance within organizations (Gellerman, 1963). For example, it has been shown that job satisfaction and productivity are not necessarily complementary (Brayfield and Crockett, 1955; Kahn, 1960). This was puzzling for a while until Herzberg, Mausner, and Snyderman (1959) demonstrated that job satisfaction itself is not a unitary concept and that certain conditions at work only prevent losses in morale but do not push toward greater motivation, while others exert strong uplifting effects upon attitudes or performance.

These developments in the study of motivation offer much promise for improved understanding of organizational behavior. Although still concerned with the effects of motivation upon the performance of individuals, most theorists give full recognition to the influence of organizational conditions upon motivation and, more important, to the effects of social motivation upon group and organizational performance.

Whereas the approach just described has focused mainly upon fitting man to the organization, another approach is more concerned with fitting the organization to man. In one way or another, theorists of the second approach see the basic problem as a conflict between the psychological needs of individuals and the formal requirements of organizations as posited by the structural theorists.

By far the most clear in his conceptualizations is Argyris (1957, 1962), who has built a complete system around the notion of the basic incompatibility of the individual and the organization. According to Argyris, this incompatibility results in frustration which can be inferred from "pathological behaviors" and "defense mechanisms" exhibited by many individuals employed in organizations. In his earlier work (1957), Argyris was mainly concerned with effects upon lower-level personnel, and his solutions involved restructuring organizations toward greater decentralization and enlarging jobs so that "self-actualization" would have more chance to blossom. In later work (1962), Argyris has addressed himself to the problems of executives, and he advocates modification of impersonal value systems and the development of "authentic" relationships.

Although he started from a somewhat different position, McGregor

(1960) based his analysis upon the same essential conflict as Argyris. McGregor began with recognition that "if there is a single assumption which pervades conventional organizational theory it is that authority is the central, indispensable means for managerial control" (1960, p. 18). McGregor then proceeded to his now-famous comparison between "Theory X" and "Theory Y." He attempted to show the limitations of authority based on role or status (Theory X) as compared with authority based on objectives, i.e., task or goal requirements (Theory Y). McGregor stressed the integration of task requirements with individual needs. However, where Argyris advocated restructuring job and organization, McGergor recognized that leadership is the means whereby the demands of the individual and the requirements of the organization can be reconciled. For him, leadership is "the creation of conditions such that members of the organization can achieve their goals *best* by directing their efforts toward the success of the enterprise" (1960, p. 49).

Several other writers (Blake and Mouton, 1964; Shepard, 1965) have stressed the importance of organizational leadership as the main integrating factor. In their view, if leaders see their organizations as organic rather than mechanistic, as adaptable rather than bounded by rigid structure, emphasis will shift from arbitration to problem solving, from delegated to shared responsibility, and from centralized to decentralized authority. Thus the needs of individuals and requirements of organizations will be reconciled.

This second approach of the Individual Theorists is important because it focuses attention upon internal processes and the ways in which human components affect them. Effectiveness within an organization requires trading and negotiation by all participants. The extent to which problems are solved and objectives are accomplished is strongly determined by the degree of accommodation that can be achieved.

As a final point, it should be noted that all of the approaches mentioned in relation to both group and individual theories tend to emphasize interpersonal and group variables as causal factors in organizational effectiveness and tend to deemphasize the cognitive processes of problem solving as equally important determinants.

DECISION THEORIES

Whereas group and individual theorists have tended to play down cognitive processes, other writers have focused squarely upon problem solving and decision making as controlling factors in organizational effectiveness. Although the study of decision making, particularly that performed by individuals, is a relatively independent area of research, it has made a significant contribution to the theory of organizations.

Theories of organizational decision making have their origin in economic theories of consumers' choice (Edwards, 1954). Classical economic theory started from an assumption that man is entirely rational in his choices. Economic man was presumed to be completely informed, infinitely sensitive, and totally rational. In his decisions, not only were the alternatives in the choice known but also each alternative was known to lead to a specific outcome. Thus classical economic theory was essentially one of decision under conditions of absolute certainty (Taylor, 1965).

Classical decision theory has undergone numerous modifications, the most notable of which occurred with the advent of game theory (von Neumann and Morgenstern, 1944). Game theory recognizes the concept of decision under uncertainty or risk; however, it still rests upon the assumption of rationality. Furthermore, game theory remains a theory of decision making by individuals.

A decision made by an individual in isolation is one thing, but that made by him in an organization is another. In the latter case, the considerations to be taken into account become much more complex. A landmark in the development of theories of decision making in organizations was Simon's book, *Administrative Behavior: A Study of Decision-Making Processes in Administrative Organization* (1947). Simon retained the idea that decision behavior within organizations is "intendedly rational" and that decisions are made by individuals within organizations and not by organizations as entities. However, he also recognized the inadequacy of classical economic theory for understanding behavior within organizations. Accordingly, he distinguished between the roles of facts and of values in decision making. Questions of value are questions of what *ought* to be. Simon contended that decision makers employ values as well as facts in making choices. Limits upon rationality in decision making are imposed by lack of all the possible facts. Therefore, in Simon's view (1957a, p. 204), the decision maker must "satisfice"—find a course of action that is "good enough"—rather than maximizing returns, as would be possible if he had full knowledge of the consequences attached to every alternative.

The contrast between economic man and Simon's administrative man emphasizes an important point. Rationality is central to behavior within an organization. However, if the members of an organization were individuals capable of the kind of objective rationality attributed to classical economic man, theories of organization would have no purpose. In Simon's words:

. . . if there were no limits to human rationality, administrative theory would be barren. It would consist of the single precept: always select that alternative, among those available, which will lead to the most complete achievement of your goals. The need for an administrative theory resides in the fact that there are practical limits to human rationality, and that these limits are not static, but depend upon the organizational environment in which the individual's decision takes place. The task of administration is so to design the environment that the individual will approach as close as practicable to rationality (judged in terms of the organization's goals) in his decisions (1957a, pp. 240–241).

The most significant point in the quotation is that decisions are influenced by the organizational environment. Internal relationships and operational processes can and do exert critical effects upon the nature and quality of decisions. Thus decisions can never be completely rational. This theme was expanded into a full theory of organization by March and Simon (1958).

In the classical economic theories and Simon's administrative theories, the decision maker is the individual. On the other hand, Cyert and March (1964) have recently formulated a theory of the organization as decision maker. Cyert and March build upon the classical model of rational behavior; however, they recognize an important fact. Organizations are constantly attempting to adapt to their external and internal environments, and completely rational adaptation is constrained by some fairly strong limits on the cognitive capacity, the computational speed, and the internal goal consistency of the organizations. To describe how organizations cope with these constraints, Cyert and March posit four critical modifications of the classical axioms of rationality. First is the quasi-resolution of conflict; organizations do not have a simple preference ordering of goals but instead exist with considerable conflicts of interest which are resolved either through compromise or sequential attention to goals. Second is uncertainty avoidance; organizations tend to avoid uncertainty rather than deal with it by calculations of expected returns as in economic theory. Third is problemistic search; decisions to search for solutions are dictated by the existence of problems rather than calculations of expected returns. In short, organizations search for answers only when problems arise. Fourth is organizational learning; organizations learn from their experiences and modify procedures over time.

The notion that numbers of people make decisions as a unit is not a new idea in group dynamics. However, in decison theory it is a relatively recent concept. When the temptation to anthropomorphize can be resisted, when it can be recognized that what is involved is a number of individuals arriving at joint decisions, the concept of organizational decision making provides possibilties for promising insights into some of the more complex aspects of organizational behavior. For example, the four modifications described in the discussion of Cyert and March, open the door to the analysis of organization in terms of ongoing processes. Where previous theories viewed decision making in terms of essentially static models, Cyert and March see it as a dynamic process occurring in response to continuous changes in the environment and constantly modified on the basis of new information. Thus, decision making is seen as an adaptive response of the organization.

The importance of viewing decision making in terms of organizational processes cannot be overemphasized. Much of the research and theory presently existent ignores the circumstances under which the decision is made and under which the decision maker is acting. Much of the work in the field makes it appear that the specific act of choosing among alternatives is the core of the decision-making process and that prior or subsequent events need not be considered. Yet, in real organizations, the events leading to the act of choice and those following are often the more critical ones. Frequently, the outcome is foreordained by the time the act of choice is reached and, often, decisions are not implemented as intended. It begins to become clear that decision making cannot be separated from other organizational processes.

One final point remains with regard to decision theories. Just as group and individual theories overstress interpersonal and motivational factors, decision theories place primary emphasis upon rational aspects of cognition and perception. Accordingly, like the group and individual approaches, decision theories offer only partial explanations of the complex phenomena encountered in organization.

SYSTEMS THEORIES

Recently there has developed a mounting dissatisfaction with approaches which concern themselves with only limited aspects of organizational behavior. A number of writers have concluded that such approaches leave some of the most critical aspects of organizational functioning untouched. For example, Bennis contends that "the main challenge confronting today's organization . . . is that of responding to changing conditions and adapting to external stress" (1966, p. 44).

In a similar vein, Selznick also concludes:

The aims of large organizations are often very broad. A certain vagueness must be accepted because it is difficult to foresee whether more specific goals will be realistic or wise. This situation presents the leader with one of his most difficult but indispensable tasks. *He must specify and recast the general aims of his organization* so as to adapt them without serious corruption to the requirements of institutional survival (1957, p. 66).

Bennis (1966, pp. 34–36) is the most articulate critic of the more customary ways of approaching organizations. He contends that the traditional approaches are "out of joint" with the emerging view of organizations as adaptive, problem-solving systems and that conventional criteria of effectiveness are not sensitive to the critical needs of the organization to cope with external stress and change. Acocrding to Bennis, the present methods of evaluating effectiveness provide static indicators of certain output characteristics (performance and satisfaction) without revealing the processes by which the organization searches for, adapts to, and solves its changing problems. Yet without understanding of these dynamic processes of problem solving, knowledge about organizational behavior is woefully inadequate.

He concludes, ". . . the methodological rules by which the organization approaches its task and 'exchanges with its environments' are the critical determinants of organizational effectiveness" (1966, p. 47).

Bennis proposes that the major concern should be with "organizational health," defined in terms of "competence," "mastery," and "problem-solving ability," rather than "effectiveness," if "effectiveness" is considered in terms solely of final outputs. He then postulates some criteria for organizational health (1966, pp. 52–54).

1. Adaptability—which coincides with problem-solving ability, which, in turn, depends upon flexibility of the organization. Flexibility is the freedom to learn through experience, to change with changing internal and external circumstances.

2. Identity—adaptability requires that an organization "know who it is and what it is to do." It needs some clearly defined identity. Identity can be examined in two ways: by determining to what extent the organizational goals are understood and accepted by the personnel; and by ascertaining to what extent the organization is perceived veridically by the personnel.

3. Reality-testing—the organization must develop adequate techniques for determining the "real properties" of the environment in which it exists. The "psychological field" of the organization contains two main boundaries, the internal organization and the boundaries with the external environment. Accurate sensing of the field is essential before adaptation can occur.

Thus Bennis views an organization as an adaptive organism, and he contends that the processes through which adaptation occurs are the proper focus of analysis.

A few other writers have recognized the potentiality of studying the problem-solving processes used by an organization. For one, Altman states:

Performance effectiveness should be viewed from a much larger perspective, to include so-called "process variables" as intrinsic antecedents of performance outputs. Thus we reject the approach to small group performance or organizational performance solely from a "black box" point of view, but propose instead a strategy of research that peers into the box and attempts to understand the sequential development of performance as it progresses from input to output (1966, p. 84).

Schein (1965) goes beyond Altman and suggests an actual sequence of activities or processes used by organizations in adapting to changes in the environment. Schein calls this sequence an *adaptive-coping cycle*. The stages of the adaptive-coping cycle are as follows:

1. Sensing a change in the internal or external environment.

2. Importing the relevant information about the change into those parts of the organization which can act upon it.

3. Changing production or conversion processes inside the organization according to the information obtained.

4. Stabilizing internal changes while reducing or managing undesired by-products (undesired changes in related systems which have resulted from the desired changes).

5. Exporting new products, services, and so on, which are more in line with the originally perceived changes in the environment.

6. Obtaining feedback on the success of the change through further sensing of the state of the external environment and the degree of integration of the internal environment . . . (1965, pp. 98–99).

Schein's adaptive-coping cycle makes it possible to identify more precisely those processes where performance may be inadequate and to specify more accurately the relative contribution of each process to overall effectiveness.

In their search for a schema which will encompass the many varied aspects of organizations, Bennis (1966), Schein (1965), and a number of other writers have turned to General Systems Theory (von Bertalanffy, 1956). In systems theory, an organization is viewed as existing in an environment with which there are more or less continuous interchanges. As a system, the organization is regarded as having inputs (resources such as material, people, and information) on which it operates a conversion process (throughput) to produce outputs (products, services, etc.). Both the inputs and outputs must take account of environmental changes and demands (Emory and Trist, 1965).

The organization simultaneously engages in two general kinds of processes: (1) those concerned with adaptation to the environment; and (2) those concerned with internal development and execution. Thus it uses its internal processes and energies to continually react to changes in its environment in order to maintain equilibrium with it.

Of particular interest to organization theorists is the concept of equifinality. According to this principle, a system can reach the same final state from different initial conditions and by a variety of paths (Katz and Kahn, 1966). It has special significance for organizations because it points up the importance of ongoing process adapted for specific situations as major determinants of outcomes. Whereas bureaucratic theories rely upon rules, policies, and precedents to dictate action and theories of decision rely on rationality to indicate the obvious solution, systems theory recognizes that actions are governed by dynamic processes through which problems are approached as they arise and in accordance with their particular nature.

One of the most fully developed approaches is that of Parsons (1960). According to Parsons, all organizations must solve four basic problems:

1. Adaptation: the accommodation of the system to the reality demands of the environment and the actual modification of the external situations. Each organization must have structures and processes that will enable it to

adapt to its environment and mobilize the necessary resources to overcome changes in the environment.

2. Goal achievement: the defining of objectives and the attaining of them. Processes are required for implementing goals, to include methods for specifying objectives, mobilizing resources, etc.

3. Integration: establishing and developing a structure of relationships among the members that will unify them and integrate their actions. The organization must develop processes aimed at commanding the loyalties of its members, motivating them, and coordinating their efforts.

4. Latency: maintenance of the organization's motivational and normative patterns over time. Consensus must be promoted on values that define and legitimatize the organization's goals and performance standards.

Parsons applies his theory to all types of social phenomena. Probably because of his interest in a theory of general social systems, he paints his analysis of formal organizations with a fairly broad brush. However, Katz and Kahn (1966) have built upon Parsons' work, together with that of Allport (1962) and Miller (1955), to develop a comprehensive, wide-ranging theory of organizations which is solidly within the systems theory tradition. Katz and Kahn attempt nothing less than a complete explanation of organizational behavior with systems theory concepts. Although certain aspects of organizations require a little forcing to fit systems concepts, the attempt seems reasonably successful in putting into proper perspective such ideas as interchange with environments, operation by process instead of procedure, and the interrelationships among functional units.

Systems theory embraces a much more comprehensive set of concepts than is possible to describe here. Accordingly, an outline provided by Schein (1965, p. 95) will serve to summarize those ideas which have the most relevance for this discussion:

1. . . . the organization must be conceived of as an open system, which means that it is in constant interaction, taking in raw materials, people, energy, and information, and transforming or converting these into products and services which are exported in the environment.

2. . . . the organization must be conceived of as a system with multiple purposes or functions which involve multiple interactions between the organization and its environment. Many of the activities of subsystems within the organization cannot be understood without considering these multiple interactions and functions.

3. . . . the organization consists of many subsystems which are in dynamic interaction with one another. Instead of analyzing organizational phenomena in terms of individual behavior, it is becoming increasingly important to analyze the behavior of such subsystems, whether they be conceived in terms of groups, roles, or some other concept.

4. . . . because the subsystems are mutually dependent, changes in one subsystem are likely to affect the behavior of other subsystems.

5. . . . the organization exists in a dynamic environment which consists of other systems, some larger, some smaller than the organization. The environment places demands upon and constrains the organization in various ways. The total functioning of the organization cannot be understood, therefore, without explicit consideration of these environmental demands and constraints.

6. . . . the multiple links between the organization and its environment make it difficult to specify clearly the boundaries of any given organization. Ultimately, a concept of organization is perhaps better given in terms of the stable *processes* of import, conversion, and export, rather than characteristics such as size, shape, function, or structure.

The swing to a process emphasis by such respected theorists as Bennis, Parsons, and Selznick signals a significant new development in ways of thinking about organizations. Where previously attention was mainly focused upon the invariant aspects of organizations—the unchanging aspects of structures, policies, and procedures—there has now been recognition that the variant aspects may be the real key to understanding and controlling performance.

Thus it has finally become apparent that, with organizations as with people, it is plainly necessary to focus attention on dynamics. Since an organization is an adaptive equilibrium-seeking organism, the processes through which adaptation occurs are a significant subject of analysis. It is, therefore, important to learn precisely how these processes affect and contribute to performance. It is equally important to understand what factors influence functioning of the organizational processes and what human variables determine, in a particular organization, whether the processes can resist disruption under pressures arising from the stresses of daily operations.

REFERENCES

Allport, F. H. 1962 A structuronomic conception of behavior: individual and collective. I. Structural theory and the master problem of social psychology. *Journal of Abnormal and Social Psychology*, 64, 3–30.

Altman, I. 1966 The small group field: implications for research on behavior in organizations. In Bowers, R. V., ed., *Studies on Behavior in Organizations: A Research Symposium*. Athens: Univ. of Georgia Press.

Argyris, C. 1957 *Personality and Organization: The Conflict Between System and Individual*. New York: Harper.

Argyris, C. 1962 *Interpersonal Competence and Organizational Effectiveness*. Homewood, Ill.: Irwin-Dorsey Press.

Barnard, C. I. 1938 *The Functions of the Executive*. Cambridge: Harvard Univ. Press.

Bennis, W. G. 1966 *Changing Organizations: Essays on the Development and Evolution of Human Organizations*. New York: McGraw-Hill.

Blake, R. R., and Mouton, J. S. 1964 *The Managerial Grid*. Houston: Gulf Publishing Company.

Brayfield, A. H., and Crockett, W. H. 1955 Employee attitudes and employee performance. *Psychological Bulletin*, 52, 396–424.

Cartwright, D. 1959 Power, a neglected variable in social psychology. In Cartwright, D., ed., *Studies in Social Power*. Ann Arbor: Institute for Social Research, Univ. of Michigan.

Coch, L., and French, J. P. R., Jr. 1948 Overcoming resistance to change. *Human Relations, 1,* 512–532.

Cyert, R. M., and March, J. G. 1964 The behavioral theory of the firm: A behavioral science–economics amalgam. In Cooper, W. W.; Leavitt, H. J.; and Shelly, M. W., eds., *New Perspectives in Organizational Research*. New York: Wiley.

Dubin, R. 1949 Decision-making by management in industrial relations. *American Journal of Sociology, 54,* 292–297.

Dubin, R. 1959 Stability of human organizations. In Haire, M., ed., *Modern Organization Theory*. New York: Wiley.

Edwards, W. 1954 The theory of decision making. *Psychological Bulletin, 51,* 380–417.

Emory, F. E., and Trist, F. L. 1965 The causal texture of organizational environments. *Human Relations, 18,* 21–32.

Gellerman, S. W. 1963 *Motivation and Productivity*. New York: American Management Association.

Herzberg, F.; Mausner, B.; and Snyderman, B. B. 1959 *The Motivation to Work*. (2nd ed.) New York: Wiley.

Homans, G. C. 1950 *The Human Group*. New York: Harcourt, Brace.

Kahn, R. L. 1960 Productivity and job satisfactions. *Personnel Psychology, 13,* 275–287.

Katz, D., and Kahn, R. L. 1952 Some recent findings in human relations research. In Swanson, E.; Newcomb, T.; and Hartley, G., eds., *Readings in Social Psychology*. New York: Holt, Rinehart and Winston.

Katz, D., and Kahn, R. L. 1966 *The Social Psychology of Organizations*. New York: Wiley.

Lewin, K.; Lippitt, R.; and White, R. K. 1939 Patterns of aggressive behavior in experimentally created "social climates." *Journal of Social Psychology, 10,* 271–299.

Lewin, K. 1947 Frontiers in group dynamics. *Human Relations, 1,* 5–42.

Likert, R. 1961 *New Patterns of Management*. New York: McGraw-Hill.

Likert, R. 1967 *The Human Organization: Its Management and Value*. New York: McGraw-Hill.

McGregor, D. 1960 *The Human Side of Enterprise*. New York: McGraw-Hill.

McGregor, D. 1967 *The Professional Manager*. New York: McGraw-Hill.

March, J. G., and Simon, H. A. 1958 *Organizations*. New York: Wiley.

Marschak, J. 1959 Efficient and viable organizational forms. In Haire, M., ed., *Modern Organization Theory*. New York: Wiley.

Mayo, E. 1933 *The Human Problem of Industrial Civilization*. New York: Macmillan.

Merton, R. K. 1940 Bureaucratic structure and personality. *Social Forces, 18,* 560–568.

Miller, J. G. 1955 Toward a general theory for the behavioral sciences. *American Psychologist, 10,* 513–531.

Parsons, T. 1960 *Structure and Process in Modern Societies*. Glencoe, Ill.: Free Press.

Pugh, D. S. 1966 Modern organizational theory: A psychological and sociological study. *Psychological Bulletin, 66,* 235–251.

Rapoport, A. 1959 A logical task as a research tool in organization theory. In Haire, M., ed., *Modern Organization Theory*. New York: Wiley.

Roethlisberger, F. J., and Dickson, W. J. 1939 *Management and the Worker*. Cambridge: Harvard Univ. Press.

Schein, E. H. 1965 *Organizational Psychology*. Englewood Cliffs, N.J.: Prentice-Hall.

Selznick, P. 1957 *Leadership in Administration: A Sociological Interpretation*. Evanston: Row, Peterson.

Shepard, H. A. 1965 Changing interpersonal and intergroup relationships in organizations. In March, J., ed., *Handbook of Organizations*. Chicago: Rand McNally.

Simon, H. A. 1947 *Administrative Behavior: A Study of Decision-Making Processes in Administrative Organization.* New York: Macmillan.

Simon, H. A. 1957 *Administrative Behavior: A Study of Decision-Making Processes in Administrative Organization.* (2nd ed.) New York: Macmillan.

Stogdill, R. M. 1966 Dimensions of organization theory. In Thompson, J. D., ed., *Approaches to Organizational Design.* Pittsburgh: Univ. of Pittsburgh Press.

Taylor, D. W. 1965 Decision making and problem solving. In March, J. G., ed., *Handbook of Organizations.* Chicago: Rand McNally.

Thompson, J. E., ed. 1966 *Approaches to Organizational Design.* Pittsburgh: Univ. of Pittsburgh Press.

von Bertalanffy, L. 1956 General systems theory. *Yearbook of the Society for General Systems Research, 1,* 1–10.

von Neuman, J., and Morgenstern, O. 1944 *Theory of Games and Economic Behavior.* Princeton: Princeton Univ. Press.

Weber, M. 1947 *The Theory of Social and Economic Organization.* (Reprinted and translated.) Glencoe, Ill.: Free Press.

Whyte, W. F. 1959 *Man and Organization.* Homewood, Ill.: Richard D. Irwin.

Whyte, W. F. 1961 *Men at Work.* Homewood, Ill.: Dorsey Press, and Richard D. Irwin.

Zaleznik, A., and Moment, D. 1964 *The Dynamics of Interpersonal Behavior.* New York: Wiley.

Part IV

THE STRUCTURE AND
USES OF AUTHORITY

EDITOR'S INTRODUCTION

Social services are characteristically provided through social agencies which have a distinctive form of governance. Power relationships and decision-making mechanisms and channels are thus organized. There is always an ultimate source of authority wherein sovereignty is lodged. The essential bases of sanction and legitimacy of social agencies are several, but always include a legal or legislative source. The particular form this social government assumes is the board of directors or trustees, or its analog. Voluntary agencies are subject to laws governing membership corporations, their charters specifying rules of organizational conduct. Public agencies have their origins in legislative enactments or administrative action, and conform to the regulations so established.

While ultimate social agency authority inheres in the board of directors, there is a parallel system of authority that organizes the actual service-giving and that defines the relationship between higher and lower participants in the agency's professional and staff structure. Thus a general system of parallel governance exists, establishing both lay and professional authority. The one consists of board members, officers, committees, the other of executives, associates, supervisors, and staff. Each is guided by its own distinctive functions and traditions and each is necessarily attached to the other in a symbiotic relationship that makes possible the achievement of organizational objectives.

There is a substantial void in the administrative and research literature on the functioning of boards, on the particular organizational forms that are most conducive to effective work, on the relationship between board leadership and membership, and on the extent to which the traditional views of board prerogatives are operationally verified. Much more has been done with respect to the ways in which professional personnel function in organizations, their styles of work, their motivation, and the supervisory relationships that guide their professional behaviors.

The conventional rhetoric suggests that, in general, boards of directors establish the policies that guide the staff in their service-giving performance—the one establishing direction, the other operationalizing. Practicing administrators know from their experience that the very process in which executives and their staff provide the essential materials to the board for such determination, in fact, gives them enormous power to skew policy in one direction or another, by the very selection they make of these materials. Experience also suggests that the very act of implementation of policy can enlarge, diminish, or distort the intent of policymakers. Identical policies often yield contradictory outcomes.

Yet there is an appropriate distinction to be made between the relevant actions expected of boards on the one hand and professional staffs on the other. Permeable though they may be, boundaries of authority and responsibility are implicit in the way social agencies go about their business in the context of a democratic, free-enterprise culture. Some of the boundary prescriptions are legally defined, others flow from the tradition and inherent logic of organizational requirements. Thus boards of directors establish the legal entity and legitimacy of the organization; establish and maintain financial integrity, solvency, and accountability; engage and evaluate the chief executive officer; manage financial investments; establish personnel policies; serve as advocates for the organization and its services; serve as communication links between the relevant community and the agency; and establish and monitor the organization's broad policies and goals.

By contrast, executive authority is directed largely to the requirements of service provision, and to the internal and external relationships that impinge on the service. It is preoccupied with engaging personnel; allocation of roles, and supervision and evaluation of performance; establishing standards of work; coordinating human and material resources; preparation of budgets and reports; maintenance of records; managing organizational maintenance requirements; managing conflict and tension; and providing professional direction to staff and informed leadership to the board.

The real skill of administrative leadership is seen in the ways in which these inherent functions and responsibilities are discharged by the parallel and coordinate channels of authority, all with respect to fulfilling the organization's purposes and objectives and maintaining the integrity of the service and the organization's response to clients' needs. While the lines of authority are parallel, every relevant level requires explicit attachments one to the other. Thus staff executive and board president inevitably develop a pattern of coordinate work that ultimately provides guidance to their respective constituencies and to the organization as a whole. Presidential authority extends through the lay structure of committees and chairpeople, just as executive authority extends through the professional staff system. These structures are perforce joined by the coordinate activity of committee and staff leadership, each accountable inherently to one another and, explicitly, to their respective structures.

A persistent problem encountered by administrators grows out of the confusion of lay and professional roles, and the resultant conflict that follows upon role invasion. The assumption of authority and behavior inappropriate to one's realm of action inevitably leads to issues of turf and propriety, and tends to become organizationally disruptive. Thus, board–executive and board–staff relationships represent important aspects of competent organizational behavior.

A. THE GOVERNING BOARDS

The selections in this section deal with this three-fold aspect of administrative behavior—governing boards, executive authority, and board–executive relationships. Mitton describes a particular structure of board committee work—what he calls a matrix-type—based on the essential functions of the board and the primary program areas of the agency. He reviews the process pursued by an organization as it sought to make maximal use of the special talents of board members and promote committed involvement. A dual-purpose committee structure was established, according to which each board member belonged to a service or treatment delivery committee, and to a committee concerned with some functional organizational requirement such as finance, personnel, etc.

Robins and Blackburn present a study of governing boards of community mental health centers, guided by their postulate that it is important to differentiate the effectiveness areas of board members from the effectiveness areas of professional staff. The key to such differentiation they locate in the distinction between program and process objectives, the former concerned with such matters as treatment, disability limitation, rehabilitation; the latter with items such as community responsiveness, availability of services, increasing community support. Whether or not one approves of the specific criteria given, the exercise in differential analysis, and the classification of process objectives and variables for measuring citizen boards are most useful.

O'Donnell and Reid explore the extent and impact of citizen and consumer participation in public welfare. Public welfare boards and committees have a long but undefined history. The study here reported is one of the most recent and extensive yet undertaken and reviews functions of boards and committees, the patterns of representation, and their impact on agency services. In spite of official public policy on citizen participation and recipient representation, the study concludes that these objectives have had only limited success. The authors observe the current federal deemphasis on such participation, and conclude that communication but not control, advice but not power, will probably continue to characterize the relationship of assistance recipients, low-income persons, and other lay citizens to the public agency in its policy-determination processes. Finally, some conditions are suggested for making such representation real rather than illusory.

B. EXECUTIVE AUTHORITY

The next four selections probe several aspects of the exercise of professional or executive authority. They focus largely on administrative skill, on internal communication processes, on the engineering of organizational compliance, and on administrative style. Kotin and Sharaf use an analysis of bureaucratic succession in a mental health agency to highlight the concept of administrative style. This is defined as the executive's professional behavior in structuring his or her role and in influencing the roles and functioning of others in the organization. In exploring *how* the executive does this they pose two contrasting polar types, "loose" and "tight," and review the virtues and shortcomings of each in the context of a particular experience in leadership change, where issues of authority, consensus, conflict, and change inevitably intruded. They conclude that executive effectiveness depends on an appropriate fit between an incumbent's administrative style and the needs of the organization at a given time. In a 1974 postscript to their original 1967 article, the authors ponder the effect of decentralization on their early formulations, and suggest areas for future study of succession, style, and organizational structure.

Fallon reviews the experience of two social agencies that were introduced to a new participative management pattern of democratic decision-making. Some characteristics of this process and the essential constraints and limitations that invariably follow are detailed. A study of perceptions and attitudes toward management orientation in one agency utilizing a modified Likert questionnaire is reported. A strong desire by the staff for participative management as opposed to exploitive-authoritarian, benevolent-authoritarian, or consultative patterns was indicated.

The case for evaluating social agency executives is strongly made by Kahle. He discusses the process of such assessment, and provides a detailed Guide for Executive Evaluation adapted from one used for evaluating social workers on the staff of the Family Counseling Service of Seattle, Washington. This includes both general and specific aspects of practice, the former exploring professional expertise and knowledge, the latter referring to service to the board, the staff, the community, and the agency program.

Herbert deals with a sadly neglected aspect of administrative practice—the minority executive. While he discusses the administrative processes of government, his argument and observations are as relevant to the voluntary social service system. After reviewing the data on federal minority employment rates, and the modest extent to which minority members are located in administrative posts (even in social programs where they tend to do best), Herbert examines the multiple role demands and dilemmas confronting minority administrators. He suggests that two basic and difficult questions inevitably call for response: responsibility to minority group people and to the needs of all the people. In negotiating this hazardous terrain, Herbert rejects value neutrality in implementing policy decisions and makes the case for the necessity to research, develop, and articulate minority group perspectives on public policy questions.

An especially grievous omission in the literature concerns the place of women in social service agency administration. One searches almost in vain for material on the problems faced by women executives, the sex-role stereotyping that is rampant, and the sexism that is implicit in the actual experience of social agencies. Resistance to the placing of women in high-status administrative positions and some of the role strains that accompany such advancement are reviewed by Hanlan. She reports the data that indicates the discriminatory practices affecting women managers in a largely "women's profession," and deals with some of the psychological dynamics reportedly responsible for the current state of affairs. Finally, Hanlan suggests some approaches to the reduction of role strain and conflict, and stereotyped habits in the profession. She makes the case for special training of women for managerial positions and ends with a plea for superseding pervasive male dominance in the organizational hierarchy.

C. BOARD–EXECUTIVE RELATIONSHIPS

The ways in which the two systems of authority intersect and interact is addressed by the remaining selections in this section. Stein looks at some realities that surround this relationship, in the course of which he examines the motivation of trustees; responsibilities of board and executive in relation to establishing agency policies; issues in the evaluation of the executive by the board; the informal structure of power of boards; board–staff relationships; and the important issue of the responsibility of voluntary and public agency boards to respond to social welfare issues, particularly those that contain elements of controversy.

Perlmutter adds an important dimension to the discussion of lay–professional relationships—in historical and contingent perspective. She concludes that the stage of development of a social agency determines the appropriateness of the respective roles of policymaker and professional. Early phases of organizational growth might call for greater assertiveness by prospective consumers and community representatives. After service structures are well established, professional authority might tend to be more prominently asserted.

A. THE GOVERNING BOARDS

9/UTILIZING THE BOARD OF TRUSTEES: A UNIQUE STRUCTURAL DESIGN

DARYL G. MITTON

The board of trustees is charged with the general stewardship of the agency. The specific professional expertise and directorship of the administrator must be combined with the diversified talents of the board. A balanced and objective board and a capable director have to interact with each other.

But how can board members become acquainted with agency operations and staff? How do they tune in on current attitudes or catch the spirit of the agency? How do they sense the psychological, sociological and physiological impact of the total program and the impact of the aura of the physical facility itself?

Further, how can one design a system that will elicit board members' talent in a manner consistent with their usual talent delivery, so as to utilize their skills effectively and foster greater enthusiasm and commitment to service?

These are questions all private agencies ask themselves over and over again. The agency of which I am a board member, the San Diego Children's Home Association, like many other agencies, has sought answers.

The agency conscientiously screens its board nominees for applicable talent and for representation and commitment. The nominees are familiarized with the general service performed and with the agency itself through selected literature and reports—the history of the agency, its bylaws, long-range plans, budget, programs, newsletters, current board membership, sample case histories and periodicals or articles relevant to agency approach. In addition, they are requested to spend 4 hours on 2 separate days in agency indoctrination—observing staff meetings, lunching with staff and children, observing ongoing programs, getting acquainted with intake procedures and meeting staff personnel.

THE USUAL TRAP

In the past, the agency has been extremely sensitive to its continually changing programs and new developments. Accordingly, much board meeting time was devoted to staff reports and demonstrations of ongoing projects—so much so that the board found itself spending all its meeting time validating administrative actions and just trying to keep abreast of agency changes. But regardless of staff diligence in keeping the board informed, the information always seemed peripheral and noninvolving.

The committees of the board operated in somewhat the same way. They were only sporadically active, with major initiation and input coming from staff. Substantive board input was largely limited to individual board member performance in contributing to specific problems—fiscal interpretation, endowment investment advice, obtaining financial support, etc. It is not without significance that all the examples cited are in the fiscal area. Traditionally, if board members have any clout, it's here. But this leaves areas of agency concern (improved client care, needed community service, agency administration effectiveness, etc.) untouched by board talent.

A BREAKTHROUGH IN APPROACH

Several years ago, a particular circumstance involving minority representation brought realization to the board that its abilities could be tapped in a more creative way. The administration and staff, anticipating community and governmental pressure for affirmative action, initiated the formulation by the board of an affirmative action statement and policy. The board recognized the worth of the suggestion and set itself to the task.

The nominating committee did not have to wait for the setting of specific policy to recommend talented minority nominees to fill recurrent board vacancies. Population parity in board representation was reached quickly. All the members were concerned about the problem, understood its ramifications and worked on it with skill and zeal. The Personnel and Service Committee roughed out the initial draft. It was received and adjusted by the Executive Committee and forwarded to an ad hoc Minority Committee comprising both board and staff. Again the draft was reviewed by the Executive Committee and sent to an ad hoc Legal Committee, then back to a joint committee review and to the board for final review and adoption.

Not only was an excellent document produced, but the involvement of board and staff was outstanding. Policy formulation and policy implementation within the agency were achieved simultaneously. Board, administration and staff worked together for a significant accomplishment.

ANOTHER BREAK

More recently the board found itself in another interesting circumstance. Consultants from the Human Interaction Research Institute, operating on a grant from the Office of Child Development of the Bureau of Social Rehabilitation Services of the Department of Health, Education and Welfare, were making a pilot study using the agency. They hoped to develop, demonstrate and make available strategies, intervention models and tools to improve the operational effectiveness of child development agencies.

The agency board invited the consultants to observe it in action, and out of this grew a program of self-examination and realignment. The board examined its interpretation of board objectives, and the individual members' interpretation of board worth and potential use to the agency. The self-analysis revealed the usual frustration resulting from a desire to serve and the helplessness of being underutilized in a ritualistic, validating manner.

An ad hoc committee was set up to study board structure and function, and eventually developed a structural design that serves both as a system of information gathering and education and as a system of emitting functional information and action.

INFORMATION-GATHERING COMMITTEES

The global overview of the agency and the board members' role revealed an urgent need for a more specific understanding of the many services the agency was performing. Gradual change and adjustment had made the agency a full-fledged, multiservice organization. But the ramifications of this change had not been acted upon, and questions went unanswered. For example: What were the overt and subtle differences in the treatment programs? What really determined these differences—client need, financial necessity or agency talent and inclination? What treatment mix best suits community needs? What treatment deserves what agency priority? What unique problems do the treatment units have?

Accordingly the board determined to set up committees related to each service or treatment unit in the agency: Residential (24 hours, 7 days a week therapy); Day (8 hours, 5 days a week special education and treatment); Satellite (24 hours, 7 days a week community treatment units); and Outreach (day care, consortium and cooperative efforts with other community, public and private agencies, pilot programs). The board felt that this type of committee setup would allow it to address directly the complex of changes in treatment patterns continually evolving within the agency. Experience has proved this to be the case. This committee structure allows for information gathering with a problem orientation. It involves the members and provides specific and utilitarian input to the board. The approach is worth consideration by any multiservice agency.

FUNCTION-EMITTING COMMITTEES

Up to this point, the board had been operating with traditional functional committees. It was decided the board needed policy-formulating, action-oriented committees, but with an emphasis on function and a makeup somewhat different than before. The obvious question was asked: What needs doing?

Pursuit of the obvious provided significant results. Functional committees matched to basic functional agency needs were set up—a structure applicable to most agencies in public service. The committees are: Finance (for getting, allocating, monitoring the utilization and management of funds); Service Appraisal (for determining community needs, reviewing programs and determining service effectiveness—the degree to which the agency is treating or merely warehousing children); Personnel (for establishing and monitoring personnel policies and practices); Management Audit (for reviewing agency operation and performance, appraising administrative structure and procedure, and monitoring resource utilization); Policy Review (for providing legal expertise and interpretation and legislative guidance, and updating bylaws).

There is also an Executive Committee, which functions in the absence of the board and addresses itself to long-range strategy and planning and public relations. In addition, there are a Nominating Committee, for recruiting and screening potential members and preparing slates of future officers, and an Affirmative Action Committee, made up of both board and staff members, to monitor minority-population parity throughout the agency.

A MATRIX ORGANIZATION

With this enlarged and dual-purpose committee structure, the board looked for some way to combine and tap effectively the information-gathering and function-emitting services. What was evolved is essentially a matrix-type organization structure applied to the board itself. Each board member is automatically a member of at least two committees—one oriented toward service or treatment delivery, the other toward a functional requirement. The concept of the matrix plan was to set up a system by which board members could achieve immediate involvement and learn about the agency while playing an active role, rather than learning about the agency and then trying to do something.

The board structure is depicted in Figure 1. Each square in the grid represents a member. The vertical dimension determines the member's service or treatment committee designation. The horizontal dimension determines his functional committee.

In the assignments for the various committees, all board members were asked to indicate their first, second and third choice of combinations of committees to serve on. There was a variety of interests wide enough so that in all but about three instances (on a 21-member board) it was possible to comply with first requests.

After the member assignments were made, a chairman and a vice chairman for each of the treatment service committees and for each of the functional committees were designated. Under the setup, each member of the board acts in some leadership capacity. As shown in Figure 1, Member A

Figure 1
The Board's Matrix Organization

Service Function	Residential	Day	Satellite	Outreach
Finance	Member A #	Member F X	Member K X	Member P O
Service Appraisal	Member B *	Member G #	Member L O	Member Q X
Personnel	Member C X	Member H O	Member M *	Member R #
Management Audit	Member D O	Member I (V.P.)	Member N X	Member S *
Policy Review	Member E X	Member J *	Member O #	Member T ⊕

* Chairman, Function Committee
x Vice Chairman, Function Committee
\# Chairman, Service Committee
o Vice Chairman, Service Committee
⊕ Group Coordinator, Service Committees

(Note: Chairmanship slots will vary from year to year, depending upon talents and interests)

Executive Committee

President, Vice President and all chairmen of Function Committees (*) and the service Group Coordinator (⊕)

Nominating Committee

Vice Chairmen of Function Committees (x)
Note: All 21 board members are in some form of leadership capacity.

---

is chairman of the Residential Committee and a member of the Finance Committee; member M is a member of the Satellite Committee and chairman of the Personnel Committee, etc.

Each service committee chairman has a liaison staff contact. The service chairmen are coordinated by a "group coordinator" (Member T, Figure 1), who is also a member of the Executive Committee. The chairmen of the functional committees are also members of the Executive Committee. The president and vice president complete the Executive Committee roster (in the old arrangements the Executive Committee consisted of the officers). The vice chairmen of the functional committees make up the Nominating Committee.

The matrix concept provides a mixed representation on all committees, for a balanced input and output of information and activity. This structure not only achieves a balance, but provides a mechanism for ongoing involvement. Each member becomes a contributing participant rather than a passive, validating observer. The majority of activity takes place outside the board meeting. Direct interaction of board members and of board and staff evolves as a work pattern in place of everything from major problems to trivia having to come before the administrator and board president for approval or coordination.

THE BOARD IN ACTION

Taking a specific problem area as an example, here is how the model works. The Finance Committee, in monitoring the budget, notices a continuing rise in the cost of care in the community treatment units. Administration is questioned and two apparent causes are uncovered: 1) relatively high staffing costs due to the special nature of the programs; and 2) limitations on occupancy in the units in the agency. The Satellite Committee undertakes the task of physical facility adjustment—exploring the possibility of remodeling to increase occupancy or selling existing homes and buying residences more suitable to needs and more consistent with city, county and state code requirements. The Policy Review Committee assists in legal interpretations and recommends legislative advocacy. The Service Appraisal Committee, its members familiar with all phases of treatment and sensitive to community needs, seeks alternatives to the high-cost community treatment concept or ways of increasing treatment cost effectiveness. The Finance Committee explores the availability of funds for any kind of physical plant or treatment adjustment to alleviate the problem.

When the issue comes before the Executive Committee, the input is real, the problem is understood and a rational solution can be attained. Neither Executive Committee nor board feels it is merely validating an administration-sponsored program.

The former procedure would have been for administrative staff to explain away the cost rise—or take an arbitrary action to solve the problem;

ask for board approval; pick someone on the board cognizant of real estate dealings to help switch properties or someone on the board cognizant of building or architecture to facilitate remodeling.

THE ULTIMATE GOAL

The use of a board as outlined here is no panacea. It is, however, food for thought for any multiservice agency. It does offer a possibility for tapping the talents of board members in ways they are used to. It provides a setting to utilize fully the time the board member gives, without usurping the administrator's authority. It demands a kind of board-member performance that makes the nonperformer uncomfortable, and therefore transient.

If a board member gives good service he will be rewarded with the recognition that he is constructively utilized. At very least, he should be able to realize that he is working with other equally committed persons and that he has a real opportunity to make the agency a little better through his service.

10/GOVERNING BOARDS IN MENTAL HEALTH: ROLES AND TRAINING NEEDS

ARTHUR J. ROBINS AND CHERYL BLACKBURN

INTRODUCTION

A concept which has guided the development of community mental health centers (CMHCs) is the importance of the participation of members of the local community in the development and operation of center programs. Chu and Trotter (1972) contend that the stress on community participation was an afterthought on the part of the NIMH policymakers. Nevertheless, many centers from their inception have recognized the need to establish the semblance, if not the substance, of community participation. Although the relevant Federal guidelines are loosely drawn, it is mandatory that a center demonstrate the requisite responsiveness to community needs by including some form of citizen participation in program planning and implementation. The individual States, exercising the discretionary powers delegated to them by the 1967 amendment to the Community Mental Health Centers Act of 1963, may specify the form that participation takes.

Traditionally, administrative volunteers have been the means for expressing the role of the local community in the development and implementation of health, education, and welfare services, under either public or voluntary auspices. Most CMHCs have some kind of board, in conformity either with State provisions or with convention.

At the same time that State-imposed constraints bring about homogeneity, even boards within the same State may vary considerably in their stated goals and authority and the nature and extent of actual power that they wield. The authority of the boards may be directive, advisory, administrative, or some combination of these. The areas for which they have authority may be circumscribed or may extend to every aspect of agency operation. Despite the formal provisions of the constitution and bylaws, they may serve primarily as a facade (Stanton 1970). Some boards serve an organization of which the center may be a minor component. For example, the university-affiliated center may have the same board that serves the entire university; the hospital-affiliated center, the same board that serves the entire medical complex.

Performance Criteria vs. Structural Criteria

The Federal injunction that CMHC boards be broadly representative of the community may lead to State requirements concerning the groups to be "represented"; still, there is no way to assure more than the achievement of token representation of various strata in the center's catchment area population. In any event, the effectiveness of boards is not ensured by provisions regarding composition and constitutional authority; rather, effectiveness is probably a function of the clarity of objectives assigned to a board, the competence of a board to achieve the explicit objectives, the formulation of objective criteria to measure achievement, and the tying of tenure of board members to achievement. The board and staff should apply the same management-by-objective approach to their respective efforts (Robins 1974). This is not to say that efforts at representativeness be abandoned; however, it may be a disappointing instrument for attaining the desired responsiveness to community needs. It would be better to achieve consensus on the specific task of the board and to select people who have characteristics believed to be relevant to successful task performance.

Program and Process Objectives

We believe that it is important to differentiate the effectiveness areas of board members from the effectiveness areas of professional staff. Good management practices should eliminate duplication and unnecessary overlap of the objectives of various components of an organization and should define clearly the output toward which the effort of any work unit is addressed. We see the professional staff as composing one general work unit; the board another. Failure to differentiate their functions may lead to conflict between the professional staff and the board, or it may lead to one or the other abdicating its responsibilities in its proper areas of effectiveness. If it is not possible to differentiate functions, then obviously one group or the other is superfluous. Indeed, the professional staff not infrequently sees its board as an unnecessary burden. This is a deplorable outcome, because we believe that organizational effectiveness depends upon a joint effort.

We see the professional staff as responsible for achieving what might be called program objectives; the board, for achieving process objectives. The former have been discussed in a paper by one of the authors (Robins 1972). Using a public health frame of reference, he classified the program goals as health promotion, specific protection, early recognition and treatment, disability limitation, or rehabilitation. The direct outcome of successful professional service is the reduction or elimination of a mental health problem of an individual, group, or community.

Process objectives have been explicated by Spaner and Windle (1971), who identify five desirable characteristics of center programs: responsiveness to community needs; availability of services to community members; continuity of services; shift of locus of care to community; increasing community support. The common theme of these objectives is their community orientation: the priority of services, the effectiveness and efficiency of the service delivery systems, and the adequacy of logistical support. The difference between program and process objectives becomes clear as one contemplates the possibility that a professional service can achieve program objectives, yet be ineffective with respect to process objectives. For example, it is conceivable that an inpatient service may be very effective in achieving its program objectives with respect to the patients who receive treatment; nonetheless, the program may not be directed toward the category of patients whose problems should receive the highest priority, according to the community's assessment of its needs. "A responsive program in one community may be quite inadequate in another" (Ozarin, Feldman, and Spaner 1971).

"Felt" Needs or "Real" Needs
Many professionals would hold that laymen do not have the competence to determine needs. (This belief probably accounts for many of the situations where the board, selected for its docility, is at best dormant.) The criticism by professionals is not easily dismissed. The concept of "felt" needs has long been a fetish of many workers in the human services. It need not lead to passivity by professionals, who should attempt to influ-

ence the selection of social goals. Professionals should educate and should undertake research that suggests policy and program directions. But the decisionmaking rights belong as much to the community as they belong to the patient.

Citizen participation in the planning of research may be crucial to utilization of findings. Limitations of objective studies need to be recognized. For example, epidemiological studies, even when the center possesses professional staff competent to execute them, cannot provide the final professional answer to program development. Our experience with the effect of social forces on human behavior must be considered in the light of human values. Value judgments must enter the process of selecting questions to which professional effort and other resources are to be committed. Professionals do not have exclusive possession of the competence to render value judgments. They can and should point out the consequences of alternative courses of action, but the values to be assigned to the outcomes are the responsibility of those who "own" the center.

The Committee on Community Mental Health, National Association of Social Workers, has flatly stated that the community must make decisions about "program priorities, deployment of resources, the interaction between staff and board, and, above all, how the community has come to grips with the social problems which contribute to social dysfunction in its citizens" (NASW 1968). The committee warned against center professional personnel's becoming an "isolated professional elite who regard themselves as the proprietors of a highly specialized establishment."

THE STUDY

An *a priori* assumption of our study, and not tested by it, was that the equity of a community in its CMHC should be expressed through a citizen board, the members of which have the power and authority to implement their responsibility for achieving specified objectives. The board's objectives are distinct from the objectives of the professional staff, although some overlap is inevitable. The study was undertaken with the idea of ascertaining goals for the training of board members that would enhance their competence to achieve those distinct objectives. It should be clear, then, that the study was not designed to derive a definition of task objectives for board members. Beginning with a preconception of what the output of a board should be, we expected to assess the extent to which these objectives were achieved and the factors that might be predictive of effectiveness, and to describe the role that board members presently play in achieving the goals of a center.

Major Questions

A study by Meyers et al. (1972) on measuring citizen board accomplishments was reviewed in order to obtain items that would be helpful in rating the achievement of process objectives. Although not explicitly addressed to the process objectives, that study derived a set of effectiveness areas which overlap the process objectives. The effectiveness areas factored out were: (1) service creation (we see this as roughly equivalent to responsiveness to community needs); (2) mobilization of outside resources dealing with the board's role in obtaining funds, but including Federal funds as well as the local sources; (3) local autonomy (roughly equivalent to a combination of the development of local funding sources and responsiveness to local needs); (4) coordination (roughly equivalent to continuity of service). The items used by Meyers to measure effectiveness areas were used in the present study, when equivalence could be assumed, to measure achievement of process objectives. A list of the process objectives and their defining variables appear in figure 1.*

At the time of our study, there were eight comprehensive CMHCs in the State and all were invited to participate. One center elected not to participate in the study; two of the centers were excluded when it was ascertained that the boards had only a token relationship to the center. The State in which these centers are located has no requirements concerning boards, their structure, or function.

After initial contact with the center directors concerning the nature of the study, the directors provided lists of board members and a copy of the constitution and bylaws. A random sample of board members of the participating five centers was selected for contact. The board president was always included, being considered best qualified to answer detailed questions about board structure and function. The total sample was 23 (the second author interviewed 20 of the 23 board members), all interviewed individually in their communities. The center directors provided data relevant to effectiveness measures.

Separate schedules were constructed for board presidents, board members, and center directors. In addition, the Community Mental Health Ideology Scale (Baker and Schulberg 1967) was administered to each board member and center director for purpose described in the findings section below. The interview schedules comprised items related to the following questions:

1. What are the characteristics of the members?
2. What are the practices relative to selection and orientation of members?
3. What does a member perceive to be his authority and responsibility?
4. How effective is the board as perceived by the member and as rated by investigators?

---

* Too late for use in our study, we learned of the work (Bass 1971) being done in the Office of Program Planning and Evaluation, NIMH, on the development of measures specific to the process objectives. This effort has since progressed rapidly. Wherever possible the Annual Inventory is being utilized as a source of items related to each process objective (Windle 1973).

FIGURE 1

PROCESS OBJECTIVES AND VARIABLES FOR MEASURING CITIZEN BOARDS*

I. Responsiveness to community need (Service creation)

1. The total number of services the board was involved in creating or improving (weighted for degree of importance and stage).
2. The average degree of involvement of the board in service-oriented activities weighted for importance.

II. Availability of services to community members

1. The length of time center has been comprehensive.
2. The number (by position) of staff members.
3. The size of the inpatient service.
4. The size of the outpatient service.
5. The size of the partial hospitalization service.
6. The total number of other services offered.
7. The size of the total budget.

III. Continuity of services (Coordination)

1. The total number of contacts by the board with service institutions weighted for kind of contact (informal to regular meetings).
2. The coordination of services with schools, clinics and hospitals, and law enforcement agencies.

IV. Increasing community support (Mobilization of outside resources and Local Autonomy)

1. The amount of money obtained by the board from the State Government.
2. The amount of money obtained by the board from the Federal Government.
3. The amount of money raised by the board from within its area.
4. Attempts to gain support from the Governor, legislature, and Commissioner of Mental Health.
5. Frequency of contact by the board with the Governor's Office of Finance or the Bureau of the Budget.
6. Attempts to write, call, and meet with State and Federal legislators.
7. The input of the board on the annual plan of the center (the greater the input the higher the score).
8. Is the board privately incorporated?
9. The board's use of mass media within its area.
10. Is there an active mental health association within the area?
11. The amount of gifts and bequests the board has obtained.
12. The amount of funds the board administers in trust.

V. Shift of locus of care to the communities

1. The number of new admissions to State hospitals from the area (in terms of the population percentage).

---

*In parentheses are the counterpart factors used in the Meyers study. The items in those categories are suggested by that study. Categories II and V were created for the present study.

FINDINGS

Characteristics of Board Members

The typical board member in the study was a 47.5 year-old, married, white, Protestant male employed as a professional or as a business executive. He had a college education and had completed some graduate work. A long time (24 years) resident of the community, he had a fairly high degree of participation in formal social organizations. Prior to joining the board, he was as likely to have had no previous interest in the field of mental health as to have had such an interest. In any case, he had not sought to serve on the board.

The Community Mental Health Ideology Scale (Baker and Schulberg 1967) was used to measure the degree to which the board members subscribed to a community mental health orientation. The major aspects of this orientation emphasize a feeling of responsibility for a total population instead of only the individual who comes for treatment, the importance of primary prevention, treatment directed toward social adjustment goals rather than basic personality change, continuity of care within an integrated network of services, and viewing the mental health specialist as only one member of a community team dealing with the mentally ill. The typical board member's score indicated a low degree of orientation to community mental health ideology, his score being similar to those obtained by criterion groups known to lack commitment to community mental health.

Recruitment and Orientation

The major criterion used to nominate him was the fact that he was deemed to be representative of the "people," or some portion of the total community, such as an organization, a profession. Other criteria were his demonstrated interests in mental health, leadership qualities, and civic mindedness. There had been no problem in finding candidates who met those broad criteria. The staff had played no role in his selection, the nominating committee having requested his services. The typical board member would be willing to serve indefinitely; in fact, he usually accepted additional terms on the board in accordance with the constitutional authorization to do so.

He was unlikely to have received any formal orientation to his role on the board. Demands on his time could be considered minimal; he attended all of the meetings per year (median number of meetings: six). The example of time devoted to fund raising gives an indication of the time required beyond attendance at regular meetings. Those who had this responsibility by reason of membership on the finance committee found that it took a nominal amount of time annually, perhaps only the time required to accompany a group on a visit to the official who held the purse strings in one county of the catchment area. A member rarely was a volunteer in service programs operated by the center.

Authority and Responsibility of Board Members

The constitution and bylaws of the centers gave comprehensive responsibility and authority to each board, and clearly indicated that ownership resided in the board. The global statements in those documents called for the board to plan, implement, and evaluate mental health services for the population of the catchment area. The usual board organization to implement this authority included an executive committee composed of chairmen of other committees, a personnel committee, a finance committee, a nominating committee and sometimes a public relations committee. This structure is consistent with the report of the members that the specific matters on which they spent the most time concerned personnel needs and overseeing the center's use of funds. Although most of the board members believed that they had administrative authority rather than advisory, almost half of the respondents thought that their actual power to influence the administration of the center was quite limited.

In response to the probing, more than half the members believed that they exercised no responsibility for program development. Most of the respondents reported that the board had nothing to do with organizational structure of the center; however, most were involved in personnel actions such as selection and evaluation of upper echelon staff. They reported responsibility for overseeing the leadership of the center and assessing its effectiveness. The data for this assessment was "feedback" from the "community." However, they tended to fulfill their liaison role with the community rather than vice versa. This is consistent with findings of the recent study of community involvement (Bloomfield 1972). Essentially, members of the board felt accountable only to each other, except for fiscal accountability to the governmental funding sources. With respect to obtaining funds, the board members played primarily a supportive role. Most of the funds came from Federal and State sources and were obtained largely through staff effort. On the other hand, the amount of money obtained from local sources, such as county and municipal governments and United Fund organizations, was believed to be a function of the persuasiveness of the board members.

Effectiveness

Most of the members believed that their center was effective in meeting the needs of the community. The response, however, to probes specific to the five process objectives elicited the fact that about two-thirds of the members felt that the center had a record of achievement in these areas. However, the same proportion did not believe that the board had contributed significantly to effectiveness in those five areas.

The work of Meyers et al. was used, when relevant, to generate effectiveness scores for each objective, and a composite score developed for each board. None of the characteristics descriptive of members was significantly related to the effectiveness of achievement of process objectives. Operational definitions of responsiveness to need, availability of service, and continuity of care were slippery and enabled us to rank the centers with respect to each other but not to assess absolute effectiveness. Measuring shift of locus of patient care from State hospitals to the community was difficult because the period since the centers had become comprehensive was too brief to expect any significant impact upon State hospital admission rates; however, each had offered most of the essential services, except for inpatient care, that could have been expected to have had some effect on those rates over the years.

The increase in local community support was assessed both in terms of annual changes in the proportion of the total budget collected from local sources and in terms of annual changes in the absolute amount. The proportion of the total budget coming from local sources showed little fluctuation prior to the centers' becoming comprehensive, but dramatically decreased after achievement of that status. Despite that proportional decrease, most of the centers achieved a substantial percentage increase in the amount of local support at about the time that they became comprehensive.

Analysis and Interpretation
The findings regarding board member characteristics are consistent with other assessments (New, Holton, and Hessler 1972) of the elitist nature of boards. Despite their apparent high status in the community, most members recognized the limitations to their power over the activities of the center with which they were affiliated. They appeared to "reign but not rule." They were not highly oriented toward the goals of a CMHC. This is not surprising, adherence to a community mental health orientation not having been a criterion for selection for board membership.

Almost none of the members had any experience as program volunteers at the center, and usually gave only a minimal amount of time to their duties as administrative volunteers. While they tended to view themselves as representatives of the community, activities directed toward the identification of community needs were meager and unsystematic.

The rhetoric of the constitution was inconsistent with the spotty activities of the board. Members did not have any well-defined set of objectives to which their activities were systematically related. One wondered whether the most important activity of the board had not been that directed toward the establishment of the center and the construction of the physical plant.

Although the members rated the center as effective in serving the community, they did not display the same unanimity in assessing the achievement of each process objective. We assume that this discrepancy was the outcome of more focused consideration of progress toward specific objectives not considered in their earlier evaluation. They were frank in assessing their lack of contribution toward the degree of effectiveness that had been achieved. Even the increase in local support may have been stimulated by the huge increase in funds from the State and Federal sources, dependence upon which had not been reduced.

The lack of relationship between factors that had been believed to be potentially related and the effectiveness of achieving process objectives may be explained in the following ways:

1. The characteristics, in fact, had no significant association with effectiveness.

2. The scores fell within a narrow range on the effectiveness scale. In other words, the centers were a homogeneous group with respect to effectiveness; they were all equally effective or not effective.

3. The operational definitions of the process objectives were inadequate.

Reliable and valid performance criteria are needed not only for research purposes but for center operations. Evaluation must become an integral component of the administrative process. Board members should make inputs into the process of establishing performance criteria for the achieving of their objectives.

Implications for Training

The difficulty of measuring effectiveness in achieving process objectives means that the selection of training objectives is dependent upon self-reported performance discrepancies and observations concerning the lack of clarity of goal definition and the unsystematic nature of programs directed to goals. We believe that the study demonstrated a need for a training program which would help the board members understand and develop values that are implicit in the community mental health movement and the goals that are appropriate to that value system. The training should be directed toward helping the board members define their unique goals as explicitly as possible. They should become familiar with the effort of the NIMH staff to utilize a center's annual inventory report as a source of data for measuring the achievement of board objectives (Bass 1971; Windle 1973). Training would help the members develop performance programs designed to achieve their goals, accept responsibility for evaluating their progress, and revise their efforts in accordance with an analysis of the outcomes.

The high motivation of board members for acquiring the relevant competence was clearly evident in the interviews. The provision of training opportunities for citizen participants is essential to fulfillment of the potential of the community mental health movement. It is gratifying to note that the Department of Mental Health of the State in which this study was done has contracted with the senior author's organization to provide training addressed to the objectives indicated above. The program will be offered to executive committee members. Participation in training may be burdensome but there is no place for the honorific board in the community mental health field. The head of the NIMH Citizen Participation Branch has unequivocally summed up the task: "The live dynamic board makes demands on its members for persistence, ingenuity, and dedication" (Rooney 1968).

REFERENCES

Baker, F., and Schulberg, H. C. The development of a community mental health ideology scale. *Community Mental Health Journal*, 3(3):216–225, 1967.

Bass, R. D. *A Method for Measuring Continuity of Care in a Community Mental Health Center.* Department of Health, Education, and Welfare Publication No. (HSM) 72–910. Washington, D.C.: Superintendent of Documents, U.S. Government Printing Office, 1971.

Bloomfield, C. *Evaluation of Community Involvement in Community Mental Health Centers.* New York: Health Policy Advisory Center, Inc., 1972.

Chu, F., and Trotter, S. *The Mental Health Complex, Part I: The Community Mental Health Centers.* Washington, D.C.: Center for Study of Responsive Law, 1972.

Meyers, W. R. et al. Methods of measuring citizen board accomplishment in mental health and retardation. *Community Mental Health Journal*, 8(4):311–310, 1972.

National Association of Social Workers. Position statement on community mental health (Mimeo.), 1968.

New, P. K.; Holton, W. E.; and Hessler, R. M. *Citizen Participation and Inter-Agency Relations: Issues and Program Implications for Community Mental Health Centers.* Boston: Department of Community Health and Social Medicine, Tufts University School of Medicine, 1972.

Ozarin, L. D.; Feldman, S.; and Spaner, F. G. Experience with mental health centers. *American Journal of Psychiatry*, 127(7):912–916, 1971.

Robins, A. J. Administrative process model for community mental health centers. *Community Mental Health Journal*, 8(3):208–219, 1972.

Robins, A. J. Management-by-objectives for community mental health programs. *Hospital and Community Psychiatry*, 25(4): April, 1974.

Rooney, H. L. Roles and functions of the advisory board. *North Carolina Journal of Mental Health*, 3(1):33–43, 1968.

Spaner, F., and Windle, C. "The Perspective of National Program Development and Administration: Program Needs and Evaluation Activities." Paper at 79th Annual Meeting of American Psychological Association, Washington, D.C., 1971.

Stanton, E. *Clients Come Last: Volunteers and Welfare Organizations.* Beverly Hills: Sage Publications Inc., 1970.

Windle, C. "The Community Mental Health Program—1971: Performance Indicators Derived From the CMHC Inventory." (Discussion draft) 1973.

11/CITIZEN PARTICIPATION ON PUBLIC WELFARE BOARDS AND COMMITTEES

EDWARD J. O'DONNELL AND OTTO M. REID

Citizen participation in general and consumer participation in particular are no longer questions of whether but of how and with what consequence. The participation of lay citizens—on boards and committees—in public welfare has a long history, and though such participation by public assistance recipients is a recent, and more problematic, phenomenon, it appears to be here to stay.[1] To date, however, the extent and impact of such participation have not been subjected to systematic study.

To shed some light on these issues, the American Public Welfare Association, in 1970, under contract to the Division of Intramural Research of the Social and Rehabilitation Service, U.S. Department of Health, Education, and Welfare, conducted a survey of local public welfare boards and committees—the most recent and most extensive study of citizen and recipient participation yet undertaken.[2] Its broad aim was to investigate the extent to which citizens—particularly low income persons and the recipient of services—are participating in the work of State and local public welfare boards and committees and the consequences of their participation. Preliminary data are now available and are the subject of this article.

Following a survey of State departments of public welfare, a sample of 750 local departments was drawn from a list of over 2,800 eligible agencies. The sample was stratified by State, the selection of local departments being proportional to the State's population and, within the State, proportional to the population of the area served. A mail questionnaire was sent to each administrator in the sample, 458 of whom completed and returned the questionnaire for a response rate of 60 percent. It is on data gathered from these responses that the present article is based.

Generally speaking, half of the States have their local welfare departments directly *administered* by the State agency through State employees. The other half are *supervised* by the State—that is, local departments are administered under State mandates. These general categorizations, of course, grossly over-simplify the complex patchwork of city, county, and district organizational arrangements; nevertheless, the extent to which local public welfare departments are State administered or State supervised does provide a useful perspective on the board-committee structures within which citizen and recipient participation takes place.

PUBLIC WELFARE BOARDS AND ADVISORY COMMITTEES

Table 1 indicates the number of boards and committees among local departments of public welfare and the distribution of such boards and committees according to whether they are State administered or State supervised. In anticipation of the data, a *board* seems to be defined in the main as a group of people who set policy for and a *committee* as a group of people who give advice to the agency. As our data will point up, this distinction is not uniformly accepted. Though major functions remain fairly constant, boards and committees will often resemble one another.

Perhaps the most striking fact shown in table 1 is that nearly a quarter (24 percent) of the agencies report that they have neither a public welfare board nor an advisory committee, though a fifth (19 percent) report having both. More than a third (36 percent) report having a board only, a fifth (20 percent) a committee only. Generally, then, more than half (55 percent) report having boards, four in 10 (39 percent) committees. More than six in 10 (62 percent) of the State-supervised agencies report having boards, in contrast to just half (50 percent) of the State-administered agencies. Some four in 10 have committees whether they are State administered (41 percent) or State supervised (42 percent). Also, proportionately more State-administered agencies have only an advisory committee, and proportionately more State-supervised agencies have both a board and a committee.

COMPARISON OF BOARDS AND COMMITTEES

What follows is a description of the activity, operation, and membership of boards and committees, together with some indication of their effect on the services of local departments of public welfare. As will become clear, these data are presented by board-committee structure (that is, by whether an agency has one or the other or both) because of the apparent differences in findings among agencies with different structures. Again, in anticipation of the data, it would seem that the usual distinctions between boards and committees do not hold consistently. For example, when agencies have only a board or only a committee, the one takes on some of the coloration of the other. Though it is difficult to generalize, it does seem that when agencies have both a board and a committee, the distinct characteristics of each are much more likely to show up than when they have only one or the other. At no time, however, does the blurring of board and committee distinctions extend to their functions—their forms may change but not their anchor functions of establishing policy for boards and giving advice for committees.

ESTABLISHMENT

More than three of every four boards were established 30 or more years ago. Committees are a much more recent phenomenon, a fourth having been established within the past year and more than half within the past 5 years. Committee age, however, varies greatly with whether a particular agency has a committee only or both a board and a committee. Among the agencies having only a committee, a third (34 percent) were established within the last 5 years, but close to half (46 percent) 10 or more years ago. Conversely, among public welfare agencies with both a board and a committee, more than eight of every 10 (85 percent) were established within the past 5 years, and fewer than one in seven (14 percent) are 10 or more years old. Apparently, in agencies without boards of public welfare, committees were formed at a much earlier point in time. Where there were such boards, however, committees were not established until relatively recently, probably in response to the increased emphasis placed on consumer participation and recipient representation in the past few years.

Most boards, nine of every 10 (90 percent), were established by statute; most committees by statute (45 percent) or administrative order (31 percent). Again, the board-committee structure makes a difference: more than six in 10 (62 percent) of the committees where no board exists were established by statute, as compared to the one in four (25 percent) established by statute where both board and committee exist. Half (50 percent) the committees where both exist were established by administrative order, as compared to the three in 10 (30 percent) similarly established where no board exists.

TABLE 1

Percent of Local Boards and Committees, by Organizational Relationship of State to Local Departments of Public Welfare

Board or Committee	Total	State Administered	State Supervised
	(Percent)	(Percent)	(Percent)
Board only	36	38	35
Committee only	20	29	15
Both board and committee	19	12	27
Neither board nor committee ...	24	21	22
Total N[1]	(458)	(196)	(215)

[1] The discrepancies in the total N's and percentages are due to the approximately 4 percent of the sample of agencies that reported an organizational arrangement other than State administered or State supervised. Though the boards and committees under this "other arrangement" are not shown in the table, they have been included in the total.

Relationship to the Agency

Administrators of local departments of public welfare work with boards and committees in various ways. In general, they are much more active with boards than with committees. Over half plan board meeting agenda (57 percent), serve the board in a staff capacity (56 percent), and work with the board chairman on setting dates for meetings and developing agenda (53 percent). Only a fourth (24 percent) serves as actual or ex officio board members. In this instance the board-committee structure makes no substantial difference (administrators work with boards in roughly the same way whether or not the agency also has a committee). Where their relationship to committees is concerned, however, the board-committee structure does seem to make a difference—at least for some of the administrators' functions. Though less than half (43 percent) the administrators work with committee chairmen to set meeting dates and develop agenda when the agency has both a committee and a board, fully seven of every 10 (70 percent) work with committee chairmen when there is no board. The administrator is much less involved with the committee than with the board in planning agenda (18 percent) and setting dates for meetings (16 percent). Yet he is more likely to serve as a regular or ex officio member of a committee (37 percent) than of a board (24 percent).

Though only a fourth (26 percent) of the boards never meet without the administrator, more than half (51 percent) the committees do. And though the department's board-committee structure does not affect whether the board meets without the administrator, it does affect committees, inasmuch as more than half (51 percent) never meet without the administrator where they operate alone, but only a third (34 percent) never meet without the administrator when they operate with boards. Moreover, though fewer than one in 10 committees (6.5 percent) frequently or always meets without the administrator when the agency has only a committee, as many as three in 10 (29 percent) of the committees with boards meet frequently or always without the administrator. In general, then, administrators are much more likely to attend board than committee meetings and much more likely to attend committee meetings when there are no boards than when there are.

Agency staff members are much less likely to provide services to boards than to committees. Though less than half (46 percent) of the boards are provided staff services, nearly seven of 10 committees (69 percent) are provided such services. In general, administrators are more likely to serve board needs, agency staff members committee needs.

Tenure

Board members serve longer terms than committee members: more than a third (35 percent) of all board members serve 3-year terms, and more than four in 10 (41 percent) 4-year or longer terms. In contrast, only a fourth

(24 percent) of the committee members serve 3-year terms, and just over one in 10 (11 percent) serve terms of 4 years or more. Again, board-committee structure makes a difference: though nearly a third (32 percent) of board members serve 5 or more years when there is no committee, less than 9 percent of members serve terms that long on boards when there is also a committee. A fifth (21 percent) of the committee members serve terms of 4 or more years when there is no board, but less than a 10th (6 percent) serve like terms when there is also a board. For both boards and committees, members serve longer terms when one or the other operates alone than when an agency has both a board and a committee.

Public officials or governing bodies—either State (39 percent) or local (33 percent) or the agency board of commissioners or supervisors (31 percent)—usually appoint board members and are also involved in appointing committee members, but to a lesser extent. Apparently, the public welfare administrator himself has relatively more responsibility for appointing committee members than he does for board members. Members of more than a fifth (22 percent) of the committees are appointed by administrators in sharp contrast to only 5 percent of the boards. Again, there is great variation according to board-committee structure—particularly for the appointment of committee members. For example, though a fifth (20 percent) of the committee members are appointed by local public officials when there is no board, nearly half (48 percent) are so appointed when there is both a committee and a board. And though a third (34 percent) of the committee members are appointed by State officials when there is no board, only 2 percent of the committee members are so appointed when there is both a committee and a board.

In general, both board and committee members are eligible for reappointment. Virtually all members are eligible for reappointment when the agency has either a board or a committee, and about nine of every 10 are eligible when the agency has both.

Most boards and committees arrange to rotate members so that terms overlap. Members of nearly eight of every 10 (79 percent) boards and seven of every 10 (67 percent) committees have overlapping terms.

Orientation and Schedule

Boards expend more effort in orienting members to their policies and procedures than committees—at least to the extent of more formal orientation. Most boards (62 percent) and committees (65 percent) orient members by providing periodic reports and other background materials. Half (52 percent) the boards, but only a quarter (25 percent) of the committees, provide manuals for their members. Altogether over a 10th of board (15 percent) and committee members (11 percent) are oriented through visits to recipients' homes with agency workers. On this issue, as with others, agency methods vary according to board-committee structure.

Board members, for example, are provided manuals by nearly six of 10 boards (58 percent) where there is no committee, but by only four of 10 boards (40 percent) where there are both. Similarly, committee members are provided manuals by nearly four of 10 committees (39 percent) where there is no board, but by only a 10th (10 percent) where there are both. When either exists alone, the local agency is much more likely to acquaint its members with agency policy and program through a board or committee manual than when both exist in the same agency.

Boards appear to be more active than committees. For instance, they meet more frequently than committees: more than seven of 10 boards (72 percent), as compared with just over half (51 percent) the committees, meet at least once every month. Though there is some variation in the frequency of meetings by board-committee structure, it is not substantial. Boards meet slightly more frequently when the agency also has a committee, and committees when they function alone.

Membership and Composition

Boards are much smaller than committees. Six of every 10 committees (61 percent) have 10 or more members; only 4 percent of the boards are as large as that. Most boards (57 percent), in fact, have five or fewer members, but nearly half (48 percent) the committees have between 10 and 15 members. Size of membership does not vary appreciably by board-committee structure.

Apparently, the composition of most boards (72 percent) and committees (81 percent) is specified; that is, certain criteria are applied in the selection of members or in achieving an appropriate mix of members. A fifth of all boards (20 percent) and committees (23 percent) are guided by certain statutes, laws, or State regulations in the appointment of members. Boards appear to be relatively more political than committees: though 16 percent of all boards require member representation from both major political parties, only 6 percent of the committees have this requirement. Moreover, though criteria regarding sex, geographic location, or occupation are applied in a fifth (20 percent) of the board appointments, they are applied in only a 10th (9 percent) of the committee appointments. Similarly, though the number of members is specified for a fifth (19 percent) of the boards, it is specified for only a 10th (11 percent) of the committees.

Perhaps the most important issue here is the differential consideration given to the necessity for consumer representation and citizen participation. Though more than a third (36 percent) of the committees specify the appointment of recipients or low income persons, hardly any (less than half of 1 percent) of the boards require such representation.

Neither committees nor boards specifically require a great deal of participation by lay citizens, though committees have such a requirement much more frequently than boards (14 percent, as opposed to 2 percent). Again, this varies according to board-committee structure—particularly among the criteria applied to committee composition.

Recipient Representation

So far our discussion has concerned only those criteria that, by report, are used by most agencies whose board and committee memberships are specified. But what of actual agency practice and, particularly, the inclusion of recipients and low income persons on boards and committees?

Data on the extent of participation by present or former public assistance recipients are presented in table 2. These figures indicate that recipient representation practices among local departments of public welfare vary considerably. Recipients are much more likely to serve on committees than on boards and most likely to serve on committees when agencies have both boards and committees. Thus, though more than six in 10 (63 percent) of the committees count present or former recipients among their members, only 6 percent of the boards do.

How can we account for this great difference? As we have just seen, though the representation of recipients or low income persons was one of the criteria used in constituting advisory committees, little or no mention was made of efforts to include recipients or low income persons on boards. And though such specification would seem to account for the differential involvement of recipients on boards and committees—at least in part—a significant difference turns up concerning the specified composition of advisory committees between agencies with only a committee and those with both a board and a committee. As pointed out, more than a third of all committees call for the representation of recipients or low income persons. But, though more than half (53 percent) of the agencies with both a board and a committee mention recipient or low income representation as one criterion for committee membership, less than a fifth (18 percent) of those

TABLE 2

Percent of Local Boards and Committees with Public Assistance Recipients, by Board-Committee Structure

Structure	Percent with Public Assistance Recipients
Boards with recipients	
Board only	4
Both board and committee	10
Committees with recipients	
Committee only	54
Both board and committee	84

TABLE 3
Percent of Local Public Welfare Administrators Who Feel Recipient
Representation Is a Good Idea, by Board-Committee Structure

Structure	Percent Saying Good Idea
Committee only	96
Both board and committee	91
Neither board or committee	86
Board only	75

with only a committee report such representation as necessary in their committee composition.

Though the administrators do not appear to be very influential in the process of selecting board and committee members, data on their attitudes toward recipient representation are, nevertheless, important.

As seen in table 3, most public welfare administrators believe that the representation of present or former recipients on boards and committees is a "good idea," principally for these reasons:

• The recipient has a better understanding of the problems involved because of his experience (29 percent).

• The board or committee becomes more aware of the problems through the participation of the recipient (19 percent).

• Better agency policies and programs result from recipient representation (14 percent).

Though most administrators seem to favor the idea, the extent to which they favor it varies according to agency board-committee structure—in this instance whether the agency has only a board, only a committee, both a board and a committee, or neither.

Table 3 shows that though more than nine of every 10 administrators of agencies with a committee favor the idea, fewer administrators whose agencies have neither a board nor a committee and only three of every four with only a board think that recipient representation is a good idea.

Participation of Low Income Persons
Data were also collected on the extent to which low income persons (excluding recipients) are included in boards and committees. The major findings are shown in table 4.

Here, again, the data indicate that low income persons are much more likely to be included on committees than boards. However, the extremes of their participation are not so evident as that of recipients. Low income persons are more likely to be included on boards than recipients, but recipients are more likely to be included on committees. In contrast to the situ-

TABLE 4
Percent of Local Boards and Committees with Low Income Persons,
by Board-Committee Structure

Structure	Percent with Low Income Persons
Boards with poor people	
Board only	25
Both board and committee	14
Committees with poor people	
Committee only	52
Both board and committee	50

ation of recipient participation when the agency has only a board, more low income persons than recipients are included on boards when the agency has both. As to participation on committees, both low income persons and recipients are represented on roughly half the committees where agencies have no boards; recipients are represented on 84 percent of the committees where agencies have both a board and a committee; but poor people are represented on only half the committees where the latter structure obtains.

The preceding section has described the extent to which recipients and low income persons are represented on boards and committees. We now turn to the actual number of recipients or low income persons represented on boards and committees, as reported by the administrators. Table 5 shows that most agencies report having no recipients or low income persons serving on their boards. The relatively few that do have one or two at most. Committees, however, are much more likely than boards to have such representation and, when they do, to have more members.

TABLE 5
Percent of Local Boards and Committees with Selected Numbers of Assistance
Recipients and Poor People, by Board-Committee Structure

| Participants | Boards | | Committees | |
	Board Only	Board and Committee	Committee Only	Committee and Board
Recipients				
None	98	92	49	16
1	2.1	5.9	18	8
2 or more	—	2.4	32	76
Low income persons				
None	76	87	57	51
1	11	8.4	16	16
2 or more	13	4.8	27	33

Again, the board-committee structure greatly affects the number of recipients participating on boards and committees. Though the number of recipients on boards is very small indeed, nearly a third (32 percent) of the committees where there are no boards and fully three of four (76 percent) committees where there is also a board include two or more recipients.

Board-committee structure does not seem to be particularly significant in determining the extent to which low income persons participate on either boards or committees. Though there are more low income persons on boards when the agency has only a board, many more low income persons participate on committees, regardless of structure: about three in 10 have two or more low income persons serving on them.

TO RECAP BRIEFLY

Low income persons and public assistance recipients in particular are not well represented on boards. In fact, low income persons serve on fewer than a fourth and recipients on fewer than a 10th of all boards. And where they do serve on boards, more often than not, they are the only such representatives. Low income persons and recipients in particular are more frequently represented on committees; more than half of all committees have such representation. Not only are recipients and low income persons more likely to serve on committees than boards, they are also more likely to serve in much greater numbers.

Compensation

The compensation available to board and committee members does not appear to be substantial. About a fifth (19 percent) of the boards and committees pay transportation expenses only. A fourth (26 percent) of the boards and almost none—six percent—of the committees provide per diem and pay transportation expenses.

Substantial or not, board members are more likely than committee members to receive compensation. Though nearly six in 10 (57 percent) boards compensate their members, just over four in 10 (42 percent) of the committees do. Moreover, of those that do compensate members, proportionately many more boards than committees compensate all members. Considering the differential involvement of recipients and low income persons in boards and committees, the lesser compensation afforded committee members no doubt discourages their further participation.

Board-committee structure seems to affect whether members are compensated, inasmuch as eight of 10 boards (79 percent) and nearly six of 10 committees (57 percent) where an agency has both compensate some or all of their members, as compared with nearly six of 10 boards (57 percent) and just over four of 10 committees (42 percent) where they operate alone.

Function
Boards and committees differ in the functions they perform. Among the
most frequently mentioned board functions are these: hiring and supervising staff members (39 percent), making policies and changes regarding
agency operations (36 percent), approving the spending of all funds (30
percent), and providing general consultation (26 percent). In sharp contrast, the most frequently mentioned functions of committees are these:
giving advice regarding agency operations (47 percent), interpreting
programs to and communicating with the public (39 percent), and reviewing and analyzing current programs and services (31 percent). These facts
add up to this conclusion—the board's primary role is to make policy, the
committee's to give advice. Though agency board-committee structure
does not affect board functions, it does affect committee functions, apparently.

A greater percentage of the committees that function without boards offer
advice and counsel (59 percent) and interpret programs for the general
public (53 percent) than the percentage of committees that function with
boards (for committees 36 and 24 percent). As to the review and analysis
of programs and services, however, a greater percentage of committees with
boards (34 percent) perform this function than those without boards (27
percent). However, the major functions performed for the agency differ
less among committees than between committees and boards.

Agency administrators were also asked whether boards and committees
should be performing these or other functions as well as making policy and
giving advice. Generally speaking, four in 10 administrators are satisfied
that boards (38 percent) and committees (43 percent) are doing what they
should be doing. Otherwise, they reconfirm boards as policymakers and
committees as interpreters—more than a 10th reinforcing these functions
for boards (15 percent) and advisory committees (13 percent).

Impact on Agency Services
Boards have had a greater effect on agency day-to-day services than committees—at least in the administrators' judgment. Though nearly seven of 10
boards (68 percent) have reportedly had a noticeable effect, less than half
the committees (46 percent) have. Moreover, though there are no differences among committees according to board-committee structure, there are
such differences among boards. Though nearly eight of 10 boards (78 percent) with both a board and a committee are judged to have a noticeable
effect, only 65 percent of the boards without committees are similarly evaluated. Very few administrators (no more than 5 percent) report any adverse
effects on agency services, but when they do report adverse effects, administrators attribute them to boards not committees—again, a reflection of
the greater power of boards.

Boards and committees also have different effects on day-to-day services—

not so much because they affect different aspects of agency operations but because boards seem to be more influential than committees "across the board." For example, though more than four in 10 boards (43 percent) have developed community interest in and support for the agency, only a third of the committees (33 percent) have developed such interest; and though nearly four in 10 boards (39 percent) have enlisted resources outside of the agency to meet recognized need, less than three in 10 (28 percent) of the committees have had the same effect. Similarly, though nearly four in 10 boards (38 percent) have been effective in supporting agency and program needs with the State legislature and governor's office, less than a fifth of the committees (18 percent) have had this same success. And, finally, though a third of the boards (34 percent) have innovated agency operations to improve services, less than a fifth of the committees (18 percent) have been similarly involved and effective.

Among the questions asked of advisory committees but not of boards are three that also bear on the issue of effectiveness. Two concern the suggestions and recommendations committees make to boards; the third concerns the effects of citizen advisory groups on State welfare programs.

The first two questions are these: Are they helpful? and Are they followed? Responses necessarily come from administrators of agencies where boards and committees both operate and, more specifically, where committee suggestions and recommendations are actually made to the board. More than nine of 10 of the 76 administrators (93 percent) who responded to this question characterize the committee suggestions and recommendations as helpful—14 percent saying they are "always helpful," only 7.1 percent saying they are "not usually helpful." Yet, though nearly three of 10 administrators (28 percent) say that such suggestions and recommendations are "very often" followed and nearly half (48 percent) that they are "fairly often" followed, nearly a quarter (24 percent) say that such suggestions and recommendations are "not very often" followed. Thus, though the bulk of committee suggestions and recommendations are characterized as helpful, they are not followed and implemented by the board to the extent of their presumed helpfulness.

The third question, that concerning the effects of citizen advisory groups on State welfare programs, in general brought positive responses. A fourth (24 percent) of the administrators say that the effect of such activity will be a better informed and understanding public, and a fifth (19 percent) say that the effects will be better policies, programs, and increased benefits. The last response varied considerably by board-committee structure, inasmuch as three of 10 administrators (30 percent) of agencies with both a board and a committee held this opinion, but only a little more than a 10th of the agency administrators with only boards (14 percent) and only committees (12 percent) had this view.

Of more pertinence, perhaps, is the fact that nearly a fifth of all administrators (18 percent), regardless of board-committee structure, think that citizen advisory groups will have little or no impact on State welfare programs.

SUMMARY AND CONCLUSIONS

Generally speaking, boards and committees are different—they have different forms and functions. The data developed in this study, as reported here, detail these differences. And though there are differences between the forms that boards take according to whether or not a committee operates in relation to them, such differences are not so great as those between committees that operate alone and those that operate in relation to a board—and perhaps none of these are so great as the fundamental differences between boards and committees.

In those agencies with a committee only, the committee often takes the form of a board and in many respects resembles one. But at no point does a committee actually take over the policymaking functions usually ascribed to the board—if anything, the committee that exists without a board is reinforced in its unique role as adviser. The committee that operates with a board is perhaps very different—certainly from the board but also often from the committee that stands alone—again, however, in form only, not function.

The differences between boards and committees in brief are these:

• Boards are older than committees.

• Boards are more often established by statute and less often by administrative order.

• Boards bear a different relationship to administrators—for board administrators more often plan agenda, set dates for meetings, and serve in a staff capacity.

• Boards are less likely to meet without the administrator present.

• Boards are less likely to be served by staff members.

• Board members serve longer terms than committee members.

• Boards are smaller than committees.

• Boards are less likely to have recipient representation and participation by poor persons.

• Boards are more likely to compensate all members and more likely to provide per diem and transportation expenses.

• Boards are more likely to have an effect on agency services and more likely to be innovative and improve agency operations.

• Boards make policy; committees make recommendations.

Of these differences the last is the most important. In this connection, it is well to recall the data given on recipient representation and the participation of low income persons on public welfare boards and committees. Though low income persons and public assistance recipients are in a position to advise and recommend, they are in no position to make policy—low income persons speak with a whisper, recipients have no voice at all.

THE FUTURE OF AN IDEA

Citizen participation and recipient representation (the more radical of the two) are ideas that have generated a corps of enthusiastic supporters and have found their way into official policy. The idea of the "maximum feasible participation" of the poor in the War on Poverty was perhaps the most celebrated and controversial implementation of these ideas, but they also found expression in directives from the Social and Rehabilitation Service of the U.S. Department of Health, Education, and Welfare, to State and local welfare department to involve public assistance recipients, low income persons, and other lay citizens in the work of their boards and committees. The present study shows the limited extent to which these ideas have been implemented to date. But is the present situation only a way station in the relentless sweep of the idea to ultimate realization, or does it already represent the high water mark, to be followed by an inevitable ebbtide?

If recipient participation means, as some of its most ardent advocates believe, that recipients will assume essential control of the organizations designed to serve them—the answer seems to be that the idea is on the ebb. The current deemphasis on such participation at the Federal level seems to be reflected in the caution public welfare agencies and administrators are exercising in ensuring that control of policy and of agency operation be retained by the appropriate "officials" and professional persons. But, if recipient participation means that more attention will be given in the future to ensuring that professional workers and the agencies in which they operate make provision for enabling the recipient to speak, at least to them, then, in our opinion, the agencies serving the public will more and more implement this idea. To what extent the recipient will be heard is still another issue. The administrators and the agencies they represent seem to us to be saying that the agency must listen to the recipient, that he can considerably improve the functioning and effectiveness of the agency, but that agency officials must be the persons who make the ultimate and critical decisions. This is the direction we guess that welfare departments, and perhaps most agencies serving the public, will be moving—at least in the immediate future.

But we may be wrong. Perhaps the public mood of caution and consolidation of social inventions and innovations is at an end. The Nation may be ready to press on—to return a measure of power to the people, in this instance poor people. Americans may be ready to turn increasingly to low income persons and recipients to provide them with real opportunity to participate in decisions that affect them deeply. But low income persons and recipients will never be decisionmakers unless they become members of boards, where decisions are made and where they can have the most impact (at least within the system). To insure that they do get on boards and that they make themselves felt, public welfare agencies must take these steps:

• They must actively seek recipients and other poor persons for positions on boards and sustain them in their roles as decisionmakers once they are on boards. It is not enough to make such opportunities passively available.

• Recipients and other poor persons must be given the means by which to participate actively and effectively—that is, it must be made as "worthwhile" for them to participate as it is for other members of such boards. In many instances they will have to receive per diem and expense money.

If public assistance recipients and other poor persons are going to "get on board," room will have to be made for them. Power is not so easily shared or surrendered—but certainly some "on board" are ready to make way. Others may yet be pushed or persuaded to move over and make room for the people they serve. May they be so persuaded!

NOTES

1. See Edward J. O'Donnell and Catherine S. Chilman, "Poor People on Public Welfare Boards and Committees: Participation in Policy-Making?" *Welfare in Review*, May–June 1969, pp. 1–10, for an analysis of the potential for such participation.
2. Virginia R. Doscher was the principal investigator at the time of the conception and design of the study. Elizabeth G. Watkins, staff associate of the American Public Welfare Association, has now assumed this responsibility. The data collection and analysis were undertaken by Opinion Research Corporation of Princeton, N.J.

B. EXECUTIVE AUTHORITY

12/MANAGEMENT SUCCESSION
AND ADMINISTRATIVE STYLE*

JOEL KOTIN AND MYRON R. SHARAF

This study of management succession is the second of two articles dealing with the events that occurred at a state mental hospital following a change of superintendents. In the first article we explored the ideological elements of the accompanying intrastaff controversy.[1] In the present study we are concerned with the interaction of social structure *and* executive personality in determining the successor's role. This is in contrast to most previous studies of management succession, which have been focused primarily on sociological factors. Conceptually, this study is part of a recent trend toward the inclusion of personality in studies of occupational roles and organizational processes.[2] We shall consider one aspect of an executive's personality, namely, his administrative style. We shall introduce the concept of tight and loose administrative styles in order to understand more fully the successor's behavior and subsequent events in the life of the institution.

PREVIOUS STUDIES

Perhaps the most significant treatment of succession in the theoretical literature is Gouldner's study of the succession of a new manager in a gyp-

* Editor's Note: "Management Succession and Administrative Style," by Joel Kotin and Myron R. Sharaf was originally published in *Psychiatry: Journal for the Study of Interpersonal Processes* in August 1967. We have now asked the authors to examine their article in the light of developments in the field since that time and share their reactions with our readers. With permission of the publisher, the original article is reprinted below. "Management Succession Revisited" follows.

sum plant.[3] Here the successor was faced with problems of communication and control. His information and authority via the existing formal system were inadequate, and he had no access to the existing informal system, especially the corps of "old lieutenants" who owed their loyalties to the former leader. These old lieutenants were under the spell of what Gouldner called the Rebecca Myth, namely, the idealization of a departed chief to whom loyalty belongs and a corresponding derogation and suspicion of the new chief.[4]

In countering this opposition, the new manager utilized two important techniques. First, he replaced some of the "old lieutenants"—some of the middle-management supervisory personnel. The replacements were loyal to the new manager and faithfully supported his policies. Gouldner calls this technique "strategic replacement." Second, he enhanced communication and control by what Gouldner calls "increased bureaucratization." As Gouldner points out,

Barred from effective use of the informal system of controls, the successor was compelled to rely more heavily upon the formal system. . . . There is a close connection between succession and a surge of bureaucratic development, particularly in the direction of formal rules.[5]

At the gypsum plant this increased bureaucratization took the form of the institution of new rules and stricter enforcement of existing ones; the introduction of required daily and weekly reports that provided the new manager with a more careful check on production results and on accidents and breakdowns; and the introduction of formal "warning notices" to be sent to delinquent workers.

Guest's study of the succession of a new manager in an automobile plant focused on how the new leader improved the plant's performance, rather than on sociological elements of the succession, but certain points can be inferred from his well-documented presentation.[6] Although the new manager did make some strategic replacements, mostly by promotion from within the organization, there was no surge of bureaucratic development; indeed, Guest describes the plant's organization as considerably looser following the succession.

Another aspect of Guest's study that contrasts sharply with Gouldner's is the description of the mythology that evolved concerning the new and departed leaders. At the automobile plant the retired manager was disliked, while the new man was immensely popular. Hodgson, Levinson, and Zaleznik suggest that these two types of response represent alternative attempts by members of the organization to deal with the loss of the departing figure and the difficulties of adjustment to a new administration. Furthermore, they add, ". . . it would appear that both types can coexist, with cyclical variations in the predominance of one over the other."[7] Thus the concept of the Rebecca Myth must be expanded to include the reverse reaction; the polarization of affect may be in either direction.

RESEARCH SETTING AND METHODS

Since the research setting has been described in detail previously,[8] we will present only a brief summary of it here. Eastern State Hospital[9] is the largest mental institution in its State, with a capacity of 2200 beds and an annual admission rate of 2000. The staff includes more than 1100 persons. Complete medical and administrative responsibility for the hospital is invested in the superintendent, under whom are an assistant superintendent and various divisions, such as medicine, nursing, and finance.

In April, 1963, Dr. Smith, eminent in psychiatry, president of various prestigious professional associations, and highly esteemed within the hospital, resigned after 17 years of service. A new superintendent, Dr. Lattimore, also of considerable renown in psychiatry, took office.

In July, 1963, the second author began recording informal observations; the research was formally begun in the spring of 1964. Between May, 1964, and August, 1965, over 100 interviews were conducted by the first author. Those interviewed included the entire senior medical staff, the heads of all major departments within the hospital, plus many others. Also interviewed were Dr. Smith and those psychiatrists and department heads who left the hospital after Dr. Lattimore's succession. However, no systematic attempt was made to interview persons in the lower levels of the organization—residents, nurses, aides, and patients. Most of the senior medical staff and many department heads were interviewed twice, with about a year intervening between the first and second interview. In addition to interviewing, the authors regularly attended numerous meetings and conferences throughout the hospital.

INITIAL PROBLEMS CONFRONTING THE SUCCESSOR

Although Dr. Smith had been concerned with developing a many-sided treatment program for the hospital, it was during his administration that the battle for psychoanalytically oriented psychotherapy had been fought and won in the state hospital. At the end of his term of office the major theoretical orientation of the hospital was psychodynamic. Psychoanalytically oriented psychotherapy was the "prestige" treatment and the core of the residency training program, even though the hospital had pioneered in an impressive number of developments in community psychiatry, including day and night hospitals, a patient employee program, and a Home Visit Unit.

Dr. Lattimore came to the hospital with a well-known interest in social psychiatry and research. Although social psychiatry and research programs had aroused little opposition during Dr. Smith's regime—in part because they never challenged the central emphasis on psychodynamics in the training program—Dr. Lattimore's increased emphasis on and more rapid implementation of these programs led to resentment in many analytically oriented staff members, who felt that individual psychotherapy was being downgraded. A good deal of controversy accompanied many of the programs, whether they were entirely new to the hospital and paid for by outside agencies or extensive modifications of existing hospital programs.[10]

There were several other complicating factors. After the arrival of Dr. Lattimore, a number of changes among the hospital's top-level personnel occurred, many of which were unrelated to the succession or the new programs. In the two-year period following Dr. Lattimore's succession, new personnel included the assistant superintendent, two successive clinical directors, the director of nurses, the head dietitian, and the head occupational therapist. Thus, the new superintendent was confronted with the loss of some key persons soon after his arrival, at a time when he was just beginning to find his way in a new social world.

In addition to the specific problems of resistance to new programs and staff turnover, Dr. Lattimore, like all successors, was faced with the general problems of communication and control. Lacking informal contacts, he could not easily find out what was going on in the system. Lacking full-hearted cooperation from some "old lieutenants," and confronted with the inertial properties of a large government institution, he found it difficult to implement change.

Finally, the prevalence of a Rebecca Myth was both a reflection of and a factor contributing to the difficulties encountered by the new superintendent. Many staff members, especially psychiatrists, were quick to note what they perceived to be flaws in Dr. Lattimore's psychiatric emphasis or his administrative methods or both. They tended to remember Dr. Smith nostalgically as the "good" superintendent and to look upon Dr. Lattimore as the "bad" one. The polarization described by Gouldner was very much in evidence.

However, the situation was not completely bleak. The "myth" did not affect all personnel. Some persons were indifferent, and others supported Dr. Lattimore and hoped that he would make needed changes. This feeling was especially strong in persons more in ideological sympathy with Dr. Lattimore than with Dr. Smith, and in persons—often the same ones—who felt that they had not received sufficient support under the old regime. Nevertheless, the dominant initial feeling was nostalgia for Dr. Smith and resentment toward Dr. Lattimore.

Like Gouldner's new manager, Dr. Lattimore approached his problems of communication and control by making numerous strategic replacements. This was facilitated by the departure of some key personnel. Dr. Lattimore was also able to use State and Federal funds to create several new positions at the middle management level, so that he could recruit new personnel without having to replace anyone. However, in some instances, the choice of a new man was heavily influenced by pressure from the old lieutenants, which tended to make the replacement less useful to Dr. Lattimore in furthering *his* plans for the hospital. As James points out, high-status professionals within an organization frequently influence the administrative decision-making process in this manner.[11]

In addition to bringing in strategic replacements from outside the hospital (assistant superintendent and clinical director), Dr. Lattimore varied the technique by making many promotions from within the hospital (several senior psychiatrists). In some instances the promoted persons were sympathetic to his aims and methods, and their promotions enhanced their enthusiasm and loyalty to the new management. When established in their new positions, they were model strategic replacements. In other instances Dr. Lattimore promoted persons who were not particularly sympathetic to his aims, but who were regarded as "entitled" to the promotion by most of the staff. Conceivably, one intent of these promotions was to win over the recalcitrant lieutenant. Very often, however, these staff members simply felt that they had received their due, and there was no increase in enthusiasm or cooperation.[12]

Strategic replacements, whatever their form, take time. As Gouldner states:

If the new manager is at all sensitive to what is going on, he does not wish to be accused of failing to give the old lieutenants a "chance" nor of seeking to install his favorites with indecent haste. He has to spend some time looking for possible allies and lining up replacements. In the meanwhile, the breakdown of upward communication to the new manager grows more acute. It is, in part, as an outgrowth of this crisis that the successor elaborates the system of "paper reports," the better to keep his finger on things and to check up on the "old lieutenants."[13]

Striking in the succession of Dr. Lattimore was the fact that he did not rely on increased "rules" or "reports." There was no "bureaucratic surge" following his succession. In order to understand this more fully, we must turn to a new concept, that of "administrative style."

TIGHT VERSUS LOOSE STYLES OF ADMINISTRATION

With the exception of Hodgson, Levinson, and Zaleznik,[14] studies of succession have emphasized sociological factors. For example, Gouldner emphasizes "the kinds of pressures and problems" which confront the successor because of his role.[15] He discusses the advantages and disadvantages of the various strategies a successor can employ. He also analyzes the particular strategies the successor of his study did in fact employ, but his analysis does not relate the successor's choice of strategies to his personality.

It is our thesis that the process of succession can be understood more fully if one examines more closely the influence of the successor's personality on his role performance and the role performances of others. We argue that the choices the successor makes reflect the influence of *both* institutional exigencies and the successor's personality. Of the many different facets of personality that might be studied, we have selected one in particular—the successor's administrative style.

Administrative style refers to an executive's professional behavior, the characteristic way in which he functions as an executive, how he structures his role, and how he influences the roles and functioning of others in the organization. It is, for the most part, unrelated to policy: it is not *what* he does, but *how* he does it. We are especially concerned here with two contrasting types, the "tight" and the "loose" administrative styles.

A tight administrative style relates to the military model, sharing with it an emphasis on hierarchical authority and communication. A tight style implies: (1) clear-cut delegation of authority and responsibility; (2) an orderly and hierarchical chain of command through which communication flows upward and downward, without skipping levels; (3) a reliance on formal communications—for example, regular meetings, reports, printed forms; (4) formal expression of power—for example, hearings, written notification of promotions and dismissals; (5) reliance on explicit, written rules, or, in their absence, on tradition.

A loose administrative style is characterized by flexibility, with fluid lines of authority and communication. A loose style implies: (1) absence, in many areas, of clearly designated authority and responsibility; (2) considerable tolerance of role ambiguity and role diffusion; (3) frequent bypassing of the chain of command, both in communication and authority; (4) informal communications; (5) informal exercise of power; (6) relatively little reliance on rules and tradition.

Using Presidents Eisenhower and Kennedy as examples, Arthur Schlesinger, Jr., illustrates some of the differences between a tight and loose administrative style:

The President [Kennedy] was in this respect very much like Roosevelt or Churchill. If he was interested in a problem like the Congo and wanted to control what was going on, he would not follow the chain of command as President Eisenhower, I gather, did. In other words, say, tell something to the Secretary of State, who would tell it to the Under Secretary of State for Political Affairs, who would tell it to the Assistant Secretary of State for Africa, who would tell it to the Congo Desk Officer, and similarly the Congo Desk Officer would reply through the same chain of command. This would often dilute the message, both ways, divesting it of any pungency of character. President Kennedy's instinct would be to call the man and ask him or tell him, and this had the effect of not only giving the President much fresher information and sharper opinion, but it also would imbue the machinery of government itself with the sense of his own purposes.[16]

Schlesinger goes on to emphasize that Kennedy used his White House staff in a very flexible way. He disliked the notion of staff assistants with fixed assignments and sharp demarcations of authority. Moreover, the boundaries between the White House staff and other governmental agencies became blurred. The Presidential assistants took an active role in defending the interests of the President and were often aggressive in invading what a particular bureaucracy regarded as its own domain. In this way the President, through his staff, could seek out those people in the government machinery who were capable of innovation and could support such persons in their own internal conflicts. It is not surprising that these efforts by the White House staff were often labeled as "meddling" and resented by officials who were wedded to the status quo.

Schlesinger emphasizes the advantages of a loose-style—for example, it gives the leader fresher information and permits him to strengthen the influence of innovative and creative persons throughout the organization. However, when Hans Morgenthau describes Kennedy's administrative style, it is difficult to realize that one is reading about the same style that Schlesinger cites so positively. Morgenthau criticizes Kennedy for the "disorderliness" of his administration:

He [Kennedy] would receive information from, and give orders to, second-level officials without informing their chiefs, and it happened that when an issue was later discussed in the formal councils of government, he had forgotten that he had already given an order contrary to his present position. From Schlesinger's discussion of Kennedy's Vietnam policy emerges a melancholy tale of ignorance, miscalculations, confusion, and absent-mindedness. The initial decision to withdraw support from Diem derived from a Presidential misunderstanding of the actual position of the different executive departments concerned. The result was confusion.[17]

Commentators tend either, like Schlesinger, totally to approve the loose style, or, like Morgenthau, totally to condemn it. The critics are more numerous than the supporters. Cumming and Cumming, in discussing administration in the mental hospital, write:

. . . The authority holder should always be alert for skipping and should try to divert communication back through the correct channels. . . . Persistent skipping always demoralizes the person skipped—first, because it cuts him out of the communication stream and, second, because it gives presumptive equality to those under him who, by other criteria such as salary and training, are not his equal.[18]

One of the few supporters of a loose style is Zaleznik, although he labels it differently. Zaleznik speaks of "bureaucratic" and "circumventive" styles of management. He writes that "bureaucracy" fosters "orderliness, equality, and proportionality," whereas "circumvention" fosters "ambiguity, competitiveness, and shifting rewards."[19] Eisenhower is his example of an executive functioning in the "bureaucratic" mode, and Franklin Roosevelt is the prototype of the "circumventive" style. Zaleznik's own sympathies are clearly with the latter, since his special concern is the fostering of innovation and initiative within an organization rather than the maintenance of order and harmony.

ADMINISTRATIVE STYLE AT ESH

At ESH one of the most outstanding characteristics of the succession was the change from a tight to a loose style of administration. Dr. Smith was widely known as an excellent administrator, and under his administration the hospital was a model of tight organization. The following excerpts from Dr. Smith's writings on hospital administration illustrate his views:

The efficiency of bureaucratic administration depends upon the reliability of its responses and its adherence to regulations.

He [the administrator] must delegate responsibilities to others. . . . the formal channels for authority will let everyone know who is responsible for what.

The good leader supports those to whom he delegates authority by avoiding *over-ruling, undercutting,* or *bypassing.*

To the best of the authors' knowledge, the hospital bureaucracy functioned as it should, with a maximum of efficiency and a minimum of nonproductive red tape. Dr. Smith delegated medical authority to his clinical director and concerned himself largely with the administrative aspects of the hospital. His personal manner was characterized by one psychiatrist as follows:

Typically Dr. Smith would get up and say, "This is our twelfth administrative meeting of the year, and I have the following to report." When changes were made, all of the appropriate people were consulted—the various levels of staff conferences, separately and together. Then there would be a barrage of memos. Then, at 12:01 A.M. on January 1, you would do it the new way.

Dr. Lattimore unquestionably had a looser administrative style. He frequently cited the remarks of a former superior:

All rules of procedure are to be neglected to a large extent. Personnel are to be taught that they are to use intuition, imagination, initiative, judgment, rather than to be constrained by rules or procedure. For example, let the nurses decide whether or not they are to wear uniforms, and the best way to get along with patients. If they want a type of ward organization, they do not need special permission, unless it unavoidably collides with something else.

We want continuing change, not by ukase but by discussion and argument, perhaps continuing for months, with respect for the opinions of all. Issues can be decided by logical debate rather than direct orders. The "High Moguls" should be willing to justify themselves to the "Low Moguls." . . . Look for capacities additional to those imparted by training or required by the role. Especially important are those qualities which are submerged, seeking outlet, but inhibited by rigidities in our system and in our thinking. . . . These concepts are not new, only the doing is new.

Dr. Lattimore's administration was characterized by flexibility and fluid lines of authority and communication. Several comments from staff members illustrate the difference in the styles:

A *psychiatrist:* The old way was to do things through regular channels; the new way is not.

A *clinical director:* With Dr. Smith there was a clear-cut assignment of roles. He was very much involved with administrative problems. With Dr. Lattimore this is not so.

A *senior psychiatrist:* I think Dr. Lattimore is much more flexible than Dr. Smith. He's younger and more flexible. He's less apt to say: "No, that's impossible," and more inclined to say: "Let see how that works out—why not go ahead and do it?" That's the main difference.

Dr. Lattimore's personal manner was folksy and equalitarian. He would sometimes begin a meeting by saying, "Does anyone have anything to get off his chest?" And in his previous job he had been nicknamed, "Hi, guys." A psychiatrist contrasted the old and new superintendents:

Dr. Smith was a very dignified, proper, distant administrator. You had to request an appointment to see him. Dr. Lattimore is sort of esaygoing, friendly, informal—more a sibling than a father image like Dr. Smith.

It is clear from the above quotations that Dr. Lattimore did *not* initiate a "surge of bureaucratic development." To do so would have run counter to his whole style of administration. The way he did proceed to solve the problems raised by his succession can be illustrated in part by his relations with his medical staff.

When Dr. Lattimore arrived at the hospital, there were two clinical directors. Both had had psychoanalytic training, and neither was especially interested in the social psychiatry or research endeavors that formed the center of Dr. Lattimore's interests. Dr. Cheever, the senior director, was clearly in charge of the clinical program and residency training. He followed in a line of clinical directors who had enjoyed considerable autonomy under Dr. Smith.

Four months after Dr. Lattimore arrived, Dr. Cheever resigned. In an interview with one of the authors he stated:

> I was used to the autonomy of my department. I was used to having my decisions backed up. Under Dr. Lattimore I couldn't make a decision, nor could I get anyone else to. My views and his about community psychiatry are at opposite poles.

The last sentence of the quotation calls attention to the sharp ideological disagreement which existed between Dr. Lattimore and Dr. Cheever.[20] Granted that difference, trouble between the superintendent and the clinical director could have been predicted, regardless of the style of the successor. However, style played a crucial role in determining how the successor handled the trouble. A successor with a tight style might have done one of several things: (1) replaced the clinical director with a man of his own choosing; (2) left the old clinical director with the autonomy he had, even though this would have meant abdicating any control over his activities; (3) increased bureaucratic measures in order to check up on the recalcitrant lieutenant and increase executive control of the organization. Gouldner suggests the likelihood of choice (3) in the initial stages of succession, since (1) would mean moving with "unseemly haste" and (2) would mean organizational ineffectiveness from the successor's viewpoint.

With his loose style Dr. Lattimore chose none of the above alternatives. Instead, he tried to "win over" Dr. Cheever through informal contact. In the meantime, since he wanted to get things moving rapidly, he preferred to "work around" his clinical director in areas where they came into opposition. For example, Dr. Lattimore started a social-psychiatric rehabilitation program even though Dr. Cheever vehemently opposed the particular form this enterprise took. The clinical director interpreted Dr. Lattimore's activities as "meddling" and as "undermining" of his authority, and, as a consequence, resigned.

In seeking a replacement, Dr. Lattimore was strongly influenced by the remaining clinical director and several senior psychiatrists. Accepting their counsel, he appointed a psychiatrist who had formerly been at ESH for some years and was at that time in psychoanalytic training. Thus, while the replacement was regarded as "legitimate" by the old lieutenants, there was some question as to how well the superintendent and the new clinical director could work together. Perhaps in realization of this fact, the new man was not given a position as *the* clinical director—a position Dr. Cheever had held—but shared authority with the remaining clinical director and a third psychiatrist, another old lieutenant who was also promoted to clinical director. In addition, a fourth psychiatrist was added to the staff at a high level, and functioned as a clinical director. He was closer to Dr. Lattimore ideologically than the other clinical directors, but his legitimacy was questioned more and he was never fully integrated as a clinical director.

During this period, Dr. Lattimore's defenses as a successor were especially apparent. He tried to woo the existing clinical directors and other old lieutenants by exchanging ideas with them and seeking their advice. At the same time he tried to maximize his own freedom by leaving the situation ambiguous and fluid, sometimes accepting their advice, sometimes moving on his own initiative where it ran counter to their wishes. Above all, he did not *fix* the authority system in any clear-cut way. To do so along previous lines might have jeopardized the possibility of moving the hospital in the direction he thought desirable. On the other hand, if he had moved decisively in his own direction, he might have shaken the equilibrium of the organization. He wished to avoid an exodus of top psychiatric personnel because (1) he valued the abilities of the old lieutenants, and (2) he realized the difficulty of recruiting staff members for state hospital positions. In short, Dr. Lattimore hoped that leadership compatible with his own interests would emerge eventually, but that he could manage not to rock the boat too much in the meantime.

Nine months after the new clinical director's arrival, he resigned. He stated in an interview:

The question is, how many clinical directors are there to be. It has varied—three, four, or five. Now the clinical directors are assigned administrative functions. Dr. Lattimore gave each a different service. He usurped, thus, the authority of the senior physicians over their services. Then the superintendent and the assistant superintendent began to deal directly with seniors, bypassing the clinical directors. . . . There is very little communication at the hospital. . . . No administration or organization.

The clinical director voiced strongly the classic complaint against the loose style—its tendency to "meddle" and to skip proper organizational levels to "deal directly" with subordinates (the "seniors"). His other complaints are also familiar: role diffusion (the assigning of administrative functions to the clinical directors), inadequate formal communication, and the lack of administrative organization.

At about this time the fourth clinical director also faded from the scene, leaving the junior clinical director from Dr. Smith's administration and the promoted old lieutenant as the two remaining clinical directors. The latter was in charge of the outpatient program while the former devoted his energies mainly to the training program; thus a *modus vivendi* was reached. Dr. Lattimore was continually criticized, however, for interfering in clinical areas and in the training program, formerly the exclusive provinces of the clinical directors.

The activities of Mr. Eisenberg, a nursing supervisor, provide another example of the working of a loose administrative style. Shortly after Dr. Lattimore's succession, Mr. Eisenberg established contact with the new administration, especially Dr. George, the new assistant superintendent. Mr. Eisenberg was supported by Dr. George in his controversial efforts to take over the family care program, a program involving the placement of patients in foster homes in the community. The social service department had jurisdiction over this particular program, but, lacking personnel and medical supervision, it had been able to run the program only on a very limited basis. Investing enormous energy and ignoring criticism from both his own superiors and other departments, Mr. Eisenberg increased the number of patients in this program from 29 to 60 in a two-year period, with nurses under his direction making the required weekly visits. In addition, Mr. Eisenberg established a community preparation ward and vigorously continued his work on the renovation of part of the aged North Side of the hospital.

The loose style of the administration was manifested in several ways. First, Mr. Eisenberg communicated directly with Dr. Lattimore and Dr. George, bypassing the nursing hierarchy and the senior psychiatrist in charge of the service. Second, departmental lines were crossed: The nursing service performed what was traditionally a social service function. Third, a subordinate with considerable talent was given support directly from the top in his conflicts both within his service and with other departments.

It is understandable that Mr. Eisenberg's superiors in the nursing service, the social service department, and the senior psychiatrist in charge of the North Side were all disgruntled at various times by Mr. Eisenberg's freewheeling activities and the support they received from the administration. In varying degrees, they felt bypassed, undermined, and, at the very least, uninformed.

Dr. Lattimore's loose style in rapidly implementing new programs, as illustrated by the support he gave to Mr. Eisenberg, led to considerable criticism of his methods by the old lieutenants, particularly the senior medical staff and some department heads. Dr. Lattimore argued that he used the tactics he did because he often could not get the cooperation of the person formally in charge of a given service or department. Those who were bypassed—some of whom had originally been somewhat critical of Dr. Lattimore's program—now focused their opposition on his "methods," complaining that they did not object to his goals but to the "way" he pursued them. Probably both interpretations held a degree of truth.

It is important to note that when Dr. Lattimore found a department head or service chief who moved energetically in directions of which the new superintendent generally approved, he fully respected the autonomy and authority of that person. In short, what was experienced as a loose or "undermining" style by some, was experienced as strong support by others. Indeed, a tighter administrative style might have prevented Dr. Lattimore from giving as much support to those he favored. He could bend the rules or break traditions in a way which fostered a rapid mobilization of resources for a project he wished to further. This ability to provide differential strong support was especially useful to Dr. Lattimore in recruiting, and helps to explain how he was able to persuade many psychiatrists to come to work at a State hospital.

DISCUSSION

As our discussion of administrative style implies, there are advantages and disadvantages to both the tight and loose styles. The gains and losses that accompany a loose style at the time of a succession are well illustrated by the course of events at ESH.

A successor's loose style permits him to avoid the Charybdis of premature direct confrontation with his recalcitrant lieutenants and the Scylla of institutional paralysis stemming from the resistance of the old lieutenants. To some extent he can impose his will on the organization by working around the recalcitrant lieutenants without forcing a showdown. He can do this by communicating with and supporting innovative and creative subordinates "down the line." At the same time he can try to win over or at least effect a working relationship with the recalcitrant lieutenants through a variety of informal means. He thus avoids drastic measures such as replacement, and formalizing measures such as the requiring of more reports and lengthier and more frequent meetings, which might fulfill the letter but not the spirit of his intentions.

The disadvantages of the loose style are also numerous. Department heads, already threatened by the coming of the successor, may feel even more insecure and undermined when the successor wheels and deals directly with subordinates. Resistance that was originally focused on the successor's aims can now be buttressed by criticism of the *way* he seeks to fulfill them, compounding the controversy. The loose style also may make it difficult to insure accountability, since working around a recalcitrant lieutenant may involve assigning an overlapping role to another person; determining who is responsible for any particular aspect of the job can remain a continuing source of ambiguity.

The advantages of a tight style for the successor have been clearly outlined by Gouldner. When confronted with inadequate communication and recalcitrant lieutenants, the successor with a tight style can rely upon formal methods of communication and control to impose his will upon the organization. We wish to add that in the face of the ideological and personal clashes that often accompany a succession, "going by the book" provides external criteria which cannot easily be challenged.

However, the absence of challenge does not necessarily mean the presence of commitment to the successor's plans. A disadvantage of the tight style is that the successor may be hampered by covert bureaucratic "sabotage" by the old lieutenants; at the same time, because of his style, he may be unable to mobilize support for his policies from sympathetic subordinates at lower levels of the organization. To the extent that he relies on the rules and the formal chain of command the successor limits his freedom and flexibility.

In addition to specific gains and losses at times of succession, there are general advantages and disadvantages to tight and loose styles. A tight style fosters responsibility and order in an organization, but can also lead to stagnation and rigidity. A loose style may nurture creativity and flexibility, but it can lead to chaos and irresponsibility.

Responsibility and creativity are both essential to the healthy growth of an organization. Conversely, stagnation and chaos must both be discouraged. We suggest that organizations "strike a balance" over time in these areas by means of alternating periods of tight and loose administration. We further speculate that the expansion phase of organizational growth may occur more frequently during periods of loose administration, while the consolidation phase may be associated more with periods of tight administration. These periods need not necessarily be associated with the term of a single top executive. As long as further tightening does not strangle the organization and further loosening does not result in disintegration, a leader with the same style as his predecessor may be tolerated. Some organizations may function well for an extremely long period of time or indefinitely with a particular style of administration. However, if and when the disadvantages of either the tight or the loose style accumulate and the losses accompanying a style of administration outweigh the gains, it becomes "time for a change." At such times a successor with a different style can provide a needed stimulus to the growth of an organization. We feel that this occurred in the succession which we are discussing.

At ESH there were signs that the organization was entering a period of stasis after 17 years of dynamic but tight leadership. Dr. Lattimore's "loosening" and "stirring things up" may indeed have provided a needed stimulus to the hospital. The new manager in Guest's study came to a plant characterized by an atmosphere of "obedience to orders, enforcement of rules, the exercise of power through the threat of punishment. . . ."[21] The new manager had a loose administrative style and his "freeing things up" reversed a trend toward constrictively tight administration. Those who appointed the new manager in Gouldner's study felt that there had been too much laxness at the plant under the old manager, and they expected the new manager to improve production. In their view the new manager's "tightening up" reversed a progressively deteriorating situation.

A final example of organization growth through an alternation of styles is provided by Eastern State Psychiatric Institute. ESPI is a small, university-affiliated psychiatric hospital which experienced a succession in 1958. The retiring superintendent, Dr. Rosenberg, had a loose administrative style, and under his leadership the hospital had achieved national prominence. However, it was felt by some of the medical staff that toward the end of Dr. Rosenberg's administration there was too much role diffusion and a lack of clear-cut authority in the organization. The new superintendent, Dr. Presley, had a tight administrative style and was known as a crisp decision-maker. He emphasized clear-cut lines of authority and delegated responsibility. His increase in bureaucratization took the form of new requirements for formal reports, formalization of the assistant clinical director's job and role, and demands for punctuality.

Thus, in Gouldner's study and at ESPI, a successor with a tight administrative style brought an increase in bureaucratization. However, at ESH and at the automobile plant described by Guest there was no "surge of bureaucratic development." We contend that a successor's administrative style is an important factor determining his responses to the exigencies of succession. A successor with a tight administrative style may rely heavily on bureaucratic methods; a successor with a loose administrative style may be unable or willing to do so. Executives with different styles may react quite differently to problems they encounter as successors. The success of the change may depend on the fit between a successor's style and the needs of the organization at a given time.

In conclusion, we would like to suggest some areas for further investigation. We have suggested that it is helpful to describe an executive's administrative styles as either tight or loose. But are there executives whose styles are neither tight nor loose—that is, executives flexible enough to realize the advantages of both styles? (Presumably an executive who seized the disadvantages of both would not long remain an executive.) Might the styles we have delineated be described better in other terms? Moreover, our characterizations of tight and loose administrative styles are very broad. What further distinctions can be made concerning the components of these styles, and what subtypes are there within the two categories? For example, is it useful to think of a tight dominating style (along the lines of de Gaulle's) in contrast to a kind of light leadership where the top executive delegates authority with little imposition of his own wishes or conceptions?

The relationship between personality, social structure, and executive functioning to a great extent remains to be explored. For example, if the tight-loose distinction proves to be useful, what are the psychological and sociological determinants of these behaviors? To what extent can a successor's style be predicted on the basis of prior knowledge of him as an individual, and to what degree is his style determined by the exigencies of his situation on a particular organizational setting? Specifically, can a given administrative style be adopted consciously as a strategy of management? Parenthetically, with regard to psychological determinants we caution against any casual association of a tight administrative style with authoritarianism or a loose administrative style with equalitarianism. Franklin Roosevelt, for example, used a loose style very effectively to keep major decision-making in his own hands, and many subordinates found his leadership very dominating.

Finally, our speculation concerning an alternation of tight and loose styles during the course of an institution's history implies that over time the disadvantages of a particular style create the need for its opposite. Other explanations are possible, however. For example, style alternation in management succession may in part reflect the need of a successor to be *different* from his predecessor, to create his own *executive identity*.

It is our conviction that research pertaining to general issues of executive functioning, as well as to the specific problem of management succession, will both expand conceptual sociopsychological knowledge and contribute practical suggestions that may help the successor in handling his often difficult problems.

NOTES

1. Joel Kotin and Myron R. Sharaf, "Intrastaff Controversy at a State Mental Hospital: An Analysis of Ideological Issues," *Psychiatry* (1967) 30:16–29.
2. Daniel J. Levinson, "Role, Personality, and Social Structure in the Organizational Setting," *J. Abnormal and Social Psychology* (1959) 58:170–180. Richard C. Hodgson, Daniel J. Levinson, and Abraham Zaleznik, *The Executive Role Constellation*; Cambridge, Mass., Division of Research, Harvard Business School, 1965. Abraham Zaleznik, *Human Dilemmas of Leadership*; New York, Harper and Row, 1966. Daniel J. Levinson and Gerald L. Klerman, "The Clinician-Executive," *Psychiatry* (1967) 30:3–15.
3. Alvin W. Gouldner, *Patterns of Industrial Bureaucracy*; Glencoe, Ill., Free Press, 1954.
4. Gouldner writes: "A common indication of the degree and source of workers' resistance to a new manager is the prevalence of what may be called the 'Rebecca Myth.' Some years ago Daphne DuMaurier wrote a novel about a young woman who married a widower, only to be plagued by the memory of his first wife, Rebecca, whose virtues were still widely extolled. One may suspect that many a past plant manager is, to some extent, idealized by the workers, even if disliked while present." See footnote 3; p. 79.
   The most dramatic example in recent times of the operation of the Rebecca Myth emerged in Lyndon Johnson's succession to the Presidency. William Manchester (*The Death of a President*; New York, Harper and Row, 1967) has documented in considerable detail the resentment of the Kennedy staff toward Johnson and his new lieutenants. He also shows how Kennedy staff members who did move vigorously to serve the new President were accused of opportunism and disloyalty by other "old lieutenants." Perhaps more significantly, not only those close to the Presidency, but also large segments of the population were soon quick to emphasize anything they regarded as "bad" about the new President and to contrast him unfavorably with the departed and now idealized Kennedy.
5. See footnote 3; pp. 93–94. Gouldner also describes two other strategies available to

a successor to increase his communication and control: "close supervision," and the use of *"gemeinschaft* techniques." Each of these, however, has considerable limitations. Close supervision of subordinates by a successor is difficult in a large organization and many arouse resentment. The use of *gemeinschaft* techniques—that is, becoming friendly with subordinates and working through the informal system—is difficult for a new man, especially if a Rebecca Myth is prevalent.

6. Robert H. Guest, *Organizational Change: The Effect of Successful Leadership;* Homewood, Ill., Irwin Dorsey Press, 1962.
7. See footnote 2; p. 249.
8. See footnote 1.
9. The names of persons and places have been altered.
10. The programs themselves plus the accompanying controversy were described previously. See footnote 1.
11. Bernard J. James, "Advanced Study for Psychiatric Administrators," *Mental Hospitals* (1964) 15:686–688.
12. Gouldner also found that promotions given to old lieutenants by the new manager were simply regarded as the "paying off" of inherited obligations; the promoted men felt they owed nothing in return.
13. See footnote 3; p. 93.
14. See footnote 2.
15. See footnote 3; p. 70.
16. "Schlesinger at the White House. A Conversation with Henry Brandon," *Harper's Magazine,* July, 1964; p. 58.
17. Hans J. Morgenthau, "Monuments to Kennedy," *New York Review of Books,* January 6, 1966; p. 8.
18. John Cumming and Elaine Cumming, *Ego and Milieu;* New York, Atherton, 1962; pp. 128–129.
19. See *Human Dilemmas of Leadership,* in footnote 2; pp. 95–96.
20. See footnote 1.
21. See footnote 6; p. 23.

MANAGEMENT SUCCESSION REVISITED

MYRON R. SHARAF AND JOEL KOTIN

We consider ourselves extremely fortunate to have had the opportunity to study Eastern State Hospital during a crucial time in its history. The problems of studying organizations in depth are manifold. Psychiatric institutions, however, afford unique possibilities for study.[1]

In our case the idea of scientific inquiry was acceptable to the administration and we were invited into all meetings, consultations, etc., as observers. Moreover, psychiatrists, we think, may be more willing than other executives to discuss their feelings openly. Furthermore, we observed Eastern State Hospital during one of the most crucial developmental periods in its 130-year history. A strong effective leader with a commitment to particular policies whose administration had lasted 17 years, was succeeded by another strong, effective leader with a different administrative style and commitment to different policies.

We were equally fortunate in having data on a similarly pivotal succession at Eastern State Psychiatric Institute for comparison. Thus, we could observe in pure culture different strategies of coping with the succession crisis, different administration styles, and the results of these interactions throughout the organizations.

Since 1967, Eastern State Hospital has undergone far-reaching changes. (Our data in this retrospective are less systematically complete and more impressionistic than in our previous effort but there has also been less turmoil and polarization in the organization.) There have been two successions to the superintendency at Eastern State Hospital since our study—in 1967 and in 1973. Even more far-reaching, however, has been the administrative decentralization of the hospital into smaller units, each serving a geographic catchment area. This change was begun by Dr. Lattimore and continued by his successors.

These two successions have not been accompanied by as much polarization in the form of a "Rebecca Myth" as the successions we studied. Several factors may be responsible, including decentralization. This step enhanced the power of the unit chiefs and decreased the power of central administration (Superintendent and department heads), with the important proviso that the Superintendent could still hire and fire the unit chiefs.

The leader who fights for decentralization represents a paradox in several ways. For one thing, the very idea of a leader surrendering power is not usually regarded as the way a strong leader behaves and is often viewed with some suspicion—as a kind of trick—by subordinates. At the same time, it takes considerable vigor on the part of the top leader to effect decentralization. The chant "power to the people" is popular on both the political left and right. But, in fact, people who have not had responsibility are often loathe to assume it, and people who have had power under a more centralized regime are not eager to relinquish it. The leader who fights for decentralization often has to utilize his authority in decisive, controversial ways that readily arouse the criticism of "dictatorship." For example, unitization of the hospital erodes the power of department chiefs; community school boards limit the authority of the central school department and, in some instances, civil service protection for teachers and principals; impounding congressionally authorized funds (in order to protect revenue sharing as a key instrument of fiscal decentralization) is, in a real sense, an attack on congressional authority.

However, once decentralization has taken firm roots, the authority of the top leader of a large organization may in fact be considerably diminished. Moreover, the process of decentralization, with increased power for unit chiefs, may reduce the emotional salience of the top leader for many members of the organization, who now see their primary loyalty as belonging to their "local" chief. In our view, this helps explain the fact that when Dr. Lattimore resigned from Eastern State Hospital in 1967 to take a more responsible position, his successor faced a much less pronounced Rebecca Myth than did Dr. Lattimore when he replaced Dr. Smith.

If decentralization was a major factor in reducing the emotional upheaval around succession, it was not the only one. A second important factor was length of tenure. Dr. Lattimore had replaced a leader who had been Superintendent for 17 years, but he himself served for only 4 years. This difference, in itself, made Dr. Lattimore's departure a less wrenching blow to the organization. Nor was his shorter tenure idiosyncratic. Today, there is much greater career mobility for psychiatrists, and there are many more prestigious positions above the level of Superintendent than there were in the 1940's and 1950's. Moreover, leaders of urban institutions, be they mayors of cities or heads of service organizations such as Eastern State Hospital, are likely to have a shorter tenure because of the crushing pressures of the job. Relatively peaceful reigns for heads of large institutions, insulated in various ways from public controversy, seem to be a thing of the past.

Another reason for the lessening of the Rebecca Myth appears to be the fact that top leaders today are increasingly involved in dealing with other organizations. Levinson and Klerman[2] have noted that the chief executive's extensive participation in "foreign relations" means that responsibility for internal operations must be delegated to subordinates, a result—we have suggested—which also flows from the current emphasis on decentralization.

Levinson and Klerman suggest that the limitation of contact between the top leader and the people who work for him produces an increase in "transference" phenomena. However, it may also reduce the emotional salience of the top leader, even if it generates an increased mythology about what this shadowy figure is like.

It might be argued that, in the situation we are describing, Rebecca Myth phenomena are simply displaced to the unit chiefs and it is their departures and arrivals which generate emotional storms for the staff. To some extent this is the case. However, several distinctions need to be made. First, unit chiefs are likely to be younger and less established persons than top administrators of the organizations. Hence, they tend to generate less intense transference phenomena than the revered or hated "old man" who was perceived as running the whole show. Second, there is more opportunity for day-to-day contact with the chief of a small unit. This permits greater working through of transference distortions in general and, in connection with succession crises, working through the splitting of feeling between the old and new leader which contributes to the Rebecca Myth.

The trend toward decentralization has stimulated in us new thoughts concerning "tight" and "loose" styles of administration. Smaller units are more likely to permit patterns of authority which include some differentiation into levels plus the possibility of jumping echelons without too much fuss. In this structure the Chief of a unit can hear the complaints of a lower-level subordinate and at the same time bring in the subordinate's supervisor so that the latter does not feel bypassed, or, if so, only temporarily. Face-to-face contact, group meetings, and the relative accessibility of the leader offer the possibility of loosening rigid organizational barriers without abandoning such principles as delegation, supervision and accountability.

W. H. Auden once wrote that social scientists dream of systems so perfect that no one has to be good. Lest we give the impression that decentralization represents that system, we hasten to note some of *its* problems. Decentralization puts a heavy premium on "good" unit chiefs. Their capricious or destructive exercise of authority can be especially devastating because of the weakening of the line of authority that previously flowed from department chiefs. The latter often served to protect representatives of their disciplines (e.g., nursing or psychology) from the abuses of the unit leader. Close monitoring of unit performance by the top leader (and *his* aides) is necessary. Which takes us back to the issues of top management where we began.

Recognition that the pendulum swings back and forth need not induce a feeling of futility about organizational progress—the search for combining the values of "tight" and "loose" styles of administration goes on apace. There is increasing experimentation in industry, as well as in human service organizations, with small, relatively unhierarchical work groups which have considerable autonomy in arranging their organizational structure. These also encourage role diffusion, e.g., the nurse does not restrict herself narrowly to nursing nor the assembly line worker to only one small part of the total operation. Yet there is also awareness of the necessity for accountability—someone outside the work group has to take a hard look at the output (cost analysis, evaluation of treatment program, and the like).

Above all, there is growing recognition of the fact that there are no easy answers. The emphasis on traditional bureaucratic virtues (such as clearcut, objectively determined criteria for hiring and promotion) may end up in the crippling straight-jacket of many civil service regulations. On the other hand, nice sounding terms such as democratic decisionmaking often serve to conceal organizational confusion and irresponsibility. As William Morris put it many years ago: "Men fight and lose the battle and then the thing they fought for comes about, but when it comes it turns out not to be what they meant and others have to fight for what they meant under a different name."

Our differentiation of tight and loose styles grew out of an attempt to understand an organization's experience of succession. Seven years after our study, our feeling remains that succession has been inadequately studied. A new leader represents both a trauma and an opportunity for growth for an organization. Further studies are needed in several directions. The vicissitudes of top- and middle-management successors in various organizations could be compared, e.g., in organizations with similar goals such as mental hospitals but with different organizational structures and philosophies. Another direction would be to study succession in different social settings e.g., when a new therapist begins treatment of an ongoing therapy group or when a school class has a new teacher.

Succession is important because it relates to profound psychological issues for the individual. These include how losses are handled, the individual's relations to authority, and the universal hope for a better tomorrow.

NOTES

1. See Hodgson, Levinson and Zaleznik, as cited in the original article.
2. Levinson, Daniel J., and Klerman, Gerald L. The clinician—executive. *Psychiatry: Journal for the Study of Interpersonal Processes*, 30(1): 3–15, 1967.

13/PARTICIPATORY MANAGEMENT: AN ALTERNATIVE IN HUMAN SERVICE DELIVERY SYSTEMS

KENNETH P. FALLON, JR.

Social service administrators have been incorporating into practice a number of methods and systems developed by business administration. These managament systems have offered the agency administrator new approaches to making maximum use of scarce resources for effective service delivery.[4] Such tools as Program Evaluation Review Technique, Planning

Program Budgeting System, and Management by Objectives have all had their impact upon social service administration. The accountability demanded of social service management by legislators, private boards, and consumers alike has been facilitated by these tools. Nevertheless, the greatest resource of management remains the personnel within the organization. Berliner suggested the benefits of full utilization of staff resources: "Happy is the administrator who has learned the virtues of, and techniques for, sharing of his power. Sharing of power leads to high staff morale, organizational effectiveness, and on-the-job education of a generation which inevitably must succeed him" (pp. 562–563).[3]

Argyris reported in the *Journal of Business:* "Studies show that participative management tends to 1) increase the degree of 'we' feeling or cohesiveness that participants have with their organization; 2) provide the participants with an overall organizational point of view instead of the traditional more 'now' departmental point of view; 3) decrease the amount of conflict, hostility and cutthroat competition of participants; 4) increase individuals' understanding of each other, which leads to increased tolerance and patience toward others; 5) increase the individual's free expression of his personality, which results in an employee who sticks with the organization because he (i.e., his personality) needs the gratifying experiences he finds while working there; and 6) develop a 'work climate' as a result of the other tendencies, in which the subordinates find opportunity to be more creative and to come up with the ideas beneficial to the organization" (pp. 1–7).[1]

Likert reported studies that indicated that "those firms or plants where System 4 (participatory management) is used show high productivity, low scrap loss, low costs, favorable attitudes, and excellent labor relations. The converse tends to be the case for companies or departments whose management system is well toward System 1 (exploitative-authoritative management)" (p. 46).[7]

Participatory management implies that staff will have a voice and a vote in those management decisions that affect their work. Employees who participate in this management style feel more highly motivated and tend to incorporate the organization's goals more readily than employees working in management organizations that are autocratic or consultative in nature. Participatory management encourages people to stay in the organization and improve their role performance.[7, 8, 9]

The writer was introduced to participatory management principles at the Alaska Children's Services, a multiservice agency in Anchorage. In the summer of 1972, the writer introduced participatory management to the North Idaho Child Development Center. In both agencies, the participatory management proposal was presented by the executive directors as a management alternative, and was adopted by vote of all staff members. Both agencies were fairly new. The staff of both agreed that participatory management practices would facilitate developing programs responsive to clients' needs.

DETAILS OF PARTICIPATORY MANAGEMENT

The proposal adopted by both staffs mandated that participatory processes be applied to all major decision-making tasks, and include all elements of the staff. Democratic decision making required that decisions that affect the work of any segment of the staff be made by them. Decisions were generally to be made by voting, except in smaller staff areas, where more liberal process (consensus) applied. The process required that, if possible, proposals to staff groups be made in writing and be available in advance to the staff.

Limitations of the Process
Limitations of the democratic process include:

1. No segment of the staff is empowered to make any decision that affects the work of another segment. (Example: A group home staff may not make a decision affecting staff in a residential treatment center.)

2. Democratic process may not invade areas that are a matter of designated expertise of specific staff members. (Example: Speech therapists may not make decisions affecting psychometric tests used by psychologists.)

3. The competence or performance of staff is not subject to the democratic process except as applied to elected staff representatives. (Example: The professional expertise of a speech therapist must be evaluated by a speech therapist, whereas the performance of an ad hoc committee, elected by the staff to study a budget question, may be subject to democratic process.)

4. Staff may not make decisions that require expenditure of funds not under their authority. (Example: Child care workers may decide how to use recreational funds available to their particular cottage, but not how recreational funds are to be used by another cottage.)

5. Agency policy decisions are reserved for the board of directors in the case of the Alaska agency, or the administrator of the Department of Environmental and Community Services in the case of the North Idaho agency. (Example: Decisions to develop a new group home, halfway house, etc., were reserved for the board of directors of the Alaska Children's Services. Decisions regarding contracts with local school districts to develop an educational program for older retardates rested with the administrator of the Department of Environmental and Community Services in the case of the North Idaho Center.)

Basil summarized these constraints: "There is one firm rule regarding participation of subordinates in the decision-making process: that the prerequisites for participation must be ability and knowledge. Participation in decision making must be restricted to individuals with ability to comprehend what is required and the knowledge to contribute to the position" (p. 159).[2]

Levels of Decision Making
Examples of decisions to be made by each level in the agency were as follows:

1. The board of directors or the administrator: (a) agencywide policy decisions; b) selection of a director; c) determinations of basic program direction, with input from the community the agency serves, the board or advisory board, and the staff.

2. The administrative group (composed of designated members of each program unit, usually those with responsibility for major program supervision): a) recommendations concerning coordination of services; b) new service recommendations to the board of directors or the administrator; c) preparation of proposals to various segments of staff.

3. Ad hoc agency committees (elected by the program units to deal with specific agencywide issues): a) all staff recommendations to the board of directors or the administrator; b) inservice training content; c) budget review for priorities; d) personnel practices such as regulations, and salary recommendations to all staff and the board of directors.

4. Program units: a) program changes within a unit; b) staff schedule; c) intake into unit; d) transfer, referral and discharge from the service; e) unit budget decisions; f) changes in use of staff and of staff patterns; g) unit routines and rules.

5. Cross-unit staff: a) exchange or sharing of staff for special team projects; b) some kinds of inservice training that may pertain to specific disciplines, programs, etc.

IMPLEMENTATION OF THE PROCESS

Determination of Client Need
In October 1972 the North Idaho Child Development Center held 14 meetings for professionals, consumers of service (parents and children), and interested citizens in eight communities to determine needs of children and families in those communities, and services the community felt would be responsive to those needs. In each meeting, the participants were requested to identify needs without establishing priority. Subsequently, the participants set up priorities and identified services that could be developed in response to the needs. Staff participated as resource persons but did not take part in identifying needs or service responses.

The staff reviewed the data gathered at these meetings, as well as other available data, and wrote proposals regarding program services. The proposals were summarized and sent to all participants in the community meetings. The participants were asked for their response by a community representative elected at the community meetings to represent them at a staff-community representative retreat. In November 1972 the staff proposals were considered at the 3-day retreat. Programs affecting all staff were voted upon. Three new programs required funds not then available: a preschool program for handicapped children in two rural communities, a life skill acquisition program for 13- to 21-year-old retardates, and a parent training program in communication skills and infant stimulation. The community representatives set the priorities for the programs; the staff had no vote on this.

Since November all of the programs have been put into operation. The first priority, the life skill acquisition program, was funded through a contract using money available through the public schools and 4-A money available to the North Idaho center. The second priority, the preschool programs for handicapped children in two rural communities, used money made available to the communities through a Title VI grant written by the Child Development Center on behalf of the school district. The third program, parent training in communication skills and infant stimulation, was developed through reallocation of existing resources within the Child Development Center and participation of AFDC recipients in infant stimulation through a special WIN program.

Full use of the participatory decision-making process allowed the North Idaho Child Development Center to develop an effective programming budget in the five-county region of North Idaho from $400,000 in fiscal 1973 to over $800,000 in fiscal 1974.

Staff Response

The initial response of staff to the participatory management practices was one of suspicion and ambivalence. As opportunities arose for the invoking of the process, staff became more committed to it. Most of those staff members who had doubts about the participatory process became committed through involvement in budget development. The give-and-take in staff's wrestling with the onerous task of developing a budget with limited funds was gratifying to both staff and management. Also, the evidence from both agencies suggests that staff are more responsible in managing their budget when they are involved in its development.

Staff are also aware that, like any other management method, democratic decision making is only as good as the administrator's intent to uphold its principles. One writer has indicated manipulatively: "An intelligent manager will, therefore, at times appoint a committee to come up with a recommendation or decision on a matter in which group deliberation is not necessary, a matter he has already decided or to which there is but one good answer. By skillful leadership or by the sheer force of facts, the group can be brought to a foregone conclusion. If the manager can avoid the appearance of 'railroading,' he is likely to obtain a stronger motivation toward acceptance in successful prosecution of a plan than if he had announced it to his subordinates without their participation" (pp. 382–383).[6]

It is unlikely that staff could long be so deluded. As Basil stated: "When a manager has already made a decision, he should never ask his subordinates to participate. The subordinates will soon recognize that the executive has made the decision and is merely attempting to placate them by discussion of alternatives" (p. 159).[2]

A method for determining what management style is current within an organization and what the staff would desire the management style to be was made available by Likert. He devised a questionnaire on organizational performance and characteristics of different management systems (pp. 223–233)[8] (pp. 14–24).[7]

This management orientation questionnaire, as modified by Comanor,[5] was administered to the staff of the North Idaho Child Development Center in June 1973. The purpose was to elicit from the staff where they thought the center was in management orientation and where the staff desired the center to be. The results of the questionnaire are shown in Fig. 1.

The respondents were 13 nonsupervisory staff and four supervisory staff. There are some parallels in the spikes and valleys in the figure between supervisory and nonsupervisory staff. In general, the nonsupervisory staff perceive the center's management system as more toward the participatory model than supervisory staff. Those areas where the spikes infringe in the benevolent-authoritarian area indicate problem areas to be overcome by management and staff, with management by participation as the goal.

The questionnaire was also broken down into responses by discipline and office location. This was useful in providing management with additional data in identifying specific areas where participatory management was working well and where problems existed.

The figure indicates that basically the management system at the center was consultative. It also indicates a strong desire by staff that the management be participatory.

DISCUSSION

Two months before the questionnaire was administered, the agency's former umbrella agency—the Idaho Department of Social and Rehabilitation Services—was merged by the Legislature on April 1 with the Department of Environmental Protection and Health. The new agency was named the Department of Environmental and Community Services. Its overall goal is to provide an integrated, comprehensive human service delivery system in a community-based service model. There was anxiety subsequent to the

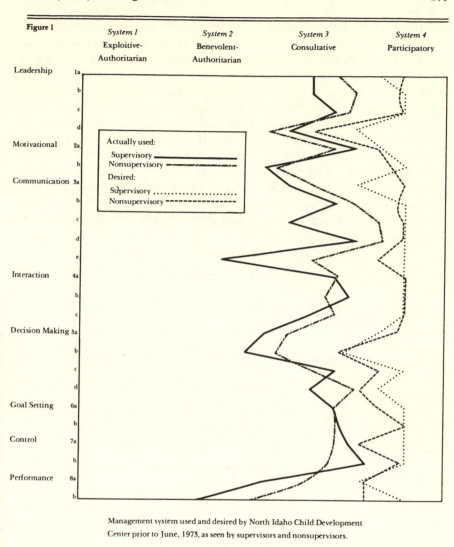

Figure 1

| | System 1 Exploitive-Authoritarian | System 2 Benevolent-Authoritarian | System 3 Consultative | System 4 Participatory |

Leadership — 1a, b, c, d

Motivational — 2a, b

Communication — 3a, b, c, d, e

Interaction — 4a, b, c

Decision Making — 5a, b, c, d

Goal Setting — 6a, b

Control — 7a, b

Performance — 8a, b

Actually used:
Supervisory ——————
Nonsupervisory ⟶⟶⟶⟶

Desired:
Supervisory ....
Nonsupervisory ----------------

Management system used and desired by North Idaho Child Development
Center prior to June, 1973, as seen by supervisors and nonsupervisors.

merger that the Child Development Center would lose its autonomy, and the participatory management system that had been operating in the agency might be lost to a less responsive, bureaucratic autocracy.

The staff was aware that even at best an agency that operates under the regulations of local, state and federal governmental agencies has difficulty in fully implementing a participatory management system. "When the top management of an enterprise is committed to System 2 (benevolent-authoritarian) and seeks to use it throughout the company, it is extremely difficult for a manager to learn System 4 (participatory management) and to shift to it" (p. 190).[7] Participatory management requires a commitment in practice by management, which will also be the watchdog and guarantor of the participatory process. If that commitment is lacking or if upper management uses an authoritarian or benevolent-authoritarian management practice, middle management will have great difficulty in implementing a participatory management system in specific areas.

The staff of the Child Development Center reaffirmed commitment to the participatory management system at a staff meeting in September 1973. At a subsequent retreat (involving representatives from the Department of Environmental and Community Services in the five northern counties of Idaho), they won unanimous adoption of a participatory management proposal affecting all staff of the newly formed department. The proposal was similar to the one adopted by the Child Development Center staff the previous year.

REFERENCES

1. Argyris, Chris. "Organizational Leadership and Participative Management," *Journal of Business*, XXVIII, 1 (January 1955).
2. Basil, Douglas C. *Managerial Skills for Executive Action*. American Management Association, 1970.
3. Berliner, A. K. "Some Pitfalls in Administrative Behavior," *Social Casework*, LII, 9 (1971).
4. Bradburd, A. W. "The Relationship of Systems Work to Administration," *Public Welfare*, XXV, 4 (1967).
5. Comanor, Al. "Program Management Workshop." Paper presented at Child Welfare League of American Northwest Regional Conference, Edmonton, Alberta, 1973.
6. Koontz, Harold, and O'Donnell, Cyril. *Principles of Management: An Analysis of Managerial Functions* (4th edition). New York: McGraw-Hill, 1968.
7. Likert, Rensis. *The Human Organization: Its Management and Value*. New York: McGraw-Hill, 1967.
8. ————. *New Patterns of Management*. New York: McGraw-Hill, 1961.
9. Litterer, Joseph A. *The Analysis of Organizations*. New York: John Wiley & Sons, 1967.

14/ASSESSING EXECUTIVE PERFORMANCE

JOSEPH H. KAHLE

Formal, written evaluation of agency executives for the purpose of improving performance has never been a common practice in the field of social work despite its widespread application to line social work staff. In fact, neither executives nor board members consider the practice a basic board responsibility, as a part of the agency's accountability to the community that supports it and to the consumers of its services. There seems to be an unspoken, mutual agreement between board and executive to avoid what both may feel would be an uncomfortable and possibly embarrassing experience. This agreement is fostered by a fictional belief that the executive will sense when his board is unhappy with him, will be able to determine the cause of this unhappiness, and will take the necessary steps to put it right—all without outside help. There is an assumption that any contact between board members and executive contains elements of evaluation and that somehow these elements will be communicated. In practice it is usual for boards to express their satisfaction by recommending salary increases and their dissatisfaction by dismissing the executive. Neither of these courses of action is really helpful to the executive or his board. Neither is a planned, open course of action. Both are reactions and usually occur "after the fact."

One might venture to say that at the present time there are few executives who either would welcome formal assessment by their boards or would even consider it particularly helpful. Perhaps experience justifies this attitude because board evaluations have been most frequently used as preliminary measures to "dumping" unwanted administrators. Used in this way, the evaluation process is a sham because the board has already made up its mind. Any pretense that the evaluation is being undertaken to help the executive under these circumstances is a distortion of a valued, professionally developed process and raises questions about the integrity of the board and the agency. However, forward-looking executives should welcome a formal evaluation process for themselves because of the help it can offer them and for the chance it can give them to judge their own positions. Since the executive's job often calls for him to walk a tight rope, it should be a relief for him to have his status made clear.

REASONS FOR EVALUATION

Because there is a lack of a systematic process of selection and preparation for administrative responsibilities, most social agency executives achieve their positions because they have demonstrated their abilities as practitioners—not as managers, planners, and leaders. Because of personal and professional interests, ambition, status, or money, many practitioners are attracted to administration. Usually they must acquire their skills ("Catch as catch can") by trial and error in a very brief period of time. Often the errors they make during the learning process are costly to them and to their agencies. Some executives attempt to acquire administrative skills through enrollment and study in management courses and workshops. Many others either do not have these resources available to them or are simply willing to subject themselves to the rigors of learning by the trial and error method. Because the social work profession has assumed little responsibility for training and educating its members for executive duties, it should at least provide a means for the administrator to gauge the quality and effectiveness of his work and offer him opportunities for improvement, if it is necessary.

Evaluation of the work of social work practitioners is an established and honored instrument for promoting professional development and has, in fact, been adopted by a number of other helping professions. The Committee on the Study of Competence of the National Association of Social Workers begins its *Guidelines for the Assessment of Professional Competence in Social Work* with the following statement: "One of the hallmarks of a profession is its willingness to set standards for its members and to have some mechanisms for designating individuals who are able to meet these norms."[1]

The report focuses on defining competence in "service activities with individuals, groups, communities, and society."[2] The committee recognized other areas of professional responsibility, among which was administration, but felt that the "feasibility and desirability of defining and assessing competence in these more indirect, implemental, professional activities are doubtful as an initial effort."[3] Since this committee completed only its initial effort in five years, it is highly unlikely that much will be done about the "indirect, implemental" areas for many years to come. With social work practice changing so rapidly, a process for evaluating administrators is needed *now*.

The literature of social work, psychology, psychiatry, medicine, education, and personnel management includes a wealth of articles on executive stress, executive failure, selection of potential executive manpower, training in various aspects of management, and ways of even eliminating unsuitable candidates for management responsibilities; there are, however, almost no references to the assessment of executive performance. Perhaps the subject is so distasteful or so foreign to us that we consciously avoid it. The lack of concern shown by our profession for the quality of its administrative leadership seems to indicate a general failure to assume legitimate professional responsibility. The Family Service Association of America recently published a guide for board members on the selection and appraisal of performance of family service agency executives.[4] Even this document, however, avoids directly confronting the issue of appraisal. It contains fifty-one pages of material closely related to selection but only two pages directly related to performance appraisal. These two pages offer the board member a number of generalizations about assessment but few specifics about how to proceed with the process.

Considering the pressures exerted on the agency executive to be a professional "jack of all trades" and to be a successful one, it is time that he received some help in building and maintaining his effectiveness as an administrator.

The executive of the voluntary agency must wear many hats and serve many masters. He must be a professional social worker, an expert office manager, a reasonably adequate accountant, a wizard at public relations, an excellent personnel officer, a top flight planner, a financial go-getter, and a chief executive.[5]

The executive must also be able to mollify his board, his staff, the agency's constituents, and the public; in addition, he must like his job in order to function effectively. If he can manage all of his responsibilities and the attendant pressures without losing his sense of perspective, he is probably performing adequately; however, he has no assurance that he is. If he cannot handle his responsibilities effectively and knows it, he would be wise to seek other work. In any case, he deserves all possible help from his board, staff, and others. Used in the same way and for the same purposes as it is with line social workers, performance evaluation can be a valuable aid to the executive in developing his administrative and leadership skills.

In addition to helping the executive measure and improve his performance, assessment serves many other less obvious but equally useful purposes. It helps to avoid situations that create conflict before they become uncontrollable. It has been said that it is easier to step on a spark before it becomes a forest fire. The saddest sights in our field are the executive who has assumed that he was functioning well and then suddenly finds himself on the brink of dismissal with no real understanding of how or why it happened and the executive who is faced by a staff revolt and is unable to understand its cause.

Every executive may become the target of a personal or professional attack for reasons over which he has no control, reasons of internal [or external] political pressures or other causes. But an executive becomes a *victim* of attack because of his own inherent weakness. If he has notions of himself that prevent a realistic assessment of his strengths, these misconceptions will allow him to compensate for weaknesses until he finds himself in a crisis situation. His illusions will cause him to falter, to lose the support he expects from trusted superiors and colleagues, and finally to lose confidence in his own ability.[6]

Despite the social agency executive's having had the advantage of social work training that presumably developed his insight and his ability to examine and weigh his own strengths and weaknesses, administrators often fall victims of their own inability to assess realistically their job effectiveness. This inability often makes the executive a "set-up" for attacks from within or from outside his own agency. Regular evaluations can serve to warn of impending trouble before it can gather enough force to overwhelm him.

ACCOUNTABILITY TO COMMUNITY

The board of directors or other governing body of a social agency is accountable to the community for the program and performance of that agency. The executive director, as its employee, is accountable to the board. As the practice of social work in agencies becomes more of an individualized professional activity, staff members assume greater responsibility for their own work. The executive needs to be somewhat less of a "controller" and more of an initiator, expediter, implementer, and coordinator. He becomes a practitioner of social work administration. As a practitioner he has a greater responsibility for accounting for his practice to his staff. It follows then that agency staff, professional colleagues, should be given opportunities to make their contributions to his evaluation just as he does to theirs. To assure that the administrator is as effective as possible, it is necessary that every agency—public and voluntary—should have as an integral part of its personnel policy a statement that the executive director will be evaluated regularly.

One view of social agency administration is that it should be responsible for initiating positive change, both within the agency as a system and within that segment of the community in which the agency exerts some influence. Too often, boards, funding bodies, and executives visualize administration in a limited way. They see the role of the executive not as a change agent but as a controller, a cost accountant, a keeper of the status quo. Because they often have limited perspectives about the function of the professional executive, agency boards may permit programs to become sterile and they may fail to keep in contact with the real and current needs of their constituents. Unless the boards are able to break away from their limited view of the executive's responsibilities, the agencies will be bypassed and will exist only as museum pieces. The role of the administrator as a change agent is a highly complicated one. If we accept the concept of administration as a tool for change as well as an instrument for management, we must also accept the responsibility for enabling the executive to develop his skills in both areas.

THE PROCESS OF ASSESSMENT

When a board undertakes to evaluate its professional executive, it will find that it is almost impossible to separate the executive from the agency. Program, effectiveness, style, relations with the community and other agencies, creativeness and relevance of the agency, and the executive become intermixed in the view of the person or organization being asked to rate the executive's competence. Although assessment of the agency may not be the primary objective of the evaluation process, it will definitely be a part of the outcome and may well have an added positive value to the board committee conducting the evaluation. It provides the committee with a view of the agency it would not ordinarily have. This view may serve as a stimulus to the board and the executive to examine, change, or reaffirm agency goals and to rally board and staff support for these goals. The process of evaluation, if board and staff are involved in meaningful ways, may bring about greater cohesiveness and unanimity among all concerned.

The process of evaluating or appraising is relatively simple although it will require considerable time and work if it is conducted properly. The first evaluation should occur no later and preferably earlier than two years after the executive begins employment. A new executive requires about two years to learn and become effective in his job. After the initial assessment, subsequent evaluations should be made at intervals of from two to five years. This policy should be made clear as a condition of employment at the time the prospective executive is being considered. Evaluations may also be initiated at any time by special request of either the board or the executive. The executive should be free to initiate an assessment when he feels it would be of value to him or when the board fails to fulfill its responsibility to complete evaluations at the specific intervals.

Although the responsibility for carrying through an evaluation lies with the full board, practicality dictates that the actual work be done by a select committee of board members thoroughly familiar with the agency's operations, programs, objectives, and goals. This committee should be selected and appointed by the board president for this specific task and should be assigned a definite deadline for the completion of its work. Before beginning the evaluation process, the board committee and the executive should have a clear agreement about the purpose of the evaluation. It should be determined if there are questions about the executive's performance and about his continued employment or if the evaluation is intended to be an aid to him.

To be meaningful to the board and helpful to the executive, the evaluation must not be limited to the observations of board or board committee members. It must make provision for the inclusion of ideas, observations, and opinions from a wide range of sources. A relatively comprehensive and unbiased view of the agency and the executive's performance can be obtained by seeking opinions not only from the agency's own board and staff but also from executives, staff, and board members of other agencies and organizations familiar with the work of the executive; such institutions as courts, schools, schools of social work, and national organizations with which the agency is affiliated; and any other meaningful and knowledgeable organizations, groups, and individuals. Finally, the executive should be expected to submit a written self-evaluation. If he is a skillful administrator, he will be honest and frank in his appraisal of his own performance.

In evaluating their staff social workers, most agencies use a guide that can readily be adapted to the tasks of the executive director. The same general headings and format that are used with other staff should be included in the executive's evaluation form. The resulting document is more easily understandable for board and staff.

The executive's job description, prepared by the board at the time he was being recruited, should be used by the committee in preparing its report. It serves as a guide for measuring the executive's progress toward accomplishing the goals set for him when he was employed. There is a danger, however, if the board committee expects rigid adherence to that job description. Jobs change as conditions in the community and the agency change. Over a period of one or two years, the executive will have modified and extended his responsibilities. If he has involved his board in the ongoing assessment of agency and community problems and conditions as well as in the ongoing activities of the agency, the modification and extension will neither constitute a threat nor evoke surprise in anyone concerned.

OUTLINE FOR AN EVALUATION

The outline for a written evaluation of the agency director was adapted from a guide used for evaluating social workers on the staff of Family Counseling Service of Seattle, Washington, and is included in the agency's staff manual. It was suggested by the executive for use by his board in conducting an evaluation of his effectiveness as the agency's chief administrator.

The written evaluation should be prepared in rough draft form and should be read by the executive and discussed with him prior to a final draft's being submitted to the board. Before the final draft is submitted, he should be given the opportunity to question, refute, amplify, and explain any areas of the document with which he disagrees or any that he feels have been overlooked. Then the final document should be prepared for the board and a copy given to the executive for his use and his personal records.

GUIDE FOR EXECUTIVE EVALUATION

  I. *The purpose of the evaluation* (This section should state briefly why the evaluation is being conducted, at whose instigation, what it proposes to accomplish, and the time interval since the last evaluation.)
 II. *Responsibilities assigned and carried* (This section should include a summary of the basic job description that was provided by the board at the time it was recruiting the executive. It should also indicate any new or ad-

ditional responsibilities that have been added or that have evolved since the beginning of his employment.)

III. *General aspects of practice* (strengths and weaknesses)

    A. What is the extent of his professional expertise? Does he attempt to increase his knowledge and keep himself informed of new developments in social work?

    B. Has he adequate working knowledge of the problems and structures and of key groups and individuals in his community?

    C. What are the quantitative aspects of his performance?

    D. How well does he organize and prepare his work?

IV. *Specific (qualitative) aspects of practice* (strengths and weaknesses)

    A. Service to the board or governing body

        1. Does he relate well to board members?

        2. Does he communicate his ideas clearly and is he receptive to communication from others?

        3. Does he involve board members meaningfully in planning, policy making, interpretation, and in the overall operations of the agency?

        4. Does he keep the board adequately informed of his activities and of the affairs of the agency?

        5. Is his general attitude acceptable to the board?

        6. Does he provide leadership in board activities?

    B. Service to the staff

        1. How well does he relate to staff?

        2. Does he understand their work and the problems that arise from their work?

        3. Does he use personnel appropriately?

        4. Does he delegate authority and responsibility appropriately?

        5. Does he communicate well with staff?

        6. Does he encourage and use staff participation in planning, policy making, and operations?

        7. Does he contribute to staff development?

        8. Is he fair in his actions relating to personnel practices?

    C. Service to the community

        1. How effective is he in his relations with funding bodies?

        2. How effective is he in his activities with planning bodies?

        3. How effective is he in his relations with other public voluntary organizations?

        4. How effective is he in community and social action?

        5. Is he effective in public relations and community education?

        6. How is he viewed by his peers in other agencies?

    D. Service to the agency program

        1. Does he plan soundly?

        2. Is he creative and innovative?

        3. Does he assume the appropriate responsibility for making decisions?

        4. Does he organize well?

        5. Does he use agency resources well?

        6. Is he effective in keeping the agency's program related to current community needs?

        7. Does he demonstrate effective leadership of the agency staff?

8. Does he understand and use the budgeting process effectively?
9. Does he demonstrate ability in developing physical and financial resources?

V. *Summary and recommendations* (This section should provide a condensation of the total evaluation; it should indicate the executive's progress toward achieving agency goals, his strengths, his problem areas, and his deficiencies. It should make recommendations for specific changes and indicate when they are expected to be accomplished. The summary should clearly state the board's satisfaction or dissatisfaction with the executive's performance.)

POSTEVALUATION PERIOD

The postevaluation period will determine whether the process has been worthwhile—whether the executive can absorb and apply what he has learned about himself. This period is a proving ground for the executive to try some new approaches to his job. He will require some time to absorb what he has learned and to put it to use. As he consciously attempts to improve his performance, he should also establish some methods for obtaining feedback about his work from board, staff, and community.

The executive may have difficulty in determining how he can use his new knowledge or how he can change some of his basic behavior patterns. In this case, he should seek a skilled professional colleague who is familiar with the problems of administration and organizational behavior—a colleague who is nonthreatening and is not in a competitive position—and use him as a "practice consultant." In fact, the use of an administrative consultant or consultants should not be limited to this situation but should be considered as a regular, problem-solving resource and used at any appropriate time. More assistance can be gained from testing ideas on an independent, unbiased, helpful consultant than can be obtained from within the executive's personal resources or from within his own organization. Although the process of undertaking an evaluation of the agency executive's performance may seem to be a weighty chore, the results in improved effectiveness for the executive, better programs and performance for the agency, and clearer understanding and improved mutual respect between board and executive should more than compensate for the effort.

REFERENCES

1. Committee on the Study of Competence, *Guidelines for the Assessment of Professional Competence in Social Work.* (New York: National Association of Social Workers, 1968), p. iii.
2. Ibid., p. 1.
3. Ibid., p. 2.
4. Family Service Association of America, *The Family Service Executive: Selection*

and Performance Appraisal (New York: Family Service Association of America, 1969).

5. Joseph H. Kahle, Structuring and Administering a Modern Voluntary Agency, *Social Work*, 14:28 (October 1969).

6. Eugene E. Jennings, The Failure-Prone Executive, *Management of Personnel Quarterly*, 5:26 (Winter 1967).

15/THE MINORITY ADMINISTRATOR: PROBLEMS, PROSPECTS, AND CHALLENGES

ADAM W. HERBERT

The first National Conference on the Role of Minorities in Urban Management and Related Fields was held in Washington, D.C., on June 10 and 11, 1973. The significance of this conference was three-fold: (1) it was the first organized national meeting of non-elected minority public administrators and educators held to discuss the problems, education, responsibilities, and needs of minority public sector professionals; (2) it represented a symbolic acknowledgement that the quest of minority groups for more responsive government must, and does now include a sophisticated concentration on the political and administrative affairs of government; and (3) its theme suggested, quite appropriately, that minority administrators do have an important and unique role to play in the public management field, which they must accept if the plight of minority (if not all) people in America is to be improved.

Since this Conference, a number of major developments around the country suggest that minority administrators, however small in number, are increasingly gaining positions from which they can respond to the universal cry for more responsive government. Five cities as diverse as Compton, California, and East Lansing, Michigan, have selected black city managers to administer their governments. Black elected administrators are leading 108 cities in all regions of the nation, including Los Angeles, Atlanta, Raleigh, and Detroit. Another 62 serve as vice mayors.[1] Data from the 1973 State and Local Information Survey (EEO-4) reveal that 18.2 percent of the total labor force in state and local governments represent minority groups (Blacks, Spanish-Surnamed Americans, Asian, American Indian, and Other). While only 6.8 percent of this group is labeled "Professional," on the surface these figures do suggest growing influence on local government policy implementation and formulation.[2]

Recent federal employment data as reflected in Table I reveal that despite the continued decline in total federal employment, minority employment has continued to increase. Total minority employment (20.4 per cent of the federal work force) expanded 1.9 per cent for the period May 1972-May 1973.[3] While the increase in the number of GS 14-15, and supergrade administrators is not significant, current hiring practices will result in greater opportunities for minorities to make inputs into agency decision-making and policy execution.

Although there has been a conscious movement toward equal employment opportunity and affirmative action in the field of public administration since the late '60s, the nature of these public sector efforts continues to be questioned in many circles. Indeed a major finding of the aforementioned Conference was that:

Minority persons are still skeptical about the willingness of governmental systems to accept them as trained professionals with the knowledge and ability to perform in administrative positions of increasing responsibility and authority.[4]

TABLE I

Net Change in Employment Under the General Schedule and Similar Pay Plan, by Grade Grouping from May 31, 1972, to May 31, 1973

Grade Grouping	Total Employ- ment Change	Minority Group Employment Change					
		Total Minority	Negro	Spanish Surnamed	American Indian	Oriental	All Other
Total, General Schedule or Similar	− 173	+11,210	+8,756	+1,913	+200	+341	−11,383
GS- 1-4	+9,159	+ 3,704	+2,797	+ 869	− 45	+ 83	+ 5,455
GS- 5-8	−6,906	+ 3,952	+3,538	+ 348	+ 48	+ 18	−10,858
GS- 9-11	−4,298	+ 2,169	+1,518	+ 434	+130	+ 87	− 6,467
GS- 12-13	+1,133	+ 961	+ 697	+ 173	+ 45	+ 46	+ 172
GS- 14-15	+ 805	+ 416	+ 199	+ 84	+ 24	+109	+ 389
GS- 16-18	− 66	+ 8	+ 7	+ 5	− 2	− 2	− 74

Source: U.S. Civil Service Commission, *Minority Groups Employment in the Federal Government* (Washington, D.C.: U.S. Government Printing Office, 1973).

This finding appears to coincide with several conclusions reached by the Civil Rights Commission in its 1969 survey of cities in seven SMSAs. While employment rates have improved for minority group administrators since this 1969 survey, some of the Commission's conclusions are worth mentioning, particularly in light of the skepticism felt by many minority group members relative to the good will of government agencies. The Commission found that:

Minority group members are denied equal access to State and local government jobs.

(a) Negroes, in general, have better success in obtaining jobs with central city governments than they do in State, county, or suburban jurisdictions and are more successful in obtaining jobs in the North than in the South.

(b) Negroes are noticeably absent from managerial and professional jobs even in those jurisdictions where they are substantially employed in the aggregate. In only two central cities, out of a total of eight surveyed, did the overall number of black employees in white-collar jobs reflect the population patterns of the cities.

(c) Access to white collar jobs in some departments is more readily available to minority group members than in others. Negroes are most likely to hold professional, managerial, and clerical jobs in health and welfare and least likely to hold these jobs in financial administration and general control.

(d) Negroes hold the large majority of laborer and general service worker jobs—jobs which are characterized by few entry skills, relatively low pay, and limited opportunity for advancement.[5]

Related to these conclusions (particularly point "C") are data from the aforementioned EEO-4 survey which indicate that while minorities do hold a number of administrative positions outside *social* agencies, most continue to work in these areas. Table II provides a summary of current local government hiring practices by functional areas. As the Civil Rights Commission indicated in 1969, minorities continued in 1973 to be assigned primarily to departments that have a "social" orientation. It is particularly significant to note that police and fire departments continue to employ significantly lower percentages of minority group people than do other governmental agencies. Financial administration also continues to be an area in which minority people have been unable to make significant inroads, although employment rates in this area are higher than in police and fire departments. It is also important to note that with the exception of housing, the percentage of professionals and officials/administrators (white collar jobs) continues to be low in all functional areas.

At the federal level, a similar pattern of minorities being hired by some agencies at much higher rates than others is evident, as reflected in Table III. Three distinguishable groups of agencies seem to be evident with reference to the percentage of minority group members employed. The first

TABLE II
Federal Government Minority Group Employment Rates, 1972–1973

Group		Per Cent Non-White Employment	Officials/ Administrators	Professionals
I	Sanitation and Sewage	38.8	12.4	8.9
	Housing	34.6	20.7	24.2
	Hospitals and Sanitariums	30.4	9.1	18.6
II	Public Welfare	23.6	11.0	15.4
	Utilities and Transport	22.7	9.4	10.6
	Other	18.9	7.9	10.0
	Employment Security	18.7	8.2	13.5
	Corrections	18.7	9.8	14.7
	Health	17.8	3.2	11.6
	Natural Resources	15.9	6.2	8.9
	Community Development	15.1	7.9	13.2
III	Streets and Highways	11.8	3.8	6.0
	Financial Administration	11.4	5.3	7.9
IV	Police	9.3	4.4	5.5
	Fire	5.0	2.2	2.8

Source: Compiled from data cited in the Equal Employment Opportunity Commission, *State and Local Government Information, EEO-4, National Statistical Summaries* (Washington, D.C.: EEOC, Office of Research, 1974).

group contains four agencies, three of which—Action, OEO, and Labor— might be labeled as "traditional." The presence of the State Department in this first group reflects a deviation from the usual governmental pattern related to minority employment. The Office of Economic Opportunity and ACTION stand out above all other federal agencies as the employers of both the greatest percentage of minority professionals at the GS 9 levels or above, and the greatest percentage of supergrade administrators. The Departments of State and Labor also have relatively high rates of minority employment overall, and particularly at the GS 9-11 levels. At the super grade levels, however, both departments have much lower minority employment rates.

The second cluster of agencies contains three departments, two of which might be labeled as "social" or "traditional" in the sense referred to by the Civil Rights Commission—Health, Education, and Welfare; and Housing and Urban Development. To some observers it may be surprising to note the presence of the Office of Management and Budget in this second group. The OMB employment figures are especially significant because of that agency's overall importance in the governmental process.

The third cluster of agencies includes Interior, Commerce, Treasury, Defense, Transportation, Justice, and Agriculture. None of these agencies are usually regarded as being social service agencies; as a consequence, the lack

TABLE III

Federal Government Minority Group Employment Rates, 1972–1973

Agencies	Total Employment Rates of Agency GS 9-18	Total Minority Employment of Agency GS 9-18	Percentage Minority Employment			
			Per Cent of Total GS 9-18	Per Cent of Total GS 9-11	Per Cent of GS 12-15	Per Cent of GS 16-18
OEO	1234	385	31.2	46.3	26.6	40.9
ACTION	946	220	23.3	30.3	19.6	18.8
State	2491	456	18.3	32.2	8.5	2.5
Labor	7568	1336	17.6	27.3	14.3	6.8
HEW	40178	5796	14.4	18.0	10.9	9.3
HUD	9912	1304	13.2	15.9	11.0	9.4
OMB	383	47	12.3	22.1	10.0	9.0
Interior	27883	2646	9.5	12.7	5.9	3.2
Commerce	16108	1434	8.9	11.7	7.3	2.3
Treasury	45133	3004	6.7	8.3	5.0	2.1
Defense	262726	16797	6.4	8.2	4.2	1.1
Transportation	46337	2578	5.6	7.9	4.3	7.0
Justice	20041	1109	5.5	7.4	3.6	3.3
Agricuture	41725	2110	5.1	6.2	3.3	2.4

Source: Compiled from data cited in the U.S. Civil Service Commission, *Minority Group Employment in the Federal Government* (Washington, D.C.: U.S. Government Printing Office, March 1974).

of substantial minority employees is not surprising. It is significant that at the federal level, as in the case of state and local governments, the percentage of minority employees decreases rapidly as decision-making responsibility (GS level) increases. The one exception to this trend is the Office of Economic Opportunity, where the percentage of supergrade administrators (40.9 per cent) is at a level comparable to those at the GS 9-11 levels (46.3 per cent) within that agency.

Although we in the public affairs field have given little attention in our literature to these data and the resulting debate, it is important to recognize that, as the number of minority professionals and administrators at all levels of government increases, the expectations of minority people for more responsive government will probably expand simultaneously. As will be argued later, the powers possessed by minorities employed in the public sector in most cases seldom are adequate to meet these expectations. As a consequence, short of a commitment on the part of administrators generally (white and non-white) to become responsive to the needs of "all" citizens, governmental agencies will continue to address on a priority basis the demands of the more powerful and affluent in our society. Where public agencies do not manifest a change in programmatic efforts which might be interpreted by minority communities as being more responsive to their needs, the tasks of minority administrators within those agencies, particularly at the local level, will become increasingly more difficult.

These difficulties will arise, in part, because of the collective perception that minority administrators understand the nature and magnitude of the problems confronting those from lower socioeconomic backgrounds. Indeed, whether one is black, brown, or red, the visible presence of an administrator with whom he/she can identify causes at least greater initial security that someone is listening who can understand the needs, realities, and perceptions being described, and who will help if at all possible.

Another factor creating the expectation among minority groups that the system will change as a result of greater "integration" of public agencies is the belief that many of these positions were made possible through community efforts. It is expected, therefore, that minority administrators and professionals will be spokesmen for other minorities out of an inherent *obligation* to speak out in their best group interest.

Perhaps the most critical factor, however, relates to bureaucratic promises made as the number of minority group members working for an agency or jurisdiction increases. In far too many cases, hiring practices are utilized to demonstrate efforts to be responsive to minority community needs. Because many agencies or governmental jurisdictions equate programmatic commitment or effort with the employment of a larger number of minorities, governmental employees from those groups can become convenient targets of protest when expectations and/or promises to the community groups are unfulfilled.

These and many other related demands and expectations create a number of major dilemmas for minority administrators to which most agencies are insensitive. In some respects many of the dilemmas and forces mentioned in this article confront all administrators, but the minority administrator seems to be subject to their weight more than most. For ultimately, every minority administrator and professional must consciously or otherwise respond to two basic and difficult questions: (1) "What responsibility do I have to minority group peoples?" (2) "What role should I attempt to play in making government more responsive to the needs of all people?"

ROLE DETERMINANTS

In addressing these questions, it is useful to consider six forces which confront the minority administrator, and which influence significantly his/her potential effectiveness and perhaps perceptions of responsibility to both the governmental agency and minority peoples more generally. Graphically these forces might be viewed as indicated in Figure 1.

A. System Demands
The first force, "system demands," refers to those expectations of public employees that a governmental system reinforces through a range of sanc-

FIGURE 1
ROLE DEMANDS ON MINORITY
ADMINISTRATORS

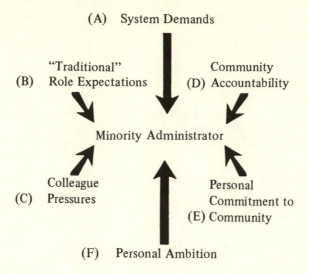

(A)   System Demands

"Traditional"   Community
(B)   Role Expectations   (D) Accountability

Minority Administrator

Colleague   Personal
(C)   Pressures   Commitment to
                                          (E) Community

(F)   Personal Ambition

tions and rewards. Bureaucratic systems are perpetuated because they demand and receive obedience to orders. The traditional model of hierarchy as described by Weber suggests that decisions are made at the top and implemented by those at lower levels within the organization. For political appointees, a failure to respond to demands made by those at the top may mean harassment, dismissal, and embarrassment. Similarly, in a civil service system, pressures are applied "to do as ordered." In cases where the civil servant "bucks" authority, intensive pressures and/or sanctions are applied (e.g., the Fitzgerald vs. Department of Defense case, as well as political pressures recently applied on the IRS, CIA, and FBI).

With regard to blacks, the system has successfully enforced its demands through a careful "weeding out" process. Only the "very best" minority group members could advance as illustrated in Sam Greenlee's novel, *The Spook Who Sat by the Door.* The techniques utilized by agencies to assure the hiring and advancement of these "outstanding" and, as Greenlee suggests, "safe" minority group members include: high education requirement, experience, oral examinations, performance tests, arrest records, probationary periods, general requirements related to residency, etc. Again, if the minority administrator is able to meet these requirements, the ongoing test that remains is that of the willingness to respond to the demands of higher-ups *without question.* Because of their historical difficulties in obtaining employment, some minority public administrators placed job security over program content or impact, and thus have become impediments to efforts to address the needs of their communities.

B. "Traditional" Role Expectations

A conventional wisdom in public administration has been that certain people do particular kinds of jobs well. Tables I and II, as well as the aforementioned Civil Rights Commission report, revealed that a large percentage of minority administrators work in specialized areas. The Civil Rights Commission noted that:

Access to white-collar jobs in some departments is more readily available to minority group members than in others. Among the seven metropolitan areas studied, the same general pattern of employment in white-collar jobs was discernable in both the North and the South. Negroes were most likely to hold jobs in health and welfare and least likely to hold them in financial administration and general control.[6]

The Commission went on to point out that:

In addition to the "old traditional jobs" for Black Americans, "new traditional jobs" appear to be emerging. These are usually jobs as staff members of human relations councils, civil right commissions, or assistants to ranking administrators. They are status jobs carrying major responsibilities and usually bring excellent salaries. But they remain almost exclusively related to minority group problems.[7]

Many of the jobs given minority administrators at both the federal and local levels have been "flack-catching" positions. As Tom Wolfe has indicated in *Radical Chic and Mau-Mauing the Flak Catcher*, during the 1960s in particular, black and brown administrators were often placed in their positions only to become sacrificial lambs in the face of community unrest.

With regard to the future, it is important that minority group members not be herded into "traditional" departments only, nor should they blindly allow themselves to be so directed. Important decisions which affect minority people are made in agencies throughout a governmental jurisdiction or agency. Minority group participation and contributions in all these decision-making processes are becoming increasingly more critical.

C. Colleague Pressures

One of the greatest dangers to the quest for governmental responsiveness remains the pressures imposed by one's peers. Peter Maas' recent book and the adopted movie, *Serpico*, clearly document the pressures which can and frequently are brought to bear on public administrators. The pressures on minority group members take many forms:

1. The minority group policeman who wants to be accepted by his peers may be forced to "bust heads" to gain acceptance, and promotions;

2. The minority welfare worker may be forced to "get tough" with welfare recipients to be regarded as a competent professional;

3. The minority school teacher is placed in the position of "blaming the victims" of the educational process to retain a place of acceptance among his/her colleagues. It is not allowed that these professionals begin to question the quality of the educational experiences of the children supposedly being served, or the unions which represent them in the quest for working conditions which may not be in the best interest of the children.

As social animals, we desire to be accepted as peers by our colleagues. It is difficult, therefore, to ward off these peer pressures. Clearly the task for the minority administrator is that of placing such collegial pressures into a perspective that does not allow them to overshadow broader program objectives and community needs.

D. Community Accountability

In recent years we have heard growing demands for greater community control, coupled with a cry for more minority group professionals who will be responsive to the needs of their people.[8] The problem historically confronting black communities in this latter regard is well described by Piven and Cloward:

Much Negro leadership exists largely by the grace of white institutions: white political parties and government agencies, white unions and businesses and professions, even white civil-rights organizations. Everything in the environment of the Negro politician, civil servant, or professional makes him attentive to white interests and perspectives.[9]

The demand is clear. Minority people want and need administrators who will listen to them, who can communicate with them, who care about them. If this is not manifested, community control becomes the ultimate demand, and perhaps a necessity.

E. Personal Commitment to Community

Of critical importance in this context is personal commitment to the community. The degree to which the administrator feels that there are obligations to fulfill and a role to be played which only he/she can fulfill can make a critical difference in public policy discussions, decisions, and ultimately, service output. It is my belief that as the number of minority administrators increases, commitment to addressing community needs will increase if only because there is more security in numbers. Equally important is the fact that a growing number of committed young minority administrators are gradually assuming more responsible positions in public agencies. They appear able to address the difficulties of balancing agency objectives with client expectations and their own personal ambitions far better than many of those who have preceded them.

F. Personal Ambition

People want to advance their careers. It is my belief that all administrators weigh important decisions not only in terms of possible programmatic consequences, but also with regard to implications for their own careers. As employment opportunities for minority group people have expanded, personal ambitions among this group have also increased. Until the early 1960s, the bureaucratic system was very effective in minimizing this desire for advancement, basically because it was clear that few opportunities for promotions into professional positions existed. As positions became more available in the 1960s, the initial result was greater competition for an apparently large but actually limited number of high-level appointments. Although employment opportunities have expanded, as mentioned above, it is still argued by some that most agencies do place limits on the numbers of minorities who will fill these positions. The challenge to minority administrators is that of seeking personal security, while simultaneously manifesting a commitment to urge greater efforts to meet governmental responsibilities more effectively.

DILEMMAS OF THE MINORITY ADMINISTRATOR

In light of the above discussion, several dilemmas stand out as being of particular significance for the minority administrator. The effective minority administrator will be one who can respond to the challenges of leadership in the quest for more responsive government in light/in spite of these obstacles:

• Governmental role expectations of minority administrators do not necessarily coincide with the minority administrator's own perceptions, goals, or expectations;

• Unresponsive public policies put minority administrators in extremely tenuous positions vis-à-vis the agency, himself/herself, and the community of which he/she is a part;

• Frequently the minority administrator is put into flack-catching positions without the capacity to make meaningful decisions, but is expected to accept the responsibilities of programmatic failures and "keep the natives calm."

• Advancement within the governmental system is generally a function of adherence to established organizational norms; one of these norms historically has been that one need not be concerned about the needs or priorities of minority communities.

• Informal pay and promotional quotas still seem to exist for minority administrators; moreover, it is assumed that they can only fill certain types of positions, usually related to social service delivery or to communication with other minority group members.

• Minority communities sometimes expect much more of the minority administrator than he/she can provide; and in most cases demand a far faster response to their demands than these administrators have developed the capacity to deliver.

• Agencies seem to search for the "super" minority administrator; and even these are frequently hired as show pieces. In other cases there has been evidence of agencies hiring individuals who clearly would be unable to do a job with the intent of showing that an effort was made but "they just can't do this kind of work."

While other dilemmas might be identified, this brief listing seems to re-enforce the argument that the task of being a minority administrator within public agencies is not an easy one. Moreover, in the short run the challenges reflected in these dilemmas may become greater in magnitude as governments at all levels fail to address in a meaningful fashion such quality of life problems as hunger, health, housing, etc.

CONCLUSION

For almost two centuries, minority groups have been systematically excluded from making inputs into the administrative processes of government as both decision makers and policy implementors. In the final analysis, it is now the responsibility of governmental leaders generally to expand opportunities for the perspectives of minority administrators to be articulated and acted upon. This responsibility derives not only from executive orders and congressional mandates, but also from the reality that there frequently is a minority perspective on public problems which policy makers should understand if public programs are to be truly responsive and effective.

Schools of public affairs also have a major charge to educate more minority administrators to assume these critical positions. The frequently criticized decrease in foundation monies previously utilized to provide financial assistance to these students must not be utilized as a cop-out to explain away lack of effort in this regard. The minority academic also has a role to play in supporting these efforts to provide the kind of professional training essential to the development of the number and caliber of top-flight minority administrators so critically needed in public agencies. They must also begin to work more closely with both minority elected officials and administrators in continuing education, and in policy research and analysis if some of the major problems facing minority group communities are to be effectively described, understood, and attacked.

Finally, to the minority administrator goes the challenge of accepting the obligation of working for the development and operation of public programs which more effectively meet the needs of *all* people. In some cases this may require an advocacy position. It may demand that the minority group perspective on public policy questions be researched, developed, and articulated. It will frequently demand the capacity and willingness to discuss policy options, directions, and needs with those who have expressed a lack of faith in the governmental process. It will demand a rejection of the argument that administrators are/must be value free and completely neutral in implementing policy decisions. Simultaneously, however, there exists the reality that public employees do work within a bureaucratic context with established procedures, job requirements, and program objectives. These neither can, nor should be ignored. Nor should minority public administrators be *expected* to present minority views, or be given positions solely because they are black, red, or brown. Public agencies, however, must begin to recognize and accept the reality that, in light of the problems confronting our society, it is in the public interest that minority administrators not forget who they are, or from whence they have come.

NOTES

1. Joint Center for Political Studies, *National Roster of Black Elected Officials* (Washington, D.C.: the Joint Center, April 1974).
2. Equal Employment Opportunity Commission, *State and Local Government Information EEO-4 National Statistical Summaries* (Washington, D.C.: Office of Research, 1974).
3. U.S. Civil Service Commission, *Minority Group Employment in the Federal Government* (Washington, D.C.: U.S. Government Printing Office, March 1974), pp. i, ii.
4. *Summary of the First National Conference on the Role of Minorities in Urban Management and Related Fields* (Washington, D.C.: Metropolitan Washington Council of Governments, 1973), p. 19.
5. U.S. Commission on Civil Rights, *For All The People . . . By All The People* (Washington, D.C.: U.S. Government Printing Office, 1968), p. 118.
6. *Ibid.*, p. 2.
7. *Ibid.*, p. 3.
8. For a representative sample of the literature describing these attitudes, see: Alan Altshular, *Community Control* (New York: Pegasus, 1970); Charles E. Wilson, "Year One at I.S. 201," *Social Policy* (May/June 1970), pp. 10–17; Sherry R. Arnstein, "Maximum Feasible Manipulation," *Public Administration Review*, Vol. XXXII (September/October 1972), pp. 377–390; and Mario Fantini and Marilyn Gittell, *Decentralization: Achieving Reform* (New York, Praeger, 1973).
9. Francis Fox Piven and Richard A. Cloward, "Black Control of Cities," in Edward S. Greenburg, et al. (eds.), *Black Politics* (New York: Holt, Rinehart and Winston, Inc., 1971), pp. 128–129.

16/WOMEN IN SOCIAL WORK ADMINISTRATION: CURRENT ROLE STRAINS

MARY S. HANLAN

Sexism in the profession of social work is an area receiving increasing attention in the seventies. Long perceived as a woman's profession, social work was felt to be somehow immune from the sex-role stereotyping that has pervaded our society and has generally escaped critical challenge in this area until recently. A perceptive exception to this view can be found in the writings of Bertha Reynolds, who, as early as 1942, cogently observed that:

Women have been discriminated against in every profession open to them at all, receiving less pay for the same work (or for more skilled and conscientious service). They have had either to struggle to the top by exceptional ability, or to be content in the role of assistant to men who were often less qualified than they.[1]

Only recently has there been much serious thought given to this problem. And only recently have studies appeared which document more precisely the lesser valuation placed on the contribution of women to social work as compared to men. These studies have related to two aspects, primarily: (1) status and salary differentials between male and female social workers,[2] and (2) different standards of health for men and women in general.[3]

It is well recognized that men have moved into higher status roles and received higher salaries within the profession, despite the fact that two-thirds of the profession are women, but data on this phenomenon have only recently been collected. Williams, Ho, and Fielder, in a study of salaries of all MSSW graduates of one school of social work (covering a period of nineteen years), assessed or controlled the variables of family commitment, career tenure, education, and, to some extent, job mobility as a way of meaningfully evaluating the differences.[4] The results indicated that large and statistically significant differences in salaries of males and females still remained when these factors were controlled in the comparisons; without such control, the differences would have been even greater. The authors felt that:

In general, the results seem to suggest that professional women do not receive lower salaries because of family obligations, inadequate education, or less career experience, or part-time work. Salary differences remain when these variables are ruled out. Rather, the results indicate that women seem to fare badly in the promotion-decision structure.[5]

Reports on two surveys among members of the National Association of Social Workers (NASW), one among all members in 1971–72 and the other among members entering the association from 1973–75 (predominantly new social work graduates), compared percentages of each sex in administration (representing a higher status) and their salaries.[6] In the 1971–72 study, 37 percent of the men and 18 percent of the women identified administration as their primary method; in the later study, the ratio was similar, with 11 percent of the men and 5 percent of the women in administration.

With the larger N in the 1971–72 data, it was possible further to categorize the female respondents as to marital and family status, as in the study by Williams et al.,[7] in order to understand better the data. Single women, and those who were previously married and had no children, showed the highest percentage in administration—22 percent; among married women with children, 14 percent; and among married women with no children, 13 percent. Thus the lower proportion of married women in administration is probably significantly influenced by the disruption of careers through family moves and/or the assumption of parental responsibility. Salaries varied similarly. Fanshel, who analyzed the data, is careful to point out, however, that although some of the sex differentiation in salaries of administrators is related to marital status and parenthood, "there is still a gap between the salaries of men and women in administration that is not explained by family characteristics."[8]

The seminal study by Broverman et al. in the late sixties has implications far beyond the issue of clinical judgments, important as that may be.[9] In their survey of seventy-nine practicing psychologists, social workers, and psychiatrists, they found a double standard of mental health being subscribed to by male and female clinicians alike. Characteristics of healthy individuals not only differed as a function of sex of the person judged, but these differences paralleled stereotypic sex-role differences (i.e., healthy, mature women are supposed to be more emotional, easily hurt, and submissive, and less independent, objective, and competitive than healthy, mature men). Even more disturbing,

behaviors and characteristics judged healthy for an adult, sex unspecified, which are presumed to reflect an ideal standard of health, will resemble behaviors judged healthy for men, but differ from behaviors judged healthy for women.[10]

As the authors point out in a later study:

If women adopt the behaviors specified as desirable for adults, they risk censure for their failure to be appropriately feminine; but if they adopt the behaviors that are designated as feminine, they are necessarily deficient with respect to general standards for adult behavior.[11]

Feminists have begun to point out the underpinnings of such judgments in the theoretical paradigms commonly used by therapists,[12] and it is clear that such paradigms have formed a large part of the basis of social work education of most current practitioners, including administrators, and have reinforced already existing stereotypes. Interestingly enough, some reassessment of such valuation of "sex-related" characteristics seems to have occurred with more recent graduates. Harris and Lucas, partially replicating the study of Broverman et al., with social work students in 1974, found that sex-role stereotypes seem to be changing among both male and female students, although females seem to be revising their views at a more rapid rate. Male and female students still had, nevertheless, a strong difference of opinion in their concepts of a healthy woman, and thus differing expectations for female competence.[13]

Given this background—the rewards of the profession (salaries and status) accruing mainly to men, and a society which has agreed with that valuation—the following statement, which recently appeared in the *NASW News*, is less surprising: "If the present trend continues, there will be no women in social work leadership positions by the year 1984."[14] Based on a survey of top administrators in four major national organizations (Family Service Association of America, Child Welfare League of America, federally funded Community Mental Health Centers, and the National Jewish Welfare Board), the statistics indicated that over the last two decades men have replaced women in administrative positions at the rate of 2 percent per year.[15]

How did it come about that a "woman's profession" is led primarily by men and, if present trends continue, will soon be completely so? Interestingly enough, some of the same kind of stereotypic thinking was involved, although then seen as a potential advantage. In the late forties and early fifties, social work, concerned with its professional image, attempted to develop a more rational, scientific (i.e., "male") base and actively recruited men into the profession. Kravetz reminds us that

women in the semiprofessions, that is, in teaching, nursing, and social work, did not reject the assumptions underlying the sexual division of labor in society; sex-role socialization effectively controlled their professional behavior and goals. They did not actively pursue higher-level positions and were more interested in direct service to clients than in broader policy and professional issues.[16]

In the next two decades, male and female social workers began to divide themselves into areas of social work most consistent with traditional roles, men going into community organization and administration (requiring independence, aggression, and ability to work with business and community leaders) in disproportionate numbers;[17] casework and group work remained feminine domains, with the emphasis on nurturing. Status and salaries divided on similar lines.

Kadushin refers to this process as a way by which males reduce the role strains inherent in practicing a profession seen as female, stating that:

Traditionally, people entering a profession that is inappropriately sex-typed for their gender have made efforts to reduce this discrepancy by specializing in an activity that is more appropriately sex-typed.[18]

And, a little later:

The procedure most frequently utilized by male minorities to reduce role strain in female professions is to move toward administrative positions. In all female professions, the administrative level of the organizational hierarchy becomes a male enclave. . . .[19]

He then argues for the functional necessity of male administrative enclaves, saying that the move to administration mitigates a number of different role strains and status inconsistencies for a male in a female profession.[20] This might have helped the male psyche and bank account and, in fact, upgraded the entire profession; but it has also clearly increased the bind of the woman social work administrator or the woman social worker who aspires to a better paying position. Currently, in our real, still sex-typed world, administration is perceived as basically a male function and the woman who aspires to this career as deviant. The "maleness" of administration is seen as overriding the "femaleness" of the profession, and social workers are being asked to protect this distinction.

Thus is posited the dilemma for women social workers who wish to enter administration or simply to increase their salaries, which may be the same thing. The same kind of sex-related role strain that has propelled men into administration and to form enclaves there has acted to inhibit women from exercising that function. It now requires an unusually competent woman, secure in her sexual identifications, to withstand the strains and contradictions currently inherent in the role of social work administrator. Ozawa, talking about women and careers in general, states:

. . . there seems to be a cultural schizophrenia in the United States that places women in a no-win situation. In an achievement-oriented society like ours, women are encouraged to succeed in their work but not to the extent they lose their femininity. If they fail in their work, they are not meeting their own standards of performance; if they succeed in it, they may not be living up to societal expectations regarding the role of women.[21]

The highest level of "success" in social work—in terms of status and salary—is in administrative posts. It is not surprising, though, that few women are lining up for such positions. Interesting exceptions to this trend are the deanships of schools of social work, where, although there are still fewer than 15 percent women deans, the proportion is increasing rather than decreasing.[22] With all the known problems of such positions in this time of shrinking funding, however, the perceived desirability of such jobs is also decreasing. Women's increased accessibility to such positions may therefore be more a function of the lessened desirability and status of deanships today than of search committees' perceptions of women candidates as being as competent as their male counterparts.

Some degree of role strain and conflict, then, remains an integral part of the leadership function for most women administrators today. Since they may be "less desirable" on some counts, generally they have had to be more competent to "make up" for it, a phenomenon well known to other minorities. Lacking many role models, women administrators also need a heavy dose of patience and a tolerancy of ambiguity to cope with all the possibilities of misunderstandings, misconceptions, and resentment which may be present.

The actual degree of role strain obviously varies according to the perceptions and status of the many role reciprocants with which the woman administrator is involved. With superiors and peers (usually male), she may initially try to be both "feminine" (in traditional terms) and extra competent, in order to develop respect for her performance without the hostility incumbent upon perceived threats to her colleagues' masculinity. Unfortunately, as writers are beginning to point out,[23] such competence often has to be demonstrated without much help from the informal structures of the organization. In fact, one of the most difficult phenomena with which women administrators often have to cope is the lack of access to nonformalized information. In a large organization, particularly, the ability to make good administrative judgments may depend upon open channels and an active informal communications network; yet access to the latter may be far more rigidly controlled by traditional thinking than are more formal avenues.

A female administrator may well need to develop her own power base, whether through access to a reference group deemed valuable by her colleagues or through the development of a separate constituency (usually external, though sometimes internal) from a particularly good or innovative program. The perception of this strength and potential value to the agency may well be the key to at least the beginning inclusion into the more informal network. However, it must be remembered that an outside power base can also be exceedingly threatening, and considerable thought must be given to timing and to the use of influence from such a base.

With subordinates, other kinds of problems can arise. Traditional values assume male administrators; thus, it takes an unusually secure male to feel comfortable in having a woman in a superordinate position. For either sex, there may also be the very real question as to whether or not a woman administrator can command as many resources as a male counterpart, given our less than androgynous world. A subordinate may feel he/she is jeopardizing his/her own position by being in a department or agency headed by a woman. There is thus additional pressure for women administrators to be more competent than their male peers in order to be, and to be seen as being, equally effective in the garnering and development of resources. Minor reminders of perceived status differentials come through from clerical staff as well: (1) male administrators' work is often finished first, and (2) written memoranda may contain titles (e.g., Dr. or Mr.) when referring to males but be omitted altogether when referring to females.

The pervasiveness of such stereotypic habits and thinking can indeed be discouraging to the neophyte woman administrator. What, then, can be done to reduce some of these role strains, so that 1984 may not really become the Year of the Big Brother in social work?

1. The notion that male administrative enclaves ought to be protected should be firmly and unequivocally rejected. The rationale for such thinking belongs to a bygone era. We can appreciate its functional value in a society committed, consciously or otherwise, to a sex division of labor but our society is no longer so committed ideologically, even though clearly we all feel its ingrown strength. In a profession committed to the innate dignity of all human beings, we should work to eliminate sexism, not apologize for it nor institutionalize it.

2. There should be specific training of women for managerial positions. Such training should include not only skills neglected during an earlier time when management was seen as male, but also discussion of women's own lingering views of themselves as less than feminine when assertive and competent, as well as to defuse some of the anxiety which results from such role conflicts.[24] Similar training and resocialization have been part of centers for continuing education for women for some time. Administrative and managerial training should also include understanding of informal organizational processes as well as the more formal ones. Much work is actually accomplished through these channels, and it is an exceedingly problematic area for a female minority in a male-dominated group.

3. Thought should be given to the possibilities of differing career patterns and their applicability to managerial and administrative positions. Sheehy's popular book *Passages* has done much to change views as to what constitutes a "normal" (i.e., male) life cycle.[25] Many women have felt too inadequate to apply for a higher status position, assuming that their "patchwork quilt" résumé will be judged against a single standard of career achievement. More flexible standards of what is considered good preparation for an administrative career might not only help women's perceptions

of themselves as adequate for such a career, but hopefully also free some men from the necessity of maintaining such a narrow track as well.

In sum, with the federal government's prohibiting discrimination in employment and the social work profession's commitment to eliminating sexism in all its aspects, the potential reality of an all-male pyramidal apex seems grossly out of step. As with other sex-role changes in our society, debating whether inner or outer constraints and incongruencies must be addressed first is almost irrelevant; they simply must be addressed.

NOTES

1. Bertha Reynolds, *Learning and Teaching in the Practise of Social Work* (New York: Farrar and Rinehart, Inc., 1942), p. 192.
2. See especially David Fanshel, "Status Differentials: Men and Women in Social Work," *Social Work* 21 (November 1976): 448–54; C. Bernard Scotch, "Sex Status in Social Work: Grist for Women's Liberation," *Social Work* 16 (July 1971): 5–11; and Martha Williams, Liz Ho, and Lucy Fielder, "Career Patterns: More Grist for Women's Liberation," *Social Work* 19 (July 1974): 463–66.
3. See especially I. K. Broverman, D. M. Broverman, R. E. Clarkson, P. Rosenkrantz, and S. R. Vogel, "Sex-Role Stereotypes and Clinical Judgments of Mental Health," *Journal of Consulting and Clinical Psychology* 34 (February 1970): 1–7; I. K. Broverman, S. R. Vogel, D. M. Broverman, F. E. Clarkson, and P. S. Rosenkrantz, "Sex-Role Stereotypes: A Current Appraisal," *Journal of Social Issues* 28 (April 1972): 59–78; and Lindo Hall Harris and Margaret Exner Lucas, "Sex-Role Stereotyping," *Social Work* 21 (September 1976): 390–395.
4. Williams et al., "Career Patterns," pp. 463–66.
5. Ibid., p. 466.
6. Fanshel, "Status Differentials," pp. 448–54.
7. Williams et al., "Career Patterns," pp. 463–66.
8. Fanshel, "Status Differentials," p. 453.
9. Broverman et al., "Sex-Role Stereotypes and Clinical Judgments of Mental Health," pp. 1–7.
10. Ibid., p. 1.
11. Broverman et al., "Sex-Role Stereotypes: A Current Appraisal," p. 75.
12. See especially Carol Wesley, "The Woman's Movement and Psychotherapy," *Social Work* 20 (March 1975): 120–24.
13. Harris and Lucas, "Sex-Role Stereotyping," pp. 390–95.
14. Juliana Szakacs, "Survey Indicates Social Work Women Losing Ground in Leadership," *NASW News* 22 (April 1977): 12.
15. Ibid.
16. Diane Kravetz, "Sexism in a Woman's Profession," *Social Work* 21 (November 1976): 422.
17. George Brager and John A. Michael, "The Sex Distribution in Social Work: Causes and Consequences," *Social Casework* 50 (December 1969): 569.
18. Alfred Kadushin, "Men in a Woman's Profession," *Social Work* 21 (November 1976): 444.
19. Ibid.
20. Ibid.
21. Martha N. Ozawa, "Women and Work," *Social Work* 21 (November 1976): 458.

22. Szakacs, "Survey Indicates Social Work Women Losing Ground In Leadership," p. 12.
23. See Barbara Stephens Brockway, "Assertive Training for Professional Women," *Social Work* 21 (November 1976): 498–505.
24. Ibid.
25. Gail Sheehy, *Passages: Predictable Crises of Adult Life* (New York: E. P. Dutton and Co., Inc., 1974).

C. BOARD–EXECUTIVE RELATIONSHIPS

17/BOARD, EXECUTIVE, AND STAFF

HERMAN D. STEIN

A good deal has been written about boards and executives and the relationship of both to staff. With most of what has been written one can take no exception. The words of Eduard Lindeman about boards and volunteers remain as sound today as they were when he first uttered them. Records of board institutes of twenty-five and thirty years ago contain useful and important lessons.[1] More recent works like Sorenson's *The Art of Board Membership*,[2] Houle's *The Effective Board*,[3] Schmidt's *The Executive and the Board in Social Welfare*[4] and Trecker's many works on administration[5] and on board membership all contain important, sound principles for useful practice. Many journal articles offer fine material.[6] What is there to add?

Two things, perhaps. One is more prodding below the surface of the principles that have been thus far developed. The other is the raising of some nagging questions about generalizations that we may regard as self-evident.

The time has passed for mere registering of complaints and wringing of hands or, for that matter, for self-congratulation on the wonders of voluntarism. We are in a period where only the most sober and hardheaded analysis of our organizational problems will do. Social welfare, voluntary or governmental, is coming increasingly into the forefront of public attention, and our responsibilities to society are deep and serious. The inner organizational relationships among board, executives, and staff represent one facet of these problems and to the extent that further analysis can improve our operations and thus the manner in which we discharge our responsibilities, this area merits continued exploration.

My task, therefore, is to examine some of the existing realities and to raise questions about some well-established tenets and assumptions.

1. THE MOTIVATION OF TRUSTEES

A decade or so ago some people were shocked to learn that eminent trustees in agencies all over the country, voluntary and public, may have had as part of their motivation for becoming trustees a prestige, political or other self-interest objective. Now we realize that excellent trustees may be utterly dedicated and altruistic or may have some degree of self-interest.

Houle reports on a survey which found that 10 percent of the members of local boards of education were extremely altruistic, 36 percent apparently altruistic, 44 percent partially self-interested, and 10 percent extremely self-interested.[7] Studies of social agency boards refer to the same phenomenon, although not in statistical terms.[8] This information should be no more surprising than the fact that some social workers come to their profession completely altruistically and some with other motivations in mind. We are far more interested in the surgeon's capacity to wield the scalpel effectively than in his dedication to surgery. What his motivations are may affect his chances of selecting and being accepted for a medical career, and how good a doctor he becomes, but the test of whether he is a good doctor lies in his performance, not in his motivations. The same is true of board members, of professional social workers, and of almost everyone else.

We have no evidence to suggest that board members are any more or any less dedicated than are professionals. We should not expect board members to be angelic any more than we expect staff members to be angelic. We have a right, however, to expect competence in their respective roles. What is essential to keep in mind is that the presence of some degree of self-interest among some proportion of trustees does not necessarily conflict with dedication to their work, and that a degree of self-interest does not necessarily impair the productive effort of a board member any more than it does that of a staff member.

2. POLICY AND EXECUTIVE; BOARD AND EXECUTIVE

If we agree that the evaluation of board member and executive behavior should be made on the basis of performance without reference to motivation, we then have to consider what comprises the job of each. We have had many words about this, and most of them have been good words. We have been told in no uncertain terms that policy determination is the responsibility of the board alone, that policy execution is the responsibility of executive and staff, that the executive ultimately is responsible for the results of agency programs. Nearly everyone understands these points and yet boards and executives have had trouble ever since there were boards and executives.

It is not, of course, only in social work that problems arise. Every field has its own version of the same underlying concerns. Note, for example, these quotes from a manual for trustees of colleges and universities, written by a retired college president some fifteen years ago:

Certainly, the president should feel free to suggest changes in policy and the trustees should give his suggestions careful consideration, but the fact remains that the control of policy is a function of the trustees and one of their most important functions. It is also one of which they very often lose sight. . . . When the trustees overlook their function of determining policies, they tend to become an official rubber stamp of the actions of the president. It is rather their duty to assure themselves that the president's administration conforms to the policies laid down by themselves.[9]

A shocking percentage of the 17,000 men and women serving as trustees, directors and members of the boards controlling our American colleges and universities know little of their responsibilities and care little about their institutions, perfunctorily attend board meetings, and approve presidential recommendations without understanding or serious consideration. On the other hand, there is no finer or more valuable group of people in the country than our able, responsible college trustees.[10]

Nothing would be gained by an attempt to analyze the nature of potential difficulties by assigning the role of villain either to board or to executive. It is more to the point to suggest that there are inherent functions and relationship problems which simply have to be understood and coped with and that good will alone will not prevent difficulties from arising. Basic to these problems is the determination of what is policy and what is execution, or professional responsibility, and the way in which this decision is made.

The matter of waiting lists offers one kind of test by which casework agencies and clinics can determine whether they are attributing a policy character or a professional character to a given type of decision. Let us take a community psychiatric clinic as an example. One could drop a psychiatric clinic almost anywhere in the country and have a waiting list within a matter of weeks. It is not only that many people want psychiatric care, but that quite a number of organizations—schools, hospitals, recreational agencies—breathe a sigh of relief when a psychiatric clinic is available and automatically refer to it clients with whom they cannot deal. As Dr. Jerome Frank has pointed out, it is one facility that breeds its own public.[11] Now some psychiatric clinics grapple with their waiting list problem by making sure that everyone is seen for at least 15 minutes or so to make sure that he is in the right place and then determine whether his situation is critical or not. If he is not in the right place, he goes somewhere else. If the situation is not critical, he is left on the waiting list, in the hope that perhaps he will get better while he is waiting. These tactics have reduced waiting lists considerably. It does mean, however, that staff is engaged in seeing more people, for fewer interviews per person and with less per capita time for interviews, so as to make sure that no emergency situation is skipped. The principle here is to provide the widest spread of service for those in need.

In other clinics, the decision is that good standards must not be jeopardized, and if someone requires intensive interviews several times a week over a period of many months or years, that is what the agency will provide. If such a policy leads to a waiting list, there is a waiting list. Another factor may be that the existence of a waiting list acts as a constant source of pressure on the financial powers that be.

If the board does not determine waiting list policy, the decision is made by the executive and staff and may never come before the board as a policy issue. If, however, the board considers intake in terms of the disposition of agency resources, the matter would become a policy question on which it would have to take a formal position. Every type of agency has these borderline issues, and I submit that in the rational determination of what is a policy matter, and who determines it, lies the true test of the board's assumption of policy responsibility.

Here is where one touches the concept of "strong" and "weak" executives. Often a "strong" executive is termed such because he basically determines as well as initiates policy and makes it easy for the board to accept his position. There are really strong executives whose strength in the executive role does not lie in sapping the strength of the board, even if it prefers to be supine. The executive in this context makes it possible for the board members to exercise their prerogatives intelligently and deliberately, and if their point of view conflicts with that of the executive, there is no loss of confidence in the executive. In other words, he helps the board to carry its own responsibilities whether it wishes to do so or not.

Sometimes a board simply cannot seem to take a policy position on an informed or dispassionate basis. Short of resigning, the executive has little choice other than to lead the board to make what he considers to be the best decision and gradually to help the board members become more aware of the preparation they need in order to make decisions themselves. For an executive to accept a policy-directing function permanently, however, even with board encouragement, is to lay the groundwork for serious agency weakness.

There were dramatic shifts in board-executive roles in an old-fashioned children's agency whose board members' favorite activity was that of running the Thanksgiving programs. There was only one trained worker, and frequent turnover made it difficult to keep the position filled. About ten years ago the board expanded to more than sixty members in order to provide for continuity. The younger members continued to review cases and hire and fire personnel, but they did not like the new executive who had been hired by the old guard. He was low-salaried, stuffy, and penurious. The younger members could not get him discharged, but they nagged him by insisting that they be allowed to read records, in accordance with the time-honored practice of this agency. The poor executive had to retain some measure of self-esteem and professional pride, and so he resigned. His replacement had excellent qualifications and demanded a good salary. He quickly established his sphere of authority, acquired good staff, worked rationally and flexibly with his board, gradually got them out of their old ways, and developed a fine board whose members understood and accepted their appropriate responsibilities. They would not dream of looking at a case record, and they were far more comfortable in this pattern than in the old. Moral: Boards can change if executives make it possible.

3. EVALUATION OF THE EXECUTIVE

Whether an agency is a small one or a large one, it is usually the executive more than any other single individual who is assumed to represent the interests, the goals, the cultural climate, and the values of the organization. In any organization, therefore, the operating premise should be that the board supports the executive since the board supports the agency as a whole. Anything which is likely to upset the security of the executive upsets the stability of the agency and is not in its interests.

Both because this is a conscious premise and because it is a natural tendency of sympathetic board members, boards tend to lean over backward not to imperil the security and stability of the executive position. This can lead to a dilemma: how can the board support the executive and yet perform one of its key functions, namely, evaluate his work.

Again, we are interested in principles. One principle is that the board should be in a position to evaluate the executive; that means that the board, or at least its officers, should have the information that will enable it to judge executive performance. Another principle is that this evaluation should be formal, and regularized, and so carried out that the position of the executive is not made untenable. If there is a formal evaluative session with the executive—as generally there should be—it would not be held in order to discover all the weaknesses of the executive and everything that has gone wrong in the agency but to consider together what the strong and weak points have been in the past and what better might be done, where executive performance bears on agency results.

If, indeed, an executive's performance is so questionable that his position is in jeopardy, this situation would, of course, have to be handled. But a formal evaluation session makes it possible to prevent minor questions or criticisms from becoming major rumors of board opposition to an executive. It makes it possible to put all these questions together in a neutral atmosphere at an appropriate and scheduled occasion. No matter how close and warm the daily interaction between the executive and the board may be, this kind of session is most wholesome, and gives both the executive and the board an opportunity to take a careful, reflective look at past achievements and weaknesses and direct their relationship in the future.

4. CLIQUES AND FRIENDSHIPS

There will usually be cliques in large boards. One way to minimize the likelihood of a clique-*ruled* board is to limit the number of board members. If a board has 100 members of whom no more than 20 or 30 usually attend meetings and only 7 or 8 participate on important committees, the likelihood is that no more than the 7 or 8 will be truly influential in making board decisions. The other board members will be on the outside looking in, either attempting to participate in meetings with middling success, or giving up and staying on the board as a necessary chore or as a desultory activity until something better comes along.

Even on medium-sized boards of fifteen to twenty-five a few members will have more influence than others. There should be some delegation of authority. The chairman should be the most important member of the board, and the executive committee should be among its most influential members. Differentiation of inner board status in this sense is not a weakness.

That friendship groups exist within the board does not mean that the body itself is weakened unless these friendships control decisions before the issues reach formal channels. Here is where the board chairman has one of his greatest responsibilities. No matter what the personal relationships may be, he must see to it that board decisions are made as part of the formal activity of the board.

Moreover, a personal relationship between some board members and the executive which interferes with business-like decisions poses a severe organizational strain and constitutes a trap for all concerned. I have made my position clear elsewhere and shall simply restate it.[12] First, I am in favor of friendship. If an executive and members of the board become personal friends, there is nothing inherently wrong with this. What is important, however, is that the informal relationship be kept as distinct as possible from the formal relationship; the larger and more complex the organization, the more important this is. It should be possible for a difference of opinion to arise at a board meeting even among friends. It should also be possible if an agency matter comes up in private conversation for one party to say, "Well, this ought to be brought to the board," instead of letting it be settled outside the board meeting so that either it will never come up before the board or will appear as a *fait accompli*. It requires self-discipline and sophistication to maintain distinct roles, but it is altogether possible; for the separation of friendship and organizational roles is achieved in many agencies.

5. BOARD-STAFF RELATIONSHIPS

Most references in the literature represent a close relationship between board and staff as a good. In other words, the more board and staff interact, the better. Sorenson states: "It is also wise to allow other senior staff members to attend board meetings with absolute freedom. Mystery is thereby dispelled and acquaintanceship promoted."[13] He suggests that other staff members may also benefit from attending board meetings as a training device and that there should be rotations in presentations by staff members to board.

The factor of size is quite important in determining what is a useful relationship between board and staff. In a small agency consisting of the executive and two professional staff members it makes sense for all the staff to know the board, and vice versa. There should be a great deal of face-to-face contact and participation on policy and direction. Quite the reverse, however, can be true of a larger, more complex organization. If one is working with 100 professional staff members, 150 nonprofessional staff members, and a board of 40 who have many other claims on their time and energies, it is both unrealistic and unnecessary to impose close and frequent interaction between board and staff.

This does not mean that staff should never see the board or vice versa. It does mean that the occasions for such meetings would be relatively formal when, for example, the program of the entire agency is being discussed, or quasi-formal when it is a matter of becoming familiar with names and faces.

So far as participation of staff members in board meetings is concerned, the central principle is that their participation should be encouraged when it is relevant to the program of the organization—not for training purposes in how to prepare a case presentation, nor to enable the board in large organizations to know the staff. It often makes sense, when particular staff members have special competence to serve on board subcommittees, for them to do so and therefore to be in rather close association with certain members of the board. However, it should be recognized that in relatively large agencies the organization does not require one-to-one contacts between board members and staff. It is usually all the board can do to take care of its immediate responsibilities adequately with the participation of the executive, and merely going through the motions of becoming acquainted with staff members is worse than useless. Staff should, nevertheless, know who board members are, should have some general occasions to meet them outside the board meeting, and through the actual policies of the organization should develop awareness and respect for their leadership.

A problem remains, and it is a serious and difficult one. In the large organization, where hierarchical lines of authority are observed, staff have no direct access to the board formally except through the executive. When all goes well, this is fine. But if trouble is brewing between executive and staff, there may be no way for the board to know it until a crisis develops. Developing board-staff lines that bypass the executive's authority will seriously weaken the organization. Ways should therefore be found for the board to satisfy itself on appropriate staff involvement in policy and on understanding staff views expressed through formal channels. It should also be possible, particularly in the large agency, for there to be a channel from staff to board available in cases of really serious disagreement between executive and staff, a channel which the executive himself keeps open. (I am glad that Houle takes this view.[14]) Even if this device is never used, its existence attests to a basic relationship of trust and confidence, and to a democratic spirit in administrative policy.

It must not be assumed, however, that distance between board and staff constitutes a problem only with voluntary agencies. While public boards are constituted under various legal arrangements and their powers are more clearly spelled out than is true of voluntary agency boards, the remoteness of some public boards from the firing line of staff activity, and their vulnerability to local political pressures, can be troublesome. In one Western state where child care institutions are under the State Board of Education, there are also local advisory bodies. Since the board could not visit the agencies, a custodial committee did so a few times a year. The committee found one children's institution in which the superintendent was concerned only with rigid economy and the children were forlorn and regimented. Consultation was secured, and it was recommended that the home become an institution for adolescents in need of group care. A new superintendent was hired, new staff, all changes were made. The State Board went on to other things, but the local advisory board did not like the looks of the "tough" youngsters who were the new clientele. They protested to the State Board. The result was, again a new superintendent, new staff, and reversion to the former policies of narrowly conceived function and stringent economy, for the State Board felt powerless to cope with local pressure.

In a second instance, jurisdiction over a state-wide public child care agency was shifted from the Board of Child Welfare to another board with different policies. The staff, who had visited their clients by means of agency cars they could garage at home, now found themselves restricted, in the name of economy, to an agency pool to which they had to come each morning. The results were fewer home visits, time unnecessarily spent each morning and evening to pick up and deposit cars, and considerable loss of morale by a devoted staff who wanted to use their time productively for their clients rather than for ferrying agency cars, and who often in the past had worked many more hours than were demanded of them. Here the distance between staff and board was so great, and so little provision was made for staff reaction and participation in policy changes, that what seemed to be a minor administrative change brought serious impairment to an entire agency service.

One of the anachronisms of modern agency life is a hangover from bygone days. In many agencies, the executive must have a trustee cosign every check; in others, only trustees can sign checks, and often two signatures are required. In one of the oldest family agencies in the country both the executive director and a member of the board had to be consulted before a staff member could grant an emergency loan in excess of $100. In one instance, when neither one could be reached, the agency was forced to call upon the Salvation Army to help a family in an overnight crisis. It might be well for agencies to reexamine how much professional responsibility is really accorded by these practices (that no business could abide), and their implications in terms of the confidence really placed by the boards in their executives and staffs.

6. BOARDS AND SOCIAL WELFARE ISSUES

The relation of voluntary agency boards to major issues in social welfare has been receiving well-merited attention.[15] The voluntary agency and the public agency differ in a number of respects. Not the least of these is the higher visibility of the public agency, and its greater vulnerability to pressure and intrusion. By contrast, the voluntary agency is far more protected, less readily called to account, its policies and practices less likely to be presented to the public gaze by the mass media even when, as is true of many children's agencies, the bulk of their operating funds come from government sources.

I shall comment on only one of the ramifications of this state of affairs: the responsibilities of voluntary agency boards to be informed of, concerned with, and actively related to, relevant social welfare issues. For the heart of the matter lies in the ease with which boards of voluntary agencies can keep themselves removed from the fierce currents of controversy in social welfare, from the attacks on those in need of social services as well as on the services themselves. From all we can observe, this strange aloofness has a frequent if not uniform pattern, with many outstanding exceptions. Indeed, in many agencies board members have taken leadership in developing new and imaginative agency policy in advance of staff thinking and despite staff trepidations. The impression many voluntary agencies convey, however, is that the Newburgh phenomenon and the attacks on ADC and on public welfare provisions generally are really none of their concern. To what do we owe this phenomenon? To a number of things:

Apathy

Ignorance of the facts

Ideological sympathy with the attacks

Absence of initiative in bringing the issues to attention

Apathy is understandable, if not acceptable. There are many competing demands on the time and energy and interest of board members. It is natural that attention would be given first to matters of immediate agency concern. The task here is to make it clear that some of these issues *are* of immediate agency concern, that no social agency in this day and age should be regarded as a privileged and autonomous sanctuary, unrelated to the entire pattern of social welfare in the country.

Ignorance is likewise understandable particularly if there is apathy, but hardly excusable as a basis for unconcern. Board members have a social responsibility to be informed, not only about the purpose and operations of their own agency, but about the social welfare context in which their agency exists.

Many a loyal and devoted board member of a family agency, community center, or even of a school of social work, may feel quite sympathetic with the position taken by Newburgh's City Manager Joseph Mitchell, with New Orleans's action on ADC, with the great concern about welfare "chiselers," with the feeling that public welfare "weakens the moral fibre"—with any or all and more of these. Now, holding such positions is any citizen's right. But something is clearly amiss if a dedicated board member does not see that the agency he supports is carrying on its work on ideological premises quite opposed to his. What is amiss in such a case is not necessarily the board member's lack of awareness, but the fact that there is nothing within the operation of the agency, the work of its staff, or, mainly, the performance of the agency's executive that leads him to feel there could possibly be an inconsistency in his point of view.

One cannot place the onus for the apathy, the ignorance, or the inconsistent point of view solely at the door of board members. It belongs as well to executives who take no initiative in bringing crucial social welfare issues to the attention of their boards, who do not realize that the much-vaunted function of "educating the board" includes education on such matters. There are three chief reasons for this lack of initiative:

1. They do not wish to rock the boat. Why raise questions that may induce board friction and conflict? The executives feel that they have enough trouble without adding to it unnecessarily.

2. They do not see such matters as relevant to the board or to the agency. "If we gave our attention to every social problem we would never get our work done."

3. They are not sufficiently convinced of the merits of the social work side of the case. This feeling is honest, if rare, but does not preclude raising the issue anyway.

None of these reasons is good enough, and it is time we placed part of the responsibility for the inaction of our lay leaders on ourselves, those of us who are in a position to work with trustees as executives, senior staff, consultants, or teachers.

I am not recommending that boards necessarily take a stand identical with that of the official social work community. We take our chances with democratic process, with the intelligence and objectivity of board members. Moreover, let us concede that if they disagree with formal social work positions, they may sometimes be right. I am simply recommending that the social work case be heard and understood.

I am not suggesting either that every agency has to be concerned with every social welfare issue at all times. Obviously, this is impossible and undesirable. On some issues information is sufficient, others call for discussion. There would have to be clear determination of relevance before the board takes a public position, and on many issues trustees may prefer to speak as private citizens rather than in their capacity as board members. It would be expected that agencies dealing with immigrants would be more concerned with immigration laws than would psychiatric clinics; settlement houses would be more concerned with delinquency than would hospital social service departments, and so forth. One could hope that across-the-board onslaughts on public welfare clients and attacks on basic decency in welfare management, however, would be considered the moral concern of all agencies.

I am not suggesting that no criticism of our public agencies should ever be made. On the contrary, all of us recognize that there is not only room for improvement, but for considerable change. But we have to earn the right to be critical, by supporting those general objectives which we all share, by identifying ourselves with these objectives and lending our strength to public agencies that are unfairly under attack, by recognizing that all of social work is being attacked when the public agencies are under fire.

Board members of voluntary agencies are vital in this conflict. They are assumed to have a special right to speak because they are social agency board members and therefore are both knowledgeable and public-spirited; their names carry weight in the community. Legislatures which hear no opposition to punitive welfare measures from agency board members would have every reason to feel that no responsible or at any rate significant opposition exists. Moreover, voluntary agencies can carry on their special functions—innovation and experimentation, for example—only by the grace of the existence of government-supported social welfare. Board members may take any position they wish on any given issue—whatever the position, it is better than apathy—but none should be unaware of this fact of life in American social work. Nor should they be unaware of the views held by our professional associations, notably the National Association of Social Workers, so that they can have some notion of the positions likely to be held, by the very social work staff in which they take pride. No greater bond can exist between board and staff than that of genuine mutual concern on fundamental matters of principle.

American society has accepted the proposition that issues of war and peace are too important to be left to the military. We seem to be arriving at the decision that policy on medical care is too serious to be left to doctors. It may therefore not be amiss to suggest that matters of social work policy are too vital to be left to social workers. As our profession moves into a position of greater authority, our need for a system of checks and balances increases. One essential element in making such a system work is to see to it that the laymen who serve on boards and presumably control policy are prepared, as many fortunately are, to exercise their responsibilities with informed intelligence and devotion to the general welfare of our society as well as to the well-being of their own agencies.

This is not to say that social workers should not contribute in the development of social policy or move toward constructive social change. On the contrary, our contribution should be stronger. We cannot and should not wish, however, to control policy. It may be fair to note that in the governmental sector of social work, the profession is generally overcontrolled, more checked than balanced. The reverse is more true of the voluntary agency field, where social work executives can have undue control, when there are weaknesses in board structure, process, commitment, or competence. These imbalances should be redressed so as to enhance the rational operation of our programs and, more basically, to enable us to be more effective and more responsive to the needs of those who require our services most, and to spur the development of needed change in organizations and policies.

As social workers, we should expect respect for our professional competence and brook no trespass. We should make our voices heard clearly on issues of social welfare. We should take leadership in the formulation of social policy. To help insure this respect, to strengthen our voices, we must have support, ideas, effective communication, and, above all, assumption of genuine responsibility by those who serve as trustees for the common good—even if we have to spur them to assume this responsibility. To those hundreds of board members who meet these expectations, we owe a great debt, whether or not they and we always see eye to eye.

REFERENCES

1. E.g., *The Board Member* (New Haven, Conn.: New Haven Council of Social Agencies, 1936).
2. Roy Sorenson, *The Art of Board Membership* (New York: Association Press, 1951).
3. Cyril O. Houle, *The Effective Board* (New York: Association Press, 1960).
4. William D. Schmidt, *The Executive and the Board in Social Welfare* (Cleveland: Howard Allen, Inc., 1959).
5. E.g., Harleigh B. Trecker, *New Understandings of Administration* (New York: Association Press, 1961).
6. Notably, Elinor K. Bernheim and Irving Brodsky. "The Realities of Board-Executive Relationships," *Journal of Jewish Communal Service*, XXXVII (1961), 381–89.
7. Houle, *op. cit.*, pp. 19–22.
8. E.g., Solomon Sutker, "The Jewish Organizational Elite of Atlanta, Georgia," *Social Forces*, XXXI (1952), 136–43.
9. Raymond M. Hughes, *A Manual for Trustees of Colleges and Universities* (Ames, Iowa: Iowa State College Press, 1945), p. 13.
10. *Ibid.*, p. 167.
11. Jerome Frank, *Persuasion and Healing: a Comparative Study of Psychotherapy* (Baltimore, Md.: Johns Hopkins Press, 1961).
12. Herman D. Stein, "Some Observations on Board-Executive Relationships in the Voluntary Agency," *Journal of Jewish Communal Service*, XXXVII (1961), 390–96.
13. Sorenson, *op. cit.*, p. 81.
14. Houle, *op. cit.*, p. 95.
15. E.g., James R. Dumpson, "Public and Voluntary Agency Partnership Responsibilities," *Child Welfare*, XLI (1962), 2–9; Joseph Walker, "Have Board Members Been Silent Too Long?" *ibid.*, XLI (1962), 168–71. Mr. Walker, president of an agency board, answers in the affirmative.

18/CITIZEN PARTICIPATION AND PROFESSIONALISM: A DEVELOPMENTAL RELATIONSHIP

FELICE PERLMUTTER

The discussion of citizen participation in policy-making, centered largely on the experience of publicly funded community programs, has raised many questions, has yielded less than satisfactory results, and has clearly indicated that the rationale for citizen involvement has been confused and frequently pragmatically or opportunistically determined (Kubey, 1970).

Furthermore, as human services have shifted in emphasis from a total concern with individual adjustment to an added concern with institutional change, much attention has been paid to the implications of this shift vis-a-vis manpower utilization. While much of the initial discussion centered on community organization programs in social work, the impact of this shift, both philosophical and practical, subsequently affected the wide spectrum of human service agencies both in the voluntary and public sector. As a result of the antidelinquency and poverty programs new professional roles were identified, such as enabler, broker, advocate, activist (Grosser, 1965). A second major concern was the utilization of nonprofessionals, and the literature is replete with discussion of the new careers programs. While the original interest was largely related to the assumption regarding the effectiveness of having people serve as helpers who were close to or had themselves experienced the problems of the client population (Perlmutter, 1965), a second and not unimportant aspect was the value of the service for the helping person himself (Reissman, 1965). In addition, the manpower implications of the new careers programs were of importance from the public policy point of view.

This paper will discuss the relationship between the nonprofessional and the professional, with a focus on the issue of citizen participation. The central thesis is that the respective roles of and relationships between the nonprofessionals, as policy makers, and the professional staff are not static and permanent but must be viewed dialectically. The experience in social welfare will be used to support the argument which is analytically framed by a model of social agency change (Perlmutter, 1969).

LAY INVOLVEMENT IN POLICY PLANNING

The involvement of nonprofessionals on the policy level in social welfare antedates the existence of the profession itself. The fact of concerned citizens organizing welfare services for various groups in need is too well documented to require further discussion. The important point to be made, however, is that the major pattern adopted in the United States is one of noblesse-oblige, in which citizens involved in the formation of social agency programs have traditionally been from the upper class; the literature calls attention to the participation of high-status citizens as the lay group involved in policy formation (Ross, 1953). A tension exists between the layman and the professional; boards are viewed as instrumentalities primarily concerned with the fiscal operation of the agency and not for their knowledge of the particular agency's technical competence which is viewed as the professional's appropriate concern (Auerbach, 1961). The consequence of this historical pattern was the establishment of a static relationship between the lay policy makers and the professionals within a traditional context of service which led to the following formulation:

. . . professionals must not become "captives" of their clientele and surrender to them the power to determine the nature of the service offered (Blau and Scott, 1962).

However, the social programs of the 1960's raised the urgent question concerning the participation of citizens in the planning of their own programs and hopefully is the legacy left by these programs (Levitan, 1969). The old roles and relationships were no longer acceptable whereby the professional unilaterally offered a service to the client; the involvement and participation of the constituents were essential.

The experience of self-help organizations provides an important field of study and can serve as a corrective to this traditional stance. There has been little examination of the experience of self-help, mutual-aid organizations as relevant to the development of professional services. The major lesson to be learned from these organizations concerns their use of professionals: *technical experts are used for specific problems as determined by the membership* (Katz, 1965, 1970). Furthermore, it is quite clear that in mutual-benefit associations (such as unions, fraternal organizations) the group is organized by the membership to meet its own interests; policies and procedures are determined by the group itself through its elected representatives. These examples of participatory democracy are consequently of heuristic value.

Since the involvement of the lay community in policy-making is traditional in social work, the major current issue in this field consequently is not the form of participation, advisory or policy-making, but rather *who* are the lay people and *what* is their role. A theoretical model of agency development accommodates important elements of both the service and the mutual-benefit organization but a differentiation in emphasis is made, appropriate to the agency's stage of development.

DETERMINING LAY AND PROFESSIONAL ROLES

An historical evolutionary model of social agency development posits three developmental stages in the life of a social agency: self-interest, professionalism and social interest. The model assumes an open system and views the agency in its social-environmental context. While the model specifies eight variables as crucial to an understanding of the agency, the variable of interest in this presentation is the "organizational elites," defined as consisting of the nonprofessional as the lay policy-makers, and the professional staff. This theoretical model suggests that the role of the two groups of elites will vary according to the stage of development of the agency as follows.

In the initial self-interest stage the elan of a social movement exists as a group of citizens respond to unsolved and pressing social problems, frequently related to a subgroup that is not accorded equal treatment.

The participation of the elites in this stage most approximates that of the self-help, mutual-benefit organizations with their emphasis on the specific needs and problems of their members. The lay board of directors is in a singular position of power for a variety of reasons: first, it has been instrumental in the formulation of the service and its definition of its mission; second, it is prestigious in relation to the community whose support is being sought; third, it selects the first administrator and staff with the intent of a clear-cut implementation of the agency's objectives in handling the pressing social problem.

Conversely, the position of the staff is weak because of the organizational requirements at this stage. The creativity and aggressive innovation rests with the board, whereas the staff operates as implementers of the agency's service. The question of professional competence is of less importance than the commitment and concern to get the job done; educational experience and training are accordingly given less attention than in the subsequent stages. For example, agencies for retarded children, primarily concerned with delivery of service rather than with quality and standards, frequently utilize nonprofessionals for their staff (Katz, 1961).

By contrast, the second stage of professionalism occurs when the pressing external problem has abated and the agency can now focus on the quality of its service, an internal rather than an external orientation. Because of the emphasis on the technical problems, the function of the elites reverses as the lay policy group *chooses* to give the ascendant role to the professional staff. The professional staff, using a body of knowledge and professional skill, operates relatively independently of the lay board of directors. (It is during this stage that the displacement of organizational goals is most likely to occur, as the professional focuses on techniques.)

The social interest or third stage of agency development occurs again within the social-economic context of the larger society. A new social problem arises directly related to that which stimulated the formation of the agency and requires that the agency reassess its position via-a-vis the larger community. It can either remain internally and professionally oriented (and fixated), or it can respond to new and urgent needs of the broader system. The requirements of the elites again change in response to the different emphasis: the lay participants on the board must now again be actively involved in decisions related to a new definition of agency mission, and cannot leave the professionals in charge.

It is crucial that the lay members of the board be selectively recruited to help the agency move into each successive stage. While pressure from external groups is important for this development as part of the changing environmental context, an elite *inside* the organization must provide the stimulus for internal change.

A relationship is thus postulated between the developmental stages of the organization and its utilization of elites.

It seems evident that the proper assignment of personnel and the diagnosis of administrative troubles will gain from a better understanding of the relation between personnel orientations and organization life history. . . . The selection of key personnel requires an understanding of the shift in problems that occurs as the organization moves from one stage of development to another. And for best results the participants should be able to recognize the phase through which they are passing (Selznick, 1957).

If an evolutionary model of social agency development were part of the knowledge base of the professional in understanding the organizational context of his practice (just as developmental personality theory underlies an understanding of the client), the role of the professional would be appropriately conceptualized and more comfortably performed. The issue of client control would not pose a problem since the role of the professional would be related to the developmental needs of the organization. Thus, in the self-interest stage the professional would be the instrumentality through which the client's objectives would be fulfilled, a relationship clearly established in self-help organizations. The lay board could then choose to move the agency system into the second, professional, stage if a more sophisticated service were desired.

For example, a community-organized medical clinic in its first stage of development would be concerned with meeting the basic needs of its community on a quantitative basis and would not wish to leave the decisions regarding the distribution of services and the organization of the program to the physicians. Once the basic needs were met and the structure of the services established, however, the needs for higher quality care would require greater professional authority.

The central point is that the stage of development of the agency would determine the appropriate role of its elites, both the policy-makers and the professionals. Rather than becoming a competitive venture based on power and conflict the choices would be more analytically and rationally determined in terms of agency direction and change.

DILEMMAS AND ISSUES

The utilization of past or potential consumers of service in self-help groups on both the policy and service delivery level has been important in retaining the vitality and flexibility of these organizations. However, it must be noted that the groups have usually been organized around specific problems of individuals at risk and are treatment oriented (e.g., Association for Retarded Children, the Polio Foundation). The utilization of these elites in agencies oriented to social and institutional change has not been sufficiently explored to justify assumptions of effectiveness.

Mogulof (1965) has suggested that lay participation in policy bodies is related to the commitment of social work to institutional change and that if "American social work will revert to the concept that presses for personal adjustment . . . rather than structural change . . . the poor will no longer be chosen for boards. . . ." This assumption must indeed be systematically tested since there is some evidence in the literature that, in fact, the opposite relationship obtains.

For example, in the San Francisco Neighborhood Legal Assistance Foundation, a Federally financed, community-controlled legal service agency, a conflict emerged between the radical white lawyers of the central office who were committed to social change and the black lawyers in the neighborhood offices who were focused on meeting the individual claims and grievances of the community clients.

The goal of community control had been institutionalized in the autonomous neighborhood offices, while the aim of institutional change was embodied in the Main Office legal staff. It was obvious that the growing antagonism between the two structures in large measure represented a conflict between the two goals. The lawyer-founders had been wrong in assuming that control by the client community was a necessary condition, let alone compatible with a program of institutional change. . . . (Carlin, 1970).

Consequently, this evolutionary model facilitates the selective recruitment of lay people based on the requirements of the agency's stage of development. Whereas the first stage of self-interest requires that the lay group which determines the mission of the agency is the ascendant elite with a vested interest in the program, the role and participation of a different group of members for lay policy-making is required in the second stage of professionalism. Similarly, in moving to the social-interest change orientation of the third stage, a more "cosmopolitan" group of policy-makers is suggested in contrast to the "local" orientation of the earlier group.

Another issue must be raised: does a program conceived, organized, and operated by professionals under public funding follow the same developmental pattern? Specifically, can the role of lay citizens be the same as that of the elites in the self-help tradition? The tension in many of the public programs (e.g., Community Mental Health Centers) can be elucidated by an application of the theoretical model as follows: whereas the community expectation is one of participation appropriate to the first, self-interest stage of organizational development, the professionals in these programs are operating in the context of the second stage of professionalism. There is an incompatibility of roles and relationships in these two different stages; consequently, an understanding of the organizational requirements would help define appropriate role performance.

CONCLUSIONS

Our rapidly changing field of human service places great demands on all parts of the system as a variety of strategies are required to meet its objectives. While decisions regarding the utilization of lay people and professionals have been haphazardly made and frequently dysfunctional to the service developed, a theoretical model of agency change can serve as the basis for decision-making in regard to the complex issues relating to policy formulation and service development.

REFERENCES

Arnold J. Auerbach. "Aspirations of Power People and Agency Goals," *Social Work*, Vol. 6, No. 1 (January 1961).

Peter M. Blau, and Richard W. Scott. *Formal Organizations* (San Francisco: Chandler Press, 1962).

Jerome E. Carlin. "Store Front Lawyers in San Francisco," *Transaction*, Vol. 7, No. 6 (April 1970).

Charles F. Grosser. "Community Development Programs Serving the Urban Poor," *Social Work*, Vol. 10, No. 3 (July 1965).

Alfred Katz. *Parents of the Handicapped* (Springfield, Ill.: Charles C Thomas Press, 1961).

Alfred Katz. "Application of Self-Help Concepts in Current Social Welfare," *Social Work*, Vol. 10, No. 3 (July 1965).

Alfred Katz. "Self-Help Organizations and Volunteer Participation," *Social Work*, Vol. 15, No. 1 (January 1970).

Sumati N. Kubey. "Community Action Programs and Citizen Participation: Issues and Confusions," *Social Work*, Vol. 15, No. 1 (January 1970).

Sar A. Levitan. *The Great Society's Poor Law: A New Approach to Poverty* (Baltimore: John Hopkins Press, 1969).

Melvin B. Mogulof. "Involving Low-Income Neighborhoods in Anti-delinquency Programs," *Social Work*, Vol. 10, No. 4 (October 1965).

Felice Perlmutter and Dorothy Durham. "Using Teenagers to Supplement Casework Service," *Social Work*, Vol. 10, No. 2 (April 1965).

Felice Perlmutter. "A Theoretical Model of Social Agency Development," *Social Casework*, Vol. 50, No. 8 (October 1969).

Frank Riessman. "The Helper Therapy Principle," *Social Work*, Vol. 10, No. 2 (April 1965).

Aileen D. Ross. "The Social Control of Philanthropy," *American Journal of Sociology*, 58 (1953).

Philip Selznick. *Leadership in Administration* (Evanston, Illinois: Row, Peterson and Co. 1957).

Part V

RESOURCES—
ALLOCATION, CONTROL,
AND ACCOUNTABILITY

EDITOR'S INTRODUCTION

Much of the interest in administration of the social services during the seventies developed as a result of official and public concern for accountability and what were considered the uncontrolled excesses of the social programs of the sixties. In substantial part this flowed from the viewpoint of the Nixon administration that these programs were failures, and that one couldn't solve social programs by "throwing money at them." The incorporation of managerial technology into public welfare programs was seen as one way to overcome the inefficiencies that were thought to be rampant. A number of government grants were made by the Social and Rehabilitation Services of DHEW to schools of social work for projects in administration. Special encouragement was given to pursue activities jointly with schools of business. Accountability and evaluation became important preoccupations of writers in the field. For some this was seen as an opportunity to develop the professional aspects of administration. For many policy-makers this was one route to containing public expenditures on public welfare.

The sharply declining resources for public and private welfare programs in the mid-seventies gave further impetus to this development. In a period of expansion, program innovation and initiative are readily encouraged. New efforts are simply added to the existing system of services with relatively little pressure to weigh alternatives or to focus on efficiency measures. The reverse is true during periods of curtailed finances. Emphasis goes to getting "the biggest bang for the buck." It is readily assumed that managerial know-how will curtail waste, cut out "fat," and yield greater efficiency of operation. A sharper look at the administration of social agencies should also make them more effective in achieving their objectives.

The complexities of modern-day funding of social service programs also call for a greater interest in administrative operations. Relatively few of these programs receive their financial substance from a single source. Increasingly over the years, governmental funds either supplemented voluntary efforts at income generation or became major sources of funds. Furthermore, funding streams tended to reflect the multiplicity of structural patterns among city, county, state, and federal departments and their legislative appropriations. Many programs now receive support from a variety of sources, each establishing requirements for evaluation and accountability. Administering social agencies requires a quality of personnel competent to deal with these complexities and the many constituencies they represent.

Finally, the recent development of both hard- and software technology applicable to organizational management calls for a degree of sophistication not previously required. New accounting procedures and the machinery that makes them possible, new patterns of word processing, and, above all, new ways of handling data and information set partial agendas for training that are becoming widespread.

A. BUDGETING

The selections in this section reflect these developments. With the exception of manuals published by some national agencies, the literature on budgeting for the social services is very meager. Gross provides a general overview of conventional budgeting for nonprofit organizations. He reviews its functions and procedures, and cites illustrations of the use of budgets as mechanisms of financial control.

B. PROGRAM BUDGETING AND COST ANALYSIS

Since the days of the Johnson administration, program budgeting in the form of Program Planning Budgeting Systems (PPBS), which the Defense Department seemed to find a revolutionary innovation, has been widely applied in and out of government. Much of its early promise has withered with experience and time. According to Wildavsky, "sufficient evidence on the operation of PPBS around the world has accumulated to permit general appraisal. PPBS has failed everywhere and at all times" (Wildavsky, 1974, p. 205). Many have held on to its rational core—a concern with specification and achievement of objectives as well as inputs into the budgetary process. Macleod presents the positive side of program budgeting. His article is essentially a case study of cost accounting and program budgeting in a complex mental health center, and suggests that it is both feasible and useful to apply these approaches to nonprofit organizations.

Levine examines the application of cost–benefit analysis to social welfare problems, and traces its relationship to PPBS and to social program evaluation. He sees cost–benefit and cost-effectiveness as essentially synonymous in practice, and suggests that their methodology fundamentally resembles competent program-effectiveness study. The ways in which cost–benefit analysis can provide useful guides for local program managers and for national or regional administrators are detailed. Levine reviews the place of theory and models in such analysis, and provides case illustrations to make his point. He finally suggests some aspects of costs and benefits in most social welfare programs where these cannot be expressed in monetary terms.

C. MANAGEMENT BY OBJECTIVES

Management by objectives (MBO) has been a major managerial tool for more than two decades. Developed initially by Peter Drucker (1954), a substantial literature has developed in both business and government. More recently, social service agencies have experimented with its use. Wiehe states the case for MBO as a helpful tool in performance appraisal and program planning in social agencies. He reviews the process, both inductive and deductive, of setting agency and individual practitioner goals and objectives, and specifies the values that grow out of staff participation in that process. While Wiehe does not deal specifically with the use of MBO for budgetary purposes, its application seems self-evident, since budgets are essentially the quantification in money terms of organizational objectives.

Raider reviews the recent experience of social agencies in applying MBO, and explores both successes and failures in its use as a management tool. After identifying indicators of potential difficulty with MBO, he provides a step-by-step series of phases essential for its effective installation. The importance of adapting an MBO approach to the particular requirements of specific agencies is stressed. Ways of dealing with expected staff resistance and to paperwork overload are indicated. Raider also stresses the importance of connecting this methodology to personal growth objectives of the agency's staff as well as to the achievement of agency goals.

D. ZERO-BASE BUDGETING

Among the newest of the innovations in budgeting, and one likely to assume increasing importance in the years ahead, is zero-base budgeting (Pyhrr, 1973). While in itself not new, the likely incorporation of ZBB into federal budgeting procedures and the experience of several states, notably Georgia while President Carter was governor, suggests that it will permeate thinking and planning of financial managers. Its essential features are in sharp contrast to conventional budgeting. In practice, traditional planning dealt with incremental changes at the margin—increasing some resources for specific items that seem to warrant expansion while reducing others. Budget justifications dealt with these marginal changes, operating on the implicit assumption that prior appropriations were given, and that only changes in amounts allocated would be rationalized. ZBB suggests that every budget year begins anew, that program planning and justification deal with total appropriations not with incremental changes alone. In the absence of a sound basis for continued operation, programs are terminated. Thus a full review of all aspects of the budget is indicated, in the course of which alternatives are probed and cost–benefit relationships are explored.

Vignola reviews briefly the main characteristics of ZBB, points to its similarities to PPBS, and suggests a series of critical comments and limitations that need to be kept in mind by budget planners as they apply this method to a variety of human resources programs. ZBB reenforces the importance of program evaluation, and specification and assessment of program objectives. The difficulty in quantifying human service objectives, with their heavy overlay of values and subjective considerations, however, presents perhaps its major challenge.

E. ACCOUNTABILITY

The hallmark of the seventies in the social services may well be the insistence on accountability, and its associated call for the evaluation of efficiency and effectiveness in service delivery and administration. The less sympathetic policy-makers became to welfare services and to welfare clients, the more they emphasized the importance of accountability. Much of the public discussion centered on two questions—accountability for what, and accountability to whom. Professional preferences for accountability to consumers of service—social welfare clients—sometimes gave way to redefinition of the client. Thus some officials in the California welfare system, joined by an academic and an official in the Department of Agriculture could write: "Who is the client for social services who must be satisfied? The critical client is the taxpayer. He pays the tabs for the programs and derives the benefits, if any, of the services. Thus he, more than the individual recipient of specific services, represents the prime target for client-satisfaction efforts. (Another important client group . . . consists of elected officials)" (Bledsoe et al., 1972, p. 800).

Hoshino reflects on the demands by Congress and the Nixon administration for greater social service accountability, and points to a series of difficulties that confront such efforts. In his view, coherence and consistency of the goals of social policy and explicit and realistic performance criteria precede the attainment of competent accountability. Contradictions in policy directions—e.g., services strategy versus work-and-training strategy—complicate operational planning and lead to confusion about goals, making evaluation problematic. Hoshino looks to the development of good program indicators, including client perceptions, as a prelude to addressing problems of identifying operational goals and selecting useful criteria of effectiveness. This is especially true under conditions of shifting policy responses to changed objective circumstances.

Perhaps one of the clearest statements in the literature on the problems and dilemmas confronting social service accountability is that of Newman and Turem. They explore the significance of limited fiscal and human resources for policy choices, and the impact of political pressures and considerations on the scale and direction of social service provision. Because the absence of market mechanisms makes political processes paramount, they suggest that credibility must be earned through appropriate focus on effectiveness and efficiency of service delivery through highlighting results, not processes. Because this has not been the case traditionally, there is a crisis of confidence and accountability which threatens the well-being of the service delivery system. A competing view might suggest that if the crisis of accountability is in substantial part related to political dynamics, the appropriate response should in fact be political. Some programs are placed in jeopardy precisely because they achieve their stated objectives. It is their political unorthodoxy and challenge of the status quo that is often questioned—i.e., Mobilization for Youth and some poverty law programs. When police programs fail to curb crime, on the other hand, greater resources tend to be allocated. Politics overcomes rationality. This is not to suggest that accountability is not an important aspect of social service planning. But difficulties in evaluating nonobjective, nonquantifiable results, and the limitations in transforming positive results into policy initiatives ought not be underestimated.

The next selection examines a neglected aspect of program evaluation and productivity—considerations of social equity. Chitwood looks at these matters from the perspective of the political scientist and governmental social services. He contrasts the concern of public officials for expenditure accountability and operational efficiency with the equitable distribution of public services. He stresses the importance of meeting minimum levels of adequacy and of ensuring entitlements of public benefits. Furthermore, social equity requires the development of a relationship between service recipients and the administering agency that reflects respect, trust, and participation.

Piliavin and McDonald analyze the often reported negative results concerning the effectiveness of social work intervention, and reflect on the "crisis in confidence" that affects social programs as a result. They indicate that, in fact, the research findings demonstrate positive as well as negative conclusions, and that in any case, social welfare programs have much to gain from examining conflicting results of well-conceived investigations. Some of the technical and methodological problems in much of the reported research are indicated. An illustration is given of a careful analysis of negative program results that led to more effective programming.

F. SYSTEMS ANALYSIS

Patti and Gruber analyze recent developments that are variously referred to as management science, systems analysis, or systems management, and view the ways in which their application to the social services, and particularly to public welfare, affects the social and political context of service delivery. Patti sees this movement as ideologically rooted, and points to the potentially negative impact they can have on clients and the agencies that serve them when indiscriminately applied. He identifies the essential features of the belief system that underlies the approach, and points to the problems and pitfalls that attend the use of the technology that they inspire. He questions the transferability of systems management to complex social welfare issues and programs. His response to the inevitable incorporation of this technology in the welfare system is to suggest approaches to the training of social administrators which include a sufficient familiarity with these technical tools, but buttressed with theoretical, empirical, and practical skills in the framework of social values and sensitivity to client needs.

Gruber takes a dim view of the incorporation of efficiency experts, systems analysts, and other management scientists into the social services, particularly in the large public bureaucracies. He suggests that preoccupation with economy and efficiency on the part of these "technocrats" can be deleterious in achieving humane objectives. He traces the continuities between Taylor's scientific management and current approaches, and points to their many failures to achieve their objectives. In Gruber's view, techniques are not neutral, tend to be mechanistic and impersonal, and should be subordinated to humane purposes. He urges a view of accountability that goes beyond technical auditing and quantitative ratios, one which considers citizen preferences at its core—a political rather than a corporate concept of efficiency.

REFERENCES

Bledsoe, Ralph C.; Denny, Dennis R.; Hobbs, Charles D.; and Long, Raymond S. "Productivity Management in the California Social Services Program." *Public Administration Review*, November/December, 1972.

Drucker, Peter. *The Practice of Management*. New York: Harper and Bros., 1954.

Pyhrr, Peter A. *Zero-Base Budgeting*. New York: John Wiley & Sons, 1973.

Wildavsky, Aaron. *The Politics of the Budgetary Process*. 2nd ed. Boston, Mass.: Little Brown and Company, 1974.

A. BUDGETING

19/THE IMPORTANCE
OF BUDGETING

MALVERN J. GROSS

A budget, like motherhood, is something very few would argue against. Yet, the art of preparing *and using* budgets in a meaningful manner is completely foreign to most nonprofit organizations. It is not that the treasurer or board is unaware of their importance, but more that they lack the skill necessary to apply budgeting techniques, and often are reluctant to use a budget as a tool to control the financial activities. The purpose of this chapter is to discuss the importance of budgeting, the art of skillfully preparing a useful budget, and equally important, the art of actually using the budget to control.

THE BUDGET: A PLAN OF ACTION

A budget is a "plan of action." It represents the organization's blueprint for the coming months, or years, expressed in monetary terms. This means the organization must know what its goals are before it can prepare a budget. If it doesn't know where it is going, obviously it is going to be very difficult for the organization to do any meaningful planning. All too often the process is reversed and it is in the process of preparing the budget that the goals are determined.

So the first function of a budget is to record, in monetary terms, what the realistic goals or objectives of the organization are for the coming year (or years). The budget is the financial plan of action which results from the board's decisions as to the program for the future.

The second function of a budget is to provide a tool to monitor the financial activities throughout the year. Properly used, the budget can provide a bench mark or comparison point which will alert the board to the first indication that their financial goals won't be met. For a budget to provide this type of information and control four elements must be present:

1. The budget must be well-conceived, and have been prepared or approved by the board.

2. The budget must be broken down into periods corresponding to the periodic financial statements.

3. Financial statements must be prepared on a timely basis throughout the year and a comparison made to the budget, right on the statements.

4. The board must be prepared to take action where the comparison with the budget indicates a significant deviation.

Each of these four elements will be discussed in this chapter.

Steps for Preparation

It was noted above that a budget should represent the end result of a periodic review by the board or by the membership of the organization's objectives or goals, expressed in monetary terms. Often the budget process is a routine "chore" handled by the treasurer to satisfy the board that the organization has a budget, which the board, in turn, routinely ratifies. Frequently, such budgets are not looked at again until the following year, at the time next year's budget is prepared. This type of budgeting serves little purpose and is worth little more than the paper it is written on. A budget, to be effective, must be a joint effort of many people. It must be a working document which forms the basis for action.

Here are the basic steps that, in one form or another, should be followed by an organization in order to prepare a well-conceived budget:

1. A list of objectives or goals of the organization for the following year should be prepared. For many organizations this process will be essentially a re-evaluation of the relative priority of the existing programs. Care should be taken, however, to avoid concluding too hastily that an existing program should continue unchanged. Our society is not static and the organization that does not constantly re-evaluate and update its program is in danger of being left behind.

2. The cost of each objective or goal listed above should be estimated. For continuing programs, last year's actual expense and last year's budget will be the starting point. For new programs or modifications of existing programs, a substantial amount of work may be necessary to accurately estimate the costs involved. This estimating process should be done in detail since elements of a particular goal or objective may involve many categories of expense and salaries.

3. The expected income of the organization should be estimated. With many organizations, contributions from members or the general public will be the principal income and careful consideration must be given to the expected economic climate in the community. A year when unem-

ployment is high or the stock market is down is a poor year to expect "increased" contributions. With other organizations the amount of income will be dependent on how successful they are in selling their program. Possibly some of the programs can be expanded if they are financially viable, or contracted if they are not. Organizations are often overly optimistic in estimating income. This can prove to be the organization's downfall if there is no margin for error, and realism must be used or the budget will have little meaning.

4. The total expected income should be compared to the expense of achieving the objectives or goals. Usually the expected expenses will exceed income, and this is where some value judgments will have to take place. What programs are most important? Where can expected costs be reduced? This process of reconciling expected income and expense is probably the most important step taken during the year because it is here that the program's blue print for the coming year is fixed.

It is important that consideration be given to the reliability of the estimated income and expense figures. Is it possible that expenses have been underestimated or that income has been overestimated? If expenses have been underestimated by 15 per cent and income has been overestimated by 10 per cent, there will be a deficit of 25 per cent, and unless the organization has substantial cash reserves it could be in serious difficulty. If the organization has small cash reserves or with little likelihood of getting additional funds quickly, then a realistic safety margin should be built into the budget.

5. The final proposed budget should be submitted to the appropriate body for ratification. This may be the full board or it may be the entire membership. This should not be just a formality but should be carefully presented to the ratifying body so that, once ratified, all persons will be firmly committed to the resulting plan of action.

The steps listed above may seem so elementary that there is no need to emphasize them here. But elementary as they are, they are often not followed and the resulting budget serves very little value to the organization.

Responsibility for Preparation

There has been very little said about "who" should follow these steps in preparing the budget. The preparation of a budget involves policy decisions. While the "treasurer" may be the person best qualified to handle the figures, he may or may not be the person to make policy decisions. For this reason, a "budget committee" should consist of persons responsible for policy decisions. Usually this means that the board should either itself act as the budget committee, or it should appoint a subcommittee of board members.

This doesn't mean that the detailed estimated cost studies for various programs can't be delegated to staff members. But the decision as to what are the goals and their relative priority has to be a board-level function.

Take, for example, a private, independent school. At first glance there might not appear to be many board-level decisions to make. The purpose of a school is to teach and it might seem that the budget would be a most routine matter. But there are many decisions that have to be made. For example:

1. Should more emphasis be placed on science courses?
2. Should the school get a small computer to help teach computer science?
3. Should the school hire a language teacher for grades 2–4?
4. Should the school increase salaries in the coming year and try to upgrade the staff?
5. Should the athletic field be resodded this year?
6. Should a fund raiser be hired?
7. Should the music program be expanded?
8. Should tuition be increased?

These questions and many more face the board. Undoubtedly they may rely on the paid staff to make recommendations, but the board is responsible for policy and the budget represents "policy." This responsibility cannot be delegated.

MONTHLY AND QUARTERLY BUDGETS

Many organizations have no real difficulty in preparing an annual budget. The real problem comes in trying to divide the budget into meaningful segments that can be compared to interim financial statements prepared on a monthly or quarterly basis. Some organizations attempt to do this by dividing the total budget by twelve and showing the resulting amounts as a monthly budget, which is then compared to actual monthly income and expense. While this is better than not making any budget comparison, it can produce misleading results when the income or expenses do not occur on a uniform basis throughout the year. Consider the following abbreviated statement of a small church:

		Three Months Ending March 31	
	Annual Budget	Annual Budget ÷ 4	Actual
Contributions	$ 120,000	$ 30,000	$ 35,000
Less Expenses	(120,000)	(30,000)	(30,000)
Excess	—	—	$ 5,000

The logical conclusion that might be drawn is that the church will have a surplus at the end of 12 months of approximately $20,000—four times the quarterly excess of $5,000. If this conclusion were reached the temptation would be to slacken off on unpaid pledge collection efforts and to be a little less careful in making purchases. This would be a very serious mistake if, in fact, the normal pattern of pledge collections were such that $36,000 should have been collected in the first quarter instead of the $35,000 actually received. A monthly or quarterly budget can produce misleading conclusions unless considerable care is taken in preparing it.

Allocating an Annual Budget to
Monthly or Quarterly Periods

One of the best and easiest ways to allocate an annual budget into shorter periods is to first analyze the actual income and expense for the prior year, and then allocate this year's budget based on last year's actual expenses.

To illustrate, assume the church's income last year was $100,000 but is expected to be $120,000 this year. A budget for the new year could be prepared as follows:

	Actual Last Year	Percent of Last Year's Total	New Budget
Income:			
First quarter	$ 30,000	30%	$ 36,000
Second quarter	25,000	25%	30,000
Third quarter	25,000	25%	30,000
Fourth quarter	20,000	20%	24,000
	$100,000	100%	$120,000

In this illustration we have assumed that the increase in income of $20,000 will be received in the same pattern as the prior year's income was received. If this assumption is not correct, then adjustment must be made for the anticipated income which will depart from past experience. For example, if it is anticipated that a single gift of $10,000 will be received in the first quarter and the other $10,000 will be received in about the same pattern as last year's income, the calculations to arrive at a new budget would be somewhat different, as shown below:

	Actual Last Year	Percent of Last Year's Total	New Budget Other Than Special	Special Gifts	Total Budget
First quarter	$ 30,000	30%	$ 33,000	$10,000	$ 43,000
Second quarter	25,000	25%	27,500	—	27,500
Third quarter	25,000	25%	27,500	—	27,500
Fourth quarter	20,000	20%	22,000	—	22,000
	$100,000	100%	$110,000	$10,000	$120,000

If at the end of the first quarter income of only 35,000 had been received compared to a budget of $43,000, it would be apparent that steps should be taken to increase contributions or the church will fall short of meeting its budget for the year.

The expense side of the budget should be handled in the same way. Generally, expenses tend to occur at a more uniform rate, although this is not always so. In many ways the expense side of the budget is more important than the income side since it is easier to increase expenditures for things that weren't budgeted than to raise additional contributions. If the budget is regularly compared to actual expenditures for deviations, it can be an effective tool to highlight unbudgeted expenditures.

The budget should probably be prepared on a monthly rather than on a quarterly basis to reduce the time lag before effective action can be taken. If a monthly basis appears to be too cumbersome, consideration could be given to bimonthly budgets and statements. However, if the organization's cash position is tight, monthly statements become almost a necessity.

ILLUSTRATIVE EXPENSE BUDGET

The Valley Country Club is a good example of an organization that has to be very careful to budget its income and expenses. While the club has a beautiful club house and a fine golf course, all of its money is tied up in these fixed assets and there is no spare cash to cover a deficit. Accordingly each fall when the board starts to wrestle with the budget for the following year it is aware that it cannot afford the luxury of a deficit. Since the budget is so important, the entire board sits as a budget committee to work out the plans for the following year. The treasurer, with the help of the club manager, prepares a worksheet in advance of the budget meeting. This worksheet indicates the actual expenses for the current year to date, the estimate of the final figures for the year, and the current year's budget to show how close the club will come. The board through discussion and debate attempts to work out a budget for the coming year. Figure 18–1 shows the worksheet for the expense budget.

In looking at this worksheet notice first that the expenses are grouped by major function so that the board can focus attention on the activities of the club. The alternative presentation would have been to list expenses by type—salaries, supplies, food, etc.—but this doesn't tell the board how much each of the major activities is costing.

There are three columns for the proposed budget—the minimum, the maximum, and the final amount. As the board considers each item it records both the minimum and the maximum it feels is appropriate. No attempt is made at the beginning to fix a "final" budget amount. Instead all budget items are considered, listed as to the minimum and maximum cost, and totals arrived at. It is only after all items have been considered, and only after a preliminary review of potential income has been made, that the board is in a position to make a judgment.

After the board has completed this worksheet showing final figures for the year, the next step is to break down the budget into monthly budgets. As with many organizations, the Valley Country Club's expenses (and income) are seasonal. In this case, the budget is broken down into monthly segments assuming that the expenses will be incurred in the same pattern as they were for the current year, in the manner discussed earlier.

TIMELY INTERIM STATEMENTS

The most carefully thought out budget will be of little value if it is not compared throughout the year with the actual results of operations. This means that the interim financial statements must be prepared on a timely basis.

What is timely? This largely depends on the organization and how much "slippage" or deviation from budget the organization can afford before serious consequences take place. If the cash balance is low an organization can't afford the luxury of not knowing where it stands on a timely basis. Guidelines are dangerous, but if an organization is unable to produce some form of abbreviated monthly or quarterly financial statement within 20 days of the end of the period the likelihood is that the information is "stale" by the time it is prepared. If twenty days is the length of time it takes then the board should plan to meet shortly after the twentieth of the month so as to be able to act on deviations while there is still time to act.

This is not to suggest that monthly financial statements are always appropriate for nonprofit organizations. But even if prepared on a bimonthly or quarterly basis, they should still be prepared on a timely basis.

Importance of Budget Comparison
The financial statement should also show the budget, and for the same period of time. Interim figures for the three months cannot easily be compared to budget figures for twelve months. The budget must also be for three months. Last year's actual figures for the same period may also be shown, although this added information could detract from the reader seeing the deviation from the current year's budget.

Figure 18–2 shows the Valley Country Club Statement of Income and Expense for both the month of June and for the 6 months, with budget comparisons to highlight deviations from the budget.

This financial statement gives the reader a great deal of information about the club's activities for the two periods. It should have the effect of alerting the reader to the fact that unless something happens, there may be a deficit for the year. For instead of having a small excess for June, there was a deficit of $6,200, and instead of having an excess of $7,500 for

THE VALLEY COUNTRY CLUB

WORKSHEET FOR PREPARING 1972 EXPENSE BUDGET
(in thousands)

	Actual Current Year				Budget for New Year		
	To Date (10 Months)	Estimate Balance Of Year	Estimate For Year	Budget Current Year	Proposed Minimum	Proposed Maximum	Final
Maintenance of greens and grounds:							
Salaries and wages..............	$ 47	$ 3	$ 50	$ 46	$ 50	$ 65	$ 55
Seeds, fertilizer and supplies......	14		14	13	14	14	14
Repairs, maintenance and other	12	2	14	10	10	15	15
Maintenance of clubhouse:							
Salaries and wages..............	20	4	24	23	24	28	26
Supplies, maintenance and repair ...	10	1	11	12	11	11	11
Golf activities:							
Salaries and wages..............	10		10	11	12	20	20
Tournament costs..............	14		14	15	15	15	15
Golf cart maintenance	8		8	5	5	5	5

Swimming pool expenses:							
Salaries and wages	4		4	4	5	10	5
Supplies and maintenance	2		2	1	2	2	2
General and administrative salaries	35	6	41	40	44	51	44
Property taxes	33	7	40	38	42	42	42
Other expenses	41	7	48	40	40	50	50
Total, excluding restaurant	250	30	280	258	274	328	304
Restaurant expenses:							
Food and beverages	96	13	109	67	110	150	130
Salaries and wages:							
Kitchen	32	6	38	30	45	60	50
Dining room	20	4	24	19	26	39	32
Bartender	11	2	13	10	14	19	16
Supplies, repairs and maintenance	13	4	17	8	15	25	18
Total restaurant	172	29	201	134	210	293	246
Total expenses	$422	$59	$481	$392	$484	$621	$550

Fig. 18–1. Worksheet used in preparing an expense budget for a country club.

VALLEY COUNTRY CLUB

STATEMENT OF INCOME AND EXPENSES, AND COMPARISON WITH BUDGET

For the Month of June and the 6 Months Ending June 30, 1972

	Month			6 Months		
	Actual	Budget	Deviation Favorable (Unfavorable)	Actual	Budget	Deviation Favorable (Unfavorable)
Income:						
Annual dues	$15,650	$17,000	($1,350)	$ 81,900	$ 90,000	($ 8,100)
Initiation fees	2,100	2,000	100	6,600	4,500	2,100
Greens fees	4,750	4,000	750	11,000	8,000	3,000
Swimming	3,300	3,000	300	2,300	2,000	300
Other	6,710	8,000	(1,290)	18,250	14,000	4,250
Total, excluding restaurant	32,510	34,000	(1,490)	120,050	118,500	1,550
Restaurant	37,850	34,000	3,850	168,500	180,000	(11,500)
Total income	70,360	68,000	2,360	288,550	298,500	(9,950)
Expenses:						
Maintenance of greens and grounds	14,650	12,000	(2,650)	37,650	36,000	(1,650)
Maintenance of clubhouse	3,450	3,000	(450)	18,100	19,000	900
Golf activities	13,500	10,000	(3,500)	19,500	16,000	(3,500)
Swimming pool	3,400	3,000	(400)	5,100	4,000	(1,100)
General and administrative	4,200	3,700	(500)	24,150	22,000	(2,150)
Payroll taxes	3,700	3,500	(200)	23,500	21,000	(2,500)
Other expenses	4,150	5,000	850	19,560	20,000	440
Total, excluding restaurant	47,050	40,200	(6,850)	147,560	138,000	(9,560)
Restaurant	29,550	27,000	(2,550)	145,650	153,000	7,350
Total expenses	76,600	67,200	(9,400)	293,210	291,000	(2,210)
Excess of income over (under) expenses	($ 6,240)	$ 800	($7,040)	($ 4,660)	$ 7,500	($12,160)

Fig. 18–2. Statement of Income and Expenses for both the month and year to date, showing a comparison to budget.

the six months, there was a deficit of almost $5,000. The board member reading the statement should be concerned about these deviations from the budget. This form of presentation makes it easy to see deviations. He can quickly pinpoint all unfavorable deviations and can then explore the reasons for them and determine the action that must be taken to prevent their recurrence.

Notice that both the current month and the year-to-date figures are shown on this statement. Both are important. The month gives a current picture of what is happening, which cannot be learned from the six-month figures. If only the six-month statements were shown the reader would have to refer to the previous month's statement showing the first five months to see what happened in June. Likewise, to show only the month, with no year-to-date figures, puts a burden on the reader. He will have to do some calculating using previous monthly statements to get his own total to see where the club stood cumulatively. Year-to-date budget comparisons are often more revealing than monthly comparisons because minor fluctuations in income and expenses tend to offset over a period of months. These fluctuations can appear rather large in any one month.

Restaurant Operation

Restaurant income and expenses have been shown "gross" in the statements. It would be equally proper for the club to show net income for the club before the restaurant operation was considered. Here is how this would look:

Income (excluding restaurant)	$ 120,050
Expenses (excluding restaurant)	147,560
Excess of expenses over income excluding restaurant	(27,510)
Restaurant	
Gross income	168,500
Expenses	(145,650)
Net restaurant income	22,850
Excess of expenses over income	$ (4,660)

Another possibility is to show only the net income of the restaurant in the statements, perhaps in the income section. In condensed form here is how the statements would look:

Income	
Other than restaurant	$ 120,050
Restaurant net income	22,850
Total income	142,900
Expenses (other than restaurant)	(147,560)
Excess of expenses over income	$ (4,660)

Either presentation, or the one in Figure 18–2, is acceptable. The appropriate presentation depends on the importance of highlighting the restaurant activities.

Variable Budget

One technique that is often used in budgeting an operation where costs increase as the volume of activity increases is to relate the budgeted costs to income. For example, the final expense budget (Figure 18–1) and the relationship to budgeted income for the restaurant operation is as follows:

	Amount	Percent of Income
Income	$290,000	100%
Food and beverages	$130,000	45%
Salaries and wages		
Kitchen	50,000	17
Dining room	32,000	11
Bartender	16,000	6
Supplies, repairs and maintenance	18,000	6
	$246,000	85%

If all costs increase proportionately as income increases, then it is a simple matter to create new budget figures each month based on actual income. Using the six-month figures shown in Figure 18–2, our budget comparison for the restaurant activity for the six month period would look like this:

	Actual	Variable Budget	Deviation from Variable Budget	Deviation from Original Budget Shown in Figure 18–2
Income	$168,500	$180,000*	$(11,500)	$(11,500)
Expenses (in total)	145,650	143,225†	(2,425)	7,350
Net	$ 22,850	$ 36,775	$(13,925)	$ (4,150)

* Original budget for six months.
† 85% of actual income for the six months, based on the relationship of budgeted expenses to budgeted income as shown above.

The significant observation here is that while the original budget comparison in Figure 18–2 showed an unfavorable deviation from budget of only $4,150, the unfavorable deviation using this variable budget is significantly higher, $13,925. Obviously if the variable budget is accurate, then the club manager has not been watching his costs carefully enough.

The financial statements would show only the variable expense budget.

The original expense budget would not be used. This kind of budget is more difficult to work with because each month the treasurer or book-keeper has to recalculate the expense figures to be used based on actual income. At the same time by doing so, a meaningful budget comparison can be made. It is very difficult otherwise for the board to judge the restaurant's results.

One final observation about this variable budget. Certain costs are not proportional to income. For example, the club cannot have less than one bartender or one chef. Accordingly, in preparing a variable budget sometimes the relationships that are developed will not be simple percentage relationships. For example, perhaps the relationship of bartender salary will be, say, $5,000 plus 5 per cent of total income over $75,000. If so, then if restaurant income is $350,000, the budget will be $18,750 ($5,000 + 5 per cent of $275,000).

Narrative Report on Deviations from Budget
It will be noted that much of the detail shown in the budget (Figure 18–1) has not been shown on the interim financial statement (Figure 18–2). If the board felt it appropriate, supporting schedules could be prepared giving as much detail as desired. Care should be taken, however, not to request details that won't be used since it obviously takes time and costs money to prepare detailed supporting schedules.

It may be that a more meaningful supporting schedule would be a narrative summary of the reasons for the deviations from budget for the major income and expense categories. The club manager, in the case of the Valley Country Club, would probably be the one to prepare this summary. The amount of detail and description that he might put in this summary would vary from account to account. Clearly the report should only discuss reasons for the major deviations. This report should accompany the financial statement so that questions raised by the statement are answered immediately. Figure 18–3 shows an example of the type of summary he might prepare to explain the expense deviations from budget (in part).

This type of report can be as informal as you want to make it as long as it conveys why there have been deviations from the original budget. But it should be in writing, both to ensure that the board knows the reasons, and to force the club manager to face squarely his responsibility to meet the projected budget. This report is a form of discipline for him.

CONCLUSION

A budget can be an extremely important and effective tool for the board in managing the affairs of the organization. However, to prepare a meaningful budget the organization must know where it is heading and its goals and objectives. Priorities change and this means that many people should

VALLEY COUNTRY CLUB
CLUB MANAGER'S REPORT TO THE BOARD
EXPENSE DEVIATIONS FROM BUDGET, JUNE 1972

Maintenance of greens and grounds ($2,650)

As you will recall, April and May were fairly wet months. This coupled with other unfavorable soil conditions required that we treat about 25% of the course with a fungicide which had not been budgeted ($1,850). We also had some unexpected repairs to the sprinkler system ($1,500). For the six months to date we have exceeded budget by only $1,650 and I am confident that our annual budget will not be exceeded.

Maintenance of clubhouse ($450)

We had scheduled painting the Clubhouse for May but because of the rains were not able to get it done until this month. Year-to-date expenses are $900 under budget.

Golf activities ($3,500)

After the budget had been approved the Board decided to have an open tournament with a view toward attracting new membership. With promotion and prizes this came to $2,850. So far the membership committee has received thirteen new applications for membership.

Fig. 18–3. An example of a narrative report prepared by the manager of a country club explaining why certain major deviations have occurred from budget.

be involved in the budget preparation and approval process to insure the resulting budget is fully supported. Once prepared, the budget must be compared to actual results on a timely basis throughout the year to insure that the board knows where deviations are occurring. Equally important, the board must promptly take corrective action if unfavorable deviations occur. The foundations of a sound financial structure are a well-conceived budget, a timely reporting system, and a willingness by the board to take corrective action.

The importance of planning into the future cannot be overemphasized. In this fast-moving age, worthy nonprofit organizations can quickly get out of step with the times, and when this happens contributions and income quickly disappear. A five-year master plan is one technique to help ensure this won't happen.

B. PROGRAM BUDGETING AND COST ANALYSIS

20/PROGRAM BUDGETING WORKS IN NONPROFIT INSTITUTIONS

RODERICK K. MACLEOD

FOREWORD

Professionals in nonprofit service organizations have long resisted the inauguration of cost accounting concepts (in many instances with good reason), but their resistance is breaking down in the face of supporters' demands for better controls over expenditure of the money, materials, and manpower they contribute. Often, however, the well-intentioned management and trustees of an institution do not know how to begin introducing cost accountability and program budgeting to their operation. In this article the author "walks" the reader through the establishment of a planning and accounting system which has resulted in much improved costing and planning at a once-drifting mental health clinic employing about 100 professionals. The same principles, he says, are applicable to other nonprofit professional activities.

A minor aspect of the honorable tradition of eleemosynary activity has been that you could not, and did not need to, account for the cost of services being provided. You could not because they were qualitative and intangible; you did not need to because funds were provided by gifts, grants, endowments, and so on. For the last several years this tradition has been called increasingly into question as the desire for cost information and accountability grows and as the control bases for cost accounting come more and more into focus. However, there has not been much recorded practical experience on which to judge the utility of cost accounting in institutional management.

This article is a record of one such practical experience—broad enough to have general application but small enough to be fully described in a few pages. It is written for businessmen who, as trustees or directors of institutions, find themselves as frustrated as I was at the inability of some administrators to deal effectively with costs or even to keep track of what was happening financially. I hope it encourages them with the thought that it can be done.

Program cost accounting is in its third year of functioning at the South Shore Mental Health Center in Quincy, Massachusetts, a community agency with about 100 professional staff members. The agency derives its funds from a variety of sources for a variety of reasons; its professional staff is employed on a variety of terms, and there is no objective or numerical measure of the value of its diversified services. It therefore has most of the cost accounting problems of nonprofit organizations.

The first two of the following sections are written for those who are not familiar with either cost accounting or program budgeting. Both are essential to understanding the utility of program cost accounting. Anyone who knows these subjects should skip to the point in the article where I describe how we put them to use. It begins with the section, "Working in the dark."

COST ACCOUNTING

Defined as a body of techniques for associating costs with the purposes for which they are incurred, cost accounting was developed primarily for determining product costs in manufacturing processes. It is also used to determine the cost of services or activities.

"Nonprofit" Uses

In profit-making enterprises cost accounting is an essential aid to maximizing profits. While this incentive is not present in nonprofit institutions, cost accounting has at least these three other important purposes: efficiency and cost control, planning and allocating resources of people and funds, and "pricing" for cost reimbursement.

Efficiency & cost control. People often (some would say always) get careless about what they are doing, and if you are paying them, that means extra costs. If you know how much it costs to do something under optimum conditions and if you can measure the output of that something fairly accurately, then you can determine actual costs per unit of output and keep track of how efficiently the job is being done.

Of course, you have to be careful that cost saving is achieved without sacrificing quality of output. This is the reason why many institutions have felt that cost accounting is a bad influence. They say that the quality of service is too precious and fragile to be subjected to the pressure of cost accountability and to the drive for efficiency.

However, cost accounting can be used to set standards and to measure performance against them in a number of institutional activities without threatening the quality of service. Clerical and record-keeping operations, library services, nursing services, and storekeeping are examples of operations involving clearly defined results and enough labor to make worthwhile the effort of directing them efficiently.

Food service is another good example. A meal is either served and eaten, or it is not, and the size of portions and nutritional value can be measured and controlled. (Cost control and efficiency are accepted goals, even though it is recognized that pleasing the person who eats the meal is a highly qualitative and subjective thing.)

Another area which has received some attention, though not as much, is maintenance, including grounds keeping and housekeeping. Most maintenance activities can be quite clearly defined and the standard of quality made explicit. It is possible, for instance, to determine the optimum time for mowing a lawn, clearing a drain, making a bed, or repairing a boiler. For the most part, these estimates are used to schedule tasks and monitor performance, but they can easily be converted into dollar casts, when there is reason to do so.

So-called "efficiency experts" have earned a deservedly bad name in some quarters, and the feeling persists that work standards constitute another technological chain fettering the human spirit. Sensibly used, they need not be. It can be far more satisfying to work toward a well-defined and attainable goal than to work under the pressure of a never-ending backlog and an unknown and never-reached standard of excellence.

Furthermore, pride in one's work can be served better by the existence of standards authorizing the worker to call for help when a deviation appears, rather than obliging him to sink or swim. Standards should be a sensible way of organizing and carrying out tasks, not a means for applying pressure to reach unnatural levels of performance.

Resource allocation. A great deal of planning is done without cost accounting, and a great many institutions survive without planning. It is generally agreed, however, that careful planning and resource allocation are important elements of good management and that precise estimates of costs are necessary for careful planning.

Costs can often be gauged accurately enough for use in planning without going through the labor of accounting for actual costs. But there is no better way to verify the accuracy of estimates than to account for actual costs and then to compare them with the estimates.

While cost accounting has to be painstakingly accurate to be useful in measuring and controlling efficiency, a much wider range of imprecision is tolerable for planning purposes. A decision to expand a facility or to move in one direction rather than another will probably be affected by a 50% change in the relevant costs, but seldom by a change of only 10% or 20%. This is why it is useful to cost professional services even though a legitimate respect for professional freedom of action requires acceptance of a substantial probability of inaccuracy.

Cost recovery pricing. The most compelling reason for undertaking the effort of cost accounting is the chance to get paid for what one does. In profit-making enterprises this incentive is obvious. In nonprofit institutions it is becoming obvious as they take on activities for which someone (usually the government) is willing to reimburse them. Medicare is one example. Another is the contract research work that many organizations undertake; cost accounting is at the heart of disputes over whether they are receiving adequate reimbursement.

When dollars change hands, accuracy is extremely important to both parties, but it is of a different order from that required for measuring efficiency. If they wish, the two parties to a cost reimbursement contract can agree on completely unrealistic or arbitrary definitions of cost. It is then necessary only to follow these agreements faithfully to obtain satisfactory reimbursement.

Usually, the simpler these agreements, the better, however much they may differ from principles of "real" cost determination. But continued use of unrealistic cost definitions ultimately makes the recipient of funds dependent on them and forces him to distort his actual experience to fit the reimbursement pattern.

Problems in Use

Associating costs with products or activities is simple enough conceptually, but in practice there are several problems for which there are no very satisfactory answers.

The most troublesome of these is what to do about costs that are common to several products or that do not vary with the amount produced. All the alternatives proposed or in use involve some means of prorating these overhead costs, joint costs, or fixed costs. The most common method is to relate these indirect costs to one or more of the direct costs, such as labor hours or labor dollars.

Whatever method is employed, users of cost data must keep in mind that the allocation is somewhat arbitrary. Troubles arise when they start thinking of these aggregates as "true" costs.

Another problem is caused by costs incurred at one point in time that underwrite activities and production over an extended period of time, such as expenditure for buildings and equipment. Plant costs are incurred before use in production, but other costs for which payment may be made in the distant future, such as employee pensions and deferred maintenance, must also be taken into account in determining the cost of current activities.

There are many theories concerning which of several methods of depreciation, amortization, or accrual is best and whether and how provisions for technological change and inflation should be made. As with overhead costs, however, all methods make somewhat arbitrary allocations.

Nonprofit institutions have traditionally ignored these capital costs, usually on the grounds that they were funded by gifts or grants. This tradition is being questioned increasingly as institutional managers try to compare costs of different activities and, particularly, as they find the government and others willing to pay for the "cost" of an activity, but demanding that the institution determine what that cost is.

Still another problem, one particularly troublesome to institutions, is determining what it is that you should compute the cost of. When you make widgets, it is easy enough to figure. In the service sector, providing meals and giving gamma globulin injections are clear-cut units of output. But it is not easy to define a satisfactory "production" unit for medical care, education, and many other kinds of social services.

There is a good deal of agonizing over this question, perhaps more than is necessary. It is useful to know the cost per patient-hour or medical treatment or the cost per student-hour of education, although they are not units of output. An hour of a doctor's care or of a professor's teaching is an input, not an output. The real output here is health or knowledge, and we do not yet know how to measure either well enough.

It is important for an organization to have accurate unit cost data for planning and evaluating the use of its resources. It is also important to be careful how the data are used for cost control. The real product could be seriously impaired by an attempt to minimize the cost per hour.

PROGRAM BUDGETING

Traditionally, budgeting in institutions has been a purely fiscal function divorced from social service planning. Customarily, about once a year the financial or accounting staff looked at the institution's expenses for heat, light, telephones, professional dues, and so on and guessed how much these might increase the next year. Sometimes the staff went so far as to ask the professionals what staff they expected to add or subtract, and at what change in cost. The result, the budget, was submitted to the board of trustees.

I wonder how many trustees have shared my experience of masking feelings of impotence and ignorance as I solemnly reviewed the lists of figures. From time to time I would ask why a figure differed from the corresponding one a year earlier.

If the income did not equal the outgo, I refused to approve the budget. But as soon as the budget was in balance, I approved it, without any real reason for knowing that the year could or should come out that way.

The process actually has worked quite well, and I do not mean to suggest that it be abandoned. After all, some sense of financial responsibility is better than none. And the trustees' review of the budget serves to remind dedicated professionals of the facts of life that they like to ignore in their pursuit of worthy social goals. Something better is available now, however.

The idea of program budgeting as an aid to planning the allocation of resources in a complex nonprofit organization is clear and very attractive. Actual practice, however, has been impeded by ignorance, caution, and preoccupation with technique.

Disciplined Thinking . . .
The principal conceptual innovation in program budgeting is disciplined thinking about what it is that an institution is producing. It follows logically that it is useful to budget the costs associated with those products and to evaluate the social benefits realized in relation to costs and alternative uses of funds and other resources.

Professionals have always thought to some degree about the programs they were engaged in, but usually without going so far as to associate costs with them. It is obvious, for example, that "patient hours" breaks down into diagnosis and prophylaxis as well as treatment and that a college's arts and sciences program includes instruction in physical sciences, social sciences, and the humanities. But professionals have generally thought it unnecessary or impossible to weigh the relative merits or costs of parts of such programs; so nobody tried. Current financial stringencies are making such "impossibilities" not only possible but also compelling.

Even rudimentary thinking about products brings useful insights. One notes that professors do not just teach students; they teach several different kinds of students, they engage in research and consulting, they publish, they help other departments, they talk, they politick, and they join in community and social service activities. The levels of capital investment and nonprofessional support services can be seen to vary from one activity to another. The interdepartmental impact of a new discipline can be glimpsed.

Sometimes, but not often, it is clear that results do not warrant the cost and that resources should be allocated elsewhere—such as converting a half-empty obstetrical ward into a geriatric ward.

In most allocation decisions, however, the relevant cost data and their relationship to the level of expected results are not at all clear. A factor even more critical to a decision is often overlooked: the implicit commitment to supply substantial additional resources in the future, as when a bequest for a new laboratory is gratefully accepted without the recipients' understanding the necessity for eventual expansion of all related and an-cillary activities.

. . . & Organization

Program budgeting permits disciplined organization of the economic data relative to a decision involving the allocation of resources. Using it, one can gather costs by program, evaluate the impact of a program's expansion or contraction on directly and indirectly related costs, and estimate with some degree of confidence the program's future economic demands.

In its highest form, as developed and advertised by the Department of Defense, program budgeting also involves measuring and comparing the value of the output of various programs in terms of social utility. This is a dazzling concept, and we can look forward with great eagerness to the day when we can gauge the value of a heart surgery unit versus that of a better cancer treatment unit or the social utility of a degree in physics versus that of a comparable degree in psychology. Nobody can do it yet. But this fact should not detract from the great contribution program budgeting can make right now.

Program budgeting offers these aids to managers of service institutions:

• The conceptual discipline for defining what the institution is doing.

• The process of sorting out expenditures so as to identify the direct and allocated costs.

• The process of relating the various types of funding to the purposes for which they were intended and of identifying the uses to which unre-stricted funds are being put.

• The means for estimating with confidence the cost consequences of expanding or contracting any program and the related impact on other programs and facilities.

• The means for examining the financial implications of a program over a span of time.

• The concept (and, sometime in the future, the means) of measuring the results of programs by some common denominator.

There are plenty of problems in employing program budgeting. Among them are getting professionals to submit to accountability, securing reli-able data, defining programs sufficiently, and finding an adequate measure of output. The discovery that these matters can be dealt with fairly di-rectly, and that it is worth doing, is the main message of this article.

WORKING IN THE DARK

The South Shore Mental Health Center began many years ago as a small children's clinic. When Dr. David Van Buskirk took over as director in 1967, it had expanded to the point where it was providing the nine communities in its area with substantially all kinds of mental health service except overnight and custodial treatment.

The services were carried out by about 100 professionals under a bewildering and seemingly unlimited variety of individual arrangements. Some of them worked full time, but most of them had other jobs or private practices.

The principal source of funds was the Commonwealth of Massachusetts, which employed physicians, psychologists, nurses, social workers, and other professionals to work at the Center in civil service "blocks" of time. The communities, represented by an association of citizens, were responsible for securing the funds for facilities and administration and, since the state salary scales were inadequate, for supplementing the professional salaries. These funds were obtained primarily through billing the communities served at a certain rate per patient-hour, and secondarily from patient fees.

The Center also enjoyed an erratic flow of money from grants and research contracts, principally through the National Institute of Mental Health. Sometimes the grants were for additional work, and the Center served merely as fiscal agent. Sometimes they were for participation in work that was the normal part of the Center's business, so that the funds served in effect to relieve the communities of part of their financial burden.

The Center also received money funded by groups or government agencies for various programs. These included community education, retarded children's schooling, a rehabilitation workshop, and several training programs.

In spite of, or perhaps because of, the complexity of the Center's operations and the funding of them, the agency's financial management prior to 1967 was extraordinarily simple. A budget was prepared annually in which each category of receipts and expenses was estimated and made to balance. Toward the end of the year, the director and his assistant adjusted their salaries (usually downward) to make the outgo equal the income.

The board of trustees had only a general idea of the way in which the Center's activities were funded and no idea at all of the important relationships among the sources of funding. Through hindsight, it appears probable that the administrators of the Center did not either. They were exceptionally dedicated people; and they paid dearly for their lack of financial acumen in the form of almost daily crises, overwork, and low salaries.

Demand-Cost Squeeze

Dr. Van Buskirk's first months at the Center must have been a time of great anxiety for him as he struggled to understand how things worked, in the face of a nearly complete lack of information. He did manage to put together figures on the number of hours given to patient diagnosis and treatment.

To develop the "cost per patient hour," a statistic widely used in the health profession, he divided the total operating cost by the number of patient-hours. The result dismayed him. It showed that costs per patient-hour were rising at a rate of about 25% a year.

Because the funds provided by the state could be expected to increase by no more than 10%, if at all, the communities served had to bear the rising costs alone. Since the nine communities had previously paid about one third of the total cost, the leverage effect was dramatic; the Center was faced with asking them to increase their appropriations to it by 65% to 75%. In a period of strong taxpayer resistance, that prospect was nearly intolerable.

The director recognized that an important reason for the soaring costs per patient-hour was the rapid expansion of other demands on the professional staff. The South Shore community was beginning to accept the long-held conviction among mental health professionals that early detection and prevention of emotional and mental problems is far better than is any amount of treatment. Instead of concentrating on seeing patients, the psychiatrists, psychologists, and social workers were beginning to spend more of their time with the front line of community social servants—school guidance counselors, teachers, police officers, court officers, and ministers.

The result was both a decline in the number of patient-hours needed for preliminary screening of applicants and an increase in the Center's total cost. Clearly, the cost per patient-hour was an inadequate and misleading statistic.

Dr. Van Buskirk had other incentives to innovate. He found that programs for which he was responsible were ballooning. The rehabilitation "sheltered workshop" project, for example, grew within a year from a small experiment to a well-established quarter-million-dollar operation, even before the board of trustees knew it existed.

Demands for new programs came from all directions and usually from persons with little interest or ability in helping to determine how they would be paid for. For example, the drug abuse problem, to which the suburban communities had awakened, began soaking up the time of the Center's professionals. "Hot line" and other counseling services were springing up all over the area, their founders assuming that the Center would take care of any and all treatment referrals.

Moreover, the professionals were asking controversial questions about the relative values of different activities. Should they give priority to services for adults or for children; to after-care and group services or to conventional doctor-patient treatment; to social services or to clinical services? There was no information available to aid the administration in evaluating any of these problems; the director was forced to make decisions solely on intuition and judgment.

DEVELOPING A SYSTEM

At about that time, a college senior came to the Center for three months as part of her work-study program. She had no accounting background or qualifications for the job Dr. Van Buskirk gave her, other than the average college student's ease with numbers and concepts. But before she left, she had helped the director install a program cost accounting system. Perhaps an important reason for this extraordinary accomplishment is that neither she nor the director was burdened with the professional accountant's knowledge of how difficult it is to set up a new system.

The first step was to define the programs that made up the Center's services. After much redrafting of lists of functions, the director settled on five main categories subdivided into a total of 26 separate programs. These main areas were clinical services, community services, retardation and rehabilitation services, training, and research. As an example of the detail involved, clinical services included five programs: children's services, adult services, after-care services, disturbed children's nursery and kindergarten, and court-requested evaluations.

For the most part, the distinctions among programs were clear. The only important artificial separation involved the training function. As in most professional service activities, nearly everything that went on had important training elements, and the trainees contributed greatly to the Center's work. Dr. Van Buskirk decided arbitrarily that trainees' direct costs would be allocated to the programs in which they worked, while the cost of time spent by professionals and teachers in instruction and guidance would be charged to training.

Staff Time

The next step was to ask the professionals to report how their time during an average week was allocated among the 26 programs. A simple form was drawn up, listing the programs and asking for the individual's estimate of the percentage of time he devoted to every one that took more than 10% of his time. Experience with this document inadvertently carried the project through three of the obstacles most commonly cited as rendering program cost accounting difficult, if not impossible:

1. It dispelled the notion that professionals simply will not hold still for rendering themselves accountable. This is no doubt the case when meticulous, detailed, and frequent reporting is required or when the ultimate value of the effort is not fully understood. However, spending 15 minutes three or four times a year with a simple form is not overly demanding, especially when a respected superior has explained the importance of the results.

The value of top professional involvement in communicating the importance of the project cannot be overemphasized, and it is a likely reason for the success of this endeavor. The Center's professional head, not the nonprofessional administrators or accountants, initiated and carried out the project. He spent at least an hour with the professionals from each program, explaining what he hoped to achieve and discussing their own needs. The professionals were understandably more willing to give him their confidence and cooperation, and he, having a well-defined goal, was able to keep the project from getting bogged down in procedural details.

2. It taught us how to deal with inaccuracy and subjectivity in the initial time estimates. It is true that an annual or even quarterly estimate is unlikely to be very accurate, and it is also true that some of the staff might report their estimates of what ought to be happening, rather than what really is happening. We found these faults tolerable for two reasons.

First, other potential inaccuracies—e.g., those introduced by overhead allocation—require a generous tolerance for imprecision in the use of the results. Also, because the estimates of the programs' social utility are necessarily vague and subjective, no other factor entering into decisions about them, such as cost, need be measured with any great precision. I must again emphasize that even a rough idea of the cost of a program is so useful that arguments about precision are reduced to the level of quibbles.

Second, every program or activity has someone responsible for it, who watches it with great professional affection and jealousy. If he understands the value of the resulting information, he can be relied on to identify gross errors of omission and commission.

He can also be relied on to respond to the test of output. The head of a program may tolerate for one or two periods, but not indefinitely, a cost allocation disproportionate to results. The Director made what amounted to a contract with each group of professionals to produce a given level and mix of services for a given level of cost, and as long as these were forthcoming and up to standard, he did not worry about the continued accuracy of the original time estimates.

3. Reporting in terms of percentages avoided problems arising from the use of other yardsticks. Accountants like to have reports prepared in precise units like hours or days, and the director had to resist the temptation to seek the orderliness inherent in using units one can measure, count, control, and balance out.

He was forced into the choice of percentages because at the Center there are too many varieties of part-time participation to permit any common denominator except "percentage of time devoted to Center activities." This choice avoided the often-heard complaint that professionals cannot report time because they do not work conventional hours. Whether a professional customarily works 18 hours a day or 4 does not affect his percentage allocation.

From the time-allocation forms, the college student made the necessary calculations for assigning the appropriate fraction of each professional's salary to the programs he was engaged in. Some of the professionals were not on the Center's payroll at all because they were assigned to training or research projects by colleges and other organizations in the area. For each of these individuals, the director computed a salary equivalent that was recorded in a memorandum account as a source of funds from his particular organization. The corresponding "cost" was then allocated among the appropriate programs.

Income & Outgo

The Center's expenses were analyzed and segregated into those that related directly to programs and those that made up general administration and overhead. The total costs turned out to be 80% program-oriented salaries, 11% other direct costs, and 9% general overhead (including administrative salaries).

Because none of the decisions to be made would hinge on a variation of cost as slight as 10%, the overhead allocation problem was determined to be insignificant. Rather than trying to refine the process, the director simply allocated the 9% of overhead costs to the 26 programs in proportion to their salary costs.

The director had a lot more trouble with allocating the portion of the Center's total cost (15%) that related to the nine separate training programs. Is training an end product of the Center, or is it a necessary element in maintaining the levels of professional skill in the other programs? It is both, of course. Also, as I have noted, it is impossible to distinguish training from the service programs where the training takes place.

We decided to treat training first as a separately accountable endeavor and secondly as an integral part of the other service programs, following the principle that a substantial element of training is essential to a high level of professional service. Each training program was therefore either assigned to the service program where it took place or prorated among the several programs to which it related. The full cost of each training program was allocated without reduction for related grants received; the grants were considered part of the income directly relating to the service programs.

The remaining step was to figure out who was paying for each program. Money received for specific purposes was first assigned to the appropriate program: grants, stipends, the "equivalent salary" of contributed workers, fees received from patients and from agencies such as school boards—all went toward the programs for which they were received. Then the appropriate fraction of the state salary paid to the professionals who had indicated participation in these programs was identified and treated as a source of funds.

The difference between the total program cost and these identified funds

EXHIBIT I

Costs and Sources of Funds for Operating the Disturbed Children's
Nursery and Kindergarten

	Amount
Costs	
Professional salaries	$18,500
Direct costs	1,950
Overhead	2,200
Training, specifically identified	3,600
Total	$26,250
Sources of money	
Wheelock College training grant	$ 3,600
State salaries, specified	12,650
State salaries, unspecified	9,500
Total	$25,750
Community funds allocated by the Center	500
Total	$26,250

had to be made up from the amounts billed to the communities served. One of the simpler examples, the finances for running the disturbed children's nursery and kindergarten, is presented in *Exhibit I*.

One other element of the new system required some thought: identifying units of service that would facilitate projections of the cost effect of a change in program. This was easy for conventional treatment services, where an interview with a patient almost invariably is scheduled to last an hour. In the school-type programs, such as the cerebral palsy nursery, we could use the traditional statistic, "full-time equivalent enrollee." The measurement of counseling and community service programs required more thought and, ultimately, presented us with another conceptual discovery.

It is a tradition in the medical profession that services are being performed only when one is face-to-face with a patient. But in a community service program, a professional can spend hours preparing material; more hours in transit to and from a community; an hour, say, with a social agency there; and then still more hours writing down the results. If he reported only the one hour spent with the agency, the record of effort—and cost—actually invested would clearly be inaccurate.

From the community's point of view, however, the unit of output received from the Center is the single hour with the professional. There has to be a distinction between time spent for costing purposes and the unit of time used for output purposes. When both are used for planning purposes, one gets a clearer picture of why community service workers' case loads seem so light compared with those of clinical workers.

What is more important, when professionals can be persuaded to report on the basis of time invested in an activity rather than on the basis of interview output, the true costs begin to appear; and clinical services are relieved of the burden of carrying part of the cost of other programs.

SOLID RESULTS

At this writing, program costing is completing its third year of operation. Since the Center's activities roughly follow the pattern of the school year and since most of the professionals work according to a pattern of commitment that changes very little during a year, it probably is unnecessary to gather information and cost it out more often than once a year, but the director does it quarterly for verification purposes. Data on output are, of course, gathered currently and compared with the budget.

It takes more than two months to pull the cost data together, but not because of clerical or computational burdens. The time elapses because the process obliges the staff to discover, discuss, examine, define, and redirect. Inadvertent shifts of effort and focus are uncovered, as are activities that seem to be taking more time than they are worth. Once accepted by the professionals, the costing effort induces an element of planning that was absent before, and also foreign to many of them.

What You Pay For, You Get

The most dramatic result of the first crude program costing effort was also the most pragmatic: the Center started assessing users for the cost of the services they demanded. This was quite a contrast with the Center's early years, when the professionals were apologetic in seeking payment for its activities.

The approach to the town finance committees and city administrators used to be, "Please help us out with x thousands of dollars." Now the Center had the information to support this position: "Here is a list of services we have been asked to provide you and the amount that each will cost. Please authorize payment, or you'll have to get along without the service."

As everyone knows who is acquainted with methods of municipal government, it is never that simple. Getting acceptance of the change in approach necessitated much demonstration, explanation, and cajoling. It was a delicate matter to explain to a community that, whereas in the past its financial support had been applied generally to the operation of the Center's programs, now these programs (many of them unfamiliar to, and typically not specifically demanded by, the community) were to be underwritten separately, or otherwise canceled.

In some cases the exigencies of politics required reversion to the time-honored procedure of raising charges per patient-hour. Nevertheless, the campaign to obtain payments for particular services rendered moved slowly ahead. The progress permitted the Center to hold the line on charge for long-established activities.

Sometimes we "found" costs that were reimbursable under one program buried in another. An example is the rehabilitation workshop whose costs are reimbursed by a state agency. Program costing turned up about $35,000 worth of unrecognized professional and nonprofessional support which was being provided by persons at the Center not specifically identified with the workshop. And this discovery served to shift the burden of reimbursement from the communities to the state agency.

Cost Data in Planning

The next most important product of the cost accounting effort was the ability to examine the cost of new demands made on the Center. In earlier days, for example, the willing response of the agency's professionals to the awakening concern over drug addiction and related mental health problems would have included little thought for the consequences—an inundation of unanswered and unanswerable calls for help, diagnosis, and treatment. Now we have the information with which to sound the alarm about needed facilities and funding while interest in the service is at a peak.

Moreover, it is now possible to think and talk about relative costs in setting priorities. Priority setting remains highly subjective; the relative importance of various activities is more or less established by the director as he listens to the demands coming from various quarters and analyzes the interests and abilities of the people available. Having cost information available leads to considerations like these:

• We could double our work with the police departments if we were willing to give up 5% of our children's clinical services.

• If we are asked to participate heavily in a drug abuse program, the resources for it cannot come from any of the programs funded by restricted money, and the nursery school and rehabilitation staffs are not qualified. So we would have to cut back on clinical or community services after determining which one would free the most money with the least loss to the communities.

• A suggestion that we join in a new community program on alcoholism must be rejected because we can foresee the amount of commitment that would be required if it were successful, and all our funds are committed to programs that seem to be more effective.

Spotlight on Funds Flows

A very important discovery was the interaction among the different kinds of funds. Before program costing and budgeting, the unrestricted money was "just used," and the forces affecting its use were unrecognized and un-controlled. When available funds were related to the costs of programs, we discovered such things as these:

• Receipt of restricted money pushes unrestricted money out of a program, making it available for other purposes.

• Loss of restricted money, even with a concurrent reduction in program, sucks up some unrestricted money, if for no other reason than the loss of contribution to overhead.

• The same service is often funded twice, thereby relieving the general demand on unrestricted funds. (For example, when a trainee—whose salary has been contributed—works on a project for which a grant was received, the portion of the grant money that otherwise would have been applied to his salary relieves the communities of part of their burden of providing the unrestricted funds for the Center.)

• Attractive service opportunities always receive "hidden funding" because they are supported by professionals who would otherwise be working on the programs for which they are being paid.

A case in point is the after-care program, which is 30% supported by community funds and requires 10% of the total community contribution. After-care is counseling and support of patients during their difficult period of adjustment after release from state mental hospitals.

Mental health professionals have long felt that an after-care program plays an extremely important part in a patient's cure, and, to the extent that he is completely rehabilitated, it is an important service to the community. However, no community has specifically contracted for an after-care program.

What, then, are the ethics of using funds appropriated for certain services to finance another service not on the list and perhaps not even known to the appropriating cities and towns? Yet if you do not do it this way, how do you get the chance to incubate new services?

There are several good answers to these questions, but the point is that you have to think of the questions before you can answer them. (In this case, we recognized "hidden funding" as a fact of life and articulated the policy that new program development is a recognized overhead cost, much like training.)

Wider Horizons

Program cost accounting has opened up some promising lines of thought that have yet to be explored. We wonder, for example, why treatment of adults seems to cost more per hour than does treatment of children, and work with school counselors more than work with courts and police. The director has not tackled these questions because he is not sure the statistics are right. The data base must grow and "season" for a while before it can be trusted to help answer such detailed questions.

Another set of interesting questions is raised by thinking about overhead costs and their relationship to programs. Perhaps most overhead items can be associated with specific programs when they are significant enough to warrant the trouble. The chief accountant and the chief engineer can make quite good estimates of where their staffs are spending their hours, and, if necessary, they can require time reports so that costs can be accounted for by program.

But why should a fully funded program bear any of the costs of the accounts receivable department? Or why should the counseling program, carried out entirely off the premises, bear as much plant and maintenance cost as do those that use the plant?

Perhaps there is not really much true overhead in any institution; perhaps most of it is really part of unidentified additional programs or additions to particular programs. Consider the college admissions office, the development office, the almuni office, the news office, the placement office, and so on; are they overhead, or is each engaged in a purposeful program of its own?

These thoughts suggest the kinds of hard questions that can be asked about overhead on the basis of the program cost concept. What is causing the overhead cost? Is it worth it? Why do we need that overhead program? Is it paying for itself? Are we asking users to share the cost of doing something unnecessary or of something for a completely unrelated beneficiary?

On a more ambitious level, the director is thinking about freeing mental health services from the encumbrances of politics and civil service by contracting for specific outputs of service at a fixed price per unit of output. He needed accurate cost accounting before he could dare propose it.

In summary, all concerned are delighted with the results of program cost accounting. The professionals do not find it burdensome, and they know much they did not know before. The administrators and the trustees are beginning to feel they understand what is going on, and they move with more confidence, both in planning and in finding the funds.

CONCLUSION

The message is not that we have found program budgeting and accounting to be a good thing; everyone knows it is. My message is that *it can be done*. Here are my recommendations for institutional administrators and trustees:

• Insist on knowing what the institution's programs are and who is paying for them.

• Insist on analysis of the costs of proposed program changes.

• Insist that the reasons for proposed changes in expenditures be stated, and in terms of output of services.

• Insist on knowing what the institution is getting for its overhead.

If you insist on all of these things, it will take a program budgeting and accounting system (at least a rudimentary one) to give you the answers.

If you are persuasive or powerful enough to move the institution in this direction, one additional admonition is in order: keep it simple. Don't let the zeal of accountants and administrators for procedural order bog down the effort in mechanics.

Your reward will be the discovery that you can be in control of the institution you are responsible for, rather than the other way around.

21/COST-BENEFIT ANALYSIS

AND SOCIAL WELFARE

PROGRAM EVALUATION

ABRAHAM S. LEVINE

BACKGROUND

For a long time cost-benefit analysis has been almost exclusively the province of the economist. Recently it has attracted attention in other circles, including public welfare, as a result of the widespread adoption of a new planning and budgeting concept which has been inaugurated in the executive branch of the federal government. Launched in August, 1965, by President Lyndon B. Johnson, the Planning-Programming-Budgeting System (PPBS) has the following objectives: (1) to identify our national goals with precision; (2) to choose among these goals the ones that are most urgent; (3) to search for alternative means of reaching these goals most effectively at the least cost; (4) to inform ourselves not merely on next year's cost—but on the second, and third, and subsequent years' costs—of our programs; and (5) to measure the performance of our programs to insure that the money is best spent.

Implicit in the statement of the last objective is an analytical process involving special studies in depth from time to time. It is here that the cost-benefit analysis approach comes into the picture.

NATURE OF COST-BENEFIT ANALYSIS

By "cost-benefit" is meant the relationship of the resources required—the cost—to attain certain goals—the benefits. It is based on the economic concept that many executive decisions involve the allocation, or best use, of limited resources among competing requirements. The allocation of available resources is determined by a comparative analysis of the current system with presumably practicable alternative systems. Thus conceived, cost-benefit analysis is a tool for the administrator confronted with the need to make choices among viable competing programs designed to achieve certain objectives. It is not a substitute for the educated judgment of the decision-maker. Rather it provides a package of relevant information on which to base certain kinds of decisions. Also, it does not favor the "cheapest" or even the "best" program, but the optimal program in terms of the available resources (money, trained personnel, facilities).

Before the federal government adopted it on a widespread basis, cost-benefit analysis had been applied primarily by economists in a large number of different contexts, such as road-building, railways, inland waterways, urban highways, urban renewal, and recreation facilities, to name but a few. Usually benefits as well as costs have been given a dollar value, and benefit over cost ratios have been computed. A ratio in excess of one indicates worthwhileness from an investment point of view—the higher the ratio, the better. Thus, a ratio of 22 indicates that $22 in benefits is being realized for every $1 expended.

When one is dealing with hardware systems it makes a great deal of sense to think of benefits as well as costs in dollar terms. But how does such a plan fit in assessing social welfare programs in which most, if not all, of the presumed payoff is in terms of the well-being of the client or the changes that take place in his attitudes and behavior? Before discussing where cost-benefit analysis fits into the social welfare research picture, it might be well to delineate the basic concepts involved.

Costs

First, there are the cost considerations. These are not easy to determine, since they depend on how they are estimated. Cost analysis is exclusively concerned with this aspect. Sometimes all that an administrator wants to know is what it costs, for example, to provide for the care of children in a number of different institutions for which he has the responsibility, and what factors account for these costs. For example, in a study by Martin Wolins[1] the cost per child in an institution was related to the degree of disturbance shown by the child and the degree of social adequacy revealed by the child's family. It was shown that the "seriously disturbed" children required more professional time than the "family-problem" children.

When the children were classified according to their tendency to avoid, or move toward or against, other children, it was noted that the children who avoided other children appeared to receive a proportionately greater amount of time from psychiatrists, psychologists, and remedial teachers.

Benefits

A cost analysis is extremely useful in identifying the costs of the various services and who received them. However, in a cost-benefit analysis we are also at least as much concerned with what these services did for recipients. "Benefits" have reference to whether the desired changes have taken place and to what extent they have occurred. Benefits are usually far more difficult to measure than are costs, for reasons that will become clearer in the discussion of the third component.

Objectives or Goals

The third essential component complex in a cost-benefit systems analysis is what may be referred to as objectives, goals, values, and the like. These are inextricably related to benefits, for they imply an agreed-upon degree and kind of change. The "objectives" constitute the criteria that determine whether a "benefit" is in fact beneficial. Usually we find that the goals or objectives are not well-defined. Unless they are clarified, there is little chance of determining the extent to which they are being, or might be, realized. Also, the objectives are often stated in broad and general terms. Before they can be useful for analytical purposes such statements must be translated into operational terms, preferably ones which are readily amenable to measurement.

Measurement

Whenever "measurement" is involved in social welfare or, for that matter, in the social sciences, there is a special kind of danger involved. This occupational hazard has its roots in the tendency we all have to do what comes most easily—in this case to measure what is most readily measurable. In order to avoid this pitfall it is necessary first to back away from the whole problem of measurement and ask the question: What should be measured and why? In order to answer this question, one must distinguish between the benefits and the outputs of a program. There is a tendency to lose sight of this difference, particularly when the real outcomes or benefits are difficult to measure. What often takes place is a relating of the costs—or "inputs"—to the services rendered to the clients—the "outputs" of the program. However, the objectives of these service programs generally are to elevate the clients and their families to a specified level of functioning or at least to maintain them at some acceptable level. In order to obtain reliable and valid measures of such "outcomes" or "benefits," it is necessary to identify clearly what they are. If the analysis is made by relating costs to outputs—for example, hours of counseling received by clients—then all that we end up with may be termed a "cost-output analysis," which is little different in principle from a cost analysis. However, in order to make certain kinds of programmatic decisions we want to know what impact this counseling had and upon whom—what behaviors were changed and how and, if possible, why? All of this is by way of saying that the benefits of a program are a function of its objectives; therefore the outputs must contribute to the realization of these objectives before they can even be regarded as being related to these benefits, if, indeed, there are any at all. Thus, in doing a proper cost-benefit analysis we must, in addition to making a cost analysis, also make what amounts to a program-effectiveness evaluation. As such, a cost-benefit analysis may be equated to a cost-effectiveness evaluation.

In the literature an attempt is sometimes made to distinguish between a cost-benefit analysis and a cost-effectiveness analysis. For our purposes, in order to avoid what is largely a semantic problem, particularly in the social welfare context, we shall equate the two as being practically, if not theoretically, synonymous.

APPLICATION TO SOCIAL WELFARE

In principle, cost-benefit analysis may be applied to social welfare problems; in practice it has not been used to any significant extent, for a number of reasons, apart from the mystique that surrounds any complicated technique. Cost-benefit analysis is usually a complex undertaking, if it is properly done, with consideration of the possible cost and relevant benefit factors in a social welfare program system.

Perhaps a partial misunderstanding is the principal reason why social researchers are reluctant to use this technique. True, the technique was developed and has been used mostly by economists in problems in which it is meaningful to express at least the major benefits in strictly economic or monetary terms. In social welfare, where many of the benefits cannot be meaningfully converted into dollar terms, a more complex approach is required. Thus, even in employment training for fathers whose families are receiving public assistance, account must be taken of such variables as the positive psychological and social effects of the improved employment status of the family head. When the end result is that a family is kept together, or that life is made more bearable for the aged and infirm, or that an infant is protected from abusive parents, there may be no clear-cut economic payoff or any basis for speculating on one. Perhaps the most important question worth asking in this frame of reference is: Which alternative programs can accomplish these end results more effectively and at lower cost? Or, perhaps more realistically, which programs are optimal in terms of the relationship of effectiveness to costs?

In general, programs whose objectives are predicted on a value system which places a high price on the integrity and well-being of the individual and family generate benefits which resist translation into monetary terms. Measurement of the intangible social and psychological benefits is one of the biggest problems in evaluating the effectiveness or efficiency of a social welfare program. It requires the skills of the social researcher competent in social science measurement, methodology, and theory.

However, there is nothing so radically new or esoteric in analyzing social welfare programs from a cost-benefit or cost-effectiveness vantage point. The research plan is very similar to that of a conventional program-effectiveness design, with the added feature that provision is made to obtain cost-analysis data of the type with which a cost accountant would be concerned. Also, even though the social and psychological benefits may be paramount and often of overriding significance, an attempt must also be made to translate the outcomes or benefits of a program into economic terms whenever it is feasible and at all meaningful. This is done in a broad systems context. For example, in evaluating the benefits derived from an employment-oriented public welfare program designed to provide its clients with work experience and training, the local labor market must be taken into account in estimating the benefits to the community as well as to the individual. Also, the long-term effects of successful employment must be estimated by using the economist's device of applying the appropriate rates of interest to discount expected future earnings. For example, one must answer such questions as: What is the present value to the individual of twenty years of increased future earnings of a given magnitude?

From the usual definitions given and from the traditional uses of cost-benefit analysis in evaluating hardware systems, it is easy to get the idea that cost-benefit analysis is a type of administrative research. It is true that, as generally used, its principal function is to help an administrator decide where a given investment in dam construction would have the biggest pay-off for the economy. It can also help decide, its proponents suggest, whether commuters would be better served by $50 million of federal funds spent on urban throughways or on mass-transit rail systems—or whether both programs offer so little benefit for the money that the $50 million should go for new schools instead. Another possibility, and one which is relevant to public welfare, is the following question: Would elderly workers whose skills are obsolete benefit more from on-the-job training or from institutional training, or would it be better simply to give them public assistance payments and use the training funds to school out-of-work teenagers? Answers to these questions are sought by the application of cost-benefit analysis in a strictly economic sense and on a global basis. The answers one gets when cost-benefit analysis is thus applied depends to a large extent upon underlying assumptions and value systems, once one leaves the purely economic domain and enters the realm of the intangibles.

The problem of quantifying intangibles plagues even highway planners who must decide which is worth more—a public park or a low-cost housing development—so they can decide which way to send the bulldozers. Transportation analysis must put a dollar value on time spent traveling so they can decide whether rapid rail systems or airplanes would be the more sensible public investment. When one has to decide between investing in a program of the care for the aged or an improved highway system, the value problem becomes truly formidable and the weight must be placed on cultural, political, and a host of other value and judgmental considerations rather than on an analytical or research technique.

ROLE OF THEORY AND MODELS

However, if one limits one's scope—not of vision, but of decision-making—cost-benefit analysis can be an extremely useful technique. Not only can it help one decide which of several child-care programs is most cost-effective, but it can also tell you why. If you know why, it is but another step to redesign any existing program so that it will do an even better job of achieving its objectives. This possibility stems from the roles of evaluation models and theory in program evaluation, whether it be the traditional program-effectiveness type or program effectiveness plus cost considerations, which may be termed "program efficiency."

In both types of program-evaluation research (effectiveness or efficiency), theory plays a central role, which is related to the measurement-of-outcomes problem. Since program outcomes in social welfare usually imply a change of behavior, it is useful to have a "change theory" or "intervention theory" to identify what constitutes the desired change to be measured. One such theoretical formulation may be that, as a program raises aspiration levels and changes perception of the opportunity structure, those individuals showing the greatest change in the appropriate direction would be most likely to seek and hold jobs. Thus, a theory provides us with clues about what to measure and why to measure it.

Good theory, by itself, is often not enough to define all the variables that should be measured. The intricate interlocking details comprising a program form too complex a system to be studied without a model. This model should serve the purpose of identifying the essential variables and their interrelationships, thereby at least implicitly incorporating the appropriate social science change theory.

A model should do something else. It should define the successive and intermediate goals and relate these to the more ultimate goals. It is particularly important to define successive and intermediate goals when the program involves a series of progressive stages which lead toward eventual success. In the work-experience-and-training projects designed primarily for public assistance recipients, stages of work preparation or literacy training may of necessity precede the skill training. It is essential here to specify meaningful intermediate milestones that may be measured as benefits. Often these constitute the basis for the client's voluntarily terminating his training because he can obtain a job.

Unless criteria of work experience and literacy are established as objectives and measured as benefits, the success of the program may be seriously underestimated. There are those, for example, who count as benefits only successful termination of either the work-experience or vocational training by the client followed by his obtaining a training-relevant job. This fallacy becomes quite apparent in review of some computer readouts on the Work Experience and Training Program (Title V of the Economic Opportunity Act of 1964). These involved some 65,000 people who entered training in projects all over the country. Either during or immediately after completing their training, 46 percent obtained employment. Thus, if immediate employment were the gauge, the success rate would be 46 percent. However, an additional 16 percent upgraded their skills and obtained employment later. If these were counted, the rate would be 62 percent. But, in addition, 6 percent of the trainees, as a result of their training, were able to move into more advanced vocational training. If these are included, the success rate is 68 percent. The 68 percent is now generally accepted as being the most valid figure.

It will be quite apparent that there is room for debate on these gauges. Who knows, for example, how many of those people would have found jobs if they had not been in the program? How many of those who dropped out of the programs before completing their assignments and obtained employment did so because of the services received, such as adult basic education and job preparation? The latter involves not only employment counseling but instruction on proper grooming, the necessity for getting to work on time, how to talk to one's supervisor and co-workers, and so on.

The central point is that a simple tabulation of relevant statistics is not enough in any kind of thoroughgoing program evaluation. It is necessary to have access to a control group, or at least data on such a group. The control group should be comparable to the group being evaluated in all relevant characteristics except that they did not receive the program services. Only by comparing these two groups can a valid estimate of the actual impact of the program be made. This point will be developed later.

To complicate the benefits-measurement picture still more, many of the trainees in the program mentioned above were mothers in the Aid to Families with Dependent Children program, who may have decided to spend their time rearing their children and to utilize the training for employment at some later date. Moreover, some very interesting things were happening in certain projects. For example, in the hill country of eastern Kentucky, when the fathers began to attend literacy training classes, the school attendance of their children improved markedly. One might ask: What is the long-term effect of the improved school attendance of these children on the nation's economy, considering the possible consequences for better employment when they grow up, the impact on intergenerational poverty, and other possible influences?

TWO ILLUSTRATIVE RESEARCH PROJECTS

All of these considerations point to the need for a model that takes into consideration the large number of interacting variables significant in evaluating the effectiveness of services in such an undertaking as the Work Experience and Training Program. The Division of Intramural Research in the Social and Rehabilitation Service is currently engaged in a number of broadly based projects, two of which are discussed here: The first is focused on the evaluation of the effectiveness of social, educational, and vocational services in AFDC programs; the second is concerned with developing a cost-benefit methodology for evaluating the spectrum of employment-oriented projects of the Title V program, which has already been mentioned.

The basic rationale of the projects dealing with the development of a program-effectiveness model leans heavily on a formation by Clarence Sherwood.[2] Program successs or effectiveness is defined in terms of impact—the difference between what happens with the intervention and what would happen without it. Measurement of this impact requires the use of a control group in order to distinguish between those outcomes which result from the program services and those changes in client behavior which occur even if no services were offered to the client population.

Such an "impact model" may be conceptualized in terms of four sets of variables. The first set, which refers to the desired outcome, is defined by the intervention. An example would be the ultimate employment of the client. The second type, or intermediate variables, must also be defined by the intervention. Examples include learning a skill and change in attitudes toward dependency. Program variables represent the third set. In the aggregate these program variables constitute the specific intervention by which it is hoped to produce changes in one or more of the intermediate variables which, in turn, should lead to impact on one or more of the outcome variables. A fourth type, population variables, is often useful, particularly in national programs in which the local projects draw upon somewhat different population-characteristics variables. Examples of these include sex, level of education, occupational history, and the like.

The model should also make provision for such practical issues as (1) comparison of alternative programs, (2) evaluation of replicated or similar programs in different community settings, (3) a research design that is not prohibitively expensive to implement, and (4) a typology which will permit generalization to the universe of projects from studies in depth of a sample of projects of each type.

The end product of this research should be a detailed statement of the general theoretical research model, the kinds of data to be obtained and from what sources, and the steps to be taken to obtain the data, including the sampling procedures to be employed. All the material necessary to data collection should be included in this package, namely, final drafts of all required data forms, interview schedules, observation recording devices, recording procedures, card formats, and the like. To permit analysis of the data, detailed statistical procedures should be formulated and the necessary computer programs developed.

The primary focus of the previous study is on the development of a general model for evaluating the effectiveness of the broad spectrum of AFDC program components. It addresses itself only in a limited sense to the cost factors in relation to outcomes. In order to develop and provide an estimate of the feasibility of using cost-benefit methodology in evaluating work-experience-and-training projects, a study in depth of a local project was undertaken. The project, administered by the Bernalillo County Welfare Department in New Mexico, has been selected as the target for the proposed research effort. The Bernalillo project, in its second year of operation, is receiving national attention for its achievements to date.

The stated objective of the project is "to upgrade skills for employability of AFDC parents and other needy persons through provision of basic education, training and work experience, in keeping with the participants' potentials and employment opportunities in the area."

Project operations involve (1) training readiness, (2) a work-experience phase, (3) adult basic education, (4) vocational training, and (5) ongoing supportive services until attainment of a full or partial self-supporting phase.

The following essential elements are involved in this research:

1. Definition of objectives (proximate and successive as well as terminal employment goals) in as operational and measurable a form as possible.

2. Identification of the program elements in the project and their inter-relationships.

3. Formulation of a method of obtaining cost data.

4. Identification of outcomes which may be defined as benefits in terms of the specified objectives.

5. Exploration of the feasibility of measuring the various kinds of social and psychological benefits.

6. Analysis of factors in the economic setting (e.g., labor market) which are functionally related to the economic benefits and the implications of this economic environment for alternative vocational training objectives.

7. Development of a system for relating cost factors to the attained

benefits for the project as a whole and analysis of benefit-cost tradeoffs of viable recombinations of program elements in the project.

8. Comparison in cost-benefit terms with a control group of AFDC recipients who did not receive Title V services.

Focus will also be placed on developing a tentative general model and set of procedures for use in analyzing several hundred similar projects across the nation. Obviously it will not be possible to generalize the findings derived from one particular project to assess the benefit-cost relationships of the entire range of work-experience-and-training projects. But these results have the potential for developing a conceptual framework for such an evaluation and permit comparison with the enrichment of the findings of the other study.

The foregoing two projects were discussed in considerable detail because they are illustrative of what kinds of considerations are involved in program-evaluation research. They also are indicative of the relationship between the program-effectiveness and the cost-benefit type of research in the evaluation of social welfare programs. It should be apparent at this stage of the discussion that both are similar in kind—involving theory and model building but differing in relative emphasis on economic factors at both the input and outcome end. Also, the program-effectiveness design places relatively greater emphasis on social science theory.

MORE ABOUT THEORY

This preoccupation with theory is not entirely necessary in evaluating programs if we are interested only in how well or efficiently a program is working. Theory is not even necessary when we want to know how good a job one program is doing compared to another with the same or similar objectives. A well-planned survey can generally give us most of the answers we need. However, as soon as we become interested in program evaluation from the point of view of program improvement through redesign and effective innovation, then the relevant scientific knowledge base usually needs a bit of stretching. The role of social science theory looms particularly large when we are interested in why something works. Usually, only by knowing the "whyness" can new applications become possible. As Alfred Kahn has said: "The *knowledge* in a given field is represented by the sum total of available theory that is considered to be highly confirmed."[3] The actual work of research—analysis of systematic observations, and testing of hypotheses—is an essential step for the designing of this kind of knowledge.

Much social theory derives from field research and laboratory experiments conducted by social scientists. But theory-building can be a two-way street. Not only does theory contribute to practice, in terms of affording better program evaluation and program improvement, but, as experience has repeatedly shown, much can be contributed to theory by the empirical findings of the social work practitioner. Theory is often refined and enriched by the interplay of social science theory and operating principles, sometimes called practice theory. Such practice theory is usually developed in the arena of program operation. These practical principles, which tell us how something works and what to do, in addition to being important in their own right, often provide the necessary clues to a breakthrough in understanding why something works.

However, there is also good reason to believe that social work will develop a solid body of practice theory only through collaborative research or interplay between social welfare practitioners and social science researchers. To use the field of medicine as an analogy or model, its giant strides became possible only when medical research involved the medically untrained biological and physical scientists, who brought to bear upon the medical problem the knowledge accumulated by their sciences. The significant aspect in the current reports of recent medical discoveries is the crucial contribution of physiologists, biochemists, physicists, and bacteriologists. If any moral can be regarded as an outcome from this medical model, it is that efforts by social workers to refine their practice theory are destined to bear meager fruits if the social sciences are ignored.

IN CONCLUSION

An apparently rather diverse number of topics have been covered in the foregoing discussion. It began with a brief discussion of the relationship of cost-benefit analysis to the planning-programming-budgeting system recently adopted by many federal agencies and now spreading to state and local governmental units. As generally used, cost-benefit analysis provides the administrator with a package of information to assist him in making a choice among alternative programs which are competing for that scarce resource—even in an affluent society—money.

Actually the uses to which such an analysis can be put by administrators vary with the level of the administrator. For the local administrator it can serve as a guide to the improvement of project operations: to remind him of the objectives and to raise the question of whether project operations have strayed from the original objectives of the program. For the administrator of a state or national program, such an analysis provides the basis for choice among programs to accomplish either the same or other important objectives in terms of the relative returns on investment.

It was pointed out that cost-benefit analysis has been successfully used in a large variety of contexts in which both costs and benefits associated with programs were expressible in monetary terms. However, in most social welfare programs this is possible only in part, if at all. What should be done in these instances? The emphasis should be placed on measuring sociopsychological outcomes as benefits in order to provide the decision-maker not only with benefit-cost ratios for those benefits which are monetarily expressible, but also to give him a "serendipity package" of sociopsychological and other important intangible benefits to use in his judgmental process. Not only a measuring methodology but also theory and models are necessary to identify significant variables and their interrelationships. Involved in this mix are the techniques and concepts employed in social research generally and, more specifically, in program-effectiveness evaluation research.

The major difference between a program-effectiveness evaluation and a cost-benefit analysis model is that the latter includes several additional sets of variables—cost-input factors and other economic variables, whenever applicable. However, in making a complete cost-benefit analysis of a social welfare program, rather than a partial one (such as, for example, measuring the success of an employment-oriented program strictly in terms of how many of the trainees entered the labor force), an enormous amount of additional useful information is obtained not only for the administrator but for the practitioner and researcher. It becomes possible to determine not only how well a program works but also why it works. The analysis provides the springboard for developing new and more effective intervention strategies and utilizing them for program redesign and improvement.

NOTES

1. Martin Wolins, *A Manual for Cost Analysis in Institutions for Children* (New York: Child Welfare League of America, 1962).
2. Clarence C. Sherwood, "Methodological, Measurement, and Social Action Considerations Related to Assessments of Large Scale Demonstration Programs" (paper presented at the 124th Annual Meeting of the American Statistical Association, Chicago, Ill., December, 1964).
3. Alfred J. Kahn, "The Nature of Social Work Knowledge," *New Directions in Social Work*, ed. Cora Kasius (New York: Harper & Bros., 1954), chap. xi, p. 205.

This article has been adapted from a speech presented at the Ninety-fourth Annual Forum of the National Conference on Social Welfare in Dallas, Texas, May 22, 1967.

C. MANAGEMENT BY OBJECTIVES

22/MANAGEMENT BY OBJECTIVES IN A FAMILY SERVICE AGENCY

VERNON R. WIEHE

What criteria are used by supervisory personnel in appraising the performance of social workers? How can creativity and enthusiasm in job performance be stimulated? Is it possible to establish short- and long-range service delivery goals in a social agency? Management by objectives, engaged in by administrative and line staff, is one answer to these questions. While management by objectives is not a panacea for management problems, it is a helpful tool in performance appraisal and in program-planning in a social agency.

DEFINITION OF TERMS

The key terms in management by objectives are *mission, objectives, goals,* and *plans.*[1] The mission is the final aim or end of action which an organization wishes to attain. The mission is generally stated in broad terms which set out the general direction the agency is attempting to achieve. The mission describes the purpose of the organization, the reason for its existence. For an agency with family and child welfare services, the mission might be stated as follows:

Middletown Family and Children's Services serves individuals, families, and groups in the community in their attempt to achieve full human potential for themselves and for others.

A sectarian agency or an agency related to a court or school system may add to its statement of mission the unique relationship or channel to the community through which it attempts to achieve its purpose for existence. The mission of such an agency might read as follows:

The Middletown Catholic Family and Children's Services, through its relationship to the parishes and schools of the Catholic community, serves individuals, families, and groups in their attempt to achieve full human potential for themselves and for others.

The objectives are the results the agency wishes to achieve in order to remain a viable organization which is fulfilling its mission. The objectives may be viewed as a further delineation or refinement of the mission of the organization. Objectives for a family and child welfare agency may include the following:

To have a balance in services between prevention and treatment.
To serve individuals and groups in their efforts to become sensitive to social issues.
To incorporate the social action function of the agency as an integral part of all agency functions.
To incorporate research as an agency function toward improving services and expanding social work knowledge.
To maintain a family-focused orientation in all agency services.
To utilize volunteers in the accomplishment of the agency mission.

The goals of a program of management by objectives are the end results to be achieved within a period of time. The period of time will vary according to the nature of the goal. The period for the attainment of a goal may be as brief as one or two months or as long as a year, the latter being equal to the annual appraisal period. In some instances long-range goals may take several years to accomplish. Both short- and long-range goals may be established by a worker, department, or agency depending on the difficulty in achieving the goals, the resources available in the attainment of the goals, and the time necessary to bring a goal to its fruition.

Examples of goals of individual workers in a family service agency may include the following:

During the coming year I intend to improve my skills in leading groups so that I may utilize group methods in working with couples requesting marital counseling.
During the next three months I plan to complete dictation on fifteen cases needing to be closed in my caseload.
During the next four months I will prepare for supervising a field work student in the agency.

The final term used in management by objectives is *plans*. Plans are the means by which goals are achieved. They are the steps, activities, projects, and tasks which must be undertaken by a worker to achieve his goals. The route to the achievement of each goal must be spelled out in terms of the plans the worker has for achieving this goal. Goals are valid and feasible only to the extent that the directions toward their achievement have been carefully thought through and defined. As conditions within an agency may change during any given period of time, plans as well as goals may need to be modified.

The goal which a family service worker may have set for himself and the plans by which to achieve this goal might be stated as follows:

Goal: During the next four months I will prepare for supervising a field work student in the agency.

Plans: Consult with the other staff at next staff meeting on reducing my caseload by 10 percent beginning one month before student's placement in the agency.

Consult with staff during the last month before placement regarding being alert at intake to specific cases for assignment to student.

Review literature in social work journals from the past three years on the supervision of students.

The formulation of plans for attaining a goal is similar to operationalizing a concept in research, wherein the researcher specifies the route he will take in measuring a concept or what he will do to quantify the concept. In management by objectives, the worker spells out in actual practice how he will attempt to reach the goal. Some goals are never accomplished because adequate or realistic plans for their attainment were not carefully developed.

A DEDUCTIVE AND INDUCTIVE PROCESS

Who determines the mission of the agency? From where do the objectives come? Do goals flow out of objectives which have been set, or do objectives arise from the plans and goals of the individual workers or departments within an agency?

In considering these questions it becomes apparent that deductive and inductive processes are involved in implementing a program of management by objectives. It may be necessary for an agency to work down (deductively) from the top (its mission) or at times to build up (inductively) from the bottom (the plans of the workers). Such processes require effort. However, out of such effort can arise a clearer perspective for the agency's board, staff, and constituency of what the agency is about, its purpose for existence, how it is working to reach this purpose, and an evaluation of its efforts.

An agency may already have a statement of mission or purpose for existence in its charter. In instances where such a statement of mission does not exist, a helpful exericse for board and staff is to have each individual formulate an encompassing statement of mission, to compare these statements, and to arrive at a commonly agreed-upon statement. What is the purpose for the existence of this agency? This is the crucial question to answer in the formulation of the statement of mission of the agency.

After a statement of mission has been determined, the objectives of the agency must be formulated. The objectives may be derived from the mission of the agency by delineating more specifically the results the agency wishes to achieve year after year—an example of deducing from the mission of the agency the objectives of the organization.

An inductive process may be used by starting with a statement of the goals and plans of the individual workers or departments of the agency. From these statements of goals the question may be asked: What common objectives are achieved by these goals? Statements of objectives may then be formulated on the basis of the accumulation of goals and plans of workers and departments in the agency. Working still further upward from the numerous objectives which have been written, a capstone statement of mission may be formulated to serve as the final aim or purpose of the organization.

There are disadvantages to using a purely deductive or inductive approach. With the use of the deductive approach of starting with the mission, an individual or the staff of a department can become too ambitious and set more goals than can be accomplished. This may not become obvious until specific plans are formulated for the attainment of the goals. The task of spelling-out in detail the plans the worker must pursue to fulfill a goal assists the individual in determining the reality of the goal in the light of such factors as time, energy, and money. When plans are not specific, goals become even more general and the route a worker must follow in the attainment of a goal becomes lost. If the inductive approach is followed in implementing management by objectives, with the worker first laying the building blocks of plans and goals he or a department wishes to attain during the coming months, the objectives may not reach a very high level of accomplishment. The objectives may only reflect the status quo of the agency rather than challenging the creativity of the organization and its personnel. Experience has shown, however, that when a department gets bogged down in trying to accomplish too much or when it must pull together to handle work because of a staff vacancy or retrenchment, it may be necessary for the department to work from the bottom up by first looking at the number of man-hours available and how intake and other demands the agency must meet can be handled with the time and resources available. After this step is done, the individual can then ask what other goals he might attempt to achieve. Thus, an individual or department may find a combination of the deductive and inductive approaches helpful in implementing management by objectives.

FITTING THE PIECES TOGETHER

Reference has been made to individual or departmental goals and plans. The implementation of management by objectives must occur on the individual, departmental, and agency levels. At this point, the old controversy of which comes first enters the picture.

An individual staff member can not set goals and plans for himself without some understanding and communication with other departmental personnel. The latter are important support systems to him in the attainment of his goals and plans. Likewise, a department can not formulate its goals without knowledge of the goals and plans of staff members whose efforts comprise the building blocks of the department. As workers within a department set goals and plans for themselves, it is necessary that communication occur within the department regarding the effect individual goals and plans will have on other staff members and on the departments as a whole. A process of fitting together into a unit the pieces of the various goals and plans of the workers is necessary in order to arrive at a statement of departmental goals. The same process is necessary on the agency level when the agency is comprised of several departments. The supervisors or departmental heads must coordinate the goals and plans of their respective departments.

The task of attempting to fit together into a mesh or unit the goals and plans of individual staff members and the goals and plans of different departments raises the following questions: Are the goals of a department merely the collection of the goals of the various workers within the department? Also, are the goals of the agency merely the collection of the goals of the various departments? The view that the whole is greater than the sum of its parts is applicable here. The goals of the various workers in a department can not merely be combined to form a departmental statement of goals, but, rather, a system of "best fit" must be achieved, a project which can be accomplished in any of several ways.

The goals of the various workers as expressed in their plans can be examined to determine if they are harmonious or at cross-purposes. One staff member in a department can not plan to carry out an activity which is directly opposed to the plans of another staff member. (Again, well-stated plans can save the day. It may be impossible to detect the opposition at the goal level.)

In arriving at the goals of an agency comprised of several departments, it is helpful to examine the common objectives under which these goals might fall. The formulation of common objectives from the goals of the various departments within an agency serves as a unifying factor in achieving the best fit possible among these goals.

VALUE OF THE PROGRAM

What is the value of a program of management by objectives? Initially it may seem to be merely a futile exercise of putting together a conceptual jigsaw puzzle. However, with time and experience in working with management by objectives, the effort takes on real meaning. There are several important values to the use of management by objectives in a social agency.

1. The implementation of management by objectives involves the participation of staff members in determining the program and course of direction of an agency. At times staff members may feel they merely respond to the policies and direction of the board and administration. Through the setting of individual and departmental goals, staff members have the opportunity to offer the administration important information from their own perspectives. This information may include the resources available to the agency in terms of staff potential, the need for shifts in service emphasis, and creative thought for new directions.

2. The discipline of writing goals and plans utilizes the initiative of the worker and recognizes his individual contribution to the agency. The worker is confronted with the question: What do I want to do with my skills this coming year within the support system of this agency? In this context workers are not regarded as private practitioners in the framework of the agency, but, rather, individual workers are given the opportunity—and even forced through the writing of goals and plans—to examine what they are contributing to the agency's program, to systematically evaluate their professional development, and to enable the agency to make effective use of their potential contribution. The accomplishment of goals which a worker has set for himself can give the individual satisfaction in job performance.

The above values of management by objectives may be viewed from the perspective of Douglas McGregor's philosophy of management, Theory X and Theory Y.[2] Theory X's assumptions are that people hate to work and that they are not ambitious and do not want to assume responsibility. Theory Y assumes the opposite. Work can be enjoyed; people like to express themselves through their work. Management by objectives allows for the expression of a Theory Y philosophy. Individuals are encouraged to participate in setting goals they themselves wish to pursue and are involved in the setting of goals and objectives for the agency.

3. As staff members within a department are forced to achieve a best fit of their goals and plans, a feeling of cohesion can develop. In this process individual staff members recognize that unless they work together as a team within a department, as well as within the agency, agency and departmental goals cannot be achieved.

4. The use of management by objectives is a tool to assist in the yearly appraisal of performance of workers. The goals and plans which a worker specifies for himself provide a basis on which performance can be appraised. Thus the worker and the supervisor can review performance in a systematic manner. There are variables, however, which are not covered if appraisal of performance is based on the goals and plans of a worker. The quality of performance is such a variable. However, using management by objectives as the framework for the appraisal of performance provides the setting and opportunity for discussion of such variables.

5. Management by objectives assists an agency in setting short- and long-range goals and prevents agency planning, for example in the area of service delivery, from being only a defensive or reactive response to requests for service. Concern for long-range planning in an agency becomes particularly important at the level of setting objectives. The objectives are the results the agency wishes to achieve in order to remain a viable organization which is fulfilling its mission. The dimension of time becomes attached to these objectives as they are delineated further in the goals of the departments. For example, as part of an objective of efficient and effective use of agency resources in the delivery of services, a long-range goal of establishing several outpost offices in parishes or neighborhood centers may be formulated. A time dimension of two, three, or four years may be attached to these objectives, based on the development of population areas in a community, the resources available to the agency, and the needed shifts in present program emphasis.

SUMMARY

Management by objectives is an effective tool for agency planning. The implementation of management by objectives makes it necessary for staff members as individuals, as a department, and as the agency to engage in short- and long-range planning. Such planning occurs through the setting of goals by individual workers, which are carefully specified in plans. Diverse goals are brought together through common objectives of the agency, which in turn are expressed in the mission or statement of purpose of the organization. The use of management by objectives assists an agency in the appraisal of performance of workers, enables staff members to participate in agency planning, and helps an agency determine short- and long-range goals.

NOTES

1. Some writers use the terms *objectives* and *goals* interchangeably.
2. Douglas McGregor, *The Human Side of Enterprise* (New York: McGraw-Hill, 1960).

23/INSTALLING MANAGEMENT BY OBJECTIVES IN SOCIAL AGENCIES

MELVYN C. RAIDER

Although Management by Objectives (MBO) has been used extensively in business and industry during the last twenty years, it is only recently that social agencies have adopted MBO. MBO has been installed in public and voluntary agencies in great numbers and based upon present indications many more agencies are planning to implement MBO in the future. Impetus to use MBO originates from several sources—pressure from boards and funding sources for accountability, for demonstrating program effectiveness, and for increasing efficiency. Regulatory bodies and other governmental agencies have also been eager to see social agencies adopt this system.[1]

MBO is a very simple system in theory. Basically, it is an approach to management in which agency staff participate in the process of specifying long-range goals and short-range objectives to be achieved within an established time period. Success in achieving these agreed upon goals and objectives is evaluated periodically.

Agencies using MBO report mixed results. There have been many successes and too many failures. Based upon the author's experience as a consultant to social work administrators in the use of this technique, it may be observed that there are three primary reasons for failure. First, agencies did not understand what they were getting into and as a consequence did not do adequate preliminary analysis and planning. Second, agencies sought to implement a model of MBO which had not been sufficiently tailored to reflect the unique needs and characteristics of social agencies. Third, a poorly conceived strategy was used to implement the system. This article offers a four-phase approach for installing MBO in social agencies.

PHASE I—SELF STUDY

Adaptation of MBO requires commitment of agency resources. During the early stages of implementing MBO, when agency personnel are learning the system, substantial expenditures of dollars as well as time must be expected. During this phase, consultants are usually utilized to orient staff to the new system and assist them to develop necessary skills in writing objectives. After the initial learning phase there are ongoing costs and time commitments. Time is usually set aside annually to assess progress relative to goal and objective attainment. Shorter periodic meetings must be held with staff in order to assess interim progress.

To avoid the commitment of such substantial agency resources to MBO only to discover that barriers to its success exist, it is first necessary to enter into a self-study to estimate prospects for success. There are a number of factors which may serve as reasonable indicators of potential difficulties with MBO. These factors are: agency instability, environmental instability, position discontinuity, and unmediated competition.[2]

Agency instability is uncertainty about the expansion or contraction of the agency. Agency instability is usually an outgrowth of funding difficulties especially when funding comes from a variety of sources. If the agency's budget is subject to frequent increases or decreases which could greatly expand or contract major programs, the agency will probably have difficulties with MBO. MBO requires a fair degree of budgetary stability because objectives and plans are usually made a year or more in advance and require accurate forecasts of resources and budgets. Frequent changes in funding require rebudgeting and consequently necessitate the formulation of new objectives and new plans, a condition which will eventually defeat the system.

Environmental instability is uncertainty about the nature of the consumers of the organization's services. It is an outgrowth of changes in the nature of the clientele, either by shifts in the catchment area or population changes within an existing catchment area. Because they require revision of objectives or the priorities assigned to objectives, unplanned changes of this kind hinder MBO. An agency serving a changing community will probably experience difficulties with MBO.

Position discontinuity is the frequent replacement of personnal or changes in duties and responsibilities of existing personnel. Accountability for achieving mutually agreed-upon objectives is an important component of MBO. Large-scale personnel changes or reassignments of job duties significantly interfere with accountability. When this condition exists, especially among administrative staff, MBO becomes almost impossible to carry out.

Unmediated competition is the lack of established channels within the agency for mediating competing goals and objectives. This is evident in an agency where there are several major service programs. Each program is administered by an individual who feels his program is most valuable and who is intent upon enhancing his program at the expense of others. Problems arise where there is no established method within the agency for resolving the competition among programs. In such situations, MBO will probably fail; goals and objectives established will often work at cross-purposes.[3]

The degree to which each of these four factors exist will determine the extent to which MBO is appropriate to an agency. In some instances it may be decided that MBO is inappropriate to an agency. In such instances it would be wise to abandon the notion of installing MBO completely; in other situations, it may be prudent to delay the installation of MBO until some of the difficulties are resolved. If MBO appears appropriate in a particular setting, analysis of the four factors will provide information which can aid in the making of a decision concerning the complexity and comprehensiveness of the MBO system which will ultimately be adopted. (This will be discussed in greater depth in Phase II.)

During the self-study phase it is also wise to collaborate with people from other agencies in which MBO is utilized. It will be very useful to learn about actual advantages and disadvantages, successes and failures from the perspective of an agency similar to your own. Many costly and frustrating errors can be avoided through such collaboration.[4]

PHASE II—IMPLEMENTATION STRATEGY

It should be recognized that installing MBO is no less than introducing major organizational change. If such change is to be long lasting, a carefully planned strategy must be developed. The first order of business is to gain the commitment of top agency administration and the board. Based upon the author's experience, significant difficulties and delays are experienced because one or both of the above groups were bypassed in the process. An agency executive will often find it easier to gain such commitment when there is a significant external or internal threat to the agency, such as of a major budget cutback. Studies of successful organizational change concluded that an organization under outside pressure is much more open to new ideas and approaches than an organization which is relatively secure.[5]

Once top management commitment is obtained, it is necessary to determine who within the agency will be charged with responsibility for implementing MBO. In many situations in which MBO was installed successfully, responsibility for installing the new system was lodged with the agency director. Lower level people in the organization such as staff development or training specialists charged with responsibility for implementing MBO have had a much more difficult time than top administrators in gaining staff commitment and in demonstrating the significance of the proposed change.[6] When responsibility for the new system is accepted by the top administration, it has been observed that participation and enthusiasm on the part of agency staff is significantly greater. It is also important that administration view MBO as a philosophy of management rather than merely a new technique.[7]

The implementation of MBO, if it is to have a good chance of being accepted, should be initially viewed as an experiment rather than something which is permanent. Staff need to proceed cautiously and to reality test the new system.[8] To feel comfortable with the new approach, they should have the freedom to contribute to modifications of the system as necessary. If MBO proves to be of no value or of negative value, staff need to feel confident that the new system will be discarded. Under these circumstances, the approach to MBO which eventually evolves will be viewed as the product and the property of staff and administration.

Since the initial use of MBO should be viewed as an experiment, it follows that MBO should be *initially* introduced on a modest scale. MBO may be implemented in a single component of the agency or only among middle-level administrators during the first phase. Success on a modest scale will provide participants with a vested interest in seeing MBO introduced on a larger scale.

Administration, the board, the staff should recognize that implementation of MBO is a lengthy process. For most social agencies, implementation of MBO represents a completely new way of doing things. Agency executives and staff members must reorient their styles of operating. A shift to MBO often means a shift from intuitive management to precise, pre-planned management. Along with MBO comes a different vocabulary and collection of concepts. For staff members most comfortable with a human behavior frame of reference, such terms as *objective, mission, program,* and *output measures* take significant time to be comprehended and even longer to be fully accepted.

Individuals experienced in training others to use MBO indicate that it takes three successive MBO cycles before expertise in formulating good goals and objectives develops. In most organizations, MBO cycles are usually one year in length; thus, it takes approximately three years to develop requisite expertise.[9]

Training

All individuals who will be using MBO will need appropriate training in writing goals and objectives. Training of this nature usually may be obtained in courses and workshops on MBO offered by most universities and community colleges. For a large agency, however, it is often less expensive to bring an instructor to the agency than to pay tuition fees for a large group of staff members. An in-service training program has the advantage that the presentation may be specifically geared to the agency. Both approaches are equally effective for acquiring the basic skills in writing goals and objectives.

Short-term contracts with management consultants are often entered into by social agencies to implement an entire MBO system. This is very expensive and, unless the consultant is chosen with care, of minimal value. It has been pointed out earlier in this article that the final form of MBO must evolve over time and be specifically tailored to the needs of the agency. If a consultant is to assist in this process he would need to work with the agency in an ongoing capacity perhaps for as long as three years. It is unlikely that a team of consultants can come into the agency for a few weeks, impose a full-blown MBO system, and then depart with expectation that the system will hold up over time. Under such circumstances the agency will most likely be the recipient of a standardized MBO model which may not have been modified to reflect the characteristics of the agency or its environment. Follow-up studies have shown that even a poor model of MBO will have positive results in the short run. These studies have demonstrated that after a year or two the positive results evaporate.[10]

PHASE III—SYSTEM DESIGN

After the self-study is completed, the degree of comprehensiveness of the MBO system to be adopted may be determined. If one or more of the indicators of potential difficulty or failure with MBO are evident to some extent, it is wise to be less ambitious when installing MBO. Under these circumstances a less complex version of MBO may be appropriate. For example, it may be determined that MBO would be used exclusively to enhance planning among administrative personnel. The system, therefore, would not encompass direct-service staff. On the other hand, conditions may be deemed favorable to apply MBO to the entire agency, involving all personnel.

Regardless of the degree of comprehensiveness chosen for the MBO system, the system needs to reflect the characteristics and organizational culture of the individual agency. There is no single model of MBO which will have universal application to all human service agencies. However, the author has identified four general guidelines for tailoring MBO to social service agencies:[11]

1. Mission Statement Consensus

A process employing consensus is desirable in formulating agency mission statements. The mission statement serves as the foundation or baseline upon which MBO is built. It specifies the reason for existence of the agency and indicates the main purposes of the organization. The mission should reflect services the community expects of the agency if the agency is to survive. Mission statements are long-range in focus and do not have a specific termination point.

In a social agency, mission statements are best developed through a process requiring the attainment of consensus among all relevant interest groups. Consensus is a process involving bargaining, trade-offs, and compromise. Staff members, administration, members of the board, and community representatives must agree upon a mission statement from their own perspectives. Subsequently, representatives from each of these interest groups would meet and attempt to formulate a unitary mission statement which would be satisfactory to all participants. Eventually it is realized that benefits for all can be realized only by mutual commitment to a unitary conception of mission.[12]

2. Inductive Goal-Setting

Use an inductive process when setting goals. From the mission statement flow several major organizational goals. A goal is a desired state of affairs. Goals are formulated to cover a long time period, usually three to five years.

Goal development should be an inductive process in a social agency. General departmental or unit goals are constructed from many specific individual worker objectives. After compiling individual worker objectives, members of the department would collectively seek to ascertain what common goals could be formulated and what plans could be developed. Advantages of the inductive method of goal formulation may be significant for a social agency. First, such a process respects the individuality of each worker and his unique contribution to the mission of the agency. Second, a more natural or humanistic system for communication and planning is encouraged. Third, participation in the formulation of goals has been shown to be a significant factor in subsequent conformity to them. And fourth, it avoids the risk of proliferation of impractical and unrealistic goals set by administrators who may be somewhat detached from actual service delivery.[13]

3. Group Objectives

Establish group objectives. Objectives are the heart of MBO. They are desired outcomes to be attained in a specific period of time. Objectives are usually measurable and always expressed in concrete terms. Objectives, to be consistent with the nature of most social agencies and the workers they employ, should be established on a departmental or group basis rather than for individual workers. Emphasis must be placed on establishing a common task to facilitate worker interaction, consultation, and mutual participation.

Establishing individual objectives often results in intense competition which may become destructive to the interests of the client. Establishing departmental objectives rather than individual objectives shifts accountability from the individual to the group; the agency climate will shift from one of competition to one of mutual support. As well as increasing agency productivity, establishing objectives in this manner may help to reduce the shortcuts and expedients which grow out of unchecked competition.[14]

4. Milestones

Use milestones to approximate objective attainment. Milestones are reasonable indicators for assessing objective attainment. Carefully selected intermediate activities are "milestones" which, in the best judgment of the agency staff, can be utilized to approximate or estimate progress toward the desired final outcome.[15] Some models of MBO require that objectives be expressed in measurable, quantifiable, concrete terms. A good objective is also expected to describe an end result or final outcome rather than an intermediate product or task that will lead to an end result.

When we seek to achieve objectives which affect people, it becomes difficult to quantify and measure objective attainment. It is very difficult to link change in the client's functioning with the service activity. Problems are encountered because "few instruments are available that validly measure before and after impact."[16] Even more significant is the fact that there is no agreement in the profession as to what to measure and how to measure it. Awaiting future development of methods which can attribute change in the client's functioning directly to the service activity (and the service activity alone), intermediate outcomes or activities, rather than end results, will have to suffice for measuring objectives in social agencies.

PHASE IV—DEVELOPING
LONG-LASTING COMMITMENT

Flexibility

If MBO is to be installed successfully in a human service setting, it must be applied to each situation in a highly flexible fashion. The process underlying MBO is substantially more important than the form that it ultimately takes. In instances where MBO was installed and great emphasis was placed on forms and procedure, MBO failed to provide the anticipated long-range benefits. Huse cites an example of an installation of MBO in industry in which the individuals charged with the responsibility of implementing MBO encountered great resistance on the part of an individual manager. The manager was strongly resisting the many forms and complex procedures which were being imposed by the installers of the MBO system. Upon closer examination it became obvious to the individuals seeking to install MBO that the resistant manager was in fact effectively using the principles of MBO without its cumbersome forms and procedures.[17]

A consistent finding in studies of MBO installations in a variety of settings is that staff resent and resist the excessive paperwork often required.[18] Unless other reports and procedures are eliminated or kept to a minimum, the paperwork associated with MBO will be regarded as an additional burden. If MBO is to be implemented successfully, care must be taken to avoid creating a paper mill. Forms used should be developed by the agency using them with the input of staff members at all levels. A form which meets the needs of one agency may be grossly inappropriate in another setting. When developing forms to be used in conjunction with MBO, it is far wiser to run the risk of devising fewer forms than too many. In some settings forms developed centrally were suggested only for those who wished to use them. Departments were free to reject or modify forms to meet their particular requirements. A narrative statement is often as effective a device for reporting progress as a series of forms while at the same time avoiding the negative attitudes associated with forms.

Freedom should also be provided to middle-level administrators and staff members with regard to the method they choose to achieve objectives. MBO is most useful in establishing targets. Plans to achieve targets should be those of the work group, not the administrator.[19] Staff should be provided with maximum flexibility to achieve objectives without undue restrictions.

In the process of implementing and using MBO, emphasis must be placed on the process and not on rigid procedures or cumbersome forms.

Personal Growth

If MBO is to be truly accepted and valued by staff, the system must relate directly to the personal growth objectives of staff. Too often MBO becomes a mechanism which facilitates the accomplishment of agency goals while ignoring the individual's need to actualize himself through his employment. Significant attention must be placed on personal and professional aspirations. Opportunities should be structured for individuals to develop on the job. Attempts should be made to make individual career goals consistent and complementary with agency goals. Harry Levinson, a psychologist, takes the position that Management by Objectives can become destructive and self-defeating unless the system emphasizes the importance of the individual's goals. Levinson states: "If a man's most powerful driving force is comprised of his needs, wishes, and personal aspirations, combined with the compelling wish to look good in his own eyes for meeting those deeply held personal goals, then Management-by-Objectives should begin with his objectives."[20]

In a human service setting there is usually a significant meshing of personal growth objectives of staff and organizational goals around the agency's emphasis on delivering quality service. Staff members aspire to a level of competency which will enable them to gain esteem and recognition from colleagues and gain the confidence of administration. Professional staff usually have the need to be reasonably autonomous and creative in their work. Personal growth objectives in social agencies will most probably have a competency focus. It is essential that personal objectives foster a climate for self-actualization.[21]

Provide Frequent Two-Way Feedback

Although the need for feedback is built into MBO, it is particularly important to schedule feedback even more frequently during the implementation phase. Staff members need to feel confident that they can make suggestions and proposals for change. It is only after these suggestions are considered and utilized that staff members begin experiencing a sense of commitment to the system.

Feedback sessions relative to objective attainment should have a problem-solving focus. Assessment of objectives, other than personal growth objectives, should be conducted on a group basis. Furthermore, the group should appraise each individual's contribution to the group effort. Criticism should be avoided. Staff need to identify obstacles which serve as barriers to the achievement of established objectives and determine ways in which these barriers may be overcome.[22]

The feedback sessions should also provide staff with the opportunity to evaluate the extent to which administration has provided input relative to achieving objectives. Here again the focus should not be to criticize but to identify administrative barriers which must be resolved.[23] If feedback and MBO itself are to serve a meaningful purpose in the agency, they must go beyond the one-to-one supervisor–staff member relationship. They must foster a partnership between staff and agency in which influence goes both ways.

NOTES

1. Jason E. Patterson, *Community Mental Health in Social Work Education* (Atlanta, Ga.: Southern Regional Education Board, 1975).
2. These factors which are discussed in a social work context are based upon an assessment of MBO installations in England. Reference may be made to J. D. Wickens, "Management by Objectives: An Appraisal," *Journal of Management Studies* 5 (October 1968):365–79.
3. See Melvyn C. Raider, "An Evaluation of Management-by-Objectives," *Social Casework* 56 (February 1975):79.
4. See Dale D. McConkey, "Implementation—The Guts of MBO," *S.A.M. Advanced Management Journal* 37 (July 1972):13–18.
5. For an interesting discussion of factors facilitating major organization change, see Larry Griener, "Patterns of Organizational Doings," *Harvard Business Review* 45 (May–June 1967):119–130.
6. See Stephen Carroll and Henry L. Tosi, Jr., *Management by Objectives* (New York: MacMillan Company, 1973).
7. Burt Scanlan and Stanley Sloan, "It Doesn't Always Work," *ASTME Vectors* 6 (1969):20.
8. Griener, "Patterns of Organizational Doings," p. 128.
9. George Morrisey, *Management by Objectives and Results* (Reading, Mass.: Addison-Wesley Publishing Co., 1970), p. 155.
10. John M. Ivancevich, "A Longitudinal Assessment of Management by Objectives," *Administrative Science Quarterly* 17 (March 1972):126–38.
11. See Melvyn C. Raider, "A Social Service Model of Management-by-Objectives," *Social Casework* 57 (October 1976):523–28.
12. The use of bargaining in the formation of organizational goals is discussed in John W. Thibalt and Harold Kelley, *The Social Psychology of Groups* (New York: John Wiley and Sons, 1959).

13. The advantages of the inductive method of developing goals are discussed in Vernon R. Weihe, *Management by Objectives in Mental Health Services* (St. Louis, MO: Monograph, 1974).
14. See Peter M. Blau, "Cooperation and Competition in a Bureaucracy," *American Journal of Sociology* 59 (May 1954):530–35.
15. The use of Milestones in the U.S. Department of Health, Education and Welfare is discussed in Rodney H. Brody, "MBO Goes to Work in the Public Sector," *Harvard Business Review* 51 (March–April 1973):65–74.
16. Edward Newman and Jerry Turem, "The Crisis of Accountability," *Social Work*, 19 (January 1974):5–16.
17. Edgar F. Huse, *Organizational Development and Change* (St. Paul: West Publishing Co. 1975), p. 189.
18. Carroll and Tosi, *Management by Objectives*, p. 123.
19. Huse, *Organizational Development*, p. 180.
20. Harry Levinson, "Management by Whose Objectives," *Harvard Business Review* 48 (July–August 1970):129.
21. Edgar Huse, "Putting in a Management Development Program That Works," *California Management Review* 9, no. 2 (Winter 1966):78.
22. For a thorough discussion of the dysfunctional effects of criticism in relation to MBO, see Edgar Huse and E. Kay, "Improving Employee Productivity Through Work Planning," in *The Personnel Job in a Changing World*, edited by J. Blood (New York: American Management Association, 1964), pp. 301–02.
23. For an excellent discussion of the group appraisal of objectives, see Levinson, "Management by Whose Objectives," p. 131.

D. ZERO-BASE BUDGETING

24/THE LATEST IN FEDERAL
SPENDING CONTROL:
ZERO-BASE BUDGETING

MARGO L. VIGNOLA

Federal Government expenditures consume about 21 percent of the gross national product. These expenditures totaled $357 billion in calendar 1975, a 19 percent growth over 1974 (compared to a 13 percent rise in 1974). Much concern has been generated by this seemingly unending rise in Government expenditures. As a result, a number of strategies have been proposed to monitor and control current increases. More recently, attention has been focused on zero-base budgeting (ZBB) as a means of effecting these goals.

THE BUDGETING MECHANISM

The allocation of Federal revenues is accomplished through a massive Federal budget, traditionally prepared by the executive branch, but greatly modified through the actions of Congress. In the past, the process was fragmented, uncoordinated, and intensely political. No one Congressional committee maintained control over either the collection of revenues or the expenditure of funds. In 1974, Congress enacted the Congressional Budget and Impoundment Control Act, legislation designed to provide some overall control and coordination in the budget process. The major features include: establishment of House and Senate budget committees; a timetable for Congressional budget activities; use of target levels for Federal expenditures; and establishment of the Congressional Budget Office to analyze the

Federal budget for Congress as the Office of Management and Budget does for the executive branch.

While the experience with the new process is fairly limited (the first full year of operation is still to be completed), most view it as highly effective. Encouraged by this apparent success, Congress is continuing to seek more control over the Federal budget. A relatively old concept, ZBB is being heralded as the next phase in Congressional budget reform. Couched in the new framework of "sunset" bills, ZBB has attracted the attention and support of numerous Federal legislators. Fifty-nine senators, Democrats and Republicans, liberals and conservatives, have joined to sponsor S. 2925, the Government Economy and Spending Reform Act, which would incorporate ZBB as the cornerstone of Federal budgeting activities. Companion legislation (H.R. 11734) has been introduced in the House and has also generated considerable interest among representatives.

The interest in ZBB is by no means confined to the Federal Government. Several states have adopted similar procedures, most notably Texas and Georgia. The procedure has received additional publicity because the Georgia program was implemented by then Gov. Jimmy Carter, now the Democratic party candidate for President. In addition, both the Democratic and Republican parties have adopted positions supporting budget reforms such as ZBB. Widespread Federal and state-level interest buttressed by recent political attention have thus combined to make a once fairly obscure concept in budgeting a major focus of Government budget reform activities.

WHY IS ZBB DIFFERENT?

The Federal Government allocates its resources, largely composed of tax revenues, to numerous Government activities. Traditionally, the Congress has relied on incremental budgeting, a process based on several assumptions about past expenditures. In particular, incremental budgeting assumes that all previous allocations were appropriate, that funds were utilized efficiently, and that only marginal changes to these basic commitments are necessary. Under this system, many programs were given automatic approval without review as to their continuing necessity. Each Congressional committee appeared to harbor its own favorite programs. In addition, several programs were favored within the Federal bureaucracy. Thus the budget became a patchwork of varying programs with diverse priorities and funding patterns, in part fostered by the budgeting process. It was the recognition of this haphazard and fragmented procedure that gave rise to legislation which produced the new Congressional budget process. However, the essential feature of the new process was review of the budget as a whole; no program-by-program review or evaluation was intended. Thus the tendency to continue what may be obsolete and duplicative programs remained. It is this failure of incremental budgeting, still maintained in the new Congressional budget process, that the zero-base technique seeks to remedy.

Zero-base budgeting is essentially a comprehensive review of all parts of the budget. No expenditure is exempted from review; no activity is sacrosanct. Budgeting proceeds without the assumption of a historical base, i.e. as if programs were starting from ground zero. The so-called "sunset provisions" carry this concept a step further: all programs are given automatic termination dates to further reliance on periodic program evaluation. Without such review and reauthorization, programs would cease to operate.

ZBB was initially the product of private enterprise, started in the late sixties at Texas Instruments. The firm applied ZBB procedures to discretionary expenditures such as marketing, advertisement, and research. The objectives of ZBB are basically to make the budget a management tool, a planning and forecasting instrument, and a primary element in evaluation of program performance. In several respects, ZBB is a partial reincarnation of another innovation of the sixties—planning, programming, budgeting system (PPBS). This technique also attempted to rationalize the budgeting process and was over-emphasized as essential to the direction of government spending. Despite brief popularity, PPBS was largely abandoned during the late sixties as cumbersome and time-consuming. ZBB, however, shares many of its characteristics, notably the evaluation of alternative spending strategies and heavy reliance on cost/benefit analysis.

THE NEED FOR MORE CONTROL MEASURES

Despite its apparent effectiveness, the new Congressional budget process was not intended to address fully some major problems in the allocation of Government resources: the tremendous overall growth in government expenditures; the rapid expansion in recent years of expenditures for programs with permanent, open-ended appropriations such as public assistance and Medicaid; the limited resources available to the Federal Government; the proliferation of Federal agencies and competing jurisdictions; and the widespread duplication of Federal programs. All of these problems have prompted continuing concern with budget reform. Several are symptomatic of the fragmented and incremental approach to budgeting partially maintained under the new Congressional budget process. Others illustrate inadequate Congressional oversight and the seeming reluctance or inability of Congress to monitor programs once enacted. As a result of these many characteristics, the Federal budget is increasingly locked into expenditures for existing programs and Congress is less able to entertain or fund new proposals. To deal with some of these problems, the program-by-program review of Federal expenditures (a "micro" versus "macro" analysis) and all other ZBB principles have been incorporated into S. 2925 and coupled with automatic termination (sunset) features.

S. 2925: GOVERNMENT ECONOMY
AND SPENDING REFORM ACT

The legislation provides for several ongoing activities, all of which would be coordinated with the existing budget schedule. First, the bill mandates automatic termination of most Government programs (and regulatory agencies) within a five-year cycle beginning in 1979. The only programs to be excluded are contributory expenditures such as Medicare, Social Security, and interest on the national debt. Even these expenditures would, however, be subject to review. All other programs would be classified by budget function and subfunction and reviewed to determine continued need and appropriate level of funding. Public assistance and health expenditures would terminate Sept. 30, 1981, without further action to reauthorize expenditures. Following the initial review, continuing programs would be authorized for a maximum of five years at which time another review would be necessary. A compilation of all programs subject to the reauthorization process would be prepared by the General Accounting Office in conjunction with the Office of Management and Budget and the Congressional Budget Office by April 1, 1977, and would include information on funding, previous expenditures, and regulatory authority.

The crux of the reauthorization process is zero-based review defined as systematic evaluation of all programs, to be prepared by the Congressional committees. A timetable for review coincident with the budget process is specified. Each committee would prepare a plan for ZBB with the input of the Government Accounting Office (GAO) and the appropriate executive agency. The plan would include identification of original program objectives and the degree to which they have been achieved; a statement of performance and accomplishments in the last four years and costs incurred; the number of persons served by the program; administrative costs; impact of the program on the national economy; degree to which program policies (such as regulations) reflect objectives; an evaluation of program management and information collection activities; and an analysis and projection of service and benefits of the program were it continued, at various funding levels. A similar procedure would be required for tax expenditures, or changes in tax policy which affect Government revenues. Committees would have considerable discretion in the scope and depth of review and establishment of priorities.

Should GAO review a program and uncover any deficiencies, it would have to reevaluate the findings at six month intervals to assure corrective action had been taken. The bill instructs the President to prepare more detailed objective statements in the executive budget to examine the feasibility of employing ZBB in all executive agencies. Finally, the bill creates a Citizen's Bicentennial Commission on the Organization and Operation of Government to examine all aspects of Government operation.

The proposed Federal legislation has attracted widespread support. In hearings held before the Senate Committee on Government Operations, Subcommittee on Intergovernment Operations, earlier this year, witnesses repeatedly praised the objectives of S. 2925, in particular the emphasis on program evaluation and review. Most indicated that such procedures would provide necessary information to undertake such efforts and would complement the new Congressional budget process. However, several operational aspects of the legislation have drawn criticism: the automatic termination of programs; the schedule of termination; the inclusion of most Government progams for zero-based review; the heavy workload placed on committees; the likely cost and complexity of review activities; and the difficulty of reviewing similar progams in different budget categories. Many subcommittee witnesses felt that the requirements specified in S. 2925 were unrealistic in scope and arbitrary in application. Several recommended that ZBB be implemented on a pilot or incremental basis, with initial evaluation of programs specified as uncontrollables given high priority. Rather than a rigid termination schedule, many suggested that review be variable, staggered over time, that programs assigned to different budget categories be reviewed simultaneously, and that the authorization period not be limited to five years.

Several witnesses questioned the impact of S. 2925 on state and local governments since many large Federal programs fund services at these levels of government. States would be forced to await Congressional reauthorizations before proceeding on their own budgeting efforts.

Finally, witnesses questioned the feasibility of S. 2925 in light of political realities. The budgeting process, even in its reformed state, remains intensely political. No budgeting procedure alone is likely to alter this fact without specific accompanying reforms designed to depoliticize the budget process. The present Congressional committee structure, frequently open to the demands of special interest groups, is not conducive to a systematic review of all Government programs. Several committees may, for example, hold joint jurisdiction over programs with similar objectives which would greatly complicate the proposed review process. The Federal bureaucracy faces similar problems; it too responds to special interests. Further, the procedure would require substantial cooperation between the legislative and executive branches of Government, a phenomenon rarely observed in recent years. Thus, S. 2925 faces major political barriers even in the best of circumstances.

While it has been reported by the Senate subcommittee, other committees must also act on the bill, and it is not expected to pass in this session.

Action on the House side has been more limited. No doubt, however, the bill will be entertained early in 1977, with special attention if Jimmy Carter is elected President (although the Republicans also favor the legislation).

HUMAN RESOURCES PROGRAMS AND ZBB

Human resource programs, including public assistance, are under intense public scrutiny. Under a ZBB scheme, particularly at the Federal level, such review would become more intense. It is within these programs that tremendous duplication was identified by GAO (228 health programs, 156 income security programs and 83 housing programs). Thus, these programs would be an appropriate target for review under any ZBB program. While few would argue that elimination of duplication is undesirable or that a review of these programs is unnecessary, their effectiveness is difficult to evaluate. The objectives of human resources programs are clear, but difficult to quantify. Under ZBB such problems would become more acute.

On the other hand, individuals and state and local government have long been frustrated with complying with numerous Federal regulations which they believe do not reflect the true program objectives. Other difficulties have been encountered in coping with overlapping and duplicative Federal programs. These problems are a clear target of ZBB. Thus, despite the possible threat of ZBB to welfare programs, such review and evaluation activities may provide some necessary reform in the administration of Federal programs.

CONCLUSION

ZBB is a very attractive concept for it seems to provide a natural framework for program evaluation, something long absent from Government budgeting. However, program review and evaluation should be one function of an ongoing activity which has the capacity to plan ahead. As presently constituted, ZBB has a more static orientation—periodic review of program effectiveness. Without some accompanying planning process, ZBB's usefulness is limited.

One major criticism of ZBB is the complexity and detail of required procedures. Even proponents recognize that the collection, compilation, and organization of massive amounts of information is costly and time-consuming; critics charge that such detail is unnecessary. In the case of Government programs, a related issue has been raised: that ZBB in its truest application is duplicating the legislative process that created the program initially. Though this process may be necessary to force a re-examination of the continued need for the program's existence, some view such activity as duplicative.

The critical argument against ZBB is not, however, directed at procedural or cost issues, but rather at the supposed capacity of the technique to effect major reform in Government spending. Critics charge that ZBB, essentially a budget tool, is being touted as something far more significant—a panacea for all budgeting problems. Most of the experience with ZBB indicates that its utility is limited. The problems the proposed Federal legislation intends to address through ZBB are very real; but without other reforms, ZBB alone in these endeavors is likely to fail. For example, at the Federal level some reorganization of agencies, commissions, and departments is necessary. And, again, the present committee structure in Congress is not suited to the demands of ZBB, even as formulated in S. 2925. The underlying goal of ZBB is program evaluation; but without provisions for information collection and adequate staffing, both in Congress and the executive agencies, the process has the potential of becoming empty routine.

E. ACCOUNTABILITY

25/SOCIAL SERVICES: THE PROBLEM OF ACCOUNTABILITY

GEORGE HOSHINO

In reporting out the 1973 appropriation bill for the Department of Health, Education, and Welfare, the Senate Appropriations Committee had the following to say about the rapidly increasing rate of expenditures for the social services authorized by the public assistance titles of the Social Security Act:

This Committee is concerned that the use of this source of Federal financing is out of any reasonable control. The Department of Health, Education, and Welfare cannot even describe to us with any precision what $2,000,000,000 of taxpayers' money is being used for. We have been informed by the Department that they intend to improve their management of this program. . . . However, until these improvements are accomplished, this Committee believes that Congress must limit the Federal liability for this largely unknown, undefined, open-ended financing mechanism . . . until convinced that these funds are being spent prudently and effectively (Note 1).

Congress responded by imposing a ceiling of $2.5 billion on federal expenditures for social services, changing the open-end grant to a closed-end grant, and prescribing that 90 percent of the funds be used for services to current recipients except for child-care services, family planning, services to the mentally retarded and drug addicts or alcoholics, and foster care for children (Note 2). The tenor of the House-Senate conference report and the thrust of the current administration's policies in respect to services indicate that accountability will be heavily stressed in the coming years.

This paper examines the implications of the demands by Congress and the administration for greater accountability and discusses the problem of accountability in the expenditure of funds for and program performance in the public welfare social services.

THE CONTEXT

The 1962 amendments to the Social Security Act, which authorized 75 percent open-ended federal sharing of expenditures for services to recipients of public assistance (subsequently extended to former recipients and persons likely to become recipients), ushered in a decade of the "social services strategy." The original rationale for the services amendments was that services provided by trained staff members would lead to the rehabilitation and self-support of recipients of public aid, with a consequent reduction in the welfare rolls and expenditures for public assistance. "Rehabilitation instead of relief" and similar slogans were the catchwords of the new thrust in public welfare policy. The catch, however, was that the decade of the 1960s saw a precipitous rise in the number of recipients of and the amount of expenditures for aid to families with dependent children (AFDC), especially in the latter half of the decade. In December 1960, recipients of AFDC numbered 3.1 million, with expenditures for the year of $9.9 million; by December 1965, recipients numbered 4.4 million and annual expenditures totaled $1.6 billion; by December 1970, the number of recipients had risen to 9.7 million and annual expenditures to $4.8 billion.

If the stated rationale for services is accepted as a basis for evaluation, the services strategy will have to be judged an unmitigated debacle. Indeed, by 1967 the handwriting was already on the wall in the form of a shift from the services strategy to a work-and-training strategy, as reflected in the Work Incentive program (WIN). The work strategy has been extended by more recent amendments, the latest being the "Talmadge amendment," which requires most adult or older recipients of AFDC to register with the manpower services. Whether the manpower services will be any more successful than the welfare services in controlling the welfare rolls remains to be seen, but it is doubtful that they will.

Many reasons have been advanced to explain the expansion of the AFDC rolls: high unemployment rates, population increases, increasing family disorganization, inadequacies of the social security system, higher assistance standards, litigation overturning restrictive policies and practices, acceptance of the view that assistance is a legal entitlement, political activity by recipient groups, and so on. The fact remains, however, that what might be called a "credibility gap" exists in respect to the public welfare social services and those who are involved in their administration and delivery.

More recently, services have been advocated in their own right. That is, the need for services is seen as independent of the need for financial aid. This view underlies the policy of separation of financial aid from social services, a policy now mandated by federal regulations[13] (Note 3). But the separation policy only puts the problem of accountability in a different way; in fact, it further highlights the problem, for, if the rationale for services is not directly to reduce the incidence of dependency on public assistance, what is the rationale for services and for what results are public welfare agencies to be held accountable?

To pose this question is to raise a litany of further questions: What is to be measured and evaluated—the effects of a program, its effectiveness, or its social impact—and against what criteria are such variables to be judged? Is the service worker to be held accountable for his activities—that is, the process—or for the results he achieves—that is, outcomes? (In systems parlance, the question is asked, "Is the emphasis on 'inputs' or 'outputs'?" The cynic might say, "Don't confuse motion with movement.") To whom is the service worker accountable—the agency or his client? Can clients really hold workers to account? By what means? What mechanisms can be used to monitor, evaluate, and control service programs, and how effective and efficient are they? How will staff react to control measures such as social service information systems, and what will be the consequences, desirable and undesirable, of their reactions? How can one evaluate the newer forms of service, such as advocacy, as well as new or combined methods such as group services and community work? Is it possible to evaluate alternative "approaches" to service delivery (as opposed to service methods and individual worker performance), especially when programs are undergoing rapid change in the face of changing conceptions of service, new federal policies, and other environmental factors?

These are incredibly difficult questions. Similar problems of account-ability were created by recent legislation that established what broadly might be termed "social policies" in respect to certain social problems or target populations. Examples of such legislation include the Economic Opportunity Act (poverty), the Older Americans Act (the aged), the Community Mental Health Center Act (mental health and retardation), and the Model Cities Act (urban problems). The United States does not have a coherent or consistent national social policy for children, but a com-prehensive child-care bill appeared to move in that direction. There is de-bate on the desirability and thrust of a population policy and a policy on drug addiction.

Legislation of this kind typically identifies the social problem or need, establishes broad goals and policies, sets down the general outlines of the system, and allocates major responsibilities for program administration, but does not usually go into program details. (In contrast, the Social Security Act provides for specific programs, such as old age, survivors, disability, and health insurance, and goes into considerable detail about benefits, eligibil-ity requirements, and methods of administration.)

Such "policy" legislation tends to emphasize planning, administrative leadership and discretion, and innovation and experimentation. Desirable as these features may be, they pose difficult problems of accountability. Agencies will be asked how effective the programs are in response to policy objectives, and what impact they have on social problems. Different kinds of performance criteria and new ways of monitoring and evaluating social welfare systems will be required (Note 4). Public welfare is faced with similar problems.

ACTIVITY, PROCESS, AND OUTCOME

It has been said that the 1960s were a decade of analysis of social welfare programs, and that the 1970s will be a decade of evaluation. That is, there will be a shift from asking, "What happened?" to asking, "How good (or effective) is what happened?"

Given that social welfare programs are components of social systems established as a consequence of social policy, it follows that staff members engaged in the provision of social services are accountable for the expendi-ture of funds and for program performance. Available information on the services program—when it exists at all—consists of little more than book-keeping reports and head counts supplemented by illustrative anecdotal material. The data usually describe program activity. Services are explained in terms of program input—so many clients served, so many interviews or home visits, so many children placed in foster homes, and so on. Such data may no longer suffice. There is increasing insistence that programs of service be justified and explained in terms of outcomes or performance related to criteria of effectiveness and stated policy goals.

The goals of public social policy, however, are seldom explicit or precise. Phrases such as "strengthening family life" or "eliminating the paradox of poverty" express values or ultimate goals, but they are of little operational usefulness. Some policy goals are potentially or actually contradictory. For example, the goal of strengthening family life is contradicted by the anti-family bias of AFDC policies, which emphasize the absence of the father. Contradictory public attitudes press on the agency. Should the demands to keep the costs of assistance under control be heeded or should staff members undertake—as does the Social Security Administration—to insure that all eligible recipients receive the maximum to which they are entitled? If the goal is to lessen the apathy of the poor and stimulate them to make their own efforts to improve their life situations, the poor are likely to perceive their problems as the unavailability of or lack of access to public aid and services. They may organize to press their demands and enlist the help of legal services. If the service worker's function is to include advocacy, his efforts on behalf of his clients may be directed to "systems change" against public agencies and even against the eligibility workers in his own agency. With separation of services and money payments, this is not an uncommon occurrence. These activities hardly square with the goal of reducing dependency on public aid, however.

PROGRAM MONITORING, EVALUATION, AND CONTROL

What are the means by which social services programs might be monitored, evaluated, and controlled? Three analogies—a cook making soup, a teacher giving an examination, and a public health officer testing the water supply of a city—illustrate several elements of a control system: a sensing or monitoring mechanism; sampling; "indicators," real or surrogate, from which inferences about quality are made; criteria or standards of quality; and a feedback system.

The cook periodically runs a ladle through the kettle of soup to secure a "representative" sample, tastes the sample, and adds this or that ingredient to bring the mixture up to his standards of taste. The teacher gives an examination and, on the basis of this small sample of the student's performance, makes certain judgments about the student's progress, capacity, and potentiality. Moreover, the teacher is likely to use the results of the examination to make adjustments in his course content or teaching methods. The public health officer, who is responsible for insuring that the city's water supply is safe and acceptable in appearance and taste, tests small samples of water periodically to determine the bacterial count and the presence of salt or other substances. If these "indicators" fall within prescribed criteria or standards, he concludes that the water is potable; if not, he takes steps to bring the water up to the desired standards. In similar fashion, one makes judgments about things and phenomena by means of techniques ranging from the cook's simple taste test to sophisticated statistical methods.

Although the same concepts can be applied to public welfare, monitoring, evaluating, and controlling social service programs present special difficulties. As already noted, social policy goals are seldom precise, and they are often contradictory. Operational criteria and measures of effectiveness or impact are difficult to establish. There are few generally accepted indicators, real or surrogate, from which the quality of social services or their outcomes can be inferred. At best, the available tools are very crude indeed.

The usual case record in family and children's work consists of a narrative or summary description of the worker's activities and the activities of the members of the family. It is a record of the casework process, an accounting of activity. There have been few efforts to evaluate the effectiveness of casework, and those few have generally failed to demonstrate statistically significant results, given the criteria used in the experiments.[2, 10] In only a few instances have the independent perceptions of clients themselves been incorporated in the evaluation data (Note 5). While it could be argued that client perceptions of services—which tend to be expressed in terms of satisfaction or dissatisfaction, or helpfulness and unhelpfulness—are not real criteria of effectiveness, nevertheless such data constitute an element of program evaluation and are essential to the concept of accountability (Note 6).

Follow-up data on client situations subsequent to the termination of service are rarely collected systematically. The lack of interest in how clients fare after their cases are closed is curious, since presumably that kind of information would be of value to agencies in evaluating their services. While many difficulties would attend the establishment of a system for collecting follow-up data on a regular basis, the methodological problems are not insurmountable.

Workers in public welfare programs have a great deal of discretion. Keeping that discretion within bounds is critical in order that the intent of policy be carried out and abuse of administrative discretion prevented. In public assistance, official behavior has been so uncontrolled as to lead some critics to characterize its administration as "lawless." Violations of legal rights and federal and state statutes are widespread, and agencies disregard their own regulations. Appeals machinery has been ineffective in holding agencies accountable for their actions. The legal services have had some success, but they cannot be expected to police the bureaucracy. Recipients cannot afford nor are they in a position to challenge the agencies through litigation. Organized recipient groups have had considerable impact, but the welfare-rights movement appears to be spending itself and bureaucracies have learned how to cope with its tactics.

A similar situation may prevail in the services programs. Indeed, controlling official behavior may be an even more difficult problem because of the discretionary powers of the worker and the fact that little of the worker's activity is directly observable. The person most acutely affected, the client, is not in a position to hold the worker or the agency accountable. (By way of contrast, consider the baseball player, whose every move is scrutinized by the umpires, his teammates, the opposition, the coaches, and the fans.) Many social services, especially the so-called hard services, such as day care, medical care, and transportation, are forms of in-kind income. Service workers are "gatekeepers" to desperately needed or wanted provisions, such as special allowances, jobs, housing, and even recreation, all of which are in short supply. The service worker's role is "functionally general" in contrast with the more limited "functionally specific" role of staff members in other fields, such as education and health. This general role, in combination with the "treatment" orientation of most social work theories, may lead the worker to intervene in virtually any aspect of the client's life. Given the vulnerable position of the low-income population, there is the danger that worker activity will be directed toward control of client behavior. Separation of aid and services may mitigate some of the more blatant uses of the recipient's dependent status to impose behavioral conformity, but there is no assurance that more subtle but no less real coercion will not accompany the social services.[5, 7] In the face of these realities, to suggest that clients of public welfare agencies can hold workers and agencies accountable to them is merely rhetoric.

The same considerations make advocacy a dubious proposition, since the concept of advocacy implies that the advocate is accountable to his client. If it is accepted, however, that poor families perceive their problems in terms of the need for "hard services," then advocacy and brokering will logically constitute the core of the service worker's role. But the worker is up against the inadequacies of social welfare programs and the shortcomings of social and economic institutions. Neither he nor the client can be expected to correct or overcome these barriers. For what results, then, can the service worker be held accountable?

Piliavin[11] (pp. 220–22) has proposed that the worker's effectiveness be assessed according to "mundane" or "lower-level" measures of performance, that is, achievement in securing the limited kinds of concrete assistance implicit in the advocate-broker role. This approach would relieve the social services of direct responsibility for altering general social problems, such as dependency and delinquency. At the same time, it would avoid the dangers inherent in the expectation that the worker effect demonstrable change in the behavior or life-styles of individuals and families, as implied in the casework approach. Thus, Piliavin suggests a much less ambitious role for the social services than might be inferred from the 1962 amendments. Services would be more responsive and accountable to the client population, and there would be a more realistic basis for evaluation.

INTENDED AND UNINTENDED CONSEQUENCES

An oft-cited expression states: "Laws do not administer themselves." Neither do administrative procedures promulgated to give effect and specificity to statutory mandates. While procedures, along with leadership and cooperation, bind an agency staff together and enable the members to work toward some common purpose, their implementation is ultimately dependent on the actions of staff members at the operating level—administrators, supervisors, and line workers. Such staff members are capable of and can usually find discretionary powers or ways to sabotage policies with which they disagree or which jeopardize their interests. Compassionate workers have ways of mitigating harsh public assistance policies, and punitive workers can pervert liberal ones. For example, employment counselors in a state employment agency reacted to changes in reporting requirements instituted to shift the agency's program in the direction desired by a new director by adjusting their activities so that the statistics would show them in their best light, with some unfortunate consequences for client services[1] (pp. 44–47). An attempt to improve the academic achievement of ghetto children by radically altering the teacher's role in an open-classroom environment failed in part because the teachers realized that their students would still be tested on reading and mathematical achievement tests, which reflected traditional subject-matter teaching.[4] The teachers returned to traditional teaching methods. Child-care administrators reacted to an amendment to a child-abuse law, which mandated reporting to law-enforcement officials of all cases of suspected child abuse, by completely subverting the intent of the amendment.[9] Although the intent was to have police investigate suspected abuse cases, virtually no change took place in local agency practice.

The "creaming" phenomenon is familiar in social welfare. If the performance of a rehabilitation counselor is rated on the number of successful placements, he is likely to look for the "best" candidates, not the ones most in need of help. Already evident are the consequences of the recent changes in WIN policies, which emphasize placement and work rather than rehabilitation and training.

The social service information systems being developed in response to the demands for better accountability may encounter similar problems. Most plans are designed to influence the behavior of the worker by requiring him to specify his activities in detail and by emphasizing results or outcomes (Note 7). However, if staff members cannot achieve the results expected or if they disagree with the intent of the procedures, they are likely to subvert the system. If outcome criteria are based on client behavioral change, the danger is that the client's vulnerability may be exploited to coerce conformity.

On the other hand, practice may be relatively unchanged by new reporting requirements alone. The tacit compliance with the requirement of the 1962 services amendments that a "social study" be made of each child receiving AFDC is a case in point. The requirement was meant to further the rehabilitation and services intent of the amendments. What happened was that thousands of workers went through the motions of filling out millions of lengthy forms in order to satisfy the requirements for the 75-percent federal funding. Very little changed in actual practice. In several agencies, supervisors were observed dutifully checking off items from stacks of case records—many from uncovered caseloads—whereupon the forms were filed and, for all practical purposes, ignored.

CONCLUSIONS

The problem of accountability points up the paradoxes of social policy and the dilemmas of social welfare administration. Until the goals of policy can be made more coherent and consistent and criteria of performance more explicit and realistic, there is little hope of attaining accountability in any real sense for either the services program as a whole or for the individual worker. Even more problematic is the question of accountability to the client population—of serving the interests of the consumers of social services as they perceive their problems and needs. Service workers need to use discretion; at the same time, that discretion can become coercive. Mechanisms of administrative control can lead to undesirable and unintended consequences or can be sabotaged by agency staff.

Given the confusion about goals and criteria of performance, it might be wiser to give priority to the development of valid and reliable indicators of program effort and output. Which indicators best reflect the critical aspects of a program, which are most efficient, how much can be inferred from them, and how are they to be interpreted and used? Will they be used to point up the need for system change or to control worker and client behavior? The combination of an array of good program indicators and systematic sampling—including client perceptions during and subsequent to the course of service—could constitute a step toward the development of more efficient programwide built-in monitoring and evaluation systems. Such a plan would not guarantee that the information generated would be used wisely, nor would it answer the questions of effectiveness and goals, but perhaps staff members would then be in a better position to address the problems of operationalizing and objectifying goals and criteria of effectiveness (Note 8).

Theoretically, goals and criteria of effectiveness against which to evaluate program performance ought to be established first. But the reality today is that policy goals and effectiveness criteria are constantly changing. Solutions in the form of management packages, blueprints, or fixed criteria or standards may be obsolete almost as soon as they are adopted. The urgent need, therefore, is to develop the capabilities of social welfare agencies—and the staff members within them—to adapt to and even anticipate rapid change in legislation, regulations, social needs, and concepts and delivery of services. Accountability systems will then become less devices through which superiors monitor employees than the means through which staff members at all levels learn how well they are doing their jobs, how to cope with change in constructive ways, and how to plan for future change.

NOTES

1. The open-ended grant formula and the extremely broad and vague definition of services under the original legislation have been exploited by the states for purposes never envisioned by Congress. It has been claimed that the services program had become a form of revenue sharing in the hands of imaginative and aggressive administrators. This partly explains the enormous jump in claims for federal reimbursement and even larger projected expenditures, which the Senate committee viewed with such alarm (see *Washington Post*, August 8, 9, 1972, and *Wall Street Journal*, August 15, 1972).
2. Title III, Pub. L. 92–512, State and Local Fiscal Assistance Act, October 20, 1972, commonly known as the general revenue-sharing act. For a brief sketch of the social services provisions from 1956 through the 1972 amendments, see *Social Service Review* (12).
3. The 1972 Social Security Act amendments provide for a new federally administered program of Supplemental Security Income (SSI) to replace the federally aided categories of aid to the aged, aid to the blind, and aid to the totally and permanently disabled. Separation will be automatically effected in the adult categories, since the service programs will remain with the states.
4. The methodological difficulties of evaluating social action programs are discussed in Cain and Hollister (3). In an ultimate sense, social policy might be said to be directed to the well-being of society as a whole, or what has come to be called "the quality of life." While the quantity and quality of public welfare services probably have something to do with "satisfaction" or "alienation" and other aspects of the quality of life in direct and indirect ways, one is hard put to be more specific.
5. See Harrison and Wright (6) for an example of the inclusion of client perceptions in the evaluation of services.
6. Student evaluation of course content and teaching is now a widespread practice, accepted more or less graciously by university faculties.
7. The much-discussed goal-oriented social services (GOSS) model proposed by the Social and Rehabilitation Service emphasized goal achievement to be accomplished by the removal of identified barriers in order to bring the client to a desired level of functioning.
8. In addition to developing ways to evaluate individual worker performance, there is a need to develop the capability of evaluating alternative "approaches" to service delivery. For example, one agency has developed a social service delivery system in

which service workers are "outposted" to schools, hospitals, the jail, and other community agencies and organizations (see Hoshino and Weber [8]). The problem of accountability is exacerbated because the usual case recording or "day sheet" reporting does not adequately reflect the activity of the workers who use a mixture of methods and approaches. The challenge is to design social service information systems that are adaptable to fluid and flexible approaches, programs, and practice methods, rather than forcing program activity into prescribed reporting schemes.

REFERENCES

1. Blau, Peter. "The Departmental Structure in a State Employment Agency." *The Dynamics of Bureaucracy*, pp. 19–117. 2d ed. Chicago: University of Chicago Press, 1963.
2. Brown, Gordon E., ed. *The Multi-Problem Dilemma*. Metuchen, N.J.: Scarecrow Press, 1968.
3. Cain, Glen G., and Hollister, Robinson G. *The Methodology of Evaluating Social Action Porgrams*. Madison, Wis.: Institute for Research on Poverty, 1969.
4. Gross, Neal; Giancquinta, Joseph B.; and Bernstein, Marilyn. *Implementing Organizational Innovations: A Sociological Analysis of Planned Educational Change.* New York: Basic Books, 1971.
5. Handler, Joel. "The Coercive Children's Officer." *New Society* 12 (October 1968): 485–87.
6. Harrison, Margaret G., and Wright, Colin R. *A Technique for Measuring the Outcomes of Social Services*. San Jose, Calif.: Department of Social Services of Santa Clara County, 1972.
7. Hoshino, George. "Money and Morality: Income Security and Personal Social Services." *Social Work* 16, no. 2 (April 1971): 16–24.
8. Hoshino, George, and Webert, Shirley. "Outposting in the Public Welfare Services." *Public Welfare* 31, no. 1 (Winter 1973): 8–14.
9. Hoshino, George, and Yoder, George Y. "Administrative Discretion in the Implementation of Child Abuse Legislation." Mimeographed. Philadelphia: School of Social Work, University of Pennsylvania, 1972.
10. Meyer, Henry J.; Borgatta, Edgar F.; and Jones, Wyatt C. *Girls at Vocational High.* New York: Russell Sage Foundation, 1965.
11. Piliavin, Irving. "Provision of Social Services to Recipients of Income Maintenance." In *Income Maintenance: Interdisciplinary Approaches to Research*, edited by L. Orr, R. Hollister, and M. Lefcowitz, pp. 214–24. Chicago: Markham Publishing Co., 1971.
12. "Sharing or Paring?" *Social Service Review* 47, no. 1 (March 1973): 95–102.
13. U.S., Social and Rehabilitation Service. "Separation of Services from Assistance Payments." *Federal Register*, vol. 37, no. 107, June 2, 1972, pt. 205, title 45.

This article is adapted from a paper presented at the Northeast Regional Conference of the American Public Welfare Association, September 6, 1972, in San Juan, Puerto Rico.

26/THE CRISIS OF
ACCOUNTABILITY

EDWARD NEWMAN AND JERRY TUREM

Accountability is an elusive concept. As addressed in this article, its terms of reference are personal social services in the broad spectrum of human services, concentrating in the main on social services available in either the public or private sector under the Social Security Act. The problems of social services that are publicly delivered or publicly supported are not necessarily different from those of services funded through other sources. However, in the case of services having governmental assistance, the problems of accountability—problems that are related to political action, ideology, policy-making, program effectiveness, and professional responsibility—are today more striking and visible. They are therefore more symptomatic of the current crisis of accountability.

This article will focus on issues that go beneath the surface of political polemics, administrative style, or intergovernmental issues to the raison d'etre of the social service profession—the problems, the goals, the means of achieving these goals, and the value of the profession's efforts according to the extent to which tasks are accomplished. Implications of accountability in social services will then be considered from the vantage point of public responsibility.

Finally, a perspective on accountability will be presented that explores why, in publicly supported programs, accountability does not simply involve accounting for the "quality of service delivery," as stated by Austin and Caulk in a paper prepared for the 1973 Delegate Assembly of the National Association of Social Workers (NASW).[1]

Indeed, that view largely misses the point that accountability comprises a series of elements ranging from problem identification to goal formulation, and it raises the central questions of efficiency and effectiveness in reducing social problems. To be accountable, in this sense, means addressing a real problem that can be remedied. It means that professional and technical work can be provided if society makes the resources available, that this work will be provided in the manner promised, and that the problem may then be effectively minimized at the least possible social cost.

Accountability is an emotionally laden issue for social workers. The profession naturally reacted vigorously when news reports of the president's former chief domestic adviser stated:

There seems to be a folk tradition around this town that it's somehow indecent to cut any social program. I don't think the second administration will be a believer in that folk tale. I think a President with a substantial mandate, who feels that the majority of the people are behind him, will feel very comfortable in saying to a vested interest group, such as the social workers, "Look, your social program of the 1960s isn't working, and we're going to dismantle it so you'll just have to go out and find honest labor somewhere else."[2]

In March 1973, Mitchell I. Ginsberg, then president of NASW, pointed out to members the unprecedented challenge presented by "program and fiscal cutbacks at all levels of government, [which] presage fewer services for those in need." Ginsberg called on NASW "to see to it that social services are not decimated, that government does not abdicate its responsibility" and to focus its efforts "on a program of professional action which will counter the erosion of services to people and the assaults on social work."[3]

Austin and Caulk recommended to the NASW Delegate Assembly program objectives and actions concentrating on political, governmental, administrative, and fiscal strategies.[4] They outlined the following roles for the federal government and the states:

• The states rather than the federal government should set priorities for social services.

• The federal government should not set forth detailed regulations and rules and keep changing them.

• The states should develop machinery to maximize rational, technically sound programs that include full participation by consumers, providers, and other individuals and groups.

• The federal government should finance the system and distribute funds to states through relatively unencumbered procedures.

These proposals reflect a concept closely allied to issues of public responsibility. Austin and Caulk seem to suggest that politically the federal government is either untrustworthy or unresponsive. Ideologically, they find a federally directed public social service strategy repugnant. Administratively, they consider federal priority-setting more aloof from the public interest than state and local priority-setting would be. Their view slides over some critical factors as to why the crisis of accountability exists.

POLITICAL AND ADMINISTRATIVE ACCOUNTABILITY

One often hears complaints that political influence is diverting the good intentions of planners and practitioners. This sounds as if planners and practitioners have a rational and comprehensive approach to developing goals—and the means to achieve them—which politicians distort or pervert. Planners tend to ignore or underrate political considerations, that is to say, the roles of power and influence. They do not realize the extent to which the political process is a means for identifying and allocating social values and for legitimating the means and resources to achieve the ends that those values define. It is in this sense that politics inevitably influences the outcome of any planning process. More strongly stated, effective planning in the public sector is always politicized.

The pluralistic American approach to services will, for the foreseeable future, be based on choices made by providers representing disparate interests who may choose to be "in" or "out" of any national scheme. So far, no interest group or coalition of like-minded interests (including the organized social work profession) has brought together sufficient influence to interest the Administration, the Congress, or other important elements of the American public in a plan to organize social services. It is particularly disconcerting that neither NASW nor professional social workers acting independently or under other auspices have successfully influenced recent decisions in more appealing directions.

A strategy that posits the states as priority-setters and orchestrators for the services within their domain moves away from a national, unified, comprehensive approach. The federal executive branch does have a point of view about services (even though social workers may not like many of its components) and has the potential power to impose decisions and make binding proposals (about which many social workers may raise questions). But the federal government is the only source from which both significant funding and comprehensive programs can develop.

The question of accountability is raised at this time because of recent events in Washington. Congress approved a ceiling of $2.5 billion on formerly open-ended public social services and narrowed the range of clients who could be served. The Administration proposed regulations that narrowed the range even further. Why has this happened and why now? What does it portend? A few years ago most social workers would have thought $2.5 billion for social services was unattainable. Now it is considered inhibiting. Why? What impelled the growth? Is there a real "crisis" in services, or are social workers reacting without even a moment's reflection? Could it be a return to normal growth after an aberrant spurt?

THE BUDGET CRISIS

When the president delivers his annual budget message some time in January, the major newspapers of the country usually greet it with a "canned" description of his recommendations for the ensuing fiscal year. Their descriptions contain summaries of the budget's major sectors—national defense, human resources, natural resources, the national interest, and "other." Their source material is provided annually in a prereleased pamphlet. The real news related to the budget announcement usually revolves around its total magnitude and legislative initiatives. Within a day or so after the president presents the message, the budget no longer is news.

In 1973, however, the budget, especially its recommendations in the human resources sector, was big news for those interested in the progress of social services.[5] Reaction to this budget generated the crisis in human services. Various groups interested in human resources agitated and formed coalitions spanning previously autonomous fields.

In most years the presentation of the budget and its appropriations processes have resulted in incremental changes in the existing budget authority and have given a slight leeway for substantial starts in any new program. As Newman and March have noted:

The complexities of institutional arrangements guard against radical departures. These complexities also make it very difficult to adjust priorities on a major scale to adjust to changing social needs.[6]

In 1973 actions on the president's budget in the human services sector involved more than incrementalism. A number of economic and administrative premises incorporated in the executive budget are difficult to attack, others go beyond substantive differences and relate to more basic political and constitutional questions of the separation of powers. The serious questions are the choices that must be made about the human services, given a relatively limited level of federal funds.

One may agree or disagree with an overall $268.7 billion maximum for fiscal year 1974. Most people would agree, though, that a budget of this magnitude will have a significant impact on prices, wages, and employment. Social workers and others may disagree with the distribution among national defense, human resources, and natural resources. Many would agree, however, that some level for defense expenditures should be preserved. They may disagree with the rise in expenditures for natural resources, although most are sympathetic to efforts to reduce air and water pollution, preserve the physical environment, and deal with the energy crisis.

The rhetoric supporting the federal government's role in promoting national priorities, while decentralizing authority and decision-making to states and local governments and moving away from central control in Washington, appeals to some social workers but not to others. Traditionally, social work support was often directed to the centralist programs of the New Deal and the Great Society. It is indeed difficult now to counteract a rationale that professes to maximize economic well-being, stresses concentration on national priorities "which really work," and justifies its humaneness on grounds that the comparative levels of defense expenditures will have decreased from 41 percent in fiscal year 1969 to a projected 30.2 percent in fiscal year 1974, while human resources will have risen from 39 percent to 46.7 percent during the same period.

In examining the human resources sector we find that of an estimated $93.9 billion proposed for fiscal year 1974, over $80 billion are tabbed for income security (mostly social security and income maintenance). These resources are allocated without regard to congressional authority to make annual appropriations and are expended from trust funds and from ostensibly uncontrollable matching funds disbursed through state and local authorities.

Responsible groups cannot ignore the implications of extending all programs under the Department of Health, Education, and Welfare (HEW) to all potential recipients. In December 1972 the secretary of HEW estimated that the department's service delivery programs, which then cost $9 billion, would cost $250 billion (about the total of the federal budget) if they were actually extended to all who could be covered.[7] Also, a recent study estimated that meeting the objectives of two major programs in compensatory education and four in social service would require the recruitment and training of an additional 6 million professionals, paraprofessionals, and volunteers.[8]

This recounting is presented neither to defend nor to scare those who may be incensed by current efforts to roll back commitments to social programs. It is meant, rather, to remind social workers that fiscal and human resources are not unlimited even in this affluent nation and that choices must be made among goals for programs.

SERVICES UNDER SOCIAL SECURITY

The treatment of the social services under the Social Security Act presents a special case of gross inconsistency between the rhetoric of decentralization and the reality of Administration proposals. Detailed federal regulations set priorities and limit eligibility and allowable services. Financial penalties for noncompliance place the states in an advocacy relationship to the federal bureaucracy. Yet Nixon's New Federalism affirms that state and local governments should have discretion in setting priorities for social programs and that the federal bureaucracy should disengage itself from handling problems that are state or local.

How closely do specific public benefits or services approximate generally accepted "rights?" For example, in the field of education, the idea that elementary and secondary education should be available to all has wide acceptability. But no such broad consensus has developed for social services, either on their parameters or on their separate components.

Services available under the Social Security Act are still generally associated with actual provision of or at least control by public welfare agencies, even though advocates of a comprehensive social service system would like it otherwise. The great growth in expenditures for social services, which some thought would reduce welfare, parallels growth in case loads and payments. Finally, and perhaps most significantly, a basic income floor under all Americans has given way as a major public issue to questions of how much income, for what categories of people, under what conditions. Some programs still include maintenance benefits as an ingredient in a plan for training or treatment. In these instances, maintenance payments may be used as incentives to continue participation in such programs.

Given lack of consensus on the scope and effectiveness of social services, along with the growth of expenditures in public assistance, changes at the federal level over the past few months are best explained as attempts to control the anticipated overall expenditures available for welfare-related services, to reduce the numbers eligible to receive such services, and to circumscribe the categories in which available resources may be expended.

Observers both within and outside the field warned, even during the early 1960s, that tying services to the goal of reducing dependence on public assistance would weaken their public credibility. At least three developments can be cited for the unhappy consequences of not heeding these warnings—all dealing with the central theme of accountability.

First, studies of service effectiveness do not convincingly show that direct service intervention, especially casework, leads to client improvement.[9] Second, federal, state, and local welfare agencies have failed to find adequate monitoring or reporting devices for separating administrative from service costs or to account adequately for the use of purchased services under the 1967 amendments to the Social Security Act. Third, state and local governments were caught short fiscally in the last few years and abused the purposes of the services amendments by replacing at least some state and local funds with federal moneys probably illegally in some instances, such as charging for social services activities properly reimbursed at the lower administrative rate authorized by the Social Security Act. Accountability was therefore increasingly challenged on grounds of effectiveness as well as evidence of inadequate responsibility to the taxpayer and intended recipients.

No one is convinced that the building blocks for social services that are clearly accountable to the public are yet available. Existing programs become exceedingly vulnerable to a cost-conscious leadership unsympathetic to unsupported claims.

What are the first steps that go beyond the political awareness necessary to make any profession responsive to societal needs? Can social workers meet the following challenge Eulau recently threw to all the humanistic professions?

. . . the professionals must bring to the treatment of public issues professionally pertinent criteria of substance and conduct that warrant their being respected for their knowledge and skills rather than for the particular ideological predilections that may be the fashion of the moment. The winds of politics are moody and have a way of changing faster than professional responses to these winds.[10]

As indicated, budget restrictions are symptomatic of a more deep-seated problem: lack of recognition of the effectiveness of social service programs. In large measure, this is because social work has not sustained the burden of proof of cost effectiveness and because service programs often operate without regard for basic accounting and the requirements of program data collection. Also, the squeeze on social service programs is part of an overall program of resource allocation within a given budget.

THE VALUE OF SERVICES

Are social work services valued? This is a question central to the concern of social workers. If services are valued, the problem of demonstrating effectiveness is easier. This is not the same as asking if they *are* effective. The term "valued" is used in the sense that someone believes services are worth spending money on them. Worth could be established by a given individual who elects to spend some of his income to purchase a service. Or it could be established by society wishing to buy a set of activities from which it gains satisfaction. This latter is a bit tricky since society may gain satisfaction from results other than what practitioners actually attain. Thus, society may indicate that it values social services by making donations to support philanthropic institutions or by providing direct tax subsidies. However, such actions may be taken primarily because they reduce social guilt rather than because they bring about change in individuals or conditions.

Consider the legal profession by analogy. The fact that people are willing to purchase unsubsidized legal services from lawyers is evidence that these services are valued in the private sector. To the extent an attorney is effective he will usually prosper. If he is ineffective, then his income will likely be less than that of his successful colleagues.

When publicly subsidized programs of legal services for the poor were established, lawyers held that the subsidies were required only for those incapable of paying. Some lawyers claimed that no such programs were necessary since there are existing societies that provide services and since many lawyers reduced their fees to the poor. The recent attack on programs of legal services for the poor did not occur because of lack of demonstrated effectiveness but because of the alleged practice of too little "personal service" law and too much "social action" law. But these are questions of emphasis and arguments as to whether government should sponsor litigation against itself, not whether people value the legal profession.

In the social services there are some, but few, comparable programs so valued. Child care, for example, can be shown to be valued; that is, one can point to programs of child care operated solely by parent subscription. Child care becomes controversial when, with government subsidy, program operators and planners develop standards that tend to price the services higher than people are willing or able to pay. The wish to subsidize, then, all "extras" for all users becomes subject to the question: What differences, if any, do these extras make?

If social work was an essentially private profession supported in the marketplace by persons willing to purchase whatever they thought gave them satisfaction, then the question of public accountability and the question of effectiveness would be less compelling. Since professional social work activities largely depend on public sources of funding, society requires some accounting. And alternative uses of limited resources will always be a major issue.

It is a simple fact, although often unappreciated by professionals, that resources expended on one person are unavailable for another—and this is true of money, time, or talent. Thus resources used for a person with a long-term, intractable problem are not available for one or two or three other persons with serious, tractable problems.

If left up to the marketplace, the problem works itself out to some extent, although one might quarrel with the distribution that results. To the extent that people perceive that they need something badly enough to spend their scarce resources to demand it, and to the extent that other people will agree to supply that amount of resources, then the allocation of resources becomes efficient. If a provider does not meet the individual's needs, a new provider is sought. To the extent that the individual is unwilling, rather than unable, to meet the provider's price, then his need cannot be said to be great in relation to other things he wants to spend his resources on. If this was the way social work operated, and if the main problem was to extend services to persons unable, rather than unwilling, to pay a price, then it would be easier to defend programs and budgets.

In the absence of a market mechanism by which individual tastes can be expressed and individual offerings may be accepted or rejected, some other way of expressing value must be developed. When the government subsidizes a program, the effect is to reduce the price to the user, thus encouraging use even by those who would not value the service enough to pay full price. When services are provided without charge, the maximum number of potential users would be expected. Without a pricing mechanism, inefficiency and ineffectiveness can be masked. Without competition among providers, there is little incentive for innovation and efficiency.

Thus, in a market context, the allocation of resources occurs through the expression of individual tastes with demanders offering a certain amount of money and suppliers offering services if an acceptable amount of money is offered. Once an equilibrium price is reached, then the exchange occurs. Without this mechanism, conscious decisions regarding allocation must be made since too few resources are available to serve everyone, especially at zero price.

One way to handle the problem of persons with low income is to have a price that varies with income. This is usually called a sliding fee. It tends to reduce the price for users, but not to zero. It requires that persons pay for some portion of their services, thereby giving an indication of how much they value them. However, with sliding fees there must either be a third-party subsidy to the provider, or else persons with higher incomes must pay enough to offset the deficit created by persons paying less than full cost. Any private practitioner realizes that, to maintain a solvent practice, full costs must be paid by someone for all clients. Charging a fee affects a program by (1) showing how those most willing to pay—presumably those in greatest need—line up for the service and (2) making additional funds available, which may permit extending the program.

The concept of pricing social services in the open market without subsidy is abhorrent to some social workers. Often, they point out, persons need services but cannot afford them. In addition, they say, "Anything that helps a person is worth the price." However, definitions of need are elusive. People have many needs they would not be willing to transform into effective demands. And not everything is "worth the price."

SCREENING AND ELIGIBILITY

It is virtually in the nature of the social work profession to try to assist an individual who lays claim to assistance, regardless of whether anything can actually be done to help. Of course a specific agency may turn away some persons seeking help because it does not provide that range of services usually identified as meeting their needs. For example, some agencies specializing in counseling may turn away persons presenting problems that require tangible resources. Some studies have indicated that the poor and minority groups are often turned away or dropped without assistance.[11] However, once a person is labeled client, there seem to be few bounds of the investment to which he can lay claim. Thus a clear conflict is evident between a professional ideology of full services to all persons in need and the practical necessity to ration scarce resources.

Suppose one thought that services should be targeted to certain individuals, or that society would be better off if certain persons were required to have services. Price screening would not be an appropriate first step, although it could be used at some point. The problem would be that all people cannot be served, either because resources are limited or because limited technology prevents help being given to some.

The usual step is to provide screening according to eligibility criteria. These may be based on income or capital resources, demographic or geographic characteristics, type of problem, or other such variables. Basically, eligibility requirements tend merely to reduce the universe of potential users rather than select among potential clients those whose utilization does most to accomplish the program's ends. Once the eligibility hurdle has been cleared, the individual is usually put on a waiting list or accepted for service and carried until closed. The first-come, first-served technique tends to be inefficient in that it does not identify the range of clients from whom those who would use the service resource most efficiently might be selected.

One can view eligibility screening as a form of tax or a price people pay to get services. For example, when government-sponsored services are free to those in the population who meet certain criteria, then persons who do not meet the criteria must pay for the services, assuming they are available in the market. Thus some people pay the total costs of such services while others pay nothing. This example is not intended to support the position that all services should be free to all people but to point out that eligibility requirements provide a way to ration scarce resources. The case has already been made against providing all things to all people. There just is not enough to go around.

If the profession operated in the marketplace, individuals could translate their preferences into demands by bidding dollars for services. Many services, such as homemaking, child care, and marital counseling, are provided in this way. When there is no market mechanism, society defines its preferences by processes that are essentially political. The rules then change drastically.

When individuals make their own way in the private sector of our society, they are accountable only to their customers, their professions, and themselves—except for certain requirements to keep fraud and dishonesty to a minimum and licensing requirements to assure some minimal level of standards. When one turns to philanthropy or taxes, then stricter requirements for accountability are imposed. Since this involves society's money, administered through its public agents (whatever one may think of them at the time), supplicants are bound to accept certain limitations as well as responsibility for their own actions. Their alternative is to abandon this source of funds or seek to change the rules by the political clout.

Accountability, at a minimum, is utilized to assure the criterion of honesty. Honesty is a necessary but not sufficient condition for a fully accountable system. When funds are misappropriated for personal use, that is clearly dishonest. When those operating programs act in capricious and discriminatory ways—that is, when they are lawless in the literal sense of having no authority to behave as they do—they are socially irresponsible. When evidence of ineffectiveness and waste is neglected or covered up, then too there is a lack of accountability. The requirements for full accountability protect everyone, in the social services, defense contracting, or whatever area. Such a system of accountability presumes having ethical persons at the top who recognize that society's resources are never adequate to meet all needs and who insist therefore that these resources should at least be expended honestly and legally.

THE CRITERION OF RESULTS

A sound system of accountability goes beyond honesty and is based on results. The techniques oriented to relationships and processes, which are the heart of the social work profession, are the most "soft" and most in need of being put in proper perspective. If credible professional accountability is to occur, casework and group work must be viewed as inputs that may or may not reduce the incidence of definable social problems, and the profession must develop a new orientation based on outputs that can be measured objectively.

Accountability, in a political system, requires a reasonable expectation that the purposes for which dollars were raised have been or could be achieved with maximum efficiency and effectiveness.

Social workers worry about accountability to clients, but there are no fiscal incentives to assure it, since clients have no market mechanism for expressing their preferences. Other mechanisms, such as having users participate on boards, are required. But to the extent that clients do not pay the bill, the focus is on the social institutions that do.

The authors are concerned with the type of accountability that argues it is wrong to continue to demand pay from society for an elegant surgical operation that impresses the interns but never saves a patient's life. The resources required might well have been used for many other untreated patients who could benefit from known procedures.

Not all outputs have to be successful nor must all interventions be measured and be statistically and methodologically precise. The concern is with accountability in a political environment in which reasonable men do not require anything resembling perfection. In vocational rehabilitation, for example, many cases are closed without attaining success. Yet a preponderance of cases are closed with a claim that clients were rehabilitated since many can be accounted for in addition to those able to meet program objectives. But these are questions of efficiency, which is but one component of accountability. In governmental policy-making it is recognized that reasonable levels of success and a reporting system that retrieves most of what actually occurs are "good enough."

GOALS AS OUTPUTS

Mogulof has noted the following with respect to goals of social work:

Our goals are couched in the kind of generalities which are unable to inform action. The actions we take are not subject to measurement, and are not conceived of as leading to goals larger than the actions themselves. In effect the instrument (Family Planning, Day Care, Counseling, etc.) becomes the ends, and our administrative energies go toward the preservation of instruments. In a sense, it is a remarkable performance by a society whose great technical achievements have come through the employment of the scientific method, where all action is potentially subject to test. We seem uninterested in viewing our social services as action probes which may or may not achieve desired states. Is it because we really don't know what these desired states are? Or is it evidence of a misguided professionalism, which develops a stake in a particular probe (e.g., Headstart) and pushes all of us (the Congress included) to see the probe as an end in itself?[12]

Characteristically, the social work profession does not define goals in terms of output, but rather input (for example, casework hours, number of persons served). One reason for emphasizing new output conventions is that better program analysts are advising decision-makers who are more sophisticated. Future decision-makers will increasingly include state and local elected officials and superagency manager-budget types. The categorical program managers at both federal and state levels will no longer define the scope of the problem and the resources needed through the traditional device of continuing to expand the programs. Tougher questions will be asked. To a greater extent, demonstrated results will be demanded because of greater exposure to a more open political process.

Social work needs an improved technology for defining goals in terms that entail not only measures of effectiveness but also measures of efficiency. There may have been a time when it was sufficient to state objectives in obscure terms, but this is no longer the case.

Seemingly, the profession is in a poor position to claim it knows best. In principle, it might be said that those providing the funds to pay the piper should call the tune, but social workers should try to be included in that essentially political process. It might also be argued that the means of achievement should be in the hands of professionals—but only as long as they are effective and do not displace or obscure the achievement of goals.

Defining goals more rigorously is so large a first step for social work practitioners and supporting scholars to develop that a concerted effort to do so would probably satisfy critics for a while. Merely redefining one set of abstractions with another may give the illusion of movement, but in fact goes nowhere. The day of reckoning comes closer with each attempt. Devising new catchwords or slogans or grasping for the latest fad in rhetoric can no longer suffice. Nor are fancy new delivery systems required. Social workers must simply define what they already do best.

Those active in the social work profession must learn to focus on the few, perhaps narrow, areas in which they can demonstrate that what they do makes a difference, a difference not possible by other means for fewer resources. They cannot afford to make promises that, given the resources, they will reduce welfare rolls, eliminate delinquency, cure the mentally ill, or educate the poor. They must learn to talk about which of how many, at what price, with what expected success, and why this is the way society should do it.

Knowledge bases and the role of schools of social work in relation to accountability have been covered by Briar.[13] To echo his views, truth, beauty, justice, and mental health are goals, but they are not useful for stimulating specific actions, and it is difficult to know when one has such a goal in hand. Systematic evaluation requires ability to state goals in objective, measurable terms. Evading such a statement leaves one open to the accusation of masking ineffectiveness or of committing a form of fraud and leads to a discounting of claims of credibility that may be sound.

If, for example, social workers claim that working with juvenile delinquents can reduce recidivism, and then recidivism is not reduced, they have demonstrated that what they were doing could not achieve the end promised. They have not made the case for the total ineffectiveness of what they were doing or denied that it accomplished some things for some people. (For example, it may have reduced the severity if not the incidence of offenses.) Nevertheless, they may have shown that it is not the best tool for reducing juvenile recidivism in general. The argument that some good was done anyway, even if it was not what was primarily intended, saves little face in the budget shop.

Delinquency has many roots: economic conditions, community and neighborhood influences, social class, the educational system, the local police and court systems, and the like. Social work cannot influence many of these factors. Therefore, the objectives should be expressed in terms of whether, for some subset of juveniles who have certain characteristics and whose offenses stem from, say inadequate parental supervision, social work can help reduce recidivism by a specified percent through working with the parents. Casting objectives in such a fashion makes headway in defining credible goals.

This approach, however, would only help determine whether the intervention worked at all. The vital questions are: Does it offer the best way? Are there alternatives that, with the same resources, would have further reduced recidivism? Or are there alternatives that would have reduced it to the same extent at less expense? Together these questions define the effectiveness and efficiency of the system of accountability.

What should be measured and how it should be measured involve a mixture of technical and political concerns. How precise the measurement should be depends on its purpose and on the person prompting it, who may be a cost-benefit expert concerned with the discount rate on future income, a politician who wants to make sure someone is really being "helped," or a program operator who wants to stay in business. The system should produce sufficient information to provide a record for audit showing that the funds were spent honestly. After that the question of how much one wishes to know to evaluate the program can vary widely. The minimum, then, is an acceptable fiscal reporting system and a management-information system covering program data.

EFFECTIVENESS AND EFFICIENCY

Briar has discussed many factors involved in the inability of social work to show effectiveness—its sliding from theory to theory, from technique to technique, but seldom grappling with the question of whether what was accomplished did the clients any good.[14] Effectiveness may be the heart of the truly legitimate question of what benefit professionals, or the profession as a whole, may be bringing clients.

If social services help people, and social workers think many of them do, then it behooves the profession to demonstrate how. Again, the authors take the hard line that case studies and case histories do not constitute evidence since they do not show controlled conditions, the influence of the intervention, the relative overall numbers of successes and failures, and the long-term effects and costs. Nor do they control for enough variables. Who asks what percentage of his clients improved? Further, how would one show it, and at what cost was the client improved? Could more have been done for others at the same cost?

As for efficiency, it would be monumental to show that any intervention worked. Before the cheers died down, one should look at the problems facing those who want to find out whether this intervention works better than another, or if the same result could be attained for less money. Efficiency in this instance does not mean that what is done is done for the lowest cost but that the ends achieved cannot be brought about in another way or at an even lower cost.

Efficiency involves weighing alternatives against costs. To a large degree, many trade-offs are not precisely comparable. For example, looking at trade-offs—say, between two techniques for reducing recidivism among inner-city delinquents—is only one way of judging efficiency. The comparisons could be between casework and group work or between counseling and manpower programs and compensatory education. Each has a different approach and different techniques, but the comparison should be with regard to degree of impact on the same measure of outcome.

Another set of issues related to efficiency deals with normative judgments as to the choice of what to do at given levels of expenditures to make society better off. Should the money go, for example, to nursing homes for the aged, foster homes for neglected children, rehabilitation of the handicapped, or services to reduce delinquency? If all are worthy, what should the mix be? When a program is fully accountable, those responsible for it can show not only that what it accomplishes is done with fiscal economy and that it is effective, but also that it does what it does better and less expensively—given quality and quantity levels—than any other program could.

SUMMARY AND CONCLUSION

The current crisis in social services is a crisis of credibility based on an inadequate system of accountability. Social programs are in trouble because they focus on processes and not results. A society with limited resources can agree on an endless catalog of needs, but its needs must be ranked to concentrate enough resources to do some good. An analogy to the marketplace indicates that when individuals translate their needs into demands by showing how much they are willing to pay, then many of the issues surrounding accountability recede. When the market mechanism is weak or missing and the support of social institutions is necessary, then political interplay influences preferences and those providing services are required to show that available resources are spent on the most pressing problems with maximum effectiveness and efficiency.

With respect to the "soft" services—those that primarily involve relationships, counseling, and process technologies—it is difficult to attribute changes in the individual's status to the service activity. Testimonials are suspect, and few instruments are available that validly measure before-and-after impact. When the bulk of activity is based on individual or group processes, changes take a long time. Experimenters and practitioners experience difficulties when they try to isolate the intervention as the key to change over time. In most cases, however, claims that the successful outcome was based on the intervention would be given benefit of doubt if the intended outcomes had been clearly specified and believable.

Occasionally one hears that programs of social work produce outcomes so subtle they cannot be measured but that somehow without them society would be worse off. When the outcome is not measurable, social workers are probably engaging in self-delusion.

At the end, these are the paramount questions: Are social workers useful? Do the programs in which they work leave society better off than it would be if the programs were abolished? In general, the authors think many aspects of society would be worse off were there no social workers and no social programs, but they hold no brief for the sacredness of any one program or any one intervention technique. It is cause for despair, however, that social workers, while indulging in rhetoric about their social responsibilities, often do not have even the most elementary regard for the mechanics of social accountability.

Many programs or specific aspects of services are in a favorable position for sophisticated defense on a limited scale, with modest claims for accomplishment. Family planning, rehabilitation, day care, homemaking, protective services, and the like, should be able to prove their worth if the necessary rigor were applied. It could be shown that other services can accomplish desired ends less expensively than alternative techniques—for example, in-home care for the retarded, the elderly, and the severely handicapped.

This article has tried to show what accountability is about, where the profession falls short, and what might be done. The rest is up to all of us in the social work profession—and time may be short.

NOTES

1. David M. Austin and Robert S. Caulk, "Issues in Social Services: A Program for NASW," *New Directions for the Seventies* (Washington, D.C.: National Association of Social Workers, 1973), p. 16.
2. John D. Erlichman, cited in James P. Gannon, "If President Wins Again, the Nation May Have a Do-Less Government," *Wall Street Journal*, October 18, 1972, pp. 1, 20.
3. Mitchell I. Ginsberg, "A Letter from Our President," *New Directions for the Seventies*, p. 1.
4. Austin and Caulk, op. cit., pp. 7–18.
5. "The United States Budget in Brief, Fiscal Year 1974" (Washington, D.C.: U.S. Government Printing Office, 1973).
6. Edward Newman and Michael S. March, "Financing Social Welfare: Governmental Allocation Procedures," *Encyclopedia of Social Work, 1971* (New York: National Association of Social Workers, 1971), p. 433.
7. Internal HEW memo.
8. Elliot L. Richardson, "Responsibility and Responsiveness," Monograph on the HEW Potential for the Seventies (Washington, D.C.: U.S. Department of Health, Education & Welfare, 1972), p. 3. (Mimeographed.)
9. See, for example, Joel Fischer, "Is Casework Effective?" *Social Work*, 18 (January 1973), pp. 5–20.
10. Heinz Eulau, "Skill Revolution and Consultive Commonwealth," *American Political Science Review*, 67 (March 1973), p. 188.
11. For a review of studies, see Richard A. Cloward and Irwin Epstein, "Private Social Welfare's Disengagement from the Poor: The Case of Family Adjustment Agencies," in Mayer Zald, ed., *Social Welfare Institutions* (New York: John Wiley & Sons, 1965), pp. 623–643; and Cloward and Frances Fox Piven, *Regulating the Poor: The Functions of Public Welfare* (New York: Pantheon Books, 1971).
12. Melvin Mogulof, "Special Revenue Sharing in Support of the Public Social Services" (Washington, D.C.: Urban Institute, March 1973). (Mimeographed.)
13. Scott Briar, "Effective Social Work Intervention in Direct Practice: Implications for Education." Paper presented at the annual meeting of the Council on Social Work Education, San Francisco, California, February 1973.
14. Ibid.

27/SOCIAL EQUITY AND SOCIAL SERVICE PRODUCTIVITY

STEPHEN R. CHITWOOD

Government spending for federal, state, and local activities currently accounts for approximately 30 percent of the Gross National Product of the United States.[1] Public decision making, therefore, controls almost a third of the monetary resources of the country and thereby determines a major portion of the goods and services provided in the economy. As government has assumed this enlarging role in American life, various managerial techniques have been promoted with the purported intent of increasing the value or benefits flowing from public expenditures. The Hoover Commissions offered performance budgeting and accrual accounting.[2] The Kennedy and Johnson Administrations promoted planning, programming, and budgeting systems (PPBS).[3] And since 1969, the Nixon Administration has emphasized program evaluation and the measurement of government productivity.[4]

This essay examines the current emphasis on increasing the productivity of government activities and briefly assesses its historical relation to earlier government management movements. This assessment illustrates how productivity measures have traditionally neglected a basic element in providing public services—the social equity accompanying the distribution of those services. Having identified this area of neglect, the important relationships between productivity measures and the determination of social equity in supplying government services are identified. This is followed by a categorization of distribution patterns and standards which may be used in measuring the social equity with which public services are provided.

PRODUCTIVITY MEASUREMENT IN GOVERNMENT

According to Harry P. Hatry of the Urban Institute:

Productivity measurement essentially means relating the amount of inputs of a service or product to the amount of outputs. Traditionally this has been expressed as a ratio such as number of units produced per man hour.[5]

Productivity measurement in government is not new. In an effort to increase the productivity of federal employees in U.S. Army arsenals in the early 1900s, managers sought to use F. W. Taylor's stopwatch, scientific management procedures—with the result that a special committee of the House of Representatives was formed to investigate the Taylor and other systems of shop management.[6] During the "good government" movement days, Herbert Simon, working with the International City Managers Association, sought procedures for measuring the unit costs of various municipal services, e.g., street cleaning, sanitation activities, etc., with the intent of designing means to reduce those costs.[7] Since 1902, the Army Corps of Engineers has had to justify proposed water resource projects with data relating benefits to costs, a measure of dollar output per dollar input.[8]

Productivity measures offer potentially valuable information to all government officials, i.e., political executives, legislators, and career public administrators. As measures of efficiency, such as work measurements or unit costs, productivity measures furnish standards for assessing actual performance and taking corresponding actions in view of the efficiency demonstrated. When productivity measures incorporate effectiveness indicators, information is also given on results achieved versus objectives stated. These data may lead to changes in objectives, alterations in program activities, or shifts in expectations of results achievable. Trend measures illustrate relative performance over time. Productivity indices provide trend information that can:

• reveal the cumulative effects of all factors which have influenced efficiency of the organization measured.

• flag the need for management action, such as plant modernization, when the trend shows signs of slowing.

• help in the determination of rational, attainable productivity improvement objectives.

• provide a means of evaluating management actions, such as the effects of installing capital improvements.[9]

From the preceding list of uses, productivity measures may be seen to offer a variety of beneficial information to participants in the governmental process. There is, however, one important dimension of government services which seldom is reflected in productivity measures. This excluded element is the distribution of services among the population, and the social equity associated with that distribution.

PRODUCTIVITY AND SOCIAL EQUITY COMPARED

Social equity and government productivity are both concerned with the final outputs of public activities. Questions of social equity, however, center upon the distribution of services and the distribution of their effects. Government productivity measures, on the other hand, focus upon the quantity or quality of output. (The distribution of services and their effects could be incorporated in productivity measures by including effectiveness indicators, but this is seldom done.) Similarly, social equity and government productivity are each concerned with accounting for resource inputs. Once again, though, social equity examines inputs in terms of the sources from which they were derived, e.g., income classes, socioeconomic groups, geographic groups; whereas government productivity measures look merely at the amount of dollar value of inputs utilized.

The magnitude of resources now under federal, state, and local government control allow these governments to bestow increasingly significant benefits or penalties on their citizenry. These benefits or penalties arise primarily from the governments' distribution of public goods and services (hereafter referred to only as public services). Thus, while expenditure accountability and efficiency of operation will continue to be prime considerations of government officials, the distribution pattern of public services must also be viewed as a basic criterion for public decision making. As a result, measures of social equity must increasingly accompany measures of productivity in order to assess the adequacy of public services.

SOCIAL EQUITY AND PUBLIC SERVICES

Proponents of the new public administration take the normative position that social equity should have a significant role in public decision making.[10] While many people share this normative orientation, recent court cases have caused the consideration of social equity to become a pragmatic as well as a philosophic and ethical matter. In the case of *Hawkins* v. *Town of Shaw* (427 F. 2d 1286 (5th Cir. 1971) *aff'd* 461 F. 2d 1171 (1972) (en banc)), evidence showed that although a range of public services in the Mississippi town was financed out of general tax revenue (without regard to assessment or property ownership), black residential areas were manifestly underserviced. The court found no constitutional justification for residents who were similarly taxed to have fewer paved streets, less sewerage service, poorer street lighting, and less police protection. The court in *Hawkins* did not consider the prevailing municipal finance scheme as such; it held only that the distribution of the services financed by that scheme was discriminatory. The facts of the case presented a clear example of discrimination, because services were distributed to the "suspect classification" of race. The Town of Shaw was therefore ordered to develop and present to the court an equitable plan for delivering public services to all the town's citizens.[11]

Reasoning similar to that in the *Hawkins* case has resulted in other local jurisdictions being required to examine the distribution pattern of their services.[12] If suits of a similar nature are upheld by future court rulings, public officials will have to consider questions of social equity for legal, if not moral, reasons. Even if the courts fail to support these earlier decisions, as the United States Supreme Court refused to sustain lower court rulings relating to inequities resulting from financing education through property taxation, political activism by various public groups will require public officials to give growing attention to matters of distributing public services.

While the movement toward considering the distribution of public services appears to be acquiring momentum, a severe hindrance to this effort lies in the vagueness of the notion of social equity.

Without criteria for measuring social equity, public officials will be unable to use this criterion for decision making. To date, no single definition of social equity has been developed. Nevertheless, several aspects or interpretations of social equity have been identified and articulated. To facilitate a clearer, and possibly more productive discussion of social equity, the more prominent aspects of this term are described in the following pages. These dimensions of social equity were deduced from past legislative, administrative, and court decisions and actions.

DIMENSIONS OF SOCIAL EQUITY

An infinite number of patterns might be used to distribute public services. Fortunately, this vast variety may be reduced to three basic distribution patterns: (1) equal services to all, (2) proportionally equal services to all, and (3) unequal services to individuals corresponding to relevant differences.[13] Each of these patterns has at some time been advocated as the only socially equitable way to distribute government services. A brief examination of each of these patterns will quickly suggest their potential usefulness for assessing the social equity of services provided by federal, state, and local governments.

Equal Services to All as a measure of social equity of allocating public services has limited applicability. Most government services cannot be equally utilized by all citizens, either because insufficient funds exist to provide them on such a broad scale or because the services are initially designed to serve the needs of a restricted clientele. Certain government services, termed pure public goods by economists, may have some limited potential for providing equal benefits to all citizens.[14] Nevertheless, the restricted range of pure public goods renders equal services to all an inadequate basis for measuring the social equity of the distribution of public services.

Proportional Equality in providing public services consists of delivering services in amounts that reflect a monotonically increasing function of a specified characteristic(s). For example, the number of uniformed policemen (public service) assigned to patrol a particular city precinct may vary in direct proportion to the crime rate (specified characteristic) of that precinct. Or the total public assistance payment (public service) made to an unemployed single head of household may increase directly with each dependent (specified characteristic) that is supported. In each instance, the quantity of service provided varies directly with changes in the amount of specified characteristic possessed by the client.

Providing public services on a proportionally equal basis seems both pragmatically and humanistically appealing. On pragmatic grounds, it provides apparently concrete, objective bases for allocating services among the populace; and on the humanistic side, it allows more services to be provided as their perceived need increases. Regardless of these apparent virtues, social equity measured on the proportionally equal basis of providing government services has several difficulties. Once a policy decision is made to provide a public service, the complex task arises of selecting the specified characteristic(s) whose magnitude determines the amount of service to be delivered. Another problem involves the proportional amount of service to be given in relation to the specified characteristic. Even when these problems have been resolved, there are the administrative difficulties of assessing the extent to which potential recipients of a service possess the specified characteristic and then providing the corresponding quantity of services. In addition, as with the equal services to all approach, this concept of social equity may also be unworkable because of insufficient funds to provide services to all eligible recipients.[15]

Unequal Public Services corresponding to relevant differences represents a third approach to defining social equity as it relates to delivering public services. With this concept, social equity in distributing public services is achieved if individuals receive services in amounts corresponding to relevant differences in some characteristic possessed by those recipients. The total services received need not be proportionate to the amount of the relevant differences present in each recipient, thus differentiating this concept of social equity from that of proportional equity.

The critical aspect of this approach to social equity is identifying the characteristic whose relevant difference among the client group will determine the quantity of services each person will receive. Two frequently used characteristics are the willingness and ability to pay for public services and the results to be achieved through those services. City libraries, parks, and other public facilities may be placed in more affluent sections of a city with the justification, usually unarticulated, that the affluent citizens have paid the most taxes and therefore deserved more service. Similarly, where public services are provided on a user charge basis, e.g., airports, cemeteries, sewer service, or sanitation collection, the relevant difference in their distribution may well be the willingness and ability of recipients to pay their costs.

Where the distribution of services depends upon individuals meeting certain minimum qualifications, criteria, or standards (other than willingness or ability to pay), each criterion represents a relevant difference which has been deemed appropriate to the receipt of the particular service. Numerous reasons exist for requiring that minimum relevant differences in characteristics or qualifications criteria, however, relate directly to the results which are to be achieved by those services.

Among the most important results sought by public services are: (1) providing services to individuals who are unable to obtain them through the free market mechanisms in the quantity or quality deemed essential by society, e.g., adequete education, police and fire protection; (2) providing services to individuals which will give them an equal opportunity to compete for and occupy all positions in society, including the most attractive ones, e.g., compensatory education, job training, physical rehabilitation; (3) providing services which insure that people will receive the benefits they are entitled to under law, e.g., public defender services, outreach activities to notify people of their rights to program benefits; and (4) providing services which allow individuals to meet approximately minimum survival needs, e.g., food stamps, public housing, cash payments.[16]

Determining the criteria for distributing the services necessary to achieve the preceding results is an extremely precarious and judgmental process. For example, what standards should be used to distribute limited, available police protection throughout a city? Should the criterion be an area's existing crime rate, with the desired results being to reduce areas of high crime? Or should the criterion be to maintain existing low crime rates in selected areas of the city by keeping those areas heavily policed? Depending on the results sought, either distribution of services could be justified as socially equitable under the unequal distribution concept.

What criteria should be used to determine the amount of services to provide individuals so they might achieve an equal opportunity to compete for and occupy all positions in society? The initial problem is to identify the different characteristics which currently exist and inhibit equal competitive opportunity among all citizens. Even when these differences are identified, and experience suggests we have often selected unimportant differences, two additional difficulties arise. First, how do you identify the level of the characteristic to which people must rise in order to have an equal opportunity? For example, if attaining a particular level of literacy is seen as necessary for equal opportunity, how is that level identified? Second, even if specific goals are established to which characteristics should be raised, how will the amount of services necessary to raise each individual to that level be determined? For example, since each individual below a set standard of literacy may have varying deficiencies, what criteria, e.g., intelligence quotient, current reading level, age, etc., should be used to determine the appropriate amount of educational services needed for each person to reach the desired level? If these problems are not solved, services will tend to be provided on an unequal basis. But to the extent the goals of equal opportunity are achieved, the initial provision of services, though unequal, will have been equitably distributed.[17]

Distribution of services so that people might meet approximate minimum living standards is another approach to social equity and shares some of the problems associated with fostering equal opportunity. The designation of the minimum living standards to be sustained is itself a relative decision, since the quality of average living standards varies even among sections of the same country. Such standards are particularly difficult to develop, since they include such a wide range of elements, e.g., diet, shelter, clothing, health care, etc. Attempting to establish minimally acceptable levels for each of these elements, assessing individuals to determine where they are in relation to these standards, and then developing programs to provide services to bring all individuals exactly to these minimal levels represent enormously complex tasks. Nevertheless, where this is done and unequal services are provided to achieve these minimal standards, a socially equitable distribution of services may be said to have occurred.

Providing services to clients to insure they will receive public benefits entitled to them by law requires: first, a delineation of the characteristics of citizens making them eligible for these benefits; second, an identification of those specific persons who meet the eligibility criteria; and third, an evaluation of what services will have to be provided to each eligible person to insure he will receive his benefits if he wants them. While the first activity is relatively simple to complete, activities two and three are more difficult and potentially quite expensive to the government. Nonetheless, if unequal services are provided in such a manner that each person entitled to and desiring public services does obtain them, the services will have been equitably distributed.

Not all qualification standards for distributing public services, however, are based on the results to be achieved by the program. Some criteria, such as residence requirements in the jurisdiction, may be designed to reduce the migration of people to that jurisdiction merely to receive public services. Other criteria, e.g., having a farm of particular size in order to receive various subsidies, may be established to reduce the administrative burden of handling numerous minor clients. Still other requirements, such as having to apply formally for benefits, may be designed to reduce the number of people who will receive them. In these cases, the criteria justifying unequal services rest not on the intrinsic results sought from the program but on obtaining or avoiding external or spillover effects related to the program.

SOCIAL EQUITY AND PUBLIC DECISION MAKING

Social equity based upoon equal, proportional, or unequal distributions of public services is in each instance justified on the grounds of how services and their benefits are ultimately apportioned among a jurisdiction's populace. Another approach to judging the social equity of a distribution of services, however, stresses the process of determining that distribution rather than the distribution pattern itself. When social equity focuses on process, any distribution pattern determined by the legitimate public decision-making process is deemed socially equitable. Any distribution pattern in conflict with that prescribed by the legitimate public decision-making process is socially inequitable.

When the process criterion is used to assess the social equity of a distribution of public services, an underlying assumption is that social equity (much as the concept of public interest) is reflected in the judgments of those groups and individuals who have access to the public decision-making process. For the pluralist school of political science, this means that whatever distributions of services emerge from the legal political processes of federal, state, and local governments, they are by definition socially equitable.[18]

In contrast to and in conflict with the pluralists are those persons who believe that social equity in providing public services require a major, and possibly controlling, influence from those receiving the services. Proponents of the citizen or client participation school of political science emphasize that social equity in providing public services requires the development of a type of relationship between the recipient of a service and the administering agency which reflects mutual trust and respect, two-way communication, and participation. Only when such a relationship is established can the provision of those public services be classified as socially equitable.[19]

VERTICAL VERSUS HORIZONTAL EQUITY

Assessing social equity in providing public services, therefore, may include both an examination of the process for establishing a distribution pattern for services and an analysis of the pattern ultimately selected. Each of the three patterns discussed earlier addressed the problem of allocating services among citizens differing in numerous characteristics, e.g., sex, age, geographic location, health, wealth, etc. These criteria for distributing services among heterogeneous people represent an attempt to achieve what might be termed vertical social equity. This term connotes the effort to devise a rationale for allocating services among individuals who possess greater and lesser degrees of various personal attributes or characteristics. To the extent such a rationale is developed and widely agreed to, vertical social equity will be thought to have been achieved. Where no rationale can be developed for apportioning services among different individuals, or where the rationale is not broadly accepted, vertical social equity will be held in question.

Accompanying vertical social equity is the idea of horizontal social equity. Horizontal equity refers to the equal treatment of equals.[20] It requires that all people possessing like amounts of a characteristic determining the provision of a particular public service should receive the same quantity of that service. A recent study by the U.S. General Accounting Office dramatized the horizontal inequities of the present welfare system. Numerous recipients who shared a similar dependency status often received quite varied dollar value benefits from several federal programs. While these individuals were basically similar in their degree of need, the qualification standards for different programs might summarily bestow benefits on one person but not another.[21] Thus, assessing social equity in providing government services must include the examination of horizontal equity as well as vertical equity and the process whereby service distribution patterns are established.

STANDARDS FOR MEASURING SOCIAL EQUITY

Even when participants in the political process can agree on a definition or criterion for identifying a socially equitable distribution of services, they often fail to use similar standards when comparing and evaluating the social equity that exists with the social equity they believe should prevail. Regardless of the criterion selected to define social equity in providing government services, each criterion may be compared to one of the following standards.[22]

First, any criterion of social equity, e.g., equal services, may be applied to the distribution of a service, and existing equity may be compared with the standard of past equity to see whether changes have occurred from previous years. Thus, as with productivity measures which compute changes in output per unit of input over time, social equity measures may also generate time series data reflecting changes in social equity in the distribution of services. A second standard is the social equity with which other governmental jurisdictions distribute their services. A third standard is a comparison of planned equity in the distribution of services with the actual equity that is finally achieved. A fourth standard is the satisfactory or satisfying level of social equity. Does the existing pattern of service distribution meet a satisfactory level of social equity as perceived by the citizenry?[23]

Numerous problems may arise when political participants cannot agree on the standards they will use to appraise existing social equity. Certain protagonists of social welfare services, e.g., aid to families with dependent children, will say that the existing social equity in the distribution of services is better than in the past and is therefore good enough. Proponents of more aid or a different distribution of services will say that the social equity of the existing distribution is inadequate compared to the services distributed by other government jurisdictions.

CONCLUSIONS

In future years, measuring the productivity of government services will continue to have high priority among the activities of public administrators. Of ascending importance, and probably of equal or greater importance, is the public administrator's responsibility for identifying the social equity with which government services are provided. As more and more benefits are generated by government programs, administrators will increasingly need to articulate their personal version of a socially equitable distribution of services. To insure that social equity considerations ultimately become as visible as matters of productivity in providing government services, a common ground for discussion of this concept is required. The preceding pages have attempted to provide a beginning for such a common ground by describing several dimensions of social equity. In addition, a suggestive set of standards is proposed which would allow a comparison and evaluation of the degree of social equity associated with different distributions of government services.

These dimensions and standards for assessing social equity should provide a theoretical departure point for students of public administration interested in investigating the social equity of existing government services. At the same time, these concepts may serve elected and appointed public officials and career administrators as a specific and concrete basis from which to legislate and administer public programs with a clear understanding of their social equity implications.

NOTES

1. "Empty Pockets on a Trillion Dollars a Year," *Time*, March 13, 1972, p. 72.
2. Arthur Smithies, "Conceptual Framework for the Program Budget," in David Novick (ed.), *Program Budgeting* (Washington, D.C.: U.S. Government Printing Office, 1964), p. 7, and Second Hoover Commission, *Budget and Accounting* (Washington, D.C.: U.S. Government Printing Office, 1955).
3. For a general description and critique of the PPB system, see Leonard Merewitz and Stephen H. Sosnick, *The Budget's New Clothes* (Chicago: Markham Publishing Company, 1971), especially chapters 1–6.
4. See Allen Schick, "From Analysis to Evaluation," *The Annals*, Vol. 394 (March 1971), p. 50; and Thomas D. Morris, William H. Corbett, and Brian L. Usilaner, "Productivity Measures in the Federal Government," *Public Administration Review*, Vol. 32 (November/December 1972), pp. 753–763.
5. Harry P. Hatry, "Issues in Productivity Measurement for Local Government," *Public Administration Review*, Vol. 32 (November/December 1972), p. 777.
6. Harwood F. Merrill (ed.), *Classics in Management* (New York: American Management Association, 1960), p. 66.
7. C. E. Ridley and Herbert A. Simon, *Measuring Municipal Activities* (Chicago: The International City Managers' Association, 1938).
8. U.S. Congress, Senate, Subcommittee on National Security and International Operations, *Hearings, Planning–Programming–Budgeting*, 90th Congress, 2nd Session, 1968, Part 3, p. 168.
9. Thomas D. Morris, *et al., op. cit.*, p. 757.
10. H. George Frederickson, "Toward a New Public Administration," in Frank Marini (ed.), *Toward a New Public Administration* (Scranton: Chandler Publishing Company, 1971), p. 311.
11. Peter Jaszi, unpublished memorandum to Howard Hallman, Center for Governmental Studies, Washington, D.C., December 13, 1972, pp. 9–10.
12. *Ibid.*, pp. 10–11.
13. Felix E. Oppenheim, "The Concept of Equality," in David L. Sills (ed.), *Interna-*

tional Encyclopedia of The Social Sciences, Vol. 5 (The Macmillan Co. and The Free Press), pp. 102–107. While not specifically phrased in terms of social equity, this article provides a useful theoretical basis from which to begin an analysis of this topic.

14. Charles L. Schultze, *The Politics and Economics of Public Spending* (Washington, D.C.: The Brookings Institution, 1968), p. 83.

15. The financial problem encountered in supplying services to clients in the amounts necessary to achieve equity and the desired effects was articulated by former Secretary of HEW Elliot L. Richardson. Secretary Richardson noted that his studies indicated that HEW's 9 billion in service programs would cost roughly 250 billion if they were "extended equitably" to all those similarly situated citizens who need them. William Greider and Nick Kotz, "Harvard Abstraction Becomes Reality," *Washington Post*, April 9, 1973, p. A–14.

16. These objectives of public expenditures are discussed in the following sources: Peter O. Steiner, "The Public Sector and The Public Interest," in Robert H. Haveman and Julius Margolis (eds.), *Public Expenditures and Policy Analysis* (Chicago: Markham Publishing Company, 1970), pp. 21–33, and Felix E. Oppenheim, *op. cit.*

17. Felix E. Oppenheim, *op. cit.*

18. The emphasis of the pluralist school is primarily on process rather than outcomes of political activities. The inference is therefore made, in a recognizably general manner, that for this school of political analysis, social equity is reflected not in political outcomes but in the nature of the political process itself. For a related critique of the process approach to political science, see Allen Schick, "Systems Politics and Systems Budgeting," *Public Administration Review*. Vol. 29 (March/April 1969), pp. 137–151.

19. Comments of Orion White as interpreted and recorded by the author during a panel discussion on "Social Equity and New Public Administration" at the ASPA 1973 National Conference on Public Administration, Los Angeles, California, April 4, 1973. See also the special issue of the *Public Administration Review* on "Curriculum Essays on Politics, Administration, and Citizen Participation," Vol. 32 (October 1972).

20. The concepts of vertical and horizontal equity have traditionally been used in relationship to governmental tax structures. These terms, however, appear equally valid for use in appraising the equity accompanying the distribution of public services. For a short discussion of vertical and horizontal equity applied to tax structures, see Otto Eckstein, *Public Finance* (Englewood Cliffs, N.J.: Prentice-Hall, Inc., 1967), p. 60.

21. George Lardner, Jr., "Hill Welfare Study Shows Inequities," *Washington Post*, March 26, 1973, p. A–1.

22. These standards are identical to several standards prescribed by Yehezkel Dror for appraising the efficacy of public policy making in *Public Policy-making Reexamined* (San Francisco: Chandler Publishing Co., 1968), pp. 58–69.

23. *Ibid.*

EVALUATIVE RESEARCH FOR

THE SOCIAL SERVICES

IRVING PILIAVIN AND THOMAS MCDONALD

The social work literature of the 1970s, at least that portion appearing in professional journals, has concentrated considerable attention on evaluation and accountability. The lines taken by this literature are diverse. Some articles exhort the profession to engage in evaluative efforts, others are concerned with optimal designs for evaluation, and still others debate the degree to which social workers need to be more accountable and to whom the accountability is owed.[1] Some reports of evaluative studies are found in this literature, and substantial controversy has developed as to whether their generally negative findings pose serious questions as to the worth of social work intervention.[2]

An important feature of this material is that the number of empirical evaluations it contains is meager. In his 1973 review of over forty years of social work literature, Fischer found only eleven controlled evaluative studies of professional social work intervention.[3] Although evaluative research activity has seemingly picked up a bit since Fischer's review, the count of empirical assessments still remains extremely low.[4] Many reasons have been put forth by social work writers to explain this seeming antipathy of the profession toward evaluative research. These will not be repeated here.[5]

Rather, this paper has two other objectives. First, it will try to establish that one major reason for social workers' coolness toward evaluation is that many members of the profession believe that evaluative research at best offers them no benefits and at worst can cause them considerable harm. Having demonstrated that this negative stance is understandable, it will then be argued that it is in error. The thesis will be presented that there are indeed rewards to agency program evaluation even for nonresearchers and even if the programs being assessed are not found effective.

THE MESSAGES OF GLOOM

Among the various messages that social workers have been receiving in regard to evaluation, two are particularly disquieting. First, there is the recurrent theme sounded most recently and perhaps most clearly by Newman and Turem that unless social workers can show that their efforts are useful to society their programs will lose public support.[6] If this message is taken seriously, and there is substantial evidence that it should be, it would move social workers to produce a plethora of research in an effort to demonstrate the worth of their activities. At the same time, however, social workers are being sent a second message regarding evaluation. This message, made very explicitly by Fischer, says essentially that professionally rendered social services have not been found effective in bringing about their stated objectives.[7] It is the authors' belief that these two communications—one demanding accountability, the other arguing no benefit—have put many social workers in a bind. They are told that in the absence of evaluative research demonstrating the utility of their efforts they and their profession have an accountability crisis. But they are also told that the few sound evaluative studies that have been done on their efforts indicate that their services are worthless.

Two responses seem predictable as a result of this bind. First, we would expect social workers to be reluctant to engage in further evaluations since these are apparently self-defeating. Second, we would expect many members of the profession to denigrate empirical research as the method for assessing their achievements. The current scene is sufficiently in accord with these predictions to suggest their validity.

Suppose, then, that social workers fear evaluation for the reasons suggested. A strong argument can be made that this fear and the beliefs on which it is based are in error. That is, there is substantial reason to conclude that evaluative research has far more rewards for social work than is generally recognized. These rewards are of two forms: (a) contrary to many beliefs, evaluation can and has found merit in some social service programs; and (b) even when evaluation indicates that a program lacks impact there are substantial benefits to be reaped from the effort. In the following discussion we will explicate these points.

POSITIVE ASSESSMENT OF SOCIAL SERVICE TYPE EFFORTS

In a recent summary of evaluations of traditional counseling and therapeutic services, Bergin concluded that these services have modest positive effects.[8] The number of projects reviewed by Bergin is large. However, they do not overlap those examined by Fischer since Fischer restricted himself to only social work services while Bergin primarily reported on the efforts of psychologists and psychiatrists. Admittedly, Bergin's findings are not unanimously agreed upon by other evaluators of psychotherapeutic programs. However, his detailed analyses and some contrasts we have been able to make suggest why his conclusions differ from those of other writers and in particularly why they differ from the conclusions of Fischer.

First, the studies reported on by Fischer almost entirely involved in voluntary recipients of service. Those examined by Bergin often involved voluntary clients. Although we know of no study demonstrating this point, it seems quite reasonable that voluntary clients would be more prepared than involuntary clients to use therapeutic services for their own benefit. Thus they would also be more likely to improve relative to controls.

Second, the methodological sophistication in the studies discussed by Fischer was often limited even though they were indeed control group studies. Obviously, however, the true merits and demerits of a program are more likely to be observed in more sophisticated evaluations. And according to Bergin, it is in the better-conducted evaluations that psychotherapy is more often found to have beneficial effects.[9] An illustration of this point is a social service study not cited by Bergin that was undertaken by the late Margaret Blenkner and that concerned protective services to the aged. Blenkner, and later Fischer, reported that, if anything, protective services seemed to have the effect of hastening death, obviously not a boost for social services. A more elaborate examination of Blenkner's data, recently reported in *Social Work*,[10] has shown that Blenkner's and Fischer's conclusions were incorrect. A more accurate statement, according to the recent analysis, is that no clear inference can be made from existing evidence on the effects of protective services. While this is not a finding to celebrate, it is obviously better than a finding of harm done.

Third, the phenomena constituting success in the Bergin-cited studies were much less profound than those used by Fischer. Almost all of Bergin's projects dealt with individuals experiencing personal tensions and anxieties. Most of Fischer's studies dealt with criminals, delinquents, welfare recipients, or people having or likely to have other problems adjusting to some social institution. While progress for Bergin's clients was generally the easing of personal symptoms, progress for Fischer's clients involved major life changes such as becoming nondelinquent, achieving economic self-sufficiency, or improving school performance. Clearly Fischer's criteria were more difficult to achieve than Bergin's.

Bergin noted numerous areas in which the evaluations he reviewed lacked specificity. He regarded these as serious weaknesses. However, these evaluations certainly score better on this criterion than those reviewed by Fischer. Specificity in an evaluative design recognizes that outcomes can vary depending upon the particular mix of treatment technology, setting, and characteristics of therapist and client. Bergin cited considerable empirical evidence of variability of outcome across diagnoses, criteria, and types of therapists.[11] It is only when we break therapy down into its components that we begin to obtain clearer results. The fact that diverse influences and processes, some probably opposite in direction to each other, are occurring in broad tests of therapy efficacy practically insures results that are difficult to interpret."[12]

In evaluating the effectiveness of casework services, Fischer encountered considerable difficulty in defining social casework. He was finally forced to adopt the definition of casework as "the services of professional case-workers."[13] In three of the eleven studies reviewed by Fischer the orientation of the caseworkers providing the treatment was listed as "undetermined." Four studies reported the major treatment approach as involving group and individualized services while three more used "intensive direct services, use of environmental resources."[14] This type of undifferentiated analysis can be expected to lead to the type of confusing results to which Bergin alluded.

Finally, the Bergin analysis found that successful treatment was associated with experienced therapists.[15] Social workers' careers generally lead them away from direct service within relatively few years of practice. Thus it is not unreasonable to speculate that the social workers whose efforts were evaluated in the Fischer projects were not as experienced as Bergin's therapists.

Aside from Bergin's comparatively optimistic findings based on evaluation of traditional forms of counseling and therapy, there are other indications that counseling services have potential benefits. This can be seen in evaluations of new forms of therapeutic endeavor, particularly behavioral methods. The data on these approaches have been reported previously by others and need not be reviewed here.[16] However, these reviews and our analysis of Bergin's findings suggest that evaluations of social service programs do not at all imply that these efforts are without value. Rather they indicate that:

1. Some kinds of clients (i.e., volunteers) may be more easily helped than others.

2. Some types of goals are more difficult to achieve than others.

3. Some forms of service are more efficacious than others.

Taken in this comparative perspective, these findings seem less the harbingers of doom than sources of information by which social workers can more constructively gear their activities.

THE BENEFITS OF NULL FINDINGS

Up to this point our remarks have been intended to indicate that social service program evaluations have not been uniformly negative. There is, however, no question that in some areas evaluative research has come up consistently with null findings. There is no reason to doubt we will find more. But even these events offer substantial benefits.

First, simply engaging in serious efforts to determine the consequences of program activities can bring monetary and status rewards. Newman and Turem imply this in their comment that social service program critics would be satisfied temporarily if program goals were merely defined more rigorously.[17] Several specific examples can be cited. The California State

Department of Corrections, the Community Service Society of New York, and the Ryther Clinic in Seattle developed reputations for quality for reasons other than effective operation in the areas of corrections, counseling, and foster care. Among these reasons was the fact that these organizations carried out numerous high-quality studies of service programs. They were seen as being accountable, serious in their efforts to serve, and nondefensive. For this they earned respect.

Second, negative results can have the positive function of informing agency staff when programs need to be dropped or how they might be modified to serve clientele better. We will illustrate this with a specific case example:

Two years ago a Milwaukee social agency (along with many other agencies across the nation) received federal funds for a summer job program for poor delinquent youths. The wage of each participant was about fifty dollars per week, and the program was ten weeks in duration. Aside from income redistribution, considered by agency personnel as an automatic benefit, it was also expected that participants would lessen their criminal activities following their program involvement. This expectation was based on the hypothesis that experience with the program would lead the delinquents to find legitimate work available and more rewarding than crime.[18] Unhappily, the evaluation of this program came up with the finding that experimentals (the program participants) and controls had similar crime patterns during the summer but that in the subsequent fall the experimentals committed crime significantly in excess of controls. The researchers argued that the postprogram crime upsurge by experimentals may have resulted from the increase in living standards these youths were provided during the summer. When their comparatively "heady" income was stopped, they increased their crime in order to maintain their new and more costly tastes. Meanwhile, controls, lacking jobs, did not vary their crime rate to any significant degree. In effect, then, the researchers argued that the summer job program was geared to backfire. Armed with this information, the agency was able to obtain money from funders for more permanent part-time employment efforts.

An important aside to this example involves the implications of these findings for similar programs nationwide. At the present time over $500 million a year is spent on summer job programs for poor youths. Many of these programs concentrate on the delinquent poor. If the Milwaukee findings are applicable elsewhere these programs may be creating new problems (crime) while attempting to mitigate others.[19]

As implied earlier, negative results from evaluative studies have the important function of making service providers more realistic about what they can accomplish and with whom. The substantial achievement claims made over the years by social workers and other human service professionals were perhaps due in large part to the absence of empirical data as to what these individuals could accomplish. Had these data been in hand, had the data we now have been obtained earlier, the claims of these workers would have been less grand. In retrospect, this would have been a positive result. But prospectively negative results will continue to have this positive function, for they will tell us where we need to limit our claims, where we need to reanalyze our methods, and where we need to articulate better which clients will not benefit from what we do. This not only puts us on more solid ground in terms of our expectations of ourselves but increases our credibility for others.

Finally, evaluative efforts can play a major role in developing and refining the tools of our profession. Earlier in the discussion, the lack of specificity in the evaluative studies reviewed by Fischer was cited as a shortcoming of these projects. However, this is not totally the result of faulty research design. The problem is much deeper than that. Many of the programs being run by social workers today can be faulted for their own lack of specificity in the goals they seek to reach, the treatment methods used, and the client population to be served.

Evaluative efforts create pressures to reduce these ambiguities. As pointed out above, a primary requisite for program assessment is the specification and operationalization of program goals. However, if the fruits of evaluation are to be maximized, the researcher must get inside the "black box" of the program. Relevant characteristics and dimensions of clients, program staff, and technologies must be specified and measured if relevant and useful evaluation is to be carried out. Evaluative research of this type allows one to go beyond the simple question of "Did it work?" to address the more important questions of "How did (or didn't) it work?" "Who benefited and who was harmed?" and "Under what conditions can it work?"

The potential for carrying out this type of research will be greatly enhanced if the research can become an integral part of the ongoing program effort. It is in this situation that one is most likely to achieve proper specification and measurement of relevant program dimensions and the maximization of information feedback that will ensure the cumulative knowledge building that results in truly progressive program change rather than simple innovation.[20]

ON FADS AND THE RETENTION OF PROGRAMS

The final section addresses a rather different function that evaluative research can have, namely, that it can lead us to retain service patterns that we might otherwise drop. Over the years social workers have retired some types of service delivery patterns, therapeutic styles, or clientele. Some clients were not sustained because they were regarded as resistant, some delivery approaches were dropped because they were said to disregard clients' rights, and some therapeutic styles were dropped because they were believed to be ineffective. But the evidence for these conclusions was virtually nonexistent. Thus whatever the stated reasons for these changes, the absence of justifying data raises the question as to whether they were warranted.

We refer to our final case in point: In the late 1960s income maintenance and social service functions were separated in most public welfare agencies. Among social workers this move received considerable support for two reasons. First, it was argued that people should not have social services imposed on them simply because they were recipients of public assistance. Second, it was said that social services would be more palatable to welfare recipients if they were supplied only when people specifically asked for them and when they were supplied by workers who did not have the alienating obligations of investigating citizens' resources and income.

While this seems reasonable, a recent evaluative study has indicated that welfare recipients *ask for* more services, believe their workers are more interested in serving them, and are less likely to believe they are inadequately helped when they receive services under the preseparation format.[21] No doubt many social workers will argue that this finding does not invalidate the appropriateness of separation. Perhaps. Perhaps not. The thing is that these findings challenge one of the important justifications for separation, and one cannot help but wonder what form separation would have taken or whether it would have taken place at all had client appreciation of the integrated service format been known. And, if we use demand as a criterion for effectiveness, a stance that many social work writers have supported, we must conclude that in the 1960s social workers argued for a service delivery system for welfare recipients that was less adequate than what they were then using. An experimental evaluation could have revealed this. And so we are led back to the basic theme of this paper. Evaluation should not be seen as the *bête noire* of social service programs. It has many rewards to offer us. We should take them rather than leave them to others.

REFERENCES

1. See, for example, George Hoshino, "Social Services: The Problem of Accountability," *Social Service Review* 47 (1973):373–83; Edward Newman and Jerry Turem, "The Crisis of Accountability," *Social Work* 10 (1974):5–17; Reed Henderson and Barbara K. Shore, "Accountability for What and to Whom?" *Social Work* 19 (1974): 387–88; Alice M. Rivlin, *Systematic Thinking for Social Action* (Washington, D.C.: Brookings Institution, 1971), pp. 120–45; Edward A. Suchman, *Evaluative Research* (New York: Russell Sage Foundation, 1967), pp. 1–26; and Carol H. Weiss, "Alternative Models of Program Evaluation," *Social Work* 19 (1974):675–81.
2. See Joel Fischer, "Is Casework Effective? A Review," *Social Work* 18 (1973):5–21, and subsequent issues of *Social Work* for commentary; Steven Paul Segal, "Research on the Outcome of Social Work Therapeutic Interventions: A Review of the literature," *Journal of Health and Social Behavior* 13 (1972):3–17; and a reply by Alan S.

Gurman, "The Efficacy of Therapeutic Interventions in Social Work: A Critical Re-Evaluation," *Journal of Health and Social Behavior* 15 (1974):136–41.
3. Fischer, "Is Casework Effective?" p. 8.
4. For example, Fischer reported that seventeen such studies exist (Joel Fischer, "Does Anything Work?" unpublished manuscript, Council on Social Work Education, New York, 1976).
5. For an excellent discussion of these issues, see Margaret Blenkner, "Obstacles to Evaluative Research on Casework: Parts I and II," *Social Casework* 31 (1950):54–60, 97–105; and Carole Austin, "Staff Resistances to Evaluation" (Paper delivered at the National Conference of Social Welfare, Washington, D.C., 1976).
6. Newman and Turem, "Crisis of Accountability," pp. 5–17.
7. Fischer, "Is Casework Effective?"
8. Allen E. Bergin, "The Evaluation of Therapeutic Outcomes," in *Handbook of Psychotherapy and Behavior Change*, ed. Allen E. Bergin and Sol L. Garfield (New York: John Wiley & Sons, 1971), pp. 217–70.
9. Ibid., p. 238.
10. Irving Piliavin and Ray Berger, "The Effect of Casework: A Research Note," *Social Work* 21 (1976):205–9.
11. Ibid., p. 249.
12. Ibid., p. 238.
13. Fischer, "Is Casework Effective?" p. 6.
14. Ibid., pp. 14–17.
15. Bergin, "Evaluation of Therapeutic Outcomes," p. 237.
16. Allen E. Bergin and Sol L. Garfield, eds., *Handbook of Psychotherapy and Behavior Change* (New York: John Wiley & Sons, 1971), pp. 543–750.
17. Newman and Turem, "Crisis of Accountability."
18. This expectation was essentially derived from the thesis proposed by Cloward and Ohlin that higher crime among lower-class adolescents is a response to the failure of society to provide these individuals with sufficient opportunities for success in legitimate economic activities (Richard Cloward and Lloyd Ohlin, *Delinquency and Opportunity* [Glencoe: Free Press, 1960]).
19. Irving Piliavin and James R. Seaberg, "The Idle Hands Thesis of Juvenile Crime: An Evaluation of the Effects of Youth Employment" (Unpublished manuscript, 1974).
20. For an excellent treatment of this issue, see Daniel Glaser, *Routinizing Evaluation: Getting Feedback of Crime and Delinquency Programs* (Rockville, Md.: National Institute of Mental Health, 1973).
21. Irving Piliavin and Allan Gross, "The Effects of Separation on AFDC Recipients' Perceptions and Uses of Social Services: Results of a Field Experiment" (Unpublished manuscript, 1976).

F. SYSTEMS ANALYSIS

29/THE NEW SCIENTIFIC MANAGEMENT: SYSTEMS MANAGEMENT FOR SOCIAL WELFARE

RINO PATTI

INTRODUCTION

In the mid-1960s when the administration was attempting to give birth to the War on Poverty, another less dramatic and seemingly innocent presidential initiative was being launched which would have far more staying power than the poverty program, and may in the long light of history, have an even greater impact on the nature of social services in the United States. This initiative was President Johnson's order that a new management approach called the Planning, Programming and Budgeting System (PPBS) be put into general usage throughout the federal bureaucracy. This system, in the president's words, had "proved its worth many times over in the Department of Defense," and would now bring to other departments and agencies of the federal government the "most advanced techniques of modern business management."[1] The optimistic rhetoric that accompanied the introduction of PPBS reflected a conviction that at long last a management technology had become available that would bring order and precision to the processes of program planning, implementation, and evaluation. It promised a set of tools that could be used with equal facility whether one was dealing with missile systems or welfare systems, and provided the advantage of imposing a common analytic framework that would enable policy makers to comparatively assess the costs and effectiveness of various programs.

A decade later, the glitter and promise that surrounded PPBS at its inception has dimmed somewhat, but the managerial ideology, the mind set that gave rise to it, has, if anything, become more pervasive. For purposes of this discussion, I shall refer to this ideology as the "New Scientific Management." I specifically use the term "ideology" to convey the assertion that the new scientific management is not distinguished as much by its technology as it is by a particular socio-political world view, characterized by certain definite (albeit often implicit) assumptions about how best to understand, control, and change organizational behavior.

In its practical expression, the new scientific management is more familiarly associated with terms like systems management, systems analysis, operations research, and systems engineering: that collection of methodologies that now enjoy increasing currency and favor in social welfare bureaucracies at every level of government. It is to this ideological and technical phenomenon, its definition, emergence, and limitations, and its implications for the social welfare enterprise, that this paper is addressed. The position I intend to argue is that the indiscriminate application of this approach in social welfare can generate negative consequences for human services agencies and the clients they serve.[2]

THE NEW SCIENTIFIC MANAGEMENT: WHAT IS IT?

It is difficult to crisply define and characterize the new scientific management without doing injustice to someone's conception of what it means. Like all management approaches, its adherents and practitioners differ markedly among themselves as to how much weight should be attached to which tenets or principles, how dogmatic or selective one should be in implementing certain strategies, and so on. Despite these variations, however, it is important to attempt a definition of this managerial phenomenon so that there can be a common referent.

Practitioners of the new scientific management, or what we shall refer to here as systems managers, are a diverse lot that come from many different academic and experiential backgrounds, including engineering, computer sciences, economics, business, the behavioral sciences, and public administration. Here and there, one even finds a social worker or a lawyer, who by virtue of personal predisposition or on-the-job training has gained entry to this coveted circle of "management scientists." What makes it possible to treat this collection of practitioners as a group, however, is not a common occupational or academic identity, but rather their adherence to a certain belief system. Committed as they are to objectifying management practices based on rigorous quantitative analysis, the belief system that directs and influences their activities tends often to be quite implicit. In day-to-day interaction it is, in fact, often difficult to discern the assumptions and values which underlie their activities, because they appear as ultimate pragmatists prepared to move in whatever direction data and logic suggest. Nevertheless, lurking below this formidable objective facade is a belief system that bears identification; among its central tenets are these:

1. *All organization systems, notwithstanding their particular histories, cultures, language, and programmatic content, can be analyzed and understood in terms of the logical relationship between means and ends.* With adequate expertise and computer hardware, information systems can ultimately be devised that will isolate and quantify all, or at least most, of the variables that are salient to an effective decision-making process.[3]

2. *The essential similarity of organizational processes, regardless of substantive content, makes it possible for the systems manager to be a pan-institutional generalist, who can apply theoretical knowledge and analytic skills with equal value in any situational context.*

3. *With adequate research technology, it is possible to define situations such that all "action relevant to environmental conditions are specifiable and predictable; and all relevant states of a system are specifiable and predictable."*[4] Organizational processes can, in short, be defined as established situations.

4. *The efficient use of material and human resources is a paramount value.* One of the major problems to contend with in this respect is the tendency for the components of a system to displace organizational goals with selfish and parochial interests. In terms of overall organizational objectives, this is defined as waste and error. To minimize these factors, the systems manager must specify activity elements and output criteria and construct an information system that allows him to monitor performance and to detect deviations so that these can be brought under control.[5]

5. *Impatience with human error motivates a constant search for ways to structure, and where possible reduce, the exercise of judgment and discretion.* The preferred approach to increasing predictability and reliability of performance is reducing the complexity of tasks performed so that activities can be routinely and consistently carried out. Human motivation and social and cultural conditioning are not considered problematic in this regard and tend to be treated as constants. The atomization of work, however, is only practicable when accompanied by well articulated systems for control and coordination.[6] Only in this way is it possible to orchestrate the universe of tasks in the service of centrally defined objectives.

6. *Consensus, bargaining, and negotiation are suspect as processes for decision making and should be replaced where possible by choices that are informed by comprehensive, rational analysis of alternatives in terms of their relative costs, effectiveness, and risks in achieving specified objectives.*[7] Organizational or subsystem survival should not be a major decision variable, nor should socio-political criteria of success.

This set of values and assumptions, as we shall see in a moment, is open to serious questions. Were these the primary tools of a systems manager, he would be vulnerable indeed. However, what makes the new scientific management such a formidable force in contemporary organizational life is not the tenets of its ideology alone, but the technology which buttresses and justifies it. The systems manager is himself skilled in, or can mobilize experts with such esoteric specialties as, cost-benefit analysis, operations research, program budgeting, network analysis, and the program evaluation review technique. This arsenal of systems analytic technologies grew out of the space and defense efforts in the post–World War II era and were collectively credited with no less lofty achievements than putting a man on the moon and bringing rationality to the Byzantine decision processes of the Department of Defense. A systems manager brings with him the credibility gained from these ventures, plus more than a little arrogance rooted in the belief that if his technology can harness problems like space travel, it should be more than equal to the task of improving the effectiveness of social welfare organizations.[8]

Thus, the new scientific management is no passing fashion that we can expect to recede quickly from the scene. It is, rather, a well articulated ideology practiced by professionals who enjoy considerable stature by virtue of a technological knowhow that gives them the image of being hardheaded realists with the ability to produce. That they should be chosen to bring some order and rationality to the muddled social welfare bureaucracy is not surprising. We turn now to how the diffusion of the new scientific management occurred in social welfare.

EMERGENCE AND DIFFUSION
OF SCIENTIFIC MANAGEMENT IN SOCIAL WELFARE

The spread of the new scientific management across institutional boundaries into domestic and, specifically for our purposes, social welfare governmental areas should first of all be placed in the economic context of the 1960s. The decade of the 1960s witnessed a growth in social welfare expenditures unparalleled in this country's history. New programs, expanded eligibility, and increased benefits, while insufficient to meet rising expectations, nevertheless resulted in a mushrooming of governmental responsibility. Between 1960 and 1973, for example, social welfare expenditures, encompassing income maintenance, health, housing, education, and social services at federal, state, and local levels increased from $52.3 to $215 billion, an increase of over 400 percent. During roughly this same period, social welfare expenditures as a percentage of the gross national product also increased dramatically, from 10.6 percent to 17.6 percent. Similarly, while federal, state, and local governments had expended 38 percent of their budgets for welfare purposes in 1960, this proportion had risen to 53 percent by 1973.[9] Thus, in both absolute and relative terms, the social welfare enterprise had expanded at a phenomenal rate. By the end of the decade it had become not only a major governmental activity but a central preoccupation of the American people and their elected officials as well.

Throughout this decade a subtle but important phenomena was occurring, namely, a gradual shrinking of the fiscal dividend. In the early 1960s it had been assumed that a continued rate of economic growth would generate a fiscal dividend sufficient to support an expanding effort to combat social problems. However, the combined effect of several tax cuts, the Viet Nam War, increased social welfare expenditures, and, more recently, inflation and a reduced rate of economic growth has served to seriously erode the surplus that might have underwritten the continued expansion of social welfare programs. It is now clear, as the Brookings Institution studies have pointed out, that there will not be sufficient resources to support all the social welfare initiatives that seemed worthwhile on their face. This will be true, one should add, even if defense expenditures are substantially cut back.[10]

The net effect of these developments has been to create a politics of scarcity where emphasis is increasingly placed on choosing from among program alternatives those that produced the greatest increment of desired social and behavioral change for the dollar expended. In this context, decision makers, both executive and legislative, increasingly look to experts who can provide them with hard information on which to base the difficult choices.

The politics of scarcity has had, and will continue to have, a profound effect on management technology and social welfare organizations. Where once the administrators of these programs had the relatively simple tasks of advocating program expansion and justifying the need for additional allocations of money and resources, by the latter part of the 1960s, they were being asked to provide detailed information about what was being done, at what cost, and with what results. Management was forced, in short, to shift from a preoccupation with program maintenance and expansion, to a concern with program description, control, and evaluation. In making this shift, social welfare organizations found themselves confronted with a gigantic skill and knowledge vacuum. The pool of career professionals and program experts that had traditionally been recruited to middle and upper management did not possess the technical know-how needed to fill this vacuum, so social welfare organizations began to import, or have imposed upon them, the technology that the new age required.

Like the social scientists who had preceded them during the early 1960s, and the psychiatrists before them, each of whom were sought to fill different vacuums, the systems analysis technicians came marching into the social welfare sector as teachers, consultants, and researchers. On the placards they carried was a new lexicon bristling with the sound of rigor and precision: management information systems (MIS); program financial plan (PFP); management by objectives (MBO); and so on. As in previous eras, social welfare professionals embraced these prophets warmly, attending endless workshops, institutes, and management seminars to learn more of this new wisdom so that it might be incorporated into their own practice repertoires.

Before long, however, it became clear that the implementation of the new management technology would require not only the infusion of knowledge but the infusion of systems managers themselves. Retraining the program-oriented, career professional was proving too difficult. The process by which this personnel succession began to occur is reflected in the study jointly conducted by the General Accounting Office and the Bureau of the Budget in 1969 to determine those factors that influenced whether sixteen federal agencies had successfully implemented PPBS. The major finding of this survey was that the attitudes of the agency head was the single most important factor in development of an agency-wide PPB system. Departments with executives who were considered indifferent to "the development of systematic analysis and planning processes . . . made less substantial progress," according to this study.[11] Note the implicit assumption here that an executive's failure to embrace PPBS was the equivalent of an indifference to systematic analysis. Perhaps more revealing is what the study concluded about the reasons for executive indifference:

. . . Wide experience in the agency's program areas: professional background which leaned toward bargaining or argument as issue resolving techniques; and finally, strong agency constituencies, whose interests would not be served by the kind of policy analysis contemplated by the PPB system.[12]

The not-so-implicit image of the PPBS resistant administrator that emerges from these "findings" is someone who is not committed to rational planning, whose vested interests in the existing program of the agency make him impervious to data suggesting the need for changes, who prefers compromise to logic as a basis for decision, and, finally, one whose consideration of alternatives is constrained by the biases and interests of groups upon whom he relies for support. One could easily come away from this characterization feeling that this group of administrators is an unprogressive, recalcitrant lot. Only a short jump in logic is necessary to conclude that if systematic analysis and planning are to be incorporated, then these administrators must be replaced by those who support PPB.

Yet looked at from another perspective, the characteristics attributed to PPB-resistant executives might well be those that are often associated with the effective administrator—i.e., an intimate acquaintance with program; an appreciation of, and ability to use, political processes in decision making; and an awareness of, and sensitivity to, agency constituencies. Needless to say, this was not the interpretation given in the study just alluded to.

The point is that once the new scientific management gained a foothold in social welfare, the program-oriented manager became a proverbial sitting duck. The process of succession was virtually assured. The mismatch between these contending forces is aptly summarized by Hoos:

Is it conceivable that anyone would logically opt for anachronistic inefficiency through horse-and-buggy means, when instead, he can invoke an arsenal of sophisticated tools that will bring efficiency? The answer to this almost rhetorical question draws strength from and strengthens the already existing ethos of efficiency, automatically accredits efficiency as a social good, and practically assures easement into the next step of the syllogism, that [social problems] need better management. It is through this logic that systems analysis has been transplanted from the realm of the military and the moon-bound to the social scene.[13]

PROBLEMS AND PITFALLS

Having asserted that the new scientific management is, and will continue to be, a potent force in social welfare, I would now like to discuss several of the problems in, and consequences of, this development. Basically, the discussion will revolve around two major points: the applicability of systems management and kindred technologies to the social welfare sector; and some of the organizational problems that will be attendant to a full-scale implementation of this management style.

On the face of it, the new scientific management and the technology it employs would seem to provide an ideal approach to solving social problems. Among other things, it suggests exhaustive fact finding regarding the problem at hand; a detailed specification of desirable goals and objectives; a comprehensive evaluation of the alternative means for achieving the desired outcomes, together with the anticipated costs and consequences of each; and, finally, the selection of those means that seem optimal for achieving goals sought. The implementation of the entire program is carefully monitored so that the decision maker is aware of how each program component is progressing toward the achievement of its subobjectives, and how its activities articulate with those of other components. Feedback is provided at periodic intervals to allow the administrator to make the necessary adjustments in the nature of the program activities, the goals, or both. At the end of a planning or budget period, the decision maker is presumably in a position to quantitatively determine the extent to which the goals set were in fact achieved.

What concerns us here is whether, in fact, this appealing scenario can be effectively applied to most social welfare organizations whose tasks and functions are influenced by a whole host of rapidly changing and difficult-to-anticipate contingencies. Systems managers argue that there is no reason why it cannot. For example, these PPB enthusiasts state:

Nothing inherent in the subject content of *any agency's program mix* [emphasis added] should impede PPB analysis. . . . It should be possible to define the benefits of a program in ways that make them susceptible to measurement.[14]

Despite this optimism, there is a growing body of opinion which suggests that the transferability of the systems management model to people serving organizations is not as simple as the advocate of PPB would lead us to believe. There are several reasons for this.

First of all, the application of systems management technology assumes certain organizational and environmental preconditions, which on examination, are found to be largely lacking in the social welfare sector. Wildavsky, for example, in his analysis of factors that facilitated the implementation of PPB in the Department of Defense, found the following factors to be essential:

1. A rising level of appropriations and program expansion which makes it possible to hire large numbers of new people who are thoroughly immersed in the new management technology.

2. A highly centralized decision-making process and a corresponding ability of those in power to control the processes of implemention.

3. Organizations that enjoy relative autonomy from their environments in the sense that they are not constrained by well-entrenched constituent groups that are likely to oppose policy decisions.

4. A situation in which a rather large margin of error is allowable—that is, where policy-making and funding bodies are willing to tolerate a substantially larger expenditure than was originally anticipated in order to solve the problem at hand.

5. A situation in which the cost of a contemplated policy or program development justifies a rather large expenditure on the implementation of systems management technology.

6. A small group of experts who have devoted to the substantive problems confronting an organization using the tools of systems management.[15]

We need not discuss each of these criteria as they apply to social welfare, since those who are familiar with human services organizations are aware that these conditions generally do not obtain in this field. Moreover, the absence of these facilitating factors becomes more marked as one considers those social welfare organizations that operate under state and local jurisdictions. What interests us here is that so little attention has been given to these preconditions that experience would indicate are necessary to properly install systems management technology. One wonders if in their eagerness to gain access to a new organizational territory, the systems technicians and managers engaged in a bit of oversell much like social workers did in the early 1960s. In any case, it appears that without adequate support, the systems management approach will find it difficult to actualize its potential.

A second and perhaps more fundamental reason for questioning the transferability of the systems management approach to social welfare is that it has proven to be most effective in situations of moderate complexity where goals are relatively clear and easily measured and the performance characteristics of the systems components are known. It deals, in other words, most effectively with those organizational processes concerned with established, routine situations.

When, however, the phenomena with which a system deals is highly complex, and influenced by an array of largely unknown and subtly independent variables, many of which cannot be observed, let alone controlled, the utility of systems management techniques declines considerably. Add to this the fact that unlike man-machine interaction, where the behavior of the worker and the responses of the machine can be specified and within limits predicted, no corresponding claim can be made for client-worker interactions in human services organizations.

Our concern, of course, is not that systems management technology cannot deal with this order of complexity, but *rather that its practitioners are likely to act as though it can.* After all, the claim of the new scientific management is based on its presumed ability to bring order and logic where disorder and confusion have previously existed. To make good on this claim, there will be a compelling tendency for systems managers to impose an artificial precision on client-worker interactions, by either selectively screening out those variables that are not amenable to measurement, or by assigning numerical values to variables no matter how imprecise or arbitrary such assignments might be.[16] The temptation will be to fill in the "black box" in the systems flow chart, impose definition where none is called for. Some will argue that such efforts, while more form than substance, are necessary at the outset in order to move toward increasingly refined measures. However, the danger is that once these data have been set into the computer and subjected to impeccable mathematical calculation, the decision makers, in their quest for hard information, will come to forget that they are dealing with the "illusion of certainty" and not the real thing.[17] Ultimately, this process has the potential for masking vast areas of ignorance and obscuring the need for real knowledge development.

Finally, the utility of systems management technology for social welfare should be questioned because of its generally simplistic view of the relationship between the organization and its environment. It is clear that policy and program development in social welfare is more characterized by its incremental and consensual nature than by its emphasis on purely rationalistic planning. In no sector of public service are there more diverse experts and interest groups who have a say in, or the ability to block, policy developments. Client groups, unions, professional associations, state and federal legislative bodies, groups of administrators, and a host of other interest factions must be considered in the development of policy and program. The potential of these groups for confounding a welfare program is substantial no matter how impeccable its design may be.[18] Because of this, it is imperative that management and social welfare organizations be sensitive to, and capable of compromising with, elements of the support environment that surround virtually all such organizations. This process may result in less than ideal programs, but it is essential to maintaining a modicum of community support. To the extent that systems managers consider these groups to be impediments in the policy development process and/or attempt to centralize decision making in the interest of gaining greater effectiveness, one would expect there to be not only a reduction of input from these groups, but an increase in resistances to proposed changes not only from those that are traditional antagonists of welfare programs, but from friends and allies as well.

In addition to those problems mentioned above, there are other limitations to the systems management approach that are likely to impede the service delivery capability of social welfare organizations. Central among these is that the assumptions and techniques which make up the new scientific management are by their nature likely to accentuate the trend to centralized decision making and control that are already pronounced in many welfare bureaucracies.[19] There are several reasons for this assertion. First of all, as we have previously pointed out, systems management tends to abhor error, uncertainty, and unreliability—i.e., those phenomena that attend the exercise of discretion and judgment by workers. To minimize these factors, the systems manager tends to divide the tasks to be performed in the organization so that each is reduced to its simplest and most routine dimension. In this way it is possible to simultaneously define and specify the nature of the work performed and to maintain better control. But the process of achieving more predictable worker performance cannot stop here because in order to avoid chaos, the atomization of tasks must be accompanied by an elaborate data retrieval and monitoring mechanism. This in turn compels the need for increasingly complex and comprehensive information systems, a sophisticated data processing capability and a sizable cadre of middle management experts who can man the hardware, analyze and interpret its output, and make the findings available to top management. The net effect of this process is that while the purview of the personnel in the lower echelons is more and more constricted, the data they generate tends increasingly to aggregate at the top. Central management comes to have a virtual monopoly on the information necessary for decisions. From the perspective of the systems manager, this may be desirable because it affords the comprehensive, holistic view that is deemed necessary to evaluate the overall performance of the organization. On the other hand, there is considerable evidence suggesting that the organizational structure and processes necessary to sustain centralized decision making generate significant undesirable consequences for staff and clients. Included among these are: stereotyped and procedure-bound staff behaviors; poor staff morale; and alienation.[20] Moreover, in a work environment which emphasizes routine and narrowly defined work parameters, one can expect that the search for innovative solutions to problematic situations will be diminished considerably.[21]

In the utopian world of the new scientific management, it is assumed that a rationally derived decision clearly communicated to subordinates will be complied with. Drawing upon experience with mechanical models, the systems manager looks upon compliance as a relatively simple process in which the component, in this case the worker, receives a message, acknowledges receipt, and proceeds to behave in a specified manner. It is true that all but the most obtuse systems technologists observe the difficulties that occur in this process, but those factors that interfere with machine-like responses tend to be lumped together as "external rational" annoyances, that cannot be understood or systematically dealt with. This kind of intellectual sleight of hand is an expensive luxury in social welfare bureaucracies, even the most elementary observations will suggest that workers have an infinite variety of ways of filtering and selectively interpreting messages from superiors, and even of undermining orders they receive. The limitation of the systems management perspective is that it is predicated on the notion that the most compelling factor motivating worker action is the rational, authoritative message. Yet rather extensive research in organizations employing well-educated, professional personnel, indicates that an overreliance on the use of authority to obtain compliance and exact obedience is likely to produce not more, but less efficient and effective worker performance.[22] The systems manager is, of course, likely to interpret this as a problem requiring yet a further set of rules, procedures, and controls.

CONCLUSIONS AND RECOMMENDATIONS

Criticism serves a useful purpose, and the new scientific management, like any major movement, deserves to receive its share. But it is one thing to criticize and quite another to suggest constructive alternatives. So, in conclusion let me suggest several ideas that I believe may be useful to the long-term development of management capability in the social welfare sector.

In the short run there seems to be no clear alternatives to the infusion of systems management perspectives and technology into social welfare. This approach is riding a crest of popularity compounded of the status borrowed from other fields of endeavor, its own salesmanship and soaring rhetoric, and the public's desperate quest for solutions to the "welfare problem." The new scientific management has promised to deliver more effective programs at less cost, and notwithstanding this assessment of its limitations, the final returns are not yet in. One suspects that the glitter of the new scientific management will begin to dim when there has been time to measure the payoff against the promise. In the meantime, the social welfare sector should actively proceed to design and implement management training programs that are specifically tailored to the distinctive organizational and political conditions that obtain in this field.

The argument for the development of specialized professional training programs in social welfare management is based primarily on the recognition that human services organizations can no longer afford to find their leadership in technicians who have developed their administrative skill through on-the-job training, nor from those trained in management skills that were developed in, and are better suited to, other substantive program areas. Social welfare is a gigantic enterprise, whose complexity, cost, and significance to the political economy of this country is such that it requires the specialized management expertise of persons whose basic educational preparation and subsequent career development occurs in the context of social welfare proper. Such persons must be identified early in their college years and groomed for a career in social welfare management, because only with lengthy, continuous, and intensive training will they be adequate to the task that confronts them. The idea that someone can spend ten years working in a direct service capacity and then be recruited to and retrained for management is an anachronism that grew out of the early days of social welfare when the nature of administration was much less well understood and the programs and policies to be administered were less complicated. Some people were able to make this transition effectively, but the vast majority were not, as evidenced by the gigantic skill vacuum that became evident in social welfare in the 1960s.

There are some who cling to the notion that the best administrators are bred in the ranks of direct practice. But if nothing else, the new scientific management has jolted most career professionals into a recognition that the task of managing an organization requires a distinctive and rigorous preparation. The persons specially trained in social welfare management should be no less sensitive to client needs, and no less steeped in social values than front-line practitioners, but they must have specialized training in the broad range of theoretical, empirical, and practical skills required of today's administrator. To detail the nature of such a training program would require yet another paper, but let me suggest some of its general dimensions.

1. *Social program managers should have substantial grounding in the cluster of technologies that we have lumped together under the phrase "systems management."* These tools have considerable value when not tied to some of the assumptions of the new scientific management and when they are selectively utilized to accomplish limited purposes. Social welfare managers should be sufficiently familiar with these technologies to know when and where they can be appropriately utilized.

2. *Social welfare managers should have substantive grounding in some*

problem-policy area within social welfare—e.g., criminal justice, poverty and income maintenance, development disabilities, or child welfare. They should be intimately familiar with the empirical and theoretical evidence pertaining to the causes and effective treatment of the problem; the community organizations and constituencies that are concerned with the problem; the legislative and administrative policy context of program delivery; the policy development processes and economic factors that contribute to and result from the particular problem phenomena.

3. *Social welfare managers should have a repertoire of interpersonal skills relevant to task group development and leadership, in-service training and staff development, and personnel management.* They should be familiar with organizational development strategies and techniques and know when they can be appropriately utilized. They should have a thorough comprehension of organizational research that suggests the interpersonal and structural conditions necessary to develop and maintain worker commitment to organizational goals.

4. *Social welfare managers should have a substantial grounding in research design and quantitative methods, especially as they relate to policy analysis and program evaluation.*

This is, of course, only the barest outline, but it is enough to suggest that the range of knowledge and skill required for the management of today's social welfare organization cannot generally be found in professional schools of engineering, business, or public administration that are currently providing much of the systems management manpower for the field of social welfare. Each has its contribution to make to the preparation of the social welfare manager, but none provides the breadth and flexibility that is required.

I believe that schools of social work should provide the leadership for this kind of training in the next decade. Significant developments in this area have been initiated in a number of schools, and enrollment in administration programs has grown substantially in the last few years.[23] While the number of graduates is still infinitesimal in relation to the need, it seems likely that these programs will continue to develop and expand. The success of such programs, if indeed they are to succeed, will depend crucially on the guidance, support, and cooperation of career professionals in social welfare who know best the urgent need for effective social welfare management and the consequences that will follow if we fail to meet this challenge.

NOTES

1. Ida Hoos, *Systems Analysis in Public Policy: A Critique* (Berkeley: University of California Press, 1972), p. 65.
2. This is not to deny the value of systems analytic technology when it is selectively

utilized for specific administrative tasks. My concern here is with those situations in which this technology and the assumptions on which it is based become the dominant management strategy in an organization.

3. See, for example, Robert J. Wolfson, "In the Hawk's Nest," *Society* 9 (April 1972): 24, 69; Hoos, *Systems Analysis in Public Policy*, p. 86–96.

4. Robert Boguslaw, *The New Utopians: A Study of System Design and Social Change* (Englewood Cliffs, N.J.: Prentice-Hall, 1965), p. 7.

5. David Clelland and William King, *Management: A Systems Approach* (New York: McGraw-Hill, 1972), pp. 395–411.

6. Boguslaw, *The New Utopians*, p. 2.

7. See, for example, discussions by Kate Archibald, "Three Views of the Experts' Role in Policy Making: Systems Analysis, Incrementation, and the Clinical Approach," *Policy Sciences* 1 (1970):77–78; and Jean Millar, "Selective Adaptations," *Policy Sciences* 3 (1972): 130–131; and Victor Thompson, *Bureaucracy and Innovation* (University: University of Alabama Press, 1969), pp. 54–55.

8. Wolfson, "In the Hawk's Nest," p. 58.

9. Alfred Skolnik and Sophie Doles, "Social Welfare Expenditures, 1970-1971," *Social Security Bulletin* 37 (January 1974):3–5.

10. Charles Schultz et al., *Setting National Priorities: The 1973 Budget* (Washington, D.C.: The Brookings Institution, 1973), pp. 394–409.

11. Keith Marvin and Andrew Rouse, "The Status of PPB in Federal Agencies: A Comparative Perspective," in *The Analysis and Evaluation of Public Expenditures: The PPBS System*, vol. 3 (Washington, D.C.: Government Printing Office, 1969), p. 808.

12. Ibid.

13. Hoos, *Systems Analysis in Public Policy*, p. 90.

14. Marvin and Rouse, "The Status of PPB in Federal Agencies," p. 814.

15. Aaron Wildavsky, "Rescuing Policy Analysis from PPBS," in *The Analysis and Evaluation of Public Expenditures: The PPB System* (Washington, D.C.: Government Printing Office, 1969), pp. 838–840.

16. Hoos, *Systems Analysis in Public Policy*, p. 70.

17. Thompson, *Bureaucracy and Innovation*, p. 57.

18. The experience with the Goal Oriented Social Services approach (GOSS), an information and evaluation system proposed by HEW for implementation on a national basis several years ago, is a good example of this. After a substantial investment in designing the system, HEW was forced to postpone implementation in the face of substantial opposition from many groups and individuals.

19. See Archibald, "Three Views of the Experts' Role in Policy Making," pp. 74–75; and Thompson, *Bureaucracy and Innovation*, pp. 29–60.

20. Gerald Hage and Michael Aiken, "Organizational Alienation: A Comparative Analysis," in *The Sociology of Formal Organizations: Basic Studies*, ed. Oscar Gursky and George Miller (New York: Free Press, 1970), pp. 517–526.

21. Thompson, *Bureau and Innovation*, pp. 9–28.

22. See, for example, Rensis Likert, *The Human Organization: Its Management and Value* (New York: McGraw-Hill, 1967), pp. 3–40.

23. Statistics available from CSWE indicate that between 1968 and 1973 the number of graduate students enrolled in programs of administration, management, and social policy in schools of social work increased approximately five-fold. *Statistics on Social Work Education, 1974*, Council on Social Work Education.

This article is based on a paper presented at the APWA Western Regional Conference, October 29, 1974, Portland, Oregon.

MURRAY GRUBER

A revolution of unknown proportions is dawning and is altering society as we know it. In the last great transformation scientific and technical knowledge were applied to improve industrial processes, and the resultant far-reaching changes in social relations were largely unplanned. In the current revolution the objects of science and technology are precisely social processes, institutions, and people.

The systems sciences, the management sciences, and the information explosion open new vistas for social management and control. Some see in these possibilities the acme of rationality and efficiency, a kind of technological utopia that blots out the last vestiges of man's irrationality and capriciousness. Others see in them a monstrous system of "total administration" that cancels out man, not through terror and brutal authoritarianism, but through gradual subjugation in the reasonable name of efficient problem-solving.[1]

Unexpectedly, even conservatives no longer dispute the existence of the welfare state. Although temporary setbacks do occur and serious gaps in programs remain, the instrumentalities of the advanced welfare state continue to expand, and there is no apparent limit in sight. With this expansion, managing resources efficiently has become a grave problem. This problem is also closely related to the longer-range trend of increasing complexity in social structures, which demands more and more control. In what is perhaps a separate "iron law of development," growing public expenditures seem to bring growing bureaucratization.

As a consequence of these conditions, the advanced welfare state moves forward in a new direction. Spiraling expenditures and spreading bureaucratization are generating a call for efficiency that both liberals and conservatives are now espousing. In the advanced welfare state the forward push thus shifts from such concerns as social equity and democratic planning to the compelling technocratic notions of "product," "output," and "getting things done efficiently."[2]

A systems perspective is at the heart of the new rationality. Applications of the systems sciences—essentially the engineering control processes that are found in systems management, systems engineering, operation research, and input-output analysis—are thus coupled with the economizing spirit, the urge to get the most for the least by rationalizing the budgetary process, allocating resources efficiently, and monitoring and evaluating social programs. The new processes of control are becoming rapidly diffused in welfare, education, health, urban planning, corrections, law enforcement, and other fields involving social management. Nor are the professions that provide direct services immune from the influence of the systems and engineering sciences.

TECHNOLOGY AND INSTITUTIONS

As the public sector of society moves toward accountability for program, finances, and management, corporate enterprise is diffusing engineering technology throughout social management. The Aerospace Systems Division of Bendix International, for example, has established an Urban/Environmental Systems Group that is involved in planning, program evaluation, data systems analysis, socioeconomic cost-benefit studies, and information requirements in the fields of criminal justice, population planning, and drug abuse. And Bendix is but one of many.

As part of this trend, the "analytic techniques and management skills of big business" are applauded as the "best hopes for bringing order to the disorderly problems of the city."[3] In municipal agencies administering health and welfare services, in city and state planning departments, as well as in federal departments and agencies, the focus is on efficient management of program, fiscal monitoring, and program evaluation.

The Rand Corporation now advises the City of New York on major questions of social administration. Private management consultant firms are assisting state governments and are bidding for contracts to design programs for the Department of Health, Education, and Welfare (HEW), the Department of Housing and Urban Development (HUD), and the Law Enforcement Assistance Administration (LEAA). Many of these firms have previously carried out research and development, feasibility studies, and planning for the Department of Defense.[4] Also crossing institutional boundaries are operations researchers and systems analysts who are trying to reorganize state departments of public welfare along the same lines used in reorganizing the U.S. Postal Service and various municipal agencies, including police and fire departments.

Thus the diffusion of technical knowledge and the movement of technicians across institutional boundaries are main characteristics of the current revolution. Even so, the present transformation does not simply hinge on new technologies of control or even their diffusion, but on the coordination of these technologies within a new framework, because the old institutional divisions have collapsed. All this adds up to a profound social transformation. Its intellectual origins and the social forces behind its start and development are important to examine.

EFFICIENCY

Systems and engineering theory, decision theory, cybernetics, information processing, game theory, linear programming, queuing theory, and scheduling and network analysis—from all these have come concepts and techniques that have been applied to management problems. They have been applied particularly to the central problem of strategic choice which involves predicting optimal outcomes of various vital decisions. The root idea of making strategic choices is simple: manage complex situations so that limited resources can be deployed for maximum benefits.

Contemporary conceptions of efficient management owe a large debt to Taylor's pre-World War I theories and precepts designed to regulate the workingman for maximum production. Using scientific principles and minute examination, Taylor urged that "things" and "hands" should be arranged to rationalize and routinize the production process, to harness labor, and to create order among the industrial masses who would then become mere unthinking components of the production system. As Taylor put it:

> . . . one of the very first requirements for a man who is fit to handle pig iron . . . is that he shall be so stupid and so phlegmatic that he more nearly resembles . . . the ox than any other type. . . . he must consequently be trained by a man more intelligent than himself.[5]

Taylorism predicated the "one best way" of doing a job and introduced to the factory the scientific time and motion study, the stop watch, and the slide rule. All planning and scheduling was taken from the work floor itself and put into a new planning department for which an engineer was responsible. Each worker received an instruction card telling in minute detail what was to be done, how done, and exactly how much time was allowed for the job. The tools for similar jobs would be standardized and so would the movements of the worker.

The ideology of efficiency did not stop at the factory. Taylor and other industrial engineers spread their gospel through industrial groups, engineering schools, and schools of business administration. From the material industries, the cult of efficiency spread to the "education industry," as some called it. Educators emphasized the importance of measuring products or results, and warned that "the school as well as other business institutions must submit to the test for efficiency." Seating plans, recitation cards, and other "labor-saving devices" for standardizing behavior were introduced to assure efficient management of the "product." Also introduced were cost accounting and cost analysis.

Taylorism spread, too, to the home, the family, and the church. Articles on home efficiency began with such questions as these: "Does your home pay? Does it make a fair return on the investment of time and money that is put into it? As a factory for the production of citizenship is it a success?" One prominent minister introduced "efficiency tests for clergymen," arguing that "if this seems to make the church something of a business establishment it is precisely what should be done."[6]

MORE SCIENTIFIC MANAGEMENT

During World War II scientific management was extended by operations research. Later in the 1950s and 1960s there were further extensions as systems analysis was developed in the Department of Defense, the aerospace industry, and the National Aeronautics and Space Administration (NASA). Sophisticated tools were devised for program and policy analysis, technological planning, managing operations, and administrative planning and control.

A variety of management techniques in the categories of systems analysis and systems engineering developed in wartime because intuitive decisions were often too costly and too ineffective. Methods were developed for describing operational problems more accurately, determining what information was needed to solve them, and examining the estimated costs and expected benefits of alternative solutions.

On the organizational side, systems engineering developed as an orderly effort to appraise and deal with a complex system of interacting elements that must carry out a predetermined function based on a set of objectives, with measures of performance related directly to those objectives. The following are among the techniques used in systems analysis and engineering that are now being used in social management: decisional analysis, which uses a variety of mathematical and logical means to solve problems; simulation and modeling, which range from informal models to formal ones that are fully computerized; and forecasting, which was originally oriented in the military toward threat analysis of a potential enemy's technological capabilities.

During the early 1960s when weapons systems had become increasingly complicated and costly, systems planning moved ahead significantly when the then Secretary of Defense Robert McNamara joined Taylor as a prophet of technology. McNamara created an Office of Deputy Assistant for Systems Analysis to introduce a new way to assess costs and choices in relation to strategy.

The planning-programming-budgeting system (PPBS) developed by the Rand Corporation replaced the line-item budget in the Department of Defense. The main objective was to assess the usefulness of different weapons systems in different kinds of programs and under different strategic choices or "scenarios." To find the cost of any weapons system and ultimately the cost of any scenario, military functions, men, equipment, and installations were grouped into common "outputs" or "functional" programs. In the end, the effectiveness of each output could be measured as a whole and related to national security. What is often referred to as "the McNamara revolution" of 1960–65 presumably represented a rationalization of government structure that used a full array of the techniques of systems management.[7]

SUCCESS AND FAILURE

Systems approaches have spread with epidemic rapidity and are now widely used in "software" types of programs (those dealing with services and people) as well as "hardware" types (those focusing on materials). It is particularly in the latter that inventory control, product flow, allocation, and scheduling have been successful. With these techniques, plus those of applied probability theory, queuing theory, and network analysis, useful solutions have been found for handling such problems as court schedules, police deployment, air traffic control, control of blood inventories, and allocation of urban fire and ambulance services.[8] In these instances the preconditions that made for success were a clear goal, a high degree of consensus, a relatively unified system, and a command type of organization.

In the extremely complex problems of management, the most stunning success has probably been the application of advanced systems design to the program of the National Aeronautics and Space Administration (NASA), which successfully integrated a great variety of people doing many different things in widely separated places. Management of the projects was an enormously difficult problem, but the program itself dealt with hardware, and compared to public welfare or educational programs there were relatively few political complexities. Space was no one's territory and NASA was a closed loop, setting its own schedule, designing its own hardware, then using the gear it designed to put men on the moon. NASA was both sponsor and user.

It is worth digging further into the effectiveness of engineering solutions for solving management problems on their own grounds, not in the social arena. There is an impressive list of failures. Probably the grandest was in the Department of Defense. There, after twelve years of "big systems management," analysis of cost effectiveness, and PPBS, not a single weapons system was delivered on time. Finally, after enormous waste, countless errors, great inefficiency, and billions of dollars in cost overruns, the General Accounting Office recommended in March 1973 that Congress and the secretary of defense strengthen their ability to determine precisely what the military need for weapons was, what they wanted each weapons system to do to meet that need, and how much was to be spent for it. One month later the post of assistant secretary of defense for systems analysis was abolished.

SYSTEMS MANAGEMENT AND PEOPLE

In practical terms systems management has fallen far short of its promises. Incontestably, abstract models and blueprints for efficient management can be built up out of systems engineering, mathematics, and economics, but neither organizations nor people automatically obey the "laws of efficiency." What then is the solution? Should one create systems that establish the priority of models based on economics and engineering, build in elaborate monitoring systems to insure that people will be subservient to rules and conform to the abstract model? That is the logical end of the input-output approach.

The systems analyst sees various kinds of resources (people, money, and the like) put into an organization, and out of the organization rolls some kind of "product"—for instance, a weapons system, trainees, students, or welfare recipients. The aim is to manage the input so that the outcome will be in the desired amount and of maximum quality.[9] The affinity with Taylorism is obvious. In fact, the techniques used in input-output analysis are largely those derived from the management of industrial processes— techniques that involve well-structured, routine, and repetitive processes.

Intellectually, input-output analysis also links with Taylorism. Both stress the impersonality of measurement. In both, human beings recede from view because they are seen as mere "cogs in the machine." The factory system and the assembly line are recreated as the conceptual ideal for all other organizations, and they reduce everything and everyone to raw material, product, input, and output.

This new managerial world view is extending its hegemony in education, health planning, the social services, and urban planning. To Enarson, Ohio State University president, the view of the university as a production unit in the knowledge industry—a specialized factory in processing human beings for strictly utilitarian ends—is a kind of "tempting heresy loose in the land." He explains this view as follows:

To the new managers the university is just another large system. It has raw material (students), a labor force (faculty and support personnel), instruments of production (classrooms, laboratories, libraries), a production schedule (academic requirements, classes admitted, and classes graduated), management (the trustees and central administration), and a production index (the cost of producing a student credit hour).[10]

In the human services the mental structure of domination and dehumanization is also running rampant, and service organizations are now thought of as "people-processing organizations." For example, Rubell, a former assistant secretary of defense and later a senior vice-president of Litton Industries, which helped plan the War on Poverty, proposed that the task of designing and running Job Corps training centers should be given to the large corporations that had designed and managed some of the most complex weapons systems for the Department of Defense. Said Rubell:

I think of the Job Corps as a complex transforming machine with many internal parts. The input—the material—that is fed into this machine is people. The output is people. It is the function of this machine to transform these people.[11]

SYSTEMS CONSULTATION

A former director of Allied Chemical Corporation, hired as assistant com-missioner of welfare for New York City, expressed the following similar view:

I visualize the department as a big paper factory. You put the client on the con-veyor belt at the beginning, and she gets off the other end with a check or some other kind of service.[12]

Engineers and business administration majors—persons concerned with productivity, time studies, utilization rates, and cost-benefit analysis—were also hired for the city's welfare department.

State departments of public welfare, which have been under pressure to reorganize, have been especially vulnerable to the lure of systems manage-ment and the efficiency experts. One of the larger consulting firms provides advice and studies for both HEW and various states. This firm is critical of the lack of standardized and measurable output and has introduced the concept of the assembly line to standardize and routinize behavior; ulti-mately habits will replace human judgments.[13]

The American Public Welfare Association (APWA), which provides similar consultation to states, also offers the "one best way" to organize, proposing a type of organization that depends on hierarchical authority and detailed specifications to machine-tool behavior. APWA explains its position as follows:

A smooth working organization . . . requires precise specification of authority and responsibility with a single source of authority and defined responsibility for each position in the agency. Otherwise, disorganization, confusion, and irre-sponsibility result. . . . Job descriptions must carry the appropriate and precise descriptions for each position.[14]

Emulating Taylor's scientific management, this new rationality in public welfare is based on specifying in minute detail what is to be done, how it is to be done, by whom, and the time allowed. The standard tools of input-output analysis are applied to the entire work-flow and the movement of clients through the system. By first charting this flow and all contingencies, the aim is to develop an integrated work-flow system and to arrange the parts, that is, people, for optimal efficiency.

Each job is broken down into the smallest possible components. Elabo-rate staffing tables are designed that include detailed job descriptions speci-fying every detail of the task to be performed.

The designers add new job designations such as entry service programmer and master service programmer. They also add new functions such as client processing, client programming, service inventory management, and more. A whole picture of carefully planned, allocated maangement—involving work-flow diagrams, elaborate job descriptions, organization charts, span of control (the specification of the number of supervisees per supervisor), the scalar principle (nonoverlapping and vertical authority system), plus computerized management information systems to monitor clients and workers—provides a stunning illusion of a rationally designed organization.[15]

HISTORY REPEATED

It is trite but nonetheless true that those who do not know history are often fated to repeat it. The "one best" organization carries the seeds of its own negation, yet its seeming rationality—together with its misleading impression of efficiency—generates an almost irresistible momentum.

The history of this form of organization is that overlapping areas of authority multiply and specializations proliferate. As they do, middle-management and white-collar levels grow, the complexities of staff relationships increase, coordination becomes more difficult, and so-called rational controls spawn more controls. Ultimately, the organization becomes mired in its own procedural specifications. A host of bureaucratic ills emerge: zealous preoccupation with rules and red tape, slowness and inefficiency, alienation, depersonalization of relationships, inflexibility, difficulty in dealing with exceptional cases, and smothered creativity. The organization is more intractable than ever.

What is the next step? One possibility is to end the quest for the engineer's rationality. The opposite is what is happening: when existing controls do not work, more are added, right down to the finely tuned ones that monitor behavior continuously. The technology for this development is already available in high-speed information systems that electronically store, process, and retrieve all kinds of personal and social data.

Now called "management information systems," data banks for overseeing human behavior are spreading rapidly. The city of Chattanooga gives the clue to this development. There the computer is used to develop client-agency service plans and the mayor applauds the city's Office of Evaluation and Management headed by a former inspector general of the Strategic Air Command. This office receives daily reports. As the mayor states:

These reports are issued in the format each administrator specifies and can include a detailed analysis of staff activities by hour and/or day and/or event and/or counseling session, etc.[16]

In a variety of contexts and under the mantle of rational planning, government agencies, information specialists, and companies that merchandise computer hardware systems are proliferating a vast telecommunications network whose transmissions crisscross the country every day. The Office of

Education, for example, funded a national data bank in Arkansas to gather educational and medical data about migrant workers' children. The objective was worthwhile, but a lack of careful planning permitted hearsay evaluations from psychologists, social workers, physicians, and teachers. Nor did the project set limits on who would have access to the data. The LEAA Project SEARCH (System for Electronic Analysis and Retrieval of Criminal Histories) has been the prototype for a National Criminal Information Center hooking together federal, state, and local data banks that in ten years could contain an estimated 22 million entries. But as one scenario puts it, "No decent American should fear monitoring."

INVASION OF SOCIAL SCIENCES

The sprawling, complex, difficult-to-manage welfare state has made many organizations and professionals vulnerable to the efficiency expert. His invasion of the social sciences began in the upper reaches of the federal government during the mid-1960s when the defense industry was in an economic slump and unemployment among engineers was mounting. The aerospace industry, seeking other growth markets, looked toward health care, child care, poverty, urban planning, education, consultation, and the like. Geneen, president of International Telephone and Telegraph Corporation (ITT), claimed conscience as well as competence in the following statement:

Now some of you may wonder why a major, profit-making corporation like ITT wants to join the war on poverty. . . . We, in industry, owe it to our society to use our resources to cure a social ill. . . . We, in industry, have the capital, the manpower, the skills, the technology . . . to get the job done.[17]

The aerospace industry enlisted in the War on Poverty, and Shriver, first director of the Office of Economic Opportunity (OEO), declared that the "advanced training methods developed by business in shooting wars are needed just as much in this new war on poverty." Former Defense Secretary Clifford presented his viewpoint as follows to the National Security Industrial Association:

I believe that we in the Department of Defense have not only a moral obligation but an opportunity to contribute far more to the social needs of our country than we have ever done before. . . . We now have a military-industrial team with unique resources of experience, engineering talent, management and problem-solving capacities, a team that must be used to help find the answers to complex domestic problems as it has found the answers to complex weapons systems.[18]

The skills and the world-view of the military-industrial complex spread rapidly. Almost hypnotically the civilian sector absorbed the counterfeit cheer word "systems" as systems analysts from the aerospace-defense-think-tank complex moved into civilian government to oversee the research and development programs of HEW, HUD, and OEO. Gorham, who made the complete circuit from the Department of Defense to HEW to The Urban Institute put it thus:

For some decades we have been providing the money and manpower to deal with the problems, for instance, of education and transportation. We put these inputs, figuratively, into a little black box, representing our society and its processes—trusting that the results would pop out the other side. Well, they did not. The results have been less than we expected.[19]

SHORTCOMINGS OF PPBS

In 1965, President Johnson hailed a revolution in government when he introduced PPBS to civilian government and transferred personnel from the Department of Defense to that sector.[20] Intellectually, PPBS is a triumph of logic and economic rationality. In practice, it improved the operations of the government system slightly, but in relation to the lofty expectations, it must be judged a failure. In the few agencies where program budgeting was seriously tried, notably HEW and OEO, the system helped decision-makers somewhat to explore costs, consequences, and alternatives, but the program budget did not affect either the allocation or the amount of money appropriated for the antipoverty program any year.

There are several reasons why economizing control processes failed in civilian government. First, civilian government faces far-flung and seemingly intractable problems embedded within a labyrinth.

Second, political processes are a necessary part of the system. This is especially true of budgetary decisions that emerge out of competing interests and the juggling of constituencies. To the systems analysts and efficiency experts, political bargaining and compromise are irrational encumbrances. As Churchman, a foremost systems analyst acknowledges, "It goes without saying that our management scientist is antipolitical, simply because so much of politics thwarts the rationality of his designs."[21]

Among others, Grosse, an analyst of national security problems in the Department of Defense, who became assistant secretary for programs systems for HEW, sought to utilize operations or systems analysis in the planning process and in budgeting decisions. Undercutting the political process by moulding it to systems designs, Grosse discovered that most bureau heads and program managers were not sympathetic to operations research and systems analysis. To Grosse, the political process debased rationality, and he looked at it as "people scheming to get more money for particular programs."[22]

"Better Management, Better Results," says a United Way of America pamphlet lauding PPBS, scientific management, the Rand Corporation, and the Department of Defense.[23] But at the federal level, PPBS and its allied tool of cost-benefit analysis are dead. They were too awkward because their goals, subgoals, programs, subcategories, and specific measures of output at each level inflicted masses of paper work of dubious value. Beyond that, applying them required a vast network of organizational controls, a superordinate management system, detailed specifications of objectives and how to attain them—all cascading downward from federal agencies. These would then be supplemented by regional, state, and municipal plans, cascading further to operating organizations—all hierarchically controlled and coordinated by a flood of new rules and regulations.

THE NEW ORDER

Government of course claims to represent the public interest and hence to have the duty of being a good manager, dispensing public funds so that they mean something and that they pay off. To the extent that management is concerned with measuring payoff it is neutral. But can government be neutral? Here is the heart of the tension between the managerial technician and the politician.

To the efficiency expert one organization is like another and government is merely an enterprise that ought to function properly. As the efficiency expert assumes an ever growing role, radical transformation of the political perspective is inevitable. Still it would be a mistake to assume that competing interests have been wiped out by management techniques and measurements. Political interests remain, but they come forward disguised as neutral and beyond politics, as if all that remained were technical problems and technical solutions. Such an illusion springs from numerous sources, not the least of them the academics. As Dahl and Lindblom noted some twenty years ago:

Whether the rapidity of innovation in new techniques of control is or is not the greatest political revolution of our times, techniques and not "isms" are the kernel of rational social action in the western world. Both socialism and capitalism are dead . . . policy in any case is technique minded.[24]

If the illusion is perpetuated by academics, technicians, and social workers, it is also carefully nourished by some politicians, who are themselves vulnerable to the myth. Few presidents have had as much faith in the efficiency of the techniques of modern management as did Nixon. His 1970 message on the reorganization of the government expressed that faith as follows: "The Domestic Council will be primarily concerned with *what* we do; the Office of Management and Budget will be concerned with *how* we do it, and *how well* we do it."[25] The executive branch became an exemplification of the tightly organized, hierarchical, chain-of-command organization.

Today the emphasis throughout government is on measuring, quantifying, and analyzing output. Management by Objectives (MBO)—a system for monitoring performance under which agencies establish their priorities and targets and report their achievements in quantified terms—is substituting for PPBS.

But neither at the federal level nor the local level is the tight chain-of-command organization or the factory model appropriate for all organizations, especially not for those in the human services. Despite this, there is an apparently relentless emphasis on technical and economic efficiency. It is assumed that this will be achieved by tightening management controls, stressing authority and hierarchical relationships, increasing specialization, and using computerized programs more extensively.

REASONS FOR WIDE APPEAL

But, if this trend carries its own negation, how and why does it have such an irresistible momentum? Among the reasons why total administration has wide appeal are these:

• The size and complexity of the social welfare structure demands some form of control and wise use of resources.

• Social processes for making decisions, planning, setting priorities, allocating resources, and choosing among alternative uses of funds are extraordinarily difficult because of the discordant preference patterns and needs in our highly pluralistic society.

• There is no single, simple way to order preferences for making social choices and for economizing.

Since such aid is lacking, economic models and engineering blueprints that purport to represent rationality and efficiency are introduced. These, in turn, create even more complexity and more controls.

Of course systems blueprints and models have no intrinsic power to compel men to obedience. But men can be made obedient. When the human factor is cancelled out and the concept of a person as a responsible agent of decision is expunged, capitulation to the blueprint follows.

Earlier, when technique was in fact represented by the machine, it was possible, as Ellul observes, to speak of "man *and* the machine." Then man could have an independent position apart from the machine.[26] Now technique progressively absorbs man. The administration of systems becomes the administration of things until man becomes a thing, an object or a component, and ultimately disappears as man. Social and health services are provided through delivery systems (a military metaphor). People are no longer people but targets, target populations, inputs, outputs, raw materials, and products.

Total administration is entrenching itself at the intersections of social structure, culture, and thought. And the fiction that techniques are neutral has reduced resistance to an evolving partnership between certain technology-intensive sectors of society—that is, multinational corporations, the aerospace-electronics industry, and computer-telecommunications firms, plus think-tanks and a phalanx of management consulting enterprises. Thus, besides increasing governmental intervention in education, health, social welfare, housing, law enforcement, and crime prevention, there is now increasing corporate intervention operating under the auspices of government. A new element has thereby been added to the administration of the advanced welfare state: the state has moved to underwrite and safeguard the private sector, first in the military-industrial sphere, now in the spheres of social welfare and urban problems.

The system begins to consolidate into a new form of collectivism, one not premised on the search for interdependence, the public interest, or genuine community, but one that subjugates the person under the new order of control and efficiency. An overarching complex seems to be in the making that is gaining power to administer society. The old words *despotism* and *totalitarianism* do not quite fit. Over a century ago de Tocqueville anticipated and thus described its effect on man as follows:

The will of man is not shattered, but softened, bent and guided. . . . Such a power does not destroy, but it prevents existence; it does not tyrannize, but it compresses, enervates, extinguishes, and stupifies a people, till each nation is reduced to nothing better than a flock of timid and industrious animals, of which the government is the shepherd.[27]

COUNTERACTION

In a turbulent world people tend to assume that systems using engineering approaches, tightly managed components, and highly impersonal techniques of efficiency will mechanically produce results. Thus they try to make behavioral programs more and more complete and to specify rules for all possible contingencies. Such systems, besides being dehumanizing, are rigid, inefficient, and change resistant. Rules are paramount.[28]

What would have to be done to revive the creative possibilities of organizational life? A central task is to begin thinking of systems in less mechanical and more organic terms. It is crucially important to devise effective processes whereby large-scale organizational decisions flow downward uninterruptedly and are in accord with group and individual preferences. Conversely, more effective means must be developed by which individual and small-group decisions build up to more satisfactory large-scale decisions.

To achieve these ends is a major task. It requires that the "one best way" to organize be scrapped in favor of open interdependencies. Processes that support creative group effort would be promoted. In effect, organizations would have to be permanently unfrozen. Task- and mission-oriented groups would develop in response to problems. Widespread sharing of power would replace authority-obedience relationships. Skills in the equalization of power, open communication, and resolution of conflict would replace formalized solutions of organizational problems.

No doubt, elements of hierarchy would remain, but organic flux with authority rotating according to mission would replace bureaucracy. Jobs would be adapted to the needs of those who performed them, rather than having people plugged into ready-made positions or shaped according to abstract principles of specialization, differentiation of labor, and economic efficiency. The system of mistrust—with subordination to rules and programs—would be replaced by the incentives that typically induce people to contribute their best efforts: loyalty, a sense of responsibility, search for the common good. Human factors would be prominent. Efficiency and good human relationships would not be regarded as separate and contradictory features of organizational life.

SOCIETAL CHANGE

At a societal level, social planners and policy-makers face similar problems, only on a much grander and more difficult scale. What is needed are social processes for planning and setting priorities. Technical program evaluation and considerations of economic efficiency must be coupled with rather than supplant citizen preferences. In our highly pluralistic society the problem is extraordinarily complicated. But it comes down to this choice: try to reform the present structures and renew the quest for more democratic forms; or abandon the search, accept the decomposition of community, and adopt engineered institutions for the achievement of control and uniformity.

A first step in refurbishing a democratic welfare state is to rescue the concept of accountability from the narrow confines of audits and counts. No matter how sophisticated they are, techniques like PPBS and MBO are simply devices for internal reckoning. Accountability in the larger sense involves the government's reckoning with the people, the organization's reckoning with the community. If social planners neglect this broader view, they will aggravate social atomization, public cynicism, and mistrust, which in turn will trigger more monitoring and more control. Thus the crux of the issue is to create community within pluralism and to restore the prerogatives of the people by reviving the political concept of accountability as distinct from the corporatist concept of efficiency.

Also, it is possible to use the newer social techniques and systems to *benefit* rather than to dehumanize man. Take for example, management information systems. Only the public's enfeeblement and its conquest by technocrats prevents the turnabout of technological controls.

Why not use high-speed telecommunications systems to give citizens the best available information about the way social institutions perform? Or is that information exclusively for the managers?

Why not devise dialogue models of planning, using the best available technology, that will provide guidelines for citizens to work with systems planners, social scientists, social work practitioners, engineers, and managers? Data gathering, data transmission, cable television, and other technical processes could surely be useful. Techniques like these could even bring meetings for public decision-making into the living room with direct citizen vote.

The possibilities for a stronger public and an informed citizenry beckon invitingly. If such opportunities are not seized, the likelihood is continued enervation of the people and then gradual envelopment in a smooth, banal tyranny that conquers not through whips and wages, but through total administration and forms of corporatist-statist oppression as yet foreseen only in imaginary technological nightmares.

NOTES

1. For contrasting views, *see* B. F. Skinner, *Beyond Freedom and Dignity* (New York: Alfred A. Knopf, 1971); Robert A. Dahl and Charles E. Lindblom, *Politics, Economics and Welfare* (New York: Harper & Row, 1956); Seymour Martin Lipset, *Political Man* (New York: Doubleday & Co., 1959); Jacques Ellul, *The Technological Society* (New York: Random House, 1964); Herbert Marcuse, *One Dimensional Man: Studies in the Ideology of Advanced Industrial Society* (Boston: Beacon Press, 1968); Jay W. Forrester, *Urban Dynamics* (Cambridge, Mass.: MIT Press, 1969); Roland N. McKean, *Efficiency in Government Through Systems Analysis* (New York: John Wiley & Sons, 1958); and Robert Boguslaw, *The New Utopians* (Englewood Cliffs, N.J.: Prentice-Hall, 1965).
2. Thorsten Veblen, *The Engineers and the Price System* (Clifton, N.J.: Augustus M. Kelley, Publishers, 1921); John K. Galbraith, *The New Industrial State* (2d rev. ed.; Boston: Houghton Mifflin Co., 1972); and Daniel Bell, *The Coming of Post-Industrial Society* (New York: Basic Books, 1973).
3. Lawrence E. Lessing, "Systems Engineering Invades the City," *Fortune*, 77 (January 1968), pp. 155–157, 217–222.
4. *See* James A. Kalish, "Flim-Flam, Double-Talk and Hustle: The Urban Problems Industry," *Washington Monthly*, 1 (November 1969), pp. 6–16.
5. Frederick W. Taylor, *Scientific Management* (New York: Harper & Bros., 1911), p. 59.
6. R. E. Callahan, *Education and the Cult of Efficiency* (Chicago: University of Chicago Press, 1962), esp. pp. 42–64.
7. *See* Charles Hitch and Ronald McKean, *The Economics of Defense in a Nuclear Age* (Washington, D.C.: Howard University Press, 1963); Robert McNamara, C. Hitch, and A. Enthoven, *A Modern Design for Defense Decision* (Washington, D.C.: Industrial College of the Armed Forces, 1966); E. S. Quade, "Some Comments on Cost-Effectiveness," paper presented at the Operations Research Symposium, Redstone Arsenal, Huntsville, Alabama, March 1965; and Quade, "Systems Analysis Techniques for Planning-Programming-Budgeting" (Santa Monica, Calif.: Rand Corporation, March 1966).

8. *See* Edward H. Blum, "The New York City Fire Project," Keith A. Stevenson, "Emergency Ambulance Transportation," Richard C. Larson, "Improving the Effectiveness of New York City's 911," Jan M. Chaiken and Richard C. Larson, "Methods for Allocating Urban Emergency Units," and John B. Jennings, "Blood Bank Inventory Control" in Alvin W. Drake et al., eds., *Analysis of Public Systems* (Cambridge, Mass.: MIT Press, 1972).

9. C. West Churchman, *The Systems Approach* (New York: Dell Publishing Co., 1968), esp. chap. 5.

10. Harold L. Enarson, "University or Knowledge Factory?" *Science,* 181 (September 7, 1972), p. 897.

11. John H. Rubell, quoted in Samuel Yette, *The Choice* (New York: G. P. Putnam's Sons, 1971), p. 47.

12. Joseph Lelyveld, "City's New View of Welfare: A Job for Businessmen," *New York Times* (February 1, 1972), p. 16.

13. Booze, Allen and Hamilton, *Purchase of Social Service: Study of the Experience of Three States in Purchase of Service by Contract Under the Provisions of the 1967 Amendments of the Social Security Act* (Washington, D.C.: National Technical Information Service, U.S. Department of Commerce, January 29, 1971).

14. *Detailed Design of a Social Service Delivery System for the Bureau of Social Welfare, Department of Health and Welfare, State of Maine* (Chicago: Technical Assistance Project, American Public Welfare Association, July 1970), p. II-1.

15. For typical examples, *see* ibid. *See also Michigan Department of Social Services Delivery System Design and Implementation Requirements Workbook,* January 1973. For an overall perspective on the formal model, *see* Jack C. Bloedorn et al., *Designing Social Service Systems* (Chicago: American Public Welfare Association, 1970).

16. Robert Kirk Walter, "Chattanooga Develops a Better Way Through the Human Service Maze," *Nation's Cities* (February 1973), p. 10.

17. Harold Geneen, president of International Telephone and Telegraph Corporation, as quoted in John McHale, "Big Business Enlists for the War on Poverty," *Transaction,* 4 (May/June 1965), p. 5.

18. Speech of Clark Clifford, former secretary of defense, reprinted in *Congressional Record,* October 3, 1968.

19. William Gorham, as quoted in Paul Dickson, *Think Tanks* (New York: Ballantine Books, 1971), pp. 232–233.

20. Executive Office of the President, *Bureau of the Budget, Bulletin No. 66–3,* October 12, 1965, and *Supplement to Bulletin No. 66–3,* February 21, 1966 (Washington, D.C.: U.S. Government Printing Office).

21. Churchman, op. cit., p. 43.

22. Robert N. Grosse. "Analysis in Health Planning," in Drake et al., eds., op. cit., p. 403.

23. A *"PPBS" Approach to Budgeting Human Service Programs for United Ways* (Alexandria, Va.: United Way of America, 1972), p. 1.

24. Dahl and Lindblom, op. cit., p. 16.

25. President Nixon quoted in John Walsh, "Office of Management and Budget: New Accent on the 'M' in OMB," *Science,* 18 (January 25, 1974), p. 286.

26. Ellul, op. cit., p. 6.

27. Alexis de Tocqueville, *Democracy in America,* Vol. 2 (New York: Vintage Books, 1957), p. 337.

28. *See* Jerald Hage and Michael Aiken, *Social Change in Complex Organizations* (New York: Random House, 1970); Tom Burns and G. M. Stalker, *The Management of Innovation* (London, England: Tavistock Publications, 1961); Michael Crozier, *The Bureaucratic Phenomenon* (London, England: Tavistock Publications, 1964).

Part VI

ADMINISTERING SOCIAL SERVICE PERSONNEL

EDITOR'S INTRODUCTION

Both the organization and deployment of personnel inevitably reflect the technology and content of service. The selections in this section deal mainly with some of the distinctive aspects of administering social service personnel. Important changes have taken place in recent years in the classification, utilization, and training of social service manpower.

For years the Master of Social Work was considered both the entry and terminal degree for professional practice. After considerable debate and discussion in and out of the professional association, in 1969 the National Association of Social Workers admitted graduates of recognized undergraduate programs into membership. This action precipitated a series of other events. Two years later the Council on Social Work Education's national committee on the length of graduate education approved advanced credit of up to one year toward the MSW degree for such graduates, but held to the two-year requirement for the degree. It followed quite naturally that the baccalaureate social work degree would become fully accepted as an entry-level preparation for practice, monitored now by the national accrediting body. Standards for accreditation of the BSW were developed and became effective on July 1, 1974. Currently there are over 200 undergraduate programs that have been certified, about two-and-a-half times as many as accredited graduate programs.

Paralleling these developments, numerous junior and community college programs were established for the preparation of social work and human service technicians. Graduates of these programs went to such positions as houseparents, child-care workers, mental health assistants, teacher aides, social service aides, and the like.

A. SOCIAL SERVICE MANPOWER

Thus, in a relatively short period of time, a new and substantial reservoir of trained social and human service manpower appeared. It was natural for social workers to direct their attention to the utilization of this many-layered personnel. The first selection in this section was prepared by a committee of the National Association of Social Workers in 1973, and represents the profession's approach to the setting of standards for social service manpower. It specifies a six-level classification of manpower, the functions properly performed at each level, and the qualifications each requires. The document forthrightly addresses issues concerned with the differential use of manpower, and lays the basis for subsequent developments which will surely come as practitioners and agencies test these guidelines and experiment with their uses.

In his critique of the manpower document, Briggs raises questions about its cogency, coherence, and utility for the profession. As an early pioneer in identifying the importance of using persons with different academic and experience preparation in the delivery of services, he supports the intent of the document as pursuing a legitimate manpower strategy. In his view, however, the categories are too severely and rigidly bounded, equate competence with achievement of academic degrees, and reflect professional rather than client interests. He does not think that, at this stage in the development of the state of the art, enough is known to codify an adequate classification scheme. A series of tasks remain before a more useful schema can effectively be produced, and these Briggs specifies. They call for changes in the profession, and considerably more attention paid to a variety of routes to the production of competent social practitioners.

Slavin and Perlmutter present a conceptual scheme for looking at the differential use of social work manpower and construct a model for education and training consistent with this approach. They differentiate professional from preprofessional roles, tasks, and knowledge, and present a case illustration of a preprofessional training program of great effectiveness in child care. The critical variables that define the hierarchy of practice task-roles are seen as complexity, autonomy, and uncertainty, which in combination determine the requirements for different levels of skill and training.

B. PERSONNEL PRACTICES

As the professional association in the field, the National Association of Social Workers was from its inception concerned with developing acceptable standards for professional practice. Successive statements of desirable personnel practices appeared through the years, the current document having been adopted in 1971. The assumptions behind these activities were that qualified staff was essential for the effective delivery of social services, and that personnel performed most adequately when they worked under favorable conditions of employment. From time to time new standards have been added and traditional practices upgraded. The document that follows covers a multitude of circumstances and contingencies, and represents a fairly exhaustive listing of significant considerations affecting the working environment of practitioners. The statements included in the standards represent guidelines for the development of personnel policies of social agencies that employ social workers. A quick reading will suggest the similarity between items included in the *Standards* and those that tend to appear in union contracts.

Having established these standards of personnel practices, the profession now has a well-defined procedure for dealing with violations of the stated practices. These are incorporated in the NASW "Procedures for Adjudication of Grievances," according to which professional practitioners who feel aggrieved because of substantial defiance of proper personnel practices can seek relief.

While not intended as an elaboration of the essential characteristics of the personnel process generic to all employing organizations, the standards deal briefly with the following:

- Selection of personnel
- Induction and orientation
- Supervision
- Training
- Evaluation
- Termination

C. AFFIRMATIVE ACTION

An increasingly important consideration in the administration of personnel concerns the ways in which affirmative action requirements are met by social agencies. This is particularly true where public resources are made available for social programs. Objectives of equal opportunity in employment are mandated by statutes and administrative regulations, and organizations are required to adhere to designated standards and procedures.

Few issues in personnel management have engendered as much discussion and anxiety as affirmative action policies, and few have occasioned more political activity and public debate. Most recently, issues defined as reverse discrimination have come to the fore as goals and timetables for action have been implemented. The policy context of equality of opportunity versus equality of results is frequently at the heart of the controversy.

Buttrick reviews the legislative history of affirmative action and examines the relationship between efforts to guarantee equal employment opportunity, unionization, and seniority. A social economy of contradiction and scarcity exacerbates competition between minority and majority and poses severe problems in achieving intergroup parity. Policy issues and dilemmas are identified and partial solutions suggested in what is surely to become an increasing preoccupation of even-handed administration.

Lovall deals with three issues that surround some of the controversial areas of affirmative action. She indicates why she feels that preferential hiring, active antidiscrimination efforts, and the reexamination of conventional quality standards and measures are necessary to overcome the apparent exclusion of women and minorities from many areas of professional employment, and particularly in advanced positions of authority.

D. LABOR RELATIONS IN SOCIAL AGENCIES

Social workers have been organized in labor unions for more than four decades. The history of this movement is dotted with conflict both within professional ranks and between workers and employers. Questions have periodically been raised about the applicability of the industrial model of unionism to social service institutions. Similarly, ethical considerations have been directed to the right to strike, particularly where matters of safety and client survival were at stake.

The profession has rather consistently maintained a policy of support for the right of employees to bargain collectively through instruments of their own choice. The *Standards for Social Work Personnel Practices of NASW* clearly states that participation in a strike "does not in itself constitute a violation of the Code of Ethics," and that the professional association "is opposed to laws or policies that prohibit strikes by employees." When a strike cannot be prevented, both management and the union are urged to staff essential services to avert threats to life and safety.

Tambor presents a case illustration of the impact of union organization on voluntary agencies in a major American city. He shows how existing power relationships can be realigned and how this could lead to new policy directions and initiatives through including new elements in agency decision-making. At the same time, budgeting and planning procedures are modified because external influences make themselves felt on existing internal relationships. Agreements to increase personnel costs can serve to limit the agency's capacity to provide services, given constant resources at its command. Alternatively, this provides pressure on agency and funding sources to broaden their appeals. The process of establishing greater financial rewards for professional services should in the long run have the effect of bringing into the service better qualified personnel.

From the perspective of a medical social service department director, Shulman looks at the background of labor organization in hospitals. He assays the compatability of professionalization and unionization; the contradiction between professional norms which serve client interests and union norms which further member interests; the move to participatory management and the place of powerlessness as a basic motivating force for collective action. Shulman suggests that the existence of a union contract in an agency creates a new structure and environment for the social work administrator. This creates a fundamental dilemma: How to extend participation in significant areas of decision without eroding authority. Dealing with the dilemma establishes an important arena for the development of administrative skill.

Hush reflects on the impact of unionization on the voluntary agency, and explores dilemmas and issues inevitably faced by administrator, board of directors, and staff. He makes the case for increased understanding of the full meaning of a union contract by all parties to the collective bargain, and concludes that the process of competent bargaining can bring benefits to clients and to the community.

A. SOCIAL SERVICE MANPOWER

31/STANDARDS FOR
SOCIAL SERVICE MANPOWER

NATIONAL ASSOCIATION OF SOCIAL WORKERS

The social work profession exists to provide humane and effective social services to individuals, families, groups, communities, and society so that social functioning may be enhanced and the quality of life improved. It is concerned with and has participated in the development of social services to meet individual and societal needs.

The social services require a variety of personnel with a range of knowledge and skills acquired through organized methods of education and experience. The necessary development and expansion of social services, the increasing complexity of services, the advances in methodology and techniques, the goal of accountability, and other factors have made necessary the rationalization of the social services "industry" and the differential use of manpower.

The Bylaws of the National Association of Social Workers (NASW) states that one of the basic functions of NASW, as the embodiment of the profession, is to "assume responsibility for manpower planning and development for the range of personnel—professional, technical, and supporting—needed in the social services." To fulfill this responsibility, NASW establishes standards for the use of social workers and related social service personnel who provide these services. Further, NASW seeks to apply its standards to social service systems to assure that the manpower is used appropriately so that the quality of service will be high and community needs will be met.

Definition of Social Work

Social work is the profession that requires the special education for providing and is specifically organized to deliver services directed to enhancing the social functioning of people. It is, therefore, the primary profession engaged in and responsible for preparing manpower to provide social services. These standards are based on the following definition of social work, adopted by the NASW Board of Directors in 1970:

Social work is the professional activity of helping individuals, groups, or communities enhance or restore their capacity for social functioning and creating societal conditions favorable to this goal. Social work practice consists of the professional application of social work values, principles, and techniques to one or more of the following ends: helping people obtain tangible services; counseling and psychotherapy with individuals, families, and groups; helping communities or groups provide or improve social and health services; and participating in relevant legislative processes. The practice of social work requires knowledge of human development and behavior; of social, economic, and cultural institutions; and of the interaction of all these factors.

"Social service manpower," as used in these standards, refers to those engaged in aspects of social work practice, which involve helping activities that do not always require specific training or education but are intimately and necessarily related to professional social work and to the accomplishment of social work objectives and services.

Objectives of Standards

These standards are designed to do the following:

1. Identify the general range of functions and tasks required in the delivery of social services.

2. Differentiate the significant requirements for practice at the various levels.

3. Relate requirements for practice to levels of competence, which are determined by experience, training, and education.

4. Establish a classification of professional and preprofessional levels of competence.

5. Encourage the application and use of this classification of social work manpower by agencies and other social service systems.

The classification scheme described in these standards is not a model for any one social service function or agency. It is a description of the various levels of social work manpower that exist in the provision of social services, that should be considered and planned for in making the optimum use of manpower, and that are relevant to planning for career development in the field.

The social work profession operates in such varied settings and carries so many disparate functions that the number of specific job titles is unknown. At the same time, there are identifiable levels of competence, regardless of the specific role, and identifiable means of achieving them. It is the purpose of these standards to establish a basic, universal scale of reference that may be applied to all settings and to which all social work and social service positions may be compared, regardless of the many individual variations of tasks and functions.

A major objective of these standards is to establish a more uniform relationship between the level of functions performed and the level of competence attained by the individual or required by the agency. It is intended that this explicit description of levels of competence will be used by individual social workers, agencies employing social service personnel, institutions training personnel, and others to define and interrelate social work manpower positions more clearly and effectively.

Another major objective of these standards is to clarify the level of educational preparation appropriate to the various levels of social work competence. Although fully appreciative of the validity and significance of life experience as an inherent aspect of the development of social work skills in the individual, NASW is convinced of the necessity for organized, accredited educational achievement as the primary basis for differentiating among levels of competence. Thus the classification plan was developed according to these concepts:

1. Different levels of complexity can be established or identified for the activities within most functions.

2. Qualitative distinctions among the levels of activity in a function require different levels of competence or skill and should be the basis for assigning the classification level.

3. Completion of defined amounts of experience, training, or education is a prerequisite to the assumption by a person of specific levels of functioning.

4. The optimum effectiveness in the provision of most social services requires the use of various levels of competence.

5. Levels of competence are more complex than can be described in a single classification scheme.

SOCIAL WORK CLASSIFICATION PLAN

A classification plan is the organization of positions into groups or classes on the basis of their duties and qualifications for the positions. This social work classification plan identifies six major classes of personnel utilized in the social services—four professional levels and two preprofessional levels—and differentiates the functions and qualifications appropriate for each.

In establishing these broad classes, there was no attempt to analyze any specific job or type of social work function, as should be done by an agency in arriving at an optimum use of manpower to accomplish its specific objectives. This plan is, however, an initial effort to provide a meaningful classification applicable to various staffing patterns.

Levels of Personnel
This classification plan recognizes six levels of competence. There are two preprofessional levels, as follows:
Social service aide. Entry is based on an assessment of the individual's maturity, appropriate life experiences, motivation, and skills required by the specific task or function.
Social service technician. Entry is based on completion of (1) a two-year educational program in one of the social services, usually granting an associate of arts degree, or (2) a baccalaureate degree in another field.
There are four professional levels, as follows:
Social worker. Entry requires a baccalaureate degree from an approved social work program.
Graduate social worker. Entry requires a master's degree from an accredited graduate school of social work.
Certified social worker. Entry requires certification by (1) the Academy of Certified Social Workers (ACSW) as being capable of autonomous, self-directed practice or (2) licensure by the state in which the person practices.
Social work fellow. Entry requires completion of a doctoral program or substantial practice in the field of specialization following certification by ACSW.

Preprofessional social work. The two levels of preprofessional social work practice have distinct levels of competence:
Social service aide. Under professionally guided supervision or as part of a team, the social service aide provides various specified duties to help clients obtain and use social and related services, including obtaining information, providing specific basic information, aiding clients in agency procedures and services, and other supportive functions. The aide classification may cover a variety of specific service-related functions other than social service, but should be integrated with the performance of duties by other social service personnel.

Responsibilities require an ability to communicate freely, to understand and describe program procedures, to interpret the concerns and needs of clients, and to provide defined, concrete assistance with the needs of living. The aide must have knowledge derived from accumulated life experiences paralleling those of the consumer community, a capacity to learn specific skills taught through on-the-job training, and motivation to serve others. The minimum educational requirement for this classification is the ability to read and count, in addition to other individual skills necessary to carry out the tasks of the particular position.

Social service technician. As part of a team or under the direction of and close supervision by a professional social worker, the social service technician performs a wide variety of duties to facilitate the knowledge and use of social services. These involve disseminating information, obtaining information from clients, assisting clients in the use of community resources, obtaining information about assessing the impact and coverage of programs, carrying out specific program activities and tasks, and in other ways applying life experiences and knowledge derived from training in working with individuals or groups.

In carrying out these responsibilities, the social service technician must be able to make inquiries discreetly, provide clear information, understand and describe agency programs, recognize general levels of anxiety or reactions of fear, maintain emotional self-control, retain values, and provide services to assist clients with defined environmental problems.

The technician must have knowledge of the fundamentals of human behavior, specific agency operations, and specific communities and their social service programs and have skills in working with people, including the ability to communicate and empathize, attitudes of respect for individual and group differences, appreciation for the capacity to change, and the ability to use social institutions on behalf of consumers. The educational requirement is an associate of arts degree in a technical program of social services or its equivalent.

Professional social work. The four levels of professional social work practice also have distinct levels of practice and preparation:

Social worker. Under supervision, the social worker is responsible for professional service designed to sustain and encourage the social functioning of individuals or groups. He assists them to appraise their situation, to identify problems and alternative solutions, and to anticipate social and environmental consequences.

The social worker is guided by professional social work values, purposes of the service, prevailing organized knowledge, societal sanctions, and social work methodology. In carrying out his responsibilities, the social worker uses methods of disciplined inquiry based on interpersonal relationships involving cause and effect; interpretation of resources and their limits; intervention with related individuals or groups, colleagues, and other disciplines and organizations; direct counseling and services; and other related activities.

The social worker must have a beginning knowledge of human behavior and development, the social and economic environment, the social service system, and the factors that contribute to normal development and social and individual abnormalities, including symptomatology. He must be able to demonstrate a conscious use of social work methods, for example, skill in the use of specific techniques, such as interviewing, diagnosis, use of self-discipline, and use of social resources. The educational prerequisites for this classification are a baccalaureate degree from an undergraduate college or university with a social welfare program approved by the Council on Social Work Education (CSWE).

Graduate social worker. The graduate social worker is responsible for providing professional, skilled social work services to individuals, groups, or larger social contexts and is capable of providing supervisory assistance to less advanced workers. Although he works under professional supervision, a significant portion of his work activity involves independent judgment and initiative.

The graduate social worker is guided by professional social work values, the purposes of the service involved, accepted theoretical and organized knowledge, societal sanctions, and social work methodology. In providing services, the graduate social worker uses methods appropriate to the situation, including a disciplined interaction based on a knowledge of interpersonal relationships of cause and effect, relevant professional literature and research to obtain necessary additional professional knowledge, the conduct of social research regarding the service or broad professional concerns, the interpretation of community resources and advocacy needed to assure the availablity of resources, intervention with related individuals and organizations, the provision of therapeutic counseling directed toward clear goals, social action to increase awareness and to work toward the resolution of professional concerns, as well as other related activities.

The graduate social worker must have a theoretical and a beginning empirical knowledge of human behavior and development, a working understanding of social and economic realities and forces, a critical knowledge of social service systems, a familiarity with the nature and causation of individual and social abnormalities, and an awareness of relevant community and professional organizations and related institutions. He must have demonstrated competence in at least one of the specialized social work methods and a knowledge of others. The educational prerequisite for this classification is the master's of social work degree from a graduate school of social work accredited by CSWE.

Certified social worker. The certified social worker is responsible for a wide range of independent social work activities requiring individual accountability for the outcome of service, including direct services to individuals, groups, or organizations; supervision of social workers and social service technicians; consultation at key points of decision-making in the social services; interdisciplinary coordination; education and in-service training; improvement and development of services; and other activities requiring sensitivity and expert judgment.

Guided by the values of professional social work, purposes of the service, prevailing organized knowledge, societal sanctions, and social work methodology, the certified social worker uses methods of basic social research and planning, interpersonal therapeutic techniques, group and social organizational relationships, education and administration, and others as required by the clients or groups served.

The certified social worker must have both theoretical and empirical knowledge of human behavior and development and be familiar with the social and economic processes, the philosophy and operations of social services systems, the nature and causation of individual and social abnormalities, and the different relationships and responsibilities of professions, organizations, and societal institutions. The educational prerequisites for this classification are a master's degree from a graduate school of social work accredited by CSWE and certification by the ACSW as being capable of autonomous, self-directed practice.

Social work fellow. The social work fellow is capable of a wide range of independent social work activities requiring individual accountability for the outcome of service and special expertise in intensive services to individuals, groups, and organizations; administration and direction of programs and organizations; specialized consultation, planning, education, and decision-making; and other activities requiring special combinations of education and experience. Having mastered the integration of social work values, the delineation of the purposes and policies of service, the integration of organized knowledge and practice, the testing of societal sanctions, and the incorporation of social work methodology, the social work fellow utilizes combinations of knowledge and skills in the following areas:

1. The direction and conduct of major research and planning efforts.
2. The application and extension of interpersonal therapeutic techniques.
3. The study and implementation of the objectives of groups or social organizations.
4. The expansion of educational and administrative theory and practice.
5. Other specialized endeavors based on social work expertise.

The social work fellow is required to have a broad knowledge of the field, with concentrations in specific areas. These areas include advanced knowledge of theories of and research in human behavior and development; the social and economic processes and their interrelationships; the nature and causation of individual and social abnormalities, and the planning of services involving the integration of professional, organization, and institutional activities. In addition, he provides leadership in the planning, development and administration of social service agencies; analysis and formulation of social policy; research and the evaluation of social service delivery systems; advanced clinical practice, and education for social service.

The educational prerequisite for this classification is (1) a doctoral degree in social work or a related social science discipline, with at least two years of experience in an area of social work specialization, or (2) certification by ACSW and two years of experience in an area of social work specialization.

GUIDELINES

These standards have been prepared by NASW to provide a basis on which local and state NASW bodies, educators of social service manpower, administrators planning for or employing social workers, personnel specialists, and individual social workers may evaluate job classifications for social work and social service personnel.

Such evaluations should have two objectives: (1) to assure that classifications of existing job functions are related to the appropriate level of competence and educational preparation and (2) to clarify and strengthen relationships among job classifications actually used to maximize the career potential in a setting or organization.

It is important to restate that the simple classification plan provided in these standards is not a substitute for the detailed and rational analysis of specific tasks required to establish accurately and professionally a staffing plan for social work manpower in an agency. It should, however, provide a means by which various staffing plans can be contrasted and interrelated for purposes of career planning and staff development.

A major purpose of these standards will be to assist in the development of curricula for social work programs appropriate to each of the defined levels. It is axiomatic that effective education requires definite educational goals. Both short-term training programs and more substantial educational programs should be directed toward specific vocational levels. Similarly, curriculum-building requires well-defined concepts of skills and competence. These standards are seen as a beginning step toward the more technically complete definitions required by educational planning. They should be adequate for general usage by personnel and staffing planners and for the administrative purposes of most agencies.

As a tool, it is hoped these standards will (1) achieve maximum effectiveness of and accountability in social service programs, (2) assure the appropriate use of qualified manpower, (3) provide opportunities for advancement in individual agencies, (4) facilitate the adaptation of workers transferring to other agencies, and (5) provide clear goals for the development of educational curricula.

Differential Use of Manpower

In applying these standards, the community social service system should be the initial focus of attention. For a comprehensive range of services to be provided in a community, a complete and appropriate use of manpower must be available. The combination of social worker classifications needed by an individual agency will be determined by the agency's size, functions, and technological development and by the available manpower. For example, in some agencies the nature of the functions would allow the use of social worker, technician, and aide levels, while in others the need for highly discretionary or technical judgments might require a greater use of the certified social worker or graduate social worker levels.

In planning for the use of all social service manpower, emphasis should be placed on permitting individual employees to contribute as much as they can, according to their ability to practice. The opportunity to make meaningful contributions to the achievement of social service goals makes the difference between motivation for professional services and mere existence on a job.

To accomplish a differential use of manpower will require individual agencies, which comprise the community social service system, to cooperate formally in implementing a career ladder. Such a ladder must have two essential characteristics: (1) it should open doors to persons wishing to find a career in the social services and provide entry at each level of competence and (2) it should provide the opportunity for career advancement, as well as for horizontal mobility. These characteristics will require programs of career recruitment, counseling, and meaningful staff development.

Job Levels

Because of the ordinal nature of this classification plan, several concepts concerning its application must be highlighted. As a general rule, a complexity-scale concept has been used. This means that an employee at any given level of competence should be capable of performing less complex functions but not be able to perform effectively those that are more complex.

Further, it should be recognized that there are qualitative differences among abilities at different levels. A social worker should be able to complete a survey schedule or interview clients for data to determine their need for agency services, while a certified social worker should be able to develop a survey design or to conduct counseling interviews involving complex marital adjustment problems. And there will be different performance levels within classifications that are dictated by such factors as length of service and demonstration of special abilities.

For a variety of reasons, agencies may find it necessary to define several grade levels within each classification level, primarily as a result of the differential activities within the agency. That is, certain clusters of work responsibilities might require unique abilities. However, additional levels should reflect two characteristics: (1) there should be a continuum of logical steps from one level to another, if possible, so that both responsibilities and opportunities for career advancement are clearly perceived and (2) opportunity for advancement to a higher level should be possible for employees who can demonstrate an ability to perform such functions and who meet the prescribed qualifications.

Finally, all classification levels should provide salary levels commensurate with the functions performed and with the employee's performance. The salary structure should be commensurate with the standards for the field and reviewed annually for equity and for comparability both within the field and to the labor market generally.

SUMMARY OF FUNCTIONS

Social Service Aide

Functions. As part of a team or other professionally guided supervision,
 • Interviews applicants for services to obtain basic data and to provide information on available services.
 • Interprets programs or services to ethnic or cultural groups and helps such groups or individuals express their needs.
 • Assists people in determining their eligibility for services and in assembling or obtaining required data or documentation.
 • Participates in neighborhood surveys, obtaining data from families or individuals.
 • Provides specific information and referral services to people seeking help.
 • Conducts case-finding activities in the community, encouraging people to use available services.
 • Provides specific instructions or directions concerning the location of services or procedures involved in obtaining help.
 • Serves as a liaison between an agency and defined groups or organizations in the community.

Qualifications.
 • Life experiences and knowledge of the community or special groups are the primary abilities required.
 • Although high school graduation is not always required and may be irrelevant, basic skills in reading, writing, and computation are important. A high school diploma may be required for certain positions.
 • A concern for people and a willingness to learn on the job are essential attitudes.

Social Service Technician

Functions. As part of a team or under close professional supervision,
 • Conducts fact-finding and referral interviews based on an awareness of generally available community resources.
 • Assists in helping individuals or groups with difficult day-to-day problems, such as finding jobs, locating sources of assistance, or organizing community groups to work on specific problems.

• Contributes to special planning studies from knowledge of a client's problems and viewpoints, as part of a project or planning unit.

• Helps assess the suitability or effectiveness of services by understanding and relating to the experiences and specific needs of a group.

• Provides coaching and special supportive role assistance to help groups or individuals use services.

• Provides specific instruction or direction to persons seeking services, as part of an outreach or orientation activity.

• Records data and helps collect information for research studies.

• Works with local agencies or workers regarding specific problems and needs of clients and agencies.

• Does emergency evaluations and provides emotional support in crises.

Qualifications.

• Completion of an organized social welfare program leading to an associate of arts degree or a bachelor of arts degree in another field.

• Motivation to help people.

Social Worker

Functions.   Using social work supervision,

• Provides social work services directed to specific, limited goals.

• Conducts workshops to promote and interpret programs or services.

• Organizes local community groups and coordinates their efforts to alleviate social problems.

• Consults with other agencies on problems of cases served in common and coordinates services among agencies helping multiproblem families.

• Conducts basic data-gathering or statistical analysis of data on social problems.

• Develops information to assist legislators and other decision-makers to understand problems and community needs.

• Serves as an advocate of those clients or groups of clients whose needs are not being met by available programs or by a specific agency.

• Works with groups to assist them in defining their needs or interests and in deciding on a course of action.

• Administers units of a program within an overall structure.

Qualifications.

• Completion of an approved social work program awarding a baccalaureate degree.

Graduate Social Worker

Functions.   Using consultative or routine supervision,

• Provides therapeutic intervention under supervision.

- Organizes a coalition of community groups to work on broad-scale problems.
    - Is the social work component on a multidisciplinary team.
    - Conducts group therapy sessions in a clinic setting.
    - Provides consultative assistance with social services to a community.
    - Develops and conducts research involving basic statistical techniques.
    - Works on program planning for a major public agency providing social services.
    - Is an instructor on a faculty of a school of social work.
    - Administers a social service program.
    - Serves as a team leader in a service unit.
    - Works in a program planning section of a social service agency.

Qualifications.
- Completion of a master's of social work program in an institution accredited by CSWE.

Certified Social Worker

Functions.   Using consultation, when appropriate,
- Serves as a team leader in a multidisciplinary therapy group.
- Provides psychotherapy to individuals and groups on an independent basis.
- Serves as a consultant to major social service and community action programs.
- Administers a social service program or agency.
- Teaches on the faculty of a school of social work.
- Plans and conducts research projects.
- Conducts program evaluation studies.
- Works as an independent consultant with industrial organizations to provide social work-oriented direction to employee service programs.
- Works as a community organizer or planner for a metropolitan coordinating body.
- Provides teaching supervision in a program providing intensive casework services.

Qualifications.
- Completion of a master's degree program in social work and certification by ACSW.

Social Work Fellow

Functions.   In accordance with professional standards,
- Administers a major social service agency or program.

- Works as an independent consultant in private practice.
- Works as a psychotherapist in private practice.
- Is a professor on the faculty of a school of social work.
- Develops and directs a research program for a consultant firm specializing in social problems.
- Conducts independent research.

Qualifications.
- Completion of a doctoral program at an accredited school of social work or in a related discipline, with two years of specialization in an area of social work or certification by ACSW and two years of social work experience in the field of specialization.

32/A CRITIQUE OF THE NASW
MANPOWER STATEMENT

THOMAS L. BRIGGS

In the fall of 1973 the National Association of Social Workers issued policy statement number four, *Standards for Social Service Manpower*, which represents the current official position of the profession on manpower matters. The document purports to identify levels of practice, each requiring various degrees of competence and then attempts to identify levels of competence based on various academic preparations and other forms of certification. The thesis of this paper is that the document fails to do either and that it is essentially useless to the conscientious educator who seeks greater specificity from the practice field regarding the "attributes" one should be educating for at each level of the continuum. The paper is divided into four parts:

1. An overall critique of the document highlighting the basic flaws that it contains.

2. A specific look at the document in terms of its utility for establishing educational objectives.

3. An analysis of underlying assumptions upon which the statement is based.

4. The state of the art—implications for differential education and practice.

A CRITIQUE OF THE POLICY STATEMENT

For many years the social work profession held the position that every social work job in the United States and Canada should be filled by a person with a master's degree.[1] Despite the acute manpower shortages that occurred in the 1960s many in the profession pursued the goal of 100 percent professional staffing of agencies. That this goal was unattainable and even more important, undesirable, was not recognized by the leadership in the profession for many years.

Despite an earlier professional myopia, many developments have occurred during the past 15 years that enabled the profession to broaden its vision and see that there were others without MSW degrees who could be performing social work functions effectively and efficiently. Among these developments were the new-careers movement ushering in paraprofessionals in large numbers, manpower research on the differential use of social work staff, the establishment of community college programs for social service technicians, and the professionalization of the baccalaureate social worker.[2]

The NASW policy statement is the *first official recognition of these developments* and for the first time states that the use of persons with different academic and experience preparation is a *legitimate manpower strategy*. This must be viewed as a positive move—unfortunately the rest of the document leaves much to be desired.

As noted by Chauncey Alexander,[3] the policy statement includes a classification plan that identifies six levels of practitioners and then attempts to define those functions and tasks that each can or should be able to perform.

The document claims that it identifies *qualitative* differences among levels of functions and tasks, and levels of competence needed to perform at that level. In arriving at the qualitative differences between functions and tasks the approach utilized is a complexity model, that is, the notion is held forth that task and functions can be identified and described in such a way as to indicate qualitative differences among levels. There are many problems encountered when one attempts to operationalize such an approach. The mere process of identifying a task or function and the way it is described greatly influences the weighting given to it. Tasks must be described verbally and the same task can be described in innumerable ways, each of which will affect how one rates it.

Another deficiency of the concept is its failure to take into account the fact that tasks do not remain static, never varying in complexity. Sometimes they are more difficult to accomplish than at other times, even though they do not appear to be so on paper. But the greatest weakness of this approach is that it places people in boxes based on labels obtained through formal academic programs and other forms of certification, encourages rigidity, and represses a dynamic use of the talent that different people bring to the service enterprise. In order to understand what has just been said, let us look at the NASW plan to see specifically how successful it is in indicating qualitative differences. In reviewing these examples the reader is reminded that *all* tasks performed by lower level staff can supposedly be performed by members of higher levels but *no* lower level person is considered able, or permitted, to perform tasks at a higher level.

For the social service aide position the document states that "the . . . aide provides various specified duties to help clients obtain and use social and related services, including obtaining information, providing specific basic information, aiding clients in agency procedures and services, and other supportive functions."[4] The duties of the social service technician appear identical: "The social service technician performs a wide variety of duties to facilitate the knowledge and use of social services. These involve disseminating information, obtaining information from clients, assisting clients in use of community resources . . . carrying out specific program activities and tasks."[5]

"Disseminating information" sounds more complicated than "providing information," but is it different? The words in the description of the tasks at the higher level are more complex, but are there qualitative differences between levels? The key to the real difference between the two positions is perhaps found in the next paragraph: "The social service technician must be able to make inquiries discreetly, provide clear information. . . ."[6] Should one assume from this statement that the aide makes indiscreet inquiries and provides garbled information? Yet these statements are held forth as the means to differentiate between the two positions.

Other attempts at differentiation appear at each level with the same results. "The social worker [BSW] uses methods of disciplined inquiry. . . ."[7] Do lesser levels use undisciplined inquiry? "The graduate social worker [MSW] uses methods appropriate to the situation. . . ."[8] Are other levels, including the BSW, expected to use inappropriate methods? Or, "the certified social worker is responsible for a wide range of independent social work activities requiring individual accountability for the outcome of service. . . ."[9] Are not the other four levels, especially the two professional ones, expected to be engaged in "independent activities" and to hold themselves "accountable?" Perhaps their supervisors will perform these functions for them!

Perhaps the most ludicrous distinction is made between the certified social worker and the social work fellow. "The social work fellow is *capable of* a wide range of independent social work activities requiring individual accountability for the outcome of service . . ." while the certified social worker is *responsible for* these same duties (italics added).[10]

Michael Austin and Philip Smith, manpower planners from Florida, commenting on the same document had this to say:

We find the use of a complexity scale for making distinctions between worker levels unacceptable. We have dealt with this problem over the past two years and have concluded that the use of a complexity scale is deficient in that it implies a continuum with the less skilled worker on one end and the most skilled worker on the other. This is problematic for several reasons. Educationally it implies that we simply teach students at graduate levels of education to perform essentially the same tasks with the distinguishing characteristics being greater proficiency at each of the next highest levels. The implication for practice is that there is nothing unique about lower level personnel other than the fact that they are less skilled than workers at higher levels. Another problem is that the complexity issue is too ambiguous. We find it difficult and furthermore inappropriate to make arbitrary distinctions about the comparative level of complexity in performing different functions. For example, a Level I aide . . . may perform an agency brokerage role with a high degree of proficiency (the literature has indicated the paraprofessionals often perform this particular role much better than the MSW). Therefore, how can we say that this worker is less skilled or less competent than a (graduate social worker)? This also points out the arbitrary nature of deciding that such a function is less complex than a similar one performed by a (graduate social worker). We would like to suggest that the concept of "unique competencies" at all levels, is a much more productive way of distinguishing between worker levels.[11]

Agreeing with Austin and Smith and stressing the need for the development of unique competencies (not lesser or greater competencies) at each educational level, Charles Guzzetta says:

Each component (level) in the continuum must be independent and furnish the graduate of that component with a legitimate occupational preparation. To be blunt, certification at each level should be marketable. Each component must have this sort of internal integrity while at the same time serving as a legitimate preparation or base for the next component. The relationship must not be between professional and non or sub (or pre) or paraprofessional, but among independent interrelated occupations. The associate of arts graduate thereby could not be the servant of, nor aide to, the human service professional but would have responsibilities different from, although related to those with other preparations. . . . The separation often seen in curriculum continuums seems to suggest that only holders of advanced degrees can be trusted with moral or ethical decisions. In effect, this is an enforced childhood and adolescence which save the independence of adulthood for others. Similarly, technical competence appropriately belongs in each component with differences more a matter of kind than degree. That is, given X as a particular technical competence, it is not properly the case that the AA person does X poorly, the baccalaureate does X adequately, the master's does X skillfully and the doctorate does X magnificently. Rather, the Associate does X skillfully, the baccalaureate does Y skillfully, the master's does Z skillfully, and the doctorate tells them all what they did wrong and right.[12]

THE PLAN AS A GUIDE TO CURRICULUM DEVELOPMENT

The policy statement declares that "a major purpose of these standards will be to assist in the development of curricula for social work programs appropriate to each of the defined levels. It is axiomatic that effective education requires definite educational goals. . . . Similarly, curriculum building requires well-defined concepts of skills and competence."[13]

Concurring with this statement and elaborating on it further, Kay Dea in another publication says:

Educational objectives require some degree of specificity and a definite focus on goals rather than processes. Since they define that point in knowledge, skill, and values that a student is expected to reach on completion of a specific course of study they must be what Loewenberg has called student-centered, activity-focused and content-specific. This means that they must explicitly describe those behaviors a student will be capable of manifesting on completion of the program.[14]

Let us turn again to the classification plan and see how helpful it is in defining the explicit behaviors needed by curriculum developers at various educational levels. In this plan, in addition to definitions of appropriate tasks and functions at each of the six levels, we find a statement related to the skills and knowledge required by the incumbent. Since knowledge of human behavior can be assumed to be a prerequisite to effective practice at all levels, let us see how the plan deals with this.

1. Social Service Aide—no mention of this item.

2. Social Service Technician—knowledge of the fundamentals of human behavior.

3. Social Worker (BSW)—beginning knowledge of human behavior and development.

4. Graduate Social Worker (MSW)—theoretical and a beginning empirical knowledge of human behavior and development.

5. Certified Social Worker (ACSW)—both theoretical and empirical knowledge of human behavior and development.

6. Social Work Fellow (DSW)—advanced knowledge of theories and research in human behavior and development.

What is the difference between "fundamentals" and "beginning knowledge?" Do these statements give the specificity that the plan claims to offer in providing a guide to help determine educational goals and terminal behaviors? Keeping in mind that in order for an educational objective to be sound, one should be able to translate it into specific behavior, let us look at one more excerpt from the statement.

The graduate social worker [MSW] must have . . . a *working* understanding of social and economic realities and forces, a *critical* knowledge of social service systems, a *familiarity* with the nature and causation of individual and social abnormalities and an *awareness* of relevant community and professional organizations and related institutions. (italics mine)[15]

Unfortunately, words and phrases such as "working understanding," "familiarity," and "awareness" are so vague as to be subject to all sorts of misunderstandings and interpretations. Just what "critical knowledge" implies escapes this author. These statements are simply not helpful to the conscientious educator who seeks guidance from the practice field as to what attributes a graduate of a particular program should possess.

In 1972, Richard Lodge, executive director of the Council on Social Work Education, addressed a group of educators representing various levels of social work education in California and had this to say: "I have pleaded at many meetings for the recognition of the need for functional manpower classifications so that educational programs can intelligently relate to them. I am beginning to think I am asking for a world that never existed."[16] Lodge's world has not changed with the issuing of the NASW statement.

AN ANALYSIS OF UNDERLYING ASSUMPTIONS

Perhaps the most serious criticism that this author can make of the policy statement has to do with some of the assumptions that underlie it, assumptions which seem to run counter to professional values. There is the assumption, for example, that the highly trained professional is the repository of ultimate competence, skill, and goodness, and has a monopoly on ethical behavior. The classification plan, in addition to expecting only ACSWs and Fellows to hold themselves accountable for their services, also mandates that the first four levels (including the MSW) must be supervised by a higher level.

The implication here is that the difference between workers at different levels is not just a question of skill. Therefore, propriety necessitates supervision at lower levels. The author finds this insinuation especially obnoxious, for it infers that workers at lower levels are potentially unethical and that the consumers of service are subject to possible harm from their behavior, while those receiving service from workers who have attained higher levels are protected against this hazard. As all professions have learned, often painfully, unethical behavior is not limited to any level of training and experience (e.g., lawyers and Watergate). Perhaps the restriction on practice can also be viewed as racist, since most paraprofessionals are members of minority groups. Why they can "do their thing" *only* under the direct supervision of a professional is left unclear.

Also, the notion of supervision for life of the lower levels of staff, including BSWs and MSWs attacks the very idea of professionalism, namely expertise and autonomy based on this expertise. Apparently the drafters of this statement were not willing to concede professional status to those who are eligible to join the professional association.

Another aspect of this statement strikes at what this author believes is a basic tenet of social work, namely the belief that people can develop and grow and ought to be afforded the opportunity to do so. Lip service is given to this concept in the following statement in the document:

In planning for the use of all social service manpower, emphasis should be placed on permitting individual employees to contribute as much as they can, according to their ability to practice. The opportunity to make meaningful contributions to the achievement of social service goals makes the difference between motivation for professional services and mere existence on a job.[17]

Apparently we do not afford our colleagues the same opportunity to grow that we do our clients. If the growth potential inherent in each individual is a matter of conviction, then why this restriction?

Although fully appreciative of the validity and significance of life experience as an inherent aspect of the development of social work skills in the individual, NASW is convinced of the necessity for organized, accredited educational achievement as the primary basis for differentiating among levels of competence.[18]

This section contains another interesting assumption. Namely, it suggests that competence can be equated with education and the way to measure it, at least in the first four levels, is exclusively by counting academic degrees. The implication is clear that regardless of how truly committed or competent a person is he should *not be allowed* to assume responsibilities appropriate to higher levels, unless, of course, he gets another degree. Who is being protected here—clients or the profession? This whole statement smacks of professional elitism and arrogance.

From the above remarks the reader may infer that the author is advocating the abandonment of social work education. Quite the contrary. Formal education is still the most predictable route to obtain the kind of socialization into the values and ethics of the profession and a mastery of the knowledge and skill base that Alexander referred to in his paper. However, this social work educator takes the position that there are other means to obtain the necessary attributes besides formal education. If only the statement had acknowledged this point.

Finally, the statement would have been less offensive to the author if it were less prescriptive (you are allowed to do only thus and so with this degree) and the examples of functions at each level illustrative. The profession does not have the functional specificity to be as definitive as the classification scheme implies.

THE STATE OF THE ART—IMPLICATIONS FOR DIFFERENTIAL EDUCATION AND PRACTICE

All professions and skilled occupations attempt to lay claim to the exclusive performance of certain functions. In addition to establishing their "turf" they also seek to establish various sanctions (legal and professional) that prevent outsiders from engaging in those functions that are viewed as their territory. A corresponding activity is the establishment of formal training programs whereby would-be practitioners may pass prescribed rites of passage in order to be accepted into the community of professionals.

Social work, as an emerging profession, has been actively engaged in the above set of activities for the past sixty years and has met with minimal success. The following list of obstacles suggests that the current manpower statement is premature at best. It also suggests that the achievement of a rational prescriptive classification plan some point in the future may be impossible unless certain changes in the profession take place.

1. The profession has not sufficiently clarified its ultimate function and in particular has not defined its boundaries or indicated what areas of involvement are beyond its realm. If all of human social welfare is within the sphere of social work, then it is assuming an obligation for virtually all human life and existence. This is too great a responsibility for any one profession, and much overlap with other human relations (or helping) professions is inevitable. Therefore, what differentiates social work from other groups similarly involved is increasingly blurred. There exists no universally accepted definition of social work that clearly establishes what it does as contrasted with other professions.

2. Failure to establish social work's functional specificity has retarded the establishment of legal recognition of the profession and a protection of its right to the performance of certain functions. The establishment of professional sanctions may be the only way of regulating the profession's practice.

3. An inability to define the profession with precision has also constituted an obstacle to defining what constitutes practice and how to assess competence for practice.

4. Difficulty in defining competence for practice makes the task of defining levels of competence a dubious activity.

5. Failure to define levels of competence has caused confusion at each level of the educational continuum as to the specific attributes (or products) that should be an end result of the educational process.

6. Lack of specificity around specific competencies at each of the educational levels has resulted in agency administrators using staff interchangeably, placing artificial restrictions on lower level staff, or avoiding the hiring of anyone without an MSW.

It is the author's impression that the issuance of the manpower statement with all its faults may be a good omen for it might force us to make a critical choice. Is this not the time for the *total* profession (including the professional organizations, the employing agencies, and educational institutions) to mount a massive reexamination of the mission of the profession as a prelude to answering the question of differential education for the differential staffing of social work programs?

NOTES

1. See for example Robert L. Barker and Thomas L. Briggs, *Differential Use of Social Work Manpower* (New York: National Association of Social Workers, 1968), p. 28.
2. For a description of these developments see Thomas L. Briggs, "Social Work Manpower: Developments and Dilemmas of the 1970s," in *Educating MSW Students to Work with Other Social Welfare Personnel*, ed. Margaret Purvine (New York: Council on Social Work Education, 1973).
3. Chauncey Alexander, "A Critique of the NASW Manpower Statement," *Journal of Education for Social Work* 11, no. 1 (Winter 1975).
4. *Standards for Social Service Manpower* (Washington, D.C.: National Association of Social Workers, 1973), p. 7.
5. *Ibid.*, p. 8.
6. *Ibid.*
7. *Ibid.*
8. *Ibid.*, p. 9.
9. *Ibid.*, p. 10.
10. *Ibid.*
11. Personal correspondence with the authors.
12. Charles Guzzetta, "The Curriculum Continuum," in *Curriculum Building for the Continuum in Social Welfare Education*, ed. Michael J. Austin et al. (Tallahassee: State University System of Florida, 1972), pp. 22, 23.
13. *Standards, op. cit.*, p. 12.
14. Kay L. Dea, "Educational Objectives and Curricula for Social Work," in *Undergraduate Social Work Education for Practice: A Report on Curriculum Content and Issues*, ed. Lester J. Glick (Syracuse, New York, and Washington, D.C.: Syracuse University and U.S. Veterans Administration, 1971), p. 29.
15. *Standards, op. cit.*, p. 9.
16. Richard Lodge, "Speech," in *Social Services Articulation Worshop Summary*, A workshop sponsored by the chancellor's office, California Community Colleges and Golden West College, Huntington Beach, California, December 6–8, 1972, p. 11.
17. *Standards, op. cit.*, p. 12.
18. *Ibid.*, p. 6.

This paper was originally presented at the CSWE 20th Annual Program Meeting held in Atlanta, March 10–13, 1974.

SIMON SLAVIN AND FELICE PERLMUTTER

ISSUES IN THE DIFFERENTIATED USE OF
SOCIAL WORK MANPOWER

Social work as a profession has for some time been concerned with the differential use of social work manpower. As early as 1959 Wolfe dealt with this issue in a National Association of Social Workers (NASW) publication, *Use of Personnel Without Professional Training in Social Service Departments*; throughout the 1960s the literature has been replete with discussion of this topic (Epstein, 1962; Farrar and Hemmy, 1963; Heyman, 1961; Weed and Denham, 1961; Wolfe, 1961).

However, in addition to the rhetoric regarding its value there exists a literature which attempts to provide an analytic basis for task and role differentiation. Blum (1966) makes a crucial point when he argues that the definition must reflect the client's interests as opposed to "a professional definition of the role." Thus it bodes well that from the outset the social work literature reflects an awareness of the dilemma of professionalism and control, a myopic bias frequently encountered in literature concerned with the professions (Rosengren and Lefton, 1970).

The complexity of this endeavor cannot be overstated; not only is the precise definition of tasks and roles a difficult one, but the additional need to define qualifications, skills, and personal attributes appropriate to their performance is complex indeed—a task of high priority for the profession (Alexander, 1972).

The components of this process have been identified:

A functional classification design derives from the program objectives of the social welfare system itself. Analysis of the objectives leads to a delineation of the tasks to be performed in fulfilling the program objectives and to a clustering of these tasks in terms of scope and range of responsibility, complexity and difficulty of performance, particular knowledge and skill required, degrees of decision-making responsibility, and extent of autonomy in practice (Wolfe, 1972, p. 21).

The task becomes one of defining the relationship between the components: scope and range of tasks, complexity and difficulty of performance, knowledge and skill, responsibility and autonomy.

Richan's model for determining roles of professional and nonprofessional workers has been frequently cited in the literature since it was one of the first attempts to discuss this issue (Richan, 1961). Moreover, it merits attention because of its clear and simple definition of conditions and responses as he specifies two crucial variables, client vulnerability and worker autonomy:

When both client vulnerability and worker autonomy are high, the greatest professional knowledge, skill and discipline are needed. When clients are highly vulnerable but set procedures and external controls are appropriate, the specialist—with technical training around specifics—can be used. When an operation essentially like that of the professional, yet with less vulnerable clientele, is called for, the person with a "preprofessional" kind of education is indicated. Finally, when external guidelines and controls are available and clients are least vulnerable, use can be made of lay persons with only brief in-service training around specifics (Richan, 1961, p. 27).

Schwartz and Sample (1972) in an experimental project concerned with the organization of work groups in a department of public assistance used three sets of criteria:

(1) presence or absence of a major social problem, (2) presence or absence of client motivation and client capacity for using service, and (3) the client's degree of social vulnerability or the extent to which he constituted an immediate threat to the public (p. 18).

The authors point out that they have expanded the "vulnerability" concept from Richan's psychological definition which focused on impact of service to include, in addition, an emphasis on the impact of the environment on the client as well as the potential threat of the client to others.

Discussions of programs which have differentiated their use of manpower can be cited. One basic guideline underpins them all: the responsibility for teaching, training, supervising, screening, and management rests with the professional (the MSW), whereas the less highly trained staff perform "the newer social and educational therapies (companionship therapy, activity group therapy, tutoring, group counseling, and retraining)" (Sobey, 1970, p. 106). Richan (1972), Carlsen (1969), and Denham and Schatz (1969) focus on the tangible services which the non-MSW can effectively provide. Barker and Briggs (1968; 1969), in discussing a series of studies which involved professional and nonprofessional staff, found that the trend is toward using the BSW as "doer" and the MSW as "director" of social work task forces of the future. While the "outer boundaries" have as yet not been reached regarding the extent of activities which can be performed by a nonprofessional, team leadership, training, and supervisory roles are appropriate for the MSW (Rivesman, 1971).

One consequence of this task differentiation is the emergence of a team approach to service delivery, "that is, a team including staff with varying levels of education . . ." (Anderson and Carlsen, 1971); this coincides with the trends identified by Pusić's discussion (1974) of administration in social welfare. While Briggs (1973) presents a different conceptual formulation for manpower differentiation and training based on an array of twelve social work roles, the administrative implications are similar: the use of a team model for social work practice which maximizes the contributions of all levels of manpower.

This brief review of the literature attempts to draw attention to a central area of concern for social work; it is not designed to be more than suggestive of the work already done and needing to be done. Although the formulations were made in relation to direct service delivery, the discussion is also applicable to the roles in research, policy, and administration presented in this volume as well as the educational model which follows.

A MODEL FOR EDUCATION AND TRAINING

Definitions
A redefinition of professional and preprofessional roles is fundamental to this discussion of an educational model for social work. Whereas the field has in the past defined professionalism as beginning at the master's level, preprofessionalism at the bachelor's level, and paraprofessionalism at the high-school level or less, a new differentiation is herein offered.

Professional social work is defined to include those who are trained for professional roles with degrees in social work at the bachelor's, master's, and doctoral levels. This specialized professional training at the university level, furthermore, provides a framework of professional ethics and social responsibility (Parsons, 1964). It should be noted that the acceptance of the bachelor's degree as the first professional degree is not unusual and occurs in education and engineering, among others.

Preprofessional social work is defined to include those who work in the field in less autonomous, more specified roles and who may have other than professional training. This includes those with bachelor of arts degrees, associate in arts certification (AA), as well as paraprofessionals. The value of this dichotomy is that it emphasizes the essential difference between professionals and nonprofessionals as one of "kind" rather than "amount" of training. NASW in 1973 worked out a similar classification for differential social work practice. The relevant characteristics of these professional and preprofessional roles are highlighted in Table 1.

Underlying Assumptions
This model is based on five assumptions which must be made explicit. First, this model aims to provide a rational system for manpower preparation in which all levels and modalities of practice are articulated and linked one to the other.

TABLE 1
Professional and Preprofessional Roles in Social Work

	Professional	Preprofessional
Role performance	Autonomous	Nonautonomous
Tasks	Diffuse	Specific
Knowledge	Conceptual, generalizable	Case-task defined
Education	Professional curriculum	University or other
Orientation	External-interdisciplinary	Internal-organizational

Should not training levels be so structured as component parts of a whole system to permit a unified system of training, and so provide opportunities for professional development as well as for promotion in the social welfare administrative hierarchy? Should not such a system of structured training accommodate the training of the volunteer and auxiliary as well as the intermediary and other senior-level positions (Gindy, 1970, p. 41)?

The systemic interrelationship of the parts cannot be overemphasized. While many programs offer a rhetoric concerning continuity and linkages, in fact the entities are discrete units. This model aims to operationalize this assumption by facilitating the progression through the various levels.

A second assumption is that education and training are interrelated components for professional preparation: professional education is viewed as providing a philosophical, conceptual, and analytic base for professional practice with knowledge that is generalizable but which will serve the specific case when needed. By contrast, training is focused on the unique and specific tasks which need to be performed to meet an organization's objectives. While the term "training" is frequently used generically, the distinction made here is of striking importance. (Though the boundaries between education and training are relatively clear, there are often elements of each in the other.)

The third assumption is that professional preparation cannot progress in a vacuum; education, training, and placement must be viewed as vital aspects of one process. This premise is based on the experience in social work education, where there is frequently a fundamental disparity between educational objectives and field needs, a problem created by both partners. For example, public welfare departments have generally failed to define the objectives of the programs in terms of reentry points into the system, and workers were put back into the same organizational slots after completing their professional education (Thompson and Riley, 1966); furthermore, the direct practice and/or clinical model of training was not appropriate for the supervisory and administrative positions obtained upon graduation (Schwartz and Sample, 1972).

A fourth assumption, which follows from the third, is that planning must become an ongoing function of educational institutions, based on continuous communication and feedback between schools and the field of practice. This is not a throwback to an earlier era when schools of social work were agency training units; rather it is an attempt to develop a rational and informed basis for institutional behavior based on an open-system model of continuous exchange between the relevant parts of that system. This is essential for the healthy performance of any professional school, be it law, medicine, engineering, or social work. Whereas to date the feedback has usually been crisis-oriented, on an *ad hoc* basis, a continuing mechanism for planning is herein assumed. A fifth and final assumption is that this, as any educational model, is not fixed and final, but flexible and formulative, to be continuously revised in relation to new findings from the field.

The model attempts to evolve a clearly articulated and linked educational system for professional and nonprofessional roles by presenting an analytic framework upon which curriculum design is based. It does not attempt to designate specific course content.

The Educational Model

This model is concerned with the two personnel groupings discussed above, preprofessional and professional.

The Paraprofessional. The first preprofessional level is primarily a practice experience. Community residents, hardly distinguishable from clients in their social characteristics, but highly motivated for service, began to play an important part in manpower development efforts of the 1960s. The similarity of cultural factors and life-style qualities made it possible to reduce social distance, create conditions of easy access and relationship, enhance communication, and make positive use of the vast knowledge that accrues to life experience, including recipient-of-service experience, in the process of providing services in a wide range of programs.

Selection of personnel at this level is based more on what people *are*, on their personal qualities, than on what they *know* of the intricacies of the helping process. Position in the community, participation in the institutional life of the area, and a feeling for people in need provide indications of potential capacity for staff roles in social programs. Readiness to learn and to accept organizational goals and educational and administrative controls figure significantly as criteria for selection.

The use of paraprofessional personnel calls for thoughtful programs of training within the agencies that employ them, and by agency personnel. Learning here is clearly prescriptive, restricted by organizational goals, procedures, and guidelines, all within the specific framework of organizational policies. Training content mirrors agency expectations and activities, and delineates performance requirements. Its focus is job-related and agency-oriented. The limits of worker discretion and initiation, as well as the realms of choice in problem-solving behavior, are significant aspects of such training. Location of accountability mechanisms and sources of professional help and supervision similarly figure importantly in program content.

While in-service training prepares personnel for effective staff functioning, encouragement to enroll in educational programs and facilitation of such activity are significant challenges to agency administrators. Several mechanisms lie at hand to further this latter objective. Some agencies provide a sequence of courses for employees that enlarge their areas of professional awareness and that constitute an internal certification system for upgrading to positions of greater responsibilities. Other agencies have arranged for courses to be given by educational institutions that carry beginning professional content, often with university credit which can be subsequently certified for credit toward the degree. Still another illustration is the move toward on-site courses by universities that serve as early inducement to engage in full-time study for eventual professional certification.

The Associate in Arts Certification. The second preprofessional level requires programs which must be carefully planned in order to be conducive to effective job performance as well as to provide a broader orientation to social work and its educational and vocational possibilities (Brawley, 1971). Education for personnel at this level must have its own integrity in order to utilize the unique competence of the preprofessional, to give job satisfaction, as well as to clarify the contribution in relation to the total welfare picture.

In a tight employment market paraprofessionals can be utilized not because of a shortage of professionals but because some agencies are unable or unwilling to meet professional salary standards. This is a very serious danger (Sobey, 1971, p. 7).

If the roles are clearly defined and the tasks clearly differentiated it will be more difficult to substitute levels inappropriately. However, the educational background is essential in providing mobility, either horizontally or vertically.

Criteria for admission into these certificate programs are still primarily the candidate's experience and interest in the human services role, now coupled with a desire for education. Candidates need not go through normal academic admissions channels. While program content is practice-oriented it is also designed to serve as an introduction or link to academic work. Thus the student can complete the program as an end in itself in order to obtain horizontal job mobility or choose to move into an academic or professional undergraduate program for vertical mobility. The following discussion provides a case illustration of an educational program for this preprofessional level.*

Prior to 1968, many child care agencies were employing untrained, poorly screened, and often psychologically unfit persons to give direct service to children. In-service training, provided by the agency, was often too little and too late, so that children suffered from the trial-and-error methods of workers in the process of acquiring new skills. In addition, the high cost of staff turnover was a major budgetary concern. Child care workers, who had the most critical role in the development of the children, had no role as members of the decision-making agency team. For a worker who had achieved a high level of competence and responsibility in one agency there was no reliable method by which he could transfer to a comparable level in another agency and no possible way he could transfer "credits" he had earned in in-service training to higher education.

Using a model for generic preservice training of child care workers, financed by the National Institute of Mental Health and made operational by an interdisciplinary faculty in the Department of Child Psychiatry at the University of Pittsburgh, Temple University began selecting and training potential child care workers in a two-year, preservice certificate program (Figure 1). Goals of the selection process were to assess the applicant's potential for the field as well as to communicate the requirements of the training program and of child care as a career choice. Areas of consideration included style, attitude, personal characteristics, and readiness (motivation, maturity). Danger signals, which become contraindications for selection, included hostility, moralistic judgments, punitiveness, and rigidity, among others.

Applicants represented wide ranges of difference in age, social and economic status, ethnic and cultural origin, educational preparation, practical judgment, and experience with children. Classes were formed with maximum heterogeneity in order that people could learn to value differences.

Many mature "certificates" have returned to the university, adding liberal arts courses to their "Introduction to the Profession" (the three-semester certificate training) to work toward a baccalaureate degree, mainly out of concern for their own developmental process. Younger, less mature trainees were often encouraged to seek a four-year educational experience before they took jobs, to compensate for their lack of practical experience of relevant life experience.

The Bachelor of Arts Degree. The third preprofessional level also provides manpower for the less complex tasks of the field. These students receive an academic background which consists mainly of theoretical and ab-

---

* This case illustration was prepared by Fran Vandivier, Director, Child Care Training Program, School of Social Administration, Temple University, Philadelphia.

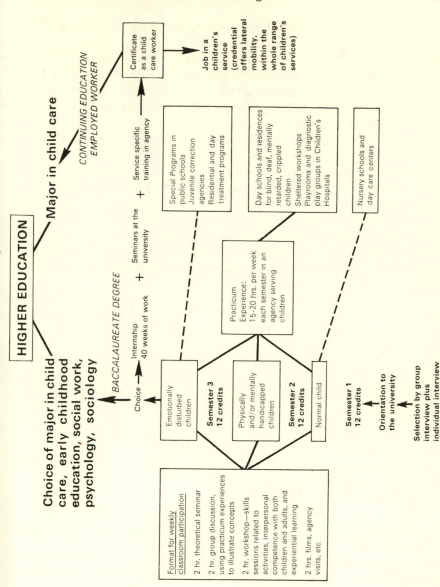

Figure 1. A Certification Program for Preprofessional Social Work

stract content, coupled with their interest and motivation to work in the field. Thus their personal qualifications are different from those of the pre-professionals, whose cultural base and personal identity are in themselves the essential qualifications. While the BA program may offer some field experience, it is a relatively superficial exposure rather than an in-depth educational experience generally, related to specific course objectives rather than to the total educational experience.

Preparation for social work performance is through in-service training and supervision in the place of work, while linkage to the educational system is through continuing education provided by the university's professional school. Linkage can also be made to the MSW professional program as a result of experience in the field.

The Bachelor of Social Work. The first professional degree must have as its basic objective preparation for the entry level of professional practice. The objectives formulated by the Council on Social Work Education are as follows:

Program objectives shall reflect the values of the profession of social work. Preparation for beginning social work practice must be a stated educational objective of an undergraduate social work program. The program shall further specify its objectives in relation to: the mission of the educational institution of which it is a part, the human needs in the region identified by the parent institution as its service area; and its student body (CSWE Doc. #73–210–1, January, 1973).

This beginning level of professional education must prepare the practitioner for the autonomy necessary in areas of direct service discussed in the section on task and role differentiation. (The profession is beginning to recognize this reality; membership in NASW has been available to bachelor's degree social workers since 1970.)

The criteria for admission are more complex than in the earlier level, combining both the standard academic university criteria and the qualitative, personal attributes of the applicant. This is a crucial point in the system's linkage, for here lies the opportunity to encourage nonprofessionals with suitable background to enter the professional stream, thus recognizing nonacademic work and training background.

As specified by the Council on Social Work Education, the program should include: (1) a liberal arts base consisting of "knowledge in the humanities, social, behavioral and biological sciences"; (2) social work content, including "practice, social welfare, policy and services, and human behavior and social environment"; and (3) "educationally directed field work" (Doc. #73–210–1). The undergraduate social work program at Temple University offers a case illustration. Approximately one third of all course work deals with professional content; the balance is divided on a two-to-one ratio between general education and professionally related courses.

Students begin a three-year professional sequence of courses in the sophomore year. The concentration on professional content increases in each successive year, with the final year essentially devoted to class and field courses in social work. Preceding and surrounding this professional concentration are courses in natural sciences, humanities, and introductory-level social and behavioral sciences which provide a broad base in general education. The third segment of this tripartite program includes professionally related content, including social research and more advanced social theory courses drawn from psychology, social psychology, political science, sociology, and economics.

Practical field experience is attached to the social work courses in the sophomore and senior years. The former is intended to introduce students to the reality of an organized service delivery system and to test interest, commitment, and capacity for professional work. There is a year-long senior seminar together with a two-day-a-week field work experience in a single social agency, where the intimate and intricate relationships between theory and practice provide the substance of student learning.

There are two ways in which this BSW program is linked to earlier levels of training. More and more students who have completed a two-year AA program have transferred to the university for full baccalaureate certification. Some come directly from the community college, others after an interregnum for work in the human services. Care needs to be given to individual assessment of content mastery so that debilitating repetition of earlier studies can be avoided. Students from preprofessional programs are helped to succeed in the BSW program through various mechanisms. Initial courses taken by these students are given by program personnel and conform to the objectives of the initial professional offerings of the undergraduate sequence. A variety of support services is provided, including counseling, intensive advising, individual and group tutoring in basic skills, study skill sessions, remedial classes, and financial aid. Other courses provided by the university as required by the BSW degree follow or are taken in tandem. In time, these students merge into the regular student body both in the undergraduate department and in the university. Thus movement from preprofessional to professional status goes on apace. Many students continue to work in their agencies, undergoing transition to student and to professional more gradually. In time, many of these students will enroll in graduate programs, including those offering MSW degrees.

It is important to recognize that graduates of these programs will be full-fledged professionals, knowledgeable and trained in direct practice, capable of performing autonomously, requiring the usual supervision. This level will in many ways be comparable to the former level of the MSW entrance position.

The Master's Degree in Social Work. This must now be viewed as the second professional degree for advanced practice in the field; it can be built on the BSW as well as on the undifferentiated BA, as at present. Entrance into the MSW must assume knowledge of social work and social welfare, including history, philosophy, social policy, and practice issues, as well as experience in direct service delivery. Flexibility in the design of the MSW program is critical in terms of this integrated and interrelated model since the needs of the BSW will differ from those of the BA. Thus the linkages between the BSW and MSW programs must be carefully constructed in order to maximize past education as the basis for advanced work. All too often MSW programs give lip service to this linkage but in fact are not prepared to offer more intensive and/or specialized content areas. An important contribution has been made by the Council on Social Work Education, which has authorized that graduates of an approved* BSW program can receive as much as a year of advanced standing in an accredited master's degree program. While each school will determine its own pattern, alternatives could include advanced standing in the MSW program and substitution of courses for greater specialization.

The program's objectives must clearly include new and advanced roles as it helps develop new expertise. These new roles and competencies, include administration, research and evaluation, policy and planning, supervision, staff development, and consultation. While some schools may include advanced training for direct practice at the master's level, we are not discussing that pattern since it has traditionally been part of the master's program.

The criteria for entrance into the program are twofold: the stringent academic criteria of graduate professional education and demonstrated competence in the practice role.

One distinctive difference in the MSW level, and one which forms the rationale for this volume, is the assumption that advanced practitioners should be experts in the functional field in which they plan to work. Consequently, in addition to general content related to service delivery, administration, and research, an in-depth knowledge of at least one field (its policies, programs, fiscal mechanisms, and social work practice) should be required.

The School of Social Work at the University of Pennsylvania, which is currently redesigning its master's degree curriculum, can serve as an illustration of one pattern of the proposed MSW. The program is designed for advanced practice, and consequently admission is based on educational background (social work undergraduate programs) and/or experience in direct practice roles in social work. The following discussion in part reflects the plans for the new program and in part reflects the authors' philosophy.

* Editor's note: Since July 1, 1974, CSWE has *accredited* baccalaureate social work programs.

The curriculum offers four specializations from which the student can select his preferred field. The four selected at Pennsylvania, which reflect the unique competencies within the school and university, are presented for illustrative purposes only; they include health, corrections, the urban family, and education.

While the field placement for this two-year program is in the student's area of specialization, the academic course work offers both general content (administration and supervision) and specialized content (legislation, programs, practice issues). The general content areas are handled during the first and fourth semesters; specialization occurs during the second and third. An independent project of the student's choice provides an opportunity for an independent in-depth study in the field of specialization in the third and fourth semesters. As Figure 2 indicates, the general and specialized contents are seen as overlapping and continuous rather than as discrete and separate areas.

As are degrees at the earlier levels, the MSW can be a terminal degree for specific practice roles in the field or it can serve as the basis for continuing on to the doctorate in social work. However, with more sophisticated and vigorous training at the MSW level, this degree should indeed serve as a sound base for practice at advanced levels in the field.

The Doctorate in Social Work. This level requires careful consideration in view of the legitimation of the BSW and the advanced specification of the MSW. What objectives are uniquely served at this level? Three can be clearly specified: teaching, research, policy-planning—all three unique in their level of expertise and technical competence. The teaching role would serve all the other levels of education, from the training of teachers for AA programs to faculty for graduate departments; the research role would be

Figure 2. An MSW Curriculum

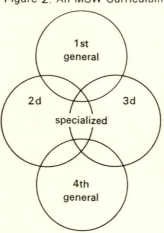

one of initiating and directing research in social work and social welfare (as opposed to the team participant role of the MSW); the policy and planning role would be in relation to major government and national level programs. Some doctoral programs will probably continue to prepare for "advanced" direct practice roles and award a clinical doctorate.

Criteria for selection must be carefully and flexibly defined to provide the possibility of selecting the best candidates on both academic and professional criteria. While there would be the obvious and direct linkage from the master's program, interest of applicants trained in other disciplines should be encouraged. Entrance into the doctoral level will assume, however, substantial knowledge in social welfare (history and philosophy, practice theory, and so forth). These content areas must be the building blocks either through the MSW or through courses taken upon admission as prerequisites. The doctoral program will then be free to focus on selected areas for academic and professional excellence.

Linkages must thus be carefully examined in order to maximize the utilization of past credits and to minimize duplication. Various patterns are possible, and one which should be given careful consideration is the "en route" master's degree. This is the usual pattern in many fields and may be appropriate in some programs, such as research specialization. The organizing principle of any doctoral program must be its thrust for a disciplined program within the university context of academic excellence.

An interdisciplinary program in social and behavioral sciences can be viewed as fundamental in doctoral level work in that it provides an internal rigor and methodology which can then be applied to the field of social welfare. The selection of social science content would depend on the interests of the student: for example, a student in administration might select sociology (organization theory); a student in policy-planning might select political science.

The emphasis of the remainder of the curriculum will vary according to the mission of the program (teaching, planning, research). Thus, for example, in a school which aims to produce educators, a second major content area would be in the field of education (curriculum design, learning theory). Similarly, the doctoral dissertations would reflect the central thrust of the program in their demonstration of the students' independent and scholarly contribution to their area of competence.

Thus the doctorate is viewed as the degree necessary for the advanced roles to be performed in an increasingly complex environment. The tension between the professional objectives versus the academic expectations is an anachronism in the present reality: both must be viewed as integral parts of a program designed to produce excellence.

Other educational functions. These too must be included in this integrated model. Continuing education, as mentioned above, is a responsibility of the professional school in helping people in the field remain *au courant* with new knowledge and skill in the field. It is particularly important in a society such as ours where rapid technological change creates profound changes in fields of knowledge. This program can be organized through short courses and institutes related to the broader educational objectives of the educational setting, as opposed to inservice training which is agency defined.

The educational model which encompasses six levels of manpower is schematically presented in Table 2.

CONCLUSIONS

In the past, the MSW was both the entry and the terminal degree. It was the center and core of professional preparation for social work practice. With the advent of the BSW as the initial mark of legitimacy for professional practice, and preprofessional training for prescribed and delimited performance roles, master's level preparation will inevitably continue to assume new and evolving characteristics.

At the other end of the continuum, some social work positions have begun to require doctoral level certification. This is increasingly true in university positions in schools of social work and in advanced research and policy-planning roles in national agencies and governmental programs. This suggests that the pivotal role of master's level education may be substantially modified, perhaps in the direction assumed by the field of education.

One can easily anticipate substantial development during the 1970s of educational and training programs at both ends of the educational continuum. Efforts that link early training programs to educational offerings at subsequent levels, and early professional education to master's and doctoral curricula, can be expected to assume the central stage in educational

TABLE 2
Social Work Level as Related to Qualifications and Work Tasks

Social Work Level	Qualifications	Work Tasks-Roles (Complexity, Autonomy, Uncertainty)
Preprofessional		
Paraprofessional	Personal	Low
AA	Personal and	
BA	Academic	Moderate
Professional		
BSW	Personal and	
MSW	Academic and	High
DSW	Professional	

planning. One can expect additional universities with graduate social work education programs to establish undergraduate departments. In the process, faculties will increasingly become integrated, and individual faculty members will become interchangeable in handling BSW, MSW, and advanced degree courses. Students, similarly, can be expected to move between course offerings on more than one level, and share courses with candidates for higher or lower degrees. The urgent task is to develop a realistic and effective system of education which can meet the various needs at the various levels.

REFERENCES

Alexander, Chauncey A. "Foreword," in Edward E. Schwartz and William C. Sample, *The Midway Office*. New York, National Association of Social Workers, 1972.

Anderson, Claire M., and Thomas Carlsen. "The Midway Project on Organization and Use of Public Assistance Personnel," in Robert L. Barker and Thomas L. Briggs, eds., *Manpower Research on the Utilization of Baccalaureate Social Workers*. Washington, D.C., Veterans Administration, 1971, pp. 17–28.

Barker, Robert L., and Thomas L. Briggs. *Differential Use of Social Work Manpower*. New York, National Association of Social Workers, 1968.

————. *Using Teams to Deliver Social Services*. Syracuse, N.Y., Syracuse University Press, 1969.

Blum, Arthur. "Differential Use of Manpower in Public Welfare," *Social Work*, XI, No. 1 (1966), 16–21.

Brawley, Edward A. *Training Preprofessional Mental Health Workers*. Philadelphia, Community College, 1971.

Briggs, Thomas L. "Needed: Differential Education for Differential Staffing—a Prerequisite for Effectiveness." Paper presented at Annual Program Meeting, Council on Social Work Education, 1973; mimeographed.

Carlsen, Thomas. *Social Work Manpower Utilization in Mental Health Programs; Proceedings of a Workshop*. Syracuse, N.Y., Syracuse University Press, 1969.

Denham, William H., and Eunice O. Shatz, "Impact of the Indigenous Nonprofessional on the Professional's Role," in Willard C. Richan, ed., *Human Services and Social Work Responsibility*, pp. 178–87. New York, National Association of Social Workers, 1969.

Epstein, Laura. "Differential Use of Staff: a Method to Expand Social Services," *Social Work*, VII, No. 4 (1962), 66–72.

Farrar, Marcella, and Mary L. Hemmy. "Use of Nonprofessional Staff in Work with the Aged," *Social Work*, VIII, No. 2 (1963), 44–50.

Fry, John, M.D. *Medicine in Three Societies*. Aylesbury, Bucks, England, Chiltern House, 1969.

Gindy, Aida. "Launching the Second Development Decade: the Challenge to Social Work Education," in *Social Work Education in the Seventies*, XVth Congress of Schools of Social Work, International Association of Schools of Social Work, 1970, pp. 29–44.

Heyman, Margaret M. "A Study of Effective Utilization of Social Workers in a Hospital Setting," *Social Work*, VI, No. 2 (1961), 36–43.

Levitan, Sar A. *The Great Society's Poor Law*, Baltimore, John Hopkins Press, 1969.

Parsons, Talcott. "The Professions and Social Structure," in *Essays in Sociological Theory*, pp. 34–39. New York, Free Press, 1964.

"Proposed Standards for the Evaluation of Undergraduate Programs in Social Work," Council on Social Work Education Document #74–210–1, Jan., 1973.

Pusić, Eugen. "The Administration of Welfare," in Felice Davidson Perlmutter, ed., *A Design for Social Work Practice*, pp. 192–209. New York, Columbia University Press, 1974.

Reich, Charles A. *The Greening of America*. New York, Bantam Books, Inc., 1971.

Richan, Willard C. "A Theoretical Scheme for Determining Roles of Professional and Nonprofessional Personnel," *Social Work*, VI, No. 4 (1961), 22–28.

——. "Indigenous Paraprofessional Staff," in F. Kaslow, ed., *Issues in Human Services*, pp. 51–71. San Francisco, Jossey-Bass, 1972.

Rivesman, Leonore. "Use of the Social Work Team with Aging Family Service Clients," in Robert L. Barker and Thomas L. Briggs, eds., *Manpower Research on the Utilization of Baccalaureate Social Workers*, pp. 63–76. Washington, D.C. Veterans Administration, 1971.

Roszak, Theodore. *The Making of a Counter Culture*. New York, Doubleday, 1969.

Rosengren, William R., and Mark Lefton. *Organizations and Clients*. Columbus, Ohio, Charles F. Merrill Publishing Co., 1970.

Schwartz, Edward E., and William C. Sample. *The Midway Office*. New York, National Association of Social Workers, 1972.

Scott, W. Richard. "Professional Employees in a Bureaucratic Structure: Social Work," in Amitai Etzioni, ed., *The Semi-Professions and Their Organization*, pp. 82–140. New York, Free Press, 1969.

Sobey, Francine. *The Nonprofessional Revolution in Mental Health*. New York, Columbia University Press, 1970.

——. "Introducing Content on Paraprofessionals in Schools of Social Work: Some Issues and Concerns for Educators," in *Workshop on Preparing Graduate Social Work Students to Work with Paraprofessionals*, pp. 3–8. New York, Council on Social Work Education, 1971.

Thompson, Jane K., and Donald P. Riley. "The Use of Professionals in Public Welfare," *Social Work*, XI, No. 1 (1966), 22–27.

Weed, Verne, and William H. Denham. "Toward More Effective Use of the Nonprofessional Worker: a Recent Experiment," *Social Work*, VI, No. 4 (1961), 29–36.

Wolfe, Corrine H. "Improving Services by Better Utilization of Staff," *Public Welfare*, XIX, No. 2 (1961), 53–57, 80–81.

——. *Use of Personnel without Professional Training in Social Service Departments*. New York, Medical Social Work Section, National Association of Social Workers, 1959.

——. "Strategies, Processes, and Resources for Achieving Needed Change in Education for the Social Professions." Paper presented at Symposium on Higher Education and the Social Professions, University of Kentucky, 1972; mimeographed.

B. PERSONNEL PRACTICES

34/NASW STANDARDS FOR SOCIAL WORK PERSONNEL PRACTICES

NATIONAL ASSOCIATION OF SOCIAL WORKERS

PERSONNEL STANDARDS

These standards are based on the principles that (1) effective social service depends on qualified staff and (2) staff members can give their best service when they work under conditions of employment that are conducive to the maintenance of high quality and quantity of production. Since the provision of responsible services to individuals and groups is the paramount concern of the social work profession, these standards are issued with the understanding that they will always be applied within the framework of this fundamental concern of the profession.

In order that social workers may function at their best, every organization employing them should have policies pertaining to personnel administration developed by an appropriate process. These policies should be in writing and should be available to all members of the staff and governing boards. Staff should participate in the development of these policies and in regular, periodic review of them. The policies should include provision for hearing staff members' grievances and other provisions substantially similar to those that follow. These policies are endorsed by the National Association of Social Workers and recommended by the association to practicing social workers, to employing agencies, and to the supporting public as being basic to good personnel administration and good social work practice.

These standards represent principles of desirable personnel policies and practices. They are not intended to substitute for the formulation by specific agencies of their own personnel policies. However, they have been formulated to serve as a guide in the development of personnel policies by social agencies and other institutions employing social workers, such as health agencies, schools, and courts. When NASW has occasion to review personnel practices in specific organizations, these standards serve as a basis for recommendations to improve them.

As part of the NASW program for improving personnel policies, procedures have been established under which the association considers complaints filed by social workers against employers alleging violations of written personnel practices.[1] When complaints are filed against an employer who does not have written personnel policies, these standards are used in the process of adjudicating the complaint.

SELECTION OF PERSONNEL

In recruiting personnel the agency shall, at the appropriate time and place, make the following known to prospective employees:

1. Specific requirements of the vacant position.
2. Qualifications sought in the candidates for the position.
3. Personnel practices and salary range applicable to the position.
4. Any anticipated changes in agency structure and function having direct bearing on the position to be filled.

The selection of personnel shall be on the basis of professional competence, which is designed to assure appointment of persons best qualified to discharge the agency's function effectively. In the selection process there shall be no discrimination because of race, color, religion, age, residence, sex, national origin, and organization membership, if unrelated to the clear and overriding needs for effective discharge of the agency's function. Any restriction of civil rights by law or governmental regulation for agency employment shall be a stated condition of employment. Employers of social workers shall recognize the right of their employees as private citizens to engage in social and political activity.

An agency recruiting to fill a vacant position shall inform members of its own staff who might be interested in and qualified for the position of its availability and allow such staff members to apply for the position, and when a merit system is in effect shall hold promotional assembled or unassembled examinations for its own staff members in addition to holding open competitive examinations.

In the course of evaluating a candidate for a position, written references shall be obtained. These shall be held in confidence by the recipient.

Appointment to a position shall be in writing, with duties, compensation, conditions of employment, and the place of the position in the general function and program of the agency set forth. After an appointment is made, any major change in the assignment or conditions of employment shall be confirmed in a letter to the employee. Letters of appointment as well as letters regarding changes in assignment or conditions of employment should be acknowledged by the employee in writing.

PROBATION

When a probationary period is required, it shall be for a specified period of time. Probation periods shall serve a dual purpose: to permit the employer and employee to evaluate the employee's performance and to provide an opportunity for the employee to assess whether the agency provides a suitable setting for effective use of his professional interests and skills. The end of such a period shall be marked by a mutual evaluation and by a clear decision by both employer and employee regarding the retention of the employee in the new position on the regular staff. Should the employee decide to terminate employment at the end of the probationary period, the opportunity to resign shall be given without adversely affecting the employee's credentials.

After satisfactory completion of the probationary period, all agency personnel policies and benefits shall apply retroactively to the date of employment with the agency.

PERSONNEL PRACTICES

Personnel practices and procedures shall appear in written form as a manual that shall be available at all times to all employees. The development and revision of these practices shall be the mutual responsibility of both administration and staff through the coordinated efforts of the governing body, a personnel policies—practices committee on which staff members serve, or other appropriate staff-represented groups that shall have channels of communication to the executive and the governing body. The executive shall have the responsibility of implementing the policies and assuring that there is effective communication between the various staff and administrative levels.

The personnel practices manual shall be furnished to all new employees. Changes in the manual shall be set forth in writing and shall be properly publicized when adopted. The manual shall include the following:

1. A description of the agency's functions, organizational structure, and administrative lines of authority and responsibility and how these are delegated or shared.

2. A clear definition of the ways in which new policies and/or practices or modifications thereof are established and implemented.

Provision shall be made for a fair and impartial hearing if the employee believes he has been unjustly affected by the agency's personnel action or policy. Such procedures shall be in writing and include the following:

1. Opportunity to confer with the immediate supervisor, the latter's supervisor, and upward to the executive and the board.

2. Provision for the protection of the employer's right to have a written statement describing the basis of the specific action giving rise to the grievance and the employee's right and responsibility to present in writing the specific basis for his dissatisfaction.

3. Opportunity for consideration of the alleged grievance by—at least—an intra-agency committee or other group capable of providing judicious review.

4. Opportunity for the employee to present testimony to the committee or board considering the alleged grievance, directly or through witnesses, and to have a representative of his own choice if he wishes.

5. A clear delineation of the person or persons having authority for final decisions.

LABOR-MANAGEMENT RELATIONS

NASW reaffirms that social workers as employees shall participate in the formulation of personnel policies and procedures. NASW further reaffirms that members of the association may participate in this formulation through whatever instruments they choose democratically and reaffirms the responsibility of management to accept and work with the means chosen by the employee group.

Employees of nonprofit organizations and public agencies should be included under the protective enactment of state labor relations laws, including provisions that guarantee collective bargaining rights. NASW supports the collective bargaining process between organized labor and management as one means of providing a rational and coherent method of solving problems inherent in employee-employer relationships and thereby achieving conditions of employment conducive to optimum service to clients.

Professional values will guide the manner in which NASW members, whether as union members or part of management, participate in collective bargaining. Management and labor should be encouraged to adopt a procedure that approaches *continuous negotiations* as a means of avoiding the trauma of deadline-determined agreements. Labor and management are responsible for understanding and utilizing effectively all the tools at the disposal of those involved in bargaining in a free society—including mediation, arbitration, and the fact-finding panel or board—as a means of finding solutions to problems when direct negotiations have failed to provide an agreement between the employer and the union. The fact of participation in a strike by a member of NASW does not in itself constitute a violation of the Code of Ethics. NASW is opposed to laws or policies that prohibit strikes by employees.

NASW as a professional association shall not engage in collective bargaining on behalf of its members or assume the technical responsibilities of mediation, independent fact-finding, or arbitration. This will not preclude use of individual social workers as mediators, fact-finders, or arbitrators. In the event of a labor dispute NASW shall use its good offices to keep communications open and should know and encourage the use of competent resources for mediation, fact-finding, and arbitration. This does not preclude NASW's taking a position for or against either party in a specific conflict situation.

The agency management has ultimate responsibility for service to clients. In the event of a work stoppage, however, both management and the union should work together to define and plan for staffing emergency services essential to the preservation of the lives and safety of people served by the agency. When there is a union contract, provision for emergency services should be included.

SALARIES

In furtherance of its purpose to promote the quality and effectiveness of social work practice through service to the individual, the group, and the community, the National Association of Social Workers seeks to develop and support policies, procedures, and programs that will help recruit and retain qualified and competent personnel to staff services. Studies indicate that there has been a continued growth in the demand for social work services. Unless social work can devise new and imaginative ways of meeting this challenge, there is a real possibility that valuable and productive community services will have to be curtailed seriously.

Of equal importance to recruiting and creating a steady stream of professionally qualified personnel is the retention of these people in the profession. Experienced and well-qualified personnel provide a basic core for the profession. Their accumulated wisdom and experience are needed to add to knowledge and skill and to raise standards of performance. These experienced workers are also essential for pre-service and in-service education and research. They provide essential leadership. At a time when additional personnel are sorely needed, well-qualified persons must not be lost to more remunerative fields because adequate compensation for years of experience is not forthcoming in social work employment.

In accordance with action by the NASW Delegate Assembly in 1958, the association has adopted a salary policy, including a suggested minimum and recommendations for classification and pay plans. This minimum is periodically reviewed by the Cabinet of the Division of Professional

Standards and is set to assure that the following are reflected: (1) changes in cost of living, (2) changes in standard of living, (3) increases in national productivity, (4) changes in salaries paid for positions requiring comparable eduction experience, and (5) assurance that the minimum represents a figure that is attainable even though it is, for the most part, not yet attained.

For the practitioner who meets the normal expectations of increased competence and responsibility, an annual increase in his salary of 6–8 percent is recommended. *As the beginning salary recommendations change, there should be corresponding increases in the salary ranges for experienced workers at different levels of responsibility.* NASW is currently engaged in the development of salary range recommendations for these workers.

Adequate salaries are necessary to attract and retain competent social workers and are an essential prerequisite to achieving the quality and quantity of social services demanded by the public. Salaries should always be based on the social worker's competence and responsibility.

Salaries paid for social work positions should compare favorably with those paid for positions in other fields, both profit and nonprofit, that require comparable education and experience and for which responsibilities assigned are of similar complexity, difficulty, and importance.

The range of salaries for professional social workers should provide a career potential. Entry level salaries should be sufficient to allow people entering the profession to maintain a standard of living appropriate for professional personnel in their community. As social workers gain experience and increase their competence and as their responsibilities are multiplied, their salaries should be increased appropriately.

Salaries for *direct service* positions of advanced complexity and responsibility that require advanced knowledge and skill should be sufficient to permit the competent practitioner to pursue, without financial sacrifice, a career in providing these basic services to individuals, groups, or communities. The budgetary situation of the employer will determine the number of positions the agency can staff, but it should not influence the salary level the agency maintains.

CLASSIFICATION AND PAY PLANS

To achieve the purpose and carry out the functions of an agency program effectively and efficiently, there should be a classification of all positions based on their relative complexity and responsibility that will clarify the duties of the positions and serve as a basis for employment interviews, equitable salary administration, and other personnel purposes. The plan should include a statement or table showing the grouping of each position with other positions of a similar level of complexity and responsibility and a statement placing this grouping or classification of positions in proper hierarchical relationship to other classifications of positions. It should be in writing and available to staff. There should be provision for continuing periodic review of positions and their classification. Whenever possible, to achieve the agency's purpose effectively, the classification structure should provide career opportunities for members of ethnic minorities and economically disadvantaged persons.

The classification plan should include the following for each position:

1. A title that accurately reflects the functions of the position.
2. A listing or description of the duties and responsibilities assigned.
3. A statement of the minimum qualifications required to perform the duties of the position.

Pay Plans

There should be a pay plan made up of a salary range for each class of position to assure that social workers receive equitable treatment in salaries and to assure efficient administration of an agency. The pay plan should

1. Cover each group of positions in the classification plan.
2. Indicate the salary range for each class of positions and the amount and frequency of increments. It should also state whether increments are periodic or based on merit.

There shall be appropriate salary differentials *within* as well as among job levels to reflect requirements of or achievements in education, training, and experience.

3. Provide for annual review.

The salary range assigned to each job classification should be high enough to attract and retain competent professional personnel. It should take into account the extent and nature of the responsibilities, qualifications required, and rates of pay for comparable positions in other agencies or fields. Salary ranges for each classification should provide enough latitude to allow a social worker to enhance performance and to continue in his position without being deprived of salary advancement or forced to take on a different assignment.

There should be a systematic progression and a logical relationship between the salary ranges assigned to different classifications. When a social worker's duties and responsibilities are changed through promotion or increased significantly through a revised job description, the job should be reclassified and the salary increased accordingly. When the agency's salary ranges overlap, the principle of increased pay for increased responsibility should still apply. This principle would prevail even if the social worker received a salary on the previous assignment equal to or higher than the minimum of the salary range for the new classification.

There should be provision in the pay plan for annual increments within each salary range. The annual increments should be a specified percentage of the social worker's salary for all positions in the salary classification plan.

The pay plan should exclude payments "in kind" as part of total salary payments.

Regular annual increments, as provided in the pay plan, should be given for satisfactory performance. Additional *merit* increments should be given for unusual and superior performance that exceeds specific agency standards.

If performance is unsatisfactory, regular increments can be withheld for a specified period not to exceed one year. Either improved performance or termination of employment in a specific position should result.

SECONDARY EMPLOYMENT

Secondary employment can provide personal satisfaction and enhance professional competence. It may strengthen community relationships and help meet a community need in the face of a chronic manpower shortage in social work.

NASW reaffirms that a social worker's remuneration from primary employment should provide him with the means to maintain a standard of living appropriate for professional personnel in his community. Secondary employment to supplement income for this purpose should, therefore, not be necessary.

The following provisions shall govern secondary employment:

After Regular Working Hours
1. An employee has the right to engage in secondary employment as long as it does not interfere in any way with his responsibilities to his primary employer. Agencies should have governing policies, including provisions that safeguard agency operations when secondary employment may entail conflict of interest or when there is evidence that it would negatively affect job performance.

2. Remuneration from secondary employment accrues solely to the employee.

3. When the primary employer's facilities and/or resources are used, the employee should obtain prior written approval. If reimbursement for such use is required by the agency, there should be a written understanding of the nature of such reimbursement.

During Regular Working Hours
Activities such as teaching, conducting seminars, and speaking engagements for which the employee is reimbursed are illustrations of this kind of secondary employment.

1. An employee has the obligation to seek advance approval of his employing agency for this kind of assignment. Although such activity may have secondary benefits to the employing agency, the agency retains final authority for approval.

2. Remuneration from this type of activity accrues to the employee.

3. Agencies should have policies governing this type of employment. If such policies include a provision for reimbursement to the primary employer for the time the employee is actually absent, it may be in the form of deductions from earnings or by requiring the employee to utilize earned compensatory, vacation, or other leave time other than sick leave.

When private practice is the secondary employment, the NASW standard for the private practice of social work—membership in the Academy of Certified Social Workers—is also to be observed.

ORIENTATION AND STAFF DEVELOPMENT

An orientation period shall be provided for any employee newly appointed to a position, whether coming from within or outside the agency, for the purpose of informing him of the specific job duties and their relationship to agency functions.

Opportunity for continued staff development shall be afforded through provision for the following:

1. Qualified supervision and consultation.

2. Professional literature.

3. Regular planned staff meetings for discussion of agency program and social work problems and methods.

4. Absence during working hours to attend conferences, institutes, workshops, or classes to advance employee skills related to the functions and goals of the employing agency. Such attendance shall result in no loss of pay or vacation time.

EVALUATIONS

As a basis for objective evaluation of performance, the agency should set forth written standards of performance for all positions in its classification plan. Such standards should describe the quality and quantity of performance expected for each job duty. The evaluation shall be made by the person or persons who directly supervise(s) the employee.

There shall be a full evaluation at such times as it is required for the professional development of the employee or the administrative needs of the agency, when there has been a significant change in the performance of the employee, or when the employee or his supervisor leaves the agency. When a probationary period is required, there shall be an evaluation at the end of that period. The evaluation shall relate specifically to the performance of the job assigned to the employee and, when indicated, to such personal behavior as is not in accord with NASW's Code of Ethics.

The time of the evaluation shall be known in advance. Evaluation shall engage the joint participation of the employee and supervisor. However, the authority of the evaluator must be recognized on both sides and final authority belongs to him.

The evaluation shall be in writing and shall cover the points discussed in the evaluation conference. The employee shall be given the opportunity to read the evaluation, to sign it (signifying that he has read it), and to file a statement covering any points with which he disagrees. A copy of the evaluation shall be furnished to the employee.

The written evaluation and the employee's statement, if any, shall become an integral part of the employee's personnel record. The personnel record shall be kept strictly confidential and be made available to authorized persons only. The record shall contain the application, contracts or agreements, a description of work assignments, service ratings, and pertinent correspondence.

The personnel record shall be available to the employee at all times with due reason except that he shall not have access to any material sent to the agency in confidence.

TEMPORARY OR PART-TIME EMPLOYMENT

Employment for a limited period for specific purposes shall not necessarily be subject to the same conditions of employment that apply to permanent staff. The length of time for which one is employed and the scope, duties, compensation, and conditions of employment pertaining to the temporary position shall be clearly defined. Regular permanent employment on a part-time basis shall be subject to the same conditions of employment that apply to full-time permanent staff.

Temporary reclassification and pay adjustment shall be provided for regular employees who, in the absence of some other staff member, are assigned duties heavier than those they usually carry when such an assignment persists for a period of time exceeding the longest compensated leave possible within the agency.

TENURE

An employee who has successfully completed the probationary period in a position for which such is required and who continues to meet the agency's standards of performance shall have the right to continue with the agency unless retrenchment or reorganization results in the abolition of the specific position. The policy of indefinite tenure shall be safeguarded by provisions for regular evaluations, specific conditions for termination of employment, and appeals procedures. Seniority (length of service) shall, along with other pertinent factors, be given due consideration when action regarding personnel is taken.

PROMOTION

In filling a vacant position the agency shall give first consideration to promotion of qualified employees within the agency. The promotion of employees shall operate under the same standards governing selection of personnel. That is, there shall be equitable consideration of all professionally qualified applicants without discrimination (except for the clear and overriding needs for effective discharge of the agency's function) on such bases as race, color, religion, age, residence, sex, national origin, or membership in a union or an organization whose primary purpose is the protection of civil rights or the improvement of living conditions and/or human relations. Procedures for promotion shall provide for evaluation of persons on the basis of professional competence, which is designed to assure appointment of persons best qualified to discharge the agency's function effectively.

Promotion shall be based on evaluation of past performance and capacity for the vacant position. When these factors are relatively equal for two or more employees, seniority shall be considered.

HOURS OF WORK

A reasonable number of hours shall be stipulated as the regular workweek. It is recommended that the workweek not exceed 37½ hours.

Overtime on a regular sustained basis shall not be expected or required. When a significant amount of overtime cannot be avoided, provision for compensation should be made.

For agencies, institutions, or resident camps requiring regular evening or weekend hours, the plan of hours shall be clearly defined with the following limitations recommended:

1. No more than two work periods per workday.
2. No more than four evening work periods per calendar week.
3. A consecutive forty-eight-hour period off in each calendar week.
4. At least one weekend of sixty consecutive hours off per month.

PARTICIPATION IN ACTIVITIES OF PROFESSIONAL ORGANIZATIONS

Social work, like other professions, has undertaken professional activities largely through the voluntary participation of its qualified members. Individual members have viewed and should view such participation as part of their professional commitment. Agencies should encourage such professional activities and make time available to social workers for them.

Since the range of professional activities is broad and varied, the agency should grant the worker time off to participate in such activities when prior discussions have concluded that the professional activity coincides with the agency's specific goals and the time off will not jeopardize the daily functioning of the agency. In those instances in which the social worker has been assigned activities; chosen to serve on such bodies as national boards, commissions, task forces, or committees; or asked to present a paper or lead a professional institute; the agency should offer no impediment to the social worker's need for time off from agency responsibility.

Time off for professional activities under these circumstances should not result in the loss of vacation, salary, or compensatory time.

LEAVE

Vacation or Annual Leave

A definite period of vacation with pay shall be earned for services performed by all regular employees. An employee shall earn vacation beginning in the first month of employment. It is recommended that such vacation be calculated on the basis of two workdays for each month of employment. Generally, annual vacations do not accrue beyond one year. However, there may be instances in which exigencies of service make it impossible for an employee to take his annual vacation. Accrual of leave under these conditions shall be the result of mutual discussion by the employee and employer. An employee leaving the agency shall be entitled to the vacation due him.

Sick Leave

A definite period of sick leave with pay shall be allowed annually. It is recommended that each employee be entitled to sick leave of at least twenty-four workdays per year. It is recommended that provision be made for accumulation of unused sick leave up to at least sixty-five workdays.

Sick leave may be used in the instance of employee illness, illness in the immediate family of the employee requiring his presence, or the death of a member of the immediate family.

Medical Leave

When an employee has used up his accrued sick leave but continues to be absent because of illness, he shall be given the opportunity to substitute vacation time. If no vacation time is accrued or if the employee chooses not to use vacation for the purpose of sick leave, he shall be granted medical leave without pay for a specified period of time. During absence on medical leave, the employee shall not accrue sick leave or vacation but shall retain his seniority rights.

Educational Leave

Provision should be made for leaves for educational purposes so that the employee may develop his skill and provide better service. Provision should be such as to make it financially feasible for employees to take such leaves.

Terms of the leave should be clearly set forth. The worker on leave is considered an employee and his seniority rights and status in the agency retirement plan should be protected.

Maternity Leave

Provision should be made for leave without pay for maternity purposes for employees who have been on the staff for one year or longer. Employees requiring maternity leave shall request it at least sixty days before the date on which the period of leave is to begin. It is recommended that maternity leave be granted for periods up to a maximum of one year. The agency shall incur the obligation of reinstating the employee returning from maternity leave to a position comparable to that which she vacated and she shall be paid at prevailing rates at such time as a suitable vacancy occurs in the staff.

Military Leave

Military leave shall be granted to men who are inducted into the armed services. Employees on military leave shall be afforded the protection of their seniority rights and their status in the agency's retirement plan and shall be reassigned promptly on return to civilian life. Provision shall be made so that employees called to individual military reserve training shall suffer no loss of regular income and no loss of vacation time owed them. When an employee chooses alternative services as a conscientious objector or is imprisoned for refusal to serve, he shall receive the same consideration as the employee who accepts military service.

Jury Duty

Leave for jury duty shall be provided so that employees called to serve on juries suffer no loss of regular income and no loss of vacation time due them.

Sabbatical Leave

It is recommended that sabbatical leave for personal and professional development be granted to employees after six consecutive years of service not interrupted by maternity leave, prolonged sick leave, or leave for study. It is recommended that sabbatical leave consist of at least three months with pay in addition to the annual vacation. Sabbatical leave should be contingent on the employee's return to the agency for a period of at least one year following the leave.

Holidays

The customary community holidays or their equivalent shall be granted. If the agency grants time off for employees to observe religious holidays, such time shall be available *equally* to all empoyees.

FINANCIAL AID FOR PROFESSIONAL EDUCATION

Financial aid programs for graduate professional education in social work play a key role in recruitment for the profession by helping qualified students attain the MSW degree. Social work agencies and other employers of social workers should support programs of financial aid either by contributing to university or community programs, developing their own programs, or supporting appropriate legislation at federal, state, or local levels designed to increase professional social work manpower.[2]

The establishment of restrictive conditions in the granting of financial aid or the imposition of employment commitments frequently limits the effectiveness of such programs. Experience and research in administration of financial aid programs have shown that social work students do not have sufficient knowledge of the range of social work methods or fields of practice or of their own skills and professional interest to choose among prospective job offerings at the beginning of their professional education. Therefore, the imposition of employment commitments should be discouraged. During the transition period until the time when no poststudy obligation will be imposed by granting agencies, the following policies should be adhered to:

Responsibility of the Applicant

Before accepting financial aid the applicant should evaluate all opportunities available to him and understand fully the terms of his agreement. He should seek the advice of a school of social work if he needs help in making his decision. Anyone who enters into an agreement with an agency in connection with a grant of financial aid for professional education has an ethical obligation to fulfill his agreement.

Responsibility of the Agency

When agencies establish programs of financial aid to students for professional education, the following practices should be observed:

1. The agency should help the applicant evaluate all opportunities available to him and help him understand fully the terms of his agreement.

2. The grant should cover the full period required for completion of the MSW degree without interruption. Agency support should be discontinued only if the student withdraws or is advised by the school of social work to withdraw from professional education or the terms of the agreement are no longer applicable.

3. The student who is an agency employee on educational leave should retain his seniority rights and his status with respect to employee benefits included in the agency personnel program.

4. A written agreement should be made between the agency and the student, taking into account the following:

a. It should include the amount of the grant and the period of time it covers.

b. Any commitment requiring the recipient of the grant to accept employment in the agency following completion of his professional education should not exceed a period of time equivalent to the period of time covered by the financial aid grant. (In cases when the student is on a work-study program and continues in active service with the agency during part of his professional education, the time spent in agency service should be credited.)

c. A clear statement should be made of conditions under which the agency may terminate the agreement, including a statement of procedures to be followed if the student does not complete his professional education or for valid or unforeseen reasons is unable to fulfill the requirements of the agreement. If financial restitution is part of the agreement, terms for repayment should be specified, usually without interest.

d. The agency is obligated to employ a person returning from educational leave at least at the same salary level as other new graduates.

5. No agreement can become final before the student has been accepted for matriculation by an accredited school of social work.

6. A grant earned by the student as a special benefit recognized in law (e.g., a G.I. educational benefit) shall not be deducted from financial aid otherwise granted to the student.

Responsibility of the School of Social Work

The school of social work has responsibility for informing applicants and students about the availability of all financial aid programs and, when appropriate, loan resources. Financial aid programs enabling students to complete graduate professional education in accredited schools of social work* take various forms, the most common of which are defined as follows:

Loan. A loan, usually small in amount, granted by school, university, voluntary agency, or federal, state, or local public agency. Usually no or low interest is charged. Repayment periods range up to ten years and there commonly is a grace period between completion of professional education and the beginning of repayment.

Fellowship. An award given in recognition of academic achievement or leadership potential. Usually financial need is not a factor in granting a fellowship.

* Editor's note: This refers to graduate social work programs that are accredited by the Council on Social Work Education. Since July 1, 1974, the Council has also accredited baccalaureate social work programs, and thus this statement applies to that level of education as well.

Scholarship. An award to an able and financially needy student that will help in substantial measure to close the gap between his personal resources and the total cost of his education. Scholastic achievement and professional promise in addition to financial need are equally determining factors in these awards.

Tuition scholarship. An award made by the school, university, or agency but limited to part or the total cost of tuition. The award may be based on financial need or on recognition of scholastic achievement and professional promise.

Fieldwork stipend. A payment made to the student by the agency in which he is placed for field instruction.

Work-study plan. A program involving some combination of full-time study and some work in which the student is paid for his work in the agency.

Educational leave. A leave for study with salary granted by an agency to an employee.

PHYSICAL CONDITIONS

Working facilities shall be of such a nature as to afford employees a reasonable degree of comfort, to insure the maintenance of health, and to make possible the discharge of duties with efficiency.

RETIREMENT

The agency shall provide for a retirement plan to be administered by a competent retirement system, insurance company, or bank. All plans should be fully funded. If the plan is a contributory one, the agency's contribution should be equal to or greater than that of the staff. It is recommended that the retirement plan include the following:

1. Provision that for all regular employees entrance into the plan be mandatory after a specified period of employment of not more than one year, with optional provision for payment retroactive to date of employment.

2. Provision for entrance into the retirement plan without a waiting period if the staff member has had retirement coverage elsewhere.

3. Provision for past service benefits for staff members who have rendered long-time service prior to adoption of the retirement plan.

4. Provision that retirement benefits from twenty-five years of cumulative service be 50 percent or more of the highest five years of employment as a base when the employee has given long-time service in one agency.

5. Provision for full and immediate credit to the staff member of equities arising from the agency's and, in case of contributory plans, staff member's contribution, thus establishing "portability" of pension rights.

6. Provision for return of the staff member's contribution plus interest if he leaves the agency and elects a cash refund or provision for return of

this contribution to the beneficiary in the event of the employee's death before retirement benefits have begun.

7. Provision for death benefits at least equal to the current annual salary if death occurs before retirement and while the employee is still on staff. This benefit should be independent of the refund referred to in 6 above.

8. Provision for election of retirement prior to or later than the planned retirement age, with appropriate adjustment of benefits.

9. Provision for retirement at full benefits prior to the planned retirement age when retirement is due to total and permanent disability.

10. Provision for change of beneficiary.

11. Provision for varied forms of optional settlement, including the joint and survivor option and guaranteed payments.

12. Provision for continuance in the retirement plan on an individual basis in the event that change in employment does not permit the individual to participate in a group retirement plan or in case of an approved leave of absence.

It is recommended that on an annual or biennial basis the staff member be apprised of benefits accrued to his account as of a given date. It is recommended that there be periodic review (at least every three years) of the entire retirement program.

INSURANCE

The agency shall finance, in whole or in part, insurance plans to help employees meet certain financial obligations. It is recommended that such insurance plans cover the following:

1. Benefits for medical and hospital expenses, including social work services.

2. Compensation (including workmen's compensation) equivalent to full salary and medical costs for a period of incapacity up to at least six months when such incapacity is a consequence of a disability incurred in the line of duty.

3. Continued compensation or disability payments for incapacity resulting from a disability incurred in the line of duty, the duration of which exceeds the six-month period referred to above.

The employer shall assist employees who wish to join together to finance sickness and accident disability insurance and other such insurance not financed in whole or in part by the agency.

If the agency requires or strongly urges employees to carry professional liability insurance, the agency shall pay the premium for such insurance or reimburse the employee for premiums paid.

The agency shall provide liability and life insurance for work-related travel.

When statutes apply, agencies shall provide coverage for unemployment insurance for all employees.

REIMBURSEMENT OF EXPENSES

Expenses incidental to the job shall be provided by the agency in addition to salary. Policies governing payment of such expenses shall be established to cover actual costs. For example, staff members shall be reimbursed for costs incurred in connection with attendance at luncheons, conferences, and the like, when they attend at the request of the agency: per diem rates shall cover actual out-of-pocket expense, mileage rates shall be sufficient to cover actual costs of operating and maintaining a car, and the employee shall be reimbursed for any extra expense incurred in purchasing liability insurance when such extra expense is a consequence of his using his car for business purposes.

TERMINATION OF EMPLOYMENT

Nature of Termination
  1. Layoff.
  a. Layoff shall be construed as removal from a position owing to the abolition of the position because of reorganization or retrenchment.
  b. When more than one employee is involved, the agency shall establish a formula governing the order in which employees shall be laid off, such formula taking into account both seniority and quality of performance. The formula shall be inversely applied if, at a later date, such employees can be rehired because of reorganization or expansion.
  c. The employee who is laid off shall receive severance pay in an amount related to length of service.
  d. The employee who is laid off shall, if he wishes, have the opportunity to resign formally and be recorded as having resigned in good standing.
  2. Demotion
  a. Demotion shall be construed as removal from a particular position with an offer of a position of lesser responsibility because of the employee's inability to perform in the position of greater responsibility or the abolition of the position of greater responsibility. (See Layoff.)
  b. When demotion is offered to more than one employee as an alternative to being laid off, a formula similar to that prescribed to govern layoff shall govern the order in which employees are demoted. The formula shall be applied inversely in the event that those so demoted can at a later date be promoted as a result of agency expansion.
  3. Dismissal
Dismissal shall be construed as the discharge of an employee from an

agency because of unsatisfactory job performance, violation of contract, or commission of certain acts defined in the personnel practices of the agency or of certain acts contrary to the Code of Ethics of the National Association of Social Workers.

4. Resignation

Resignation shall be construed as termination of employment at the volition of the employee. A resignation requested by the employer as an alternative to dismissal shall, insofar as employer-employee rights and responsibilities are concerned, be construed as equivalent to dismissal.

5. Retirement

Retirement shall be construed as the termination of employment under a defined retirement plan in effect in an agency at such time as the employee has reached retirement age and no longer wishes to work or is no longer able to work.

Notice Required

1. Termination of employment by employer action

a. The employer who terminates the employment of an employee shall give him a reasonable amount of notice. It is recommended that the permanent employee be given at least thirty days' notice and the probationary employee two weeks' notice, except that when a probationary employee is laid off he shall be entitled to thirty days' notice.

b. Pay in lieu of notice may be granted at the discretion of the employer.

c. The employer shall give written notice of the action and the reasons for the action, and the employee shall acknowledge such notice in writing.

2. Termination of employment through planned retirement

a. As employees approach retirement age, there should be consultation services available to assist them in making the necessary transitional adjustment to retirement.

b. The retirement policy should state the planned retirement age and contain provisions for retirement prior to the planned retirement age or the continuation of employment beyond such age.

c. The executive or designated person should be charged with the responsibility for determining with the individual the plan for his retirement or continued employment. Such planning should be initiated six months to a year prior to the planned retirement date. The final decision to continue employment beyond the planned retirement age is the responsibility of the employer.

d. There should be a written confirmation of the plan agreed on.

3. Termination of employment by employee action

a. The agency shall specify the amount of advance written notice required in instances of resignation and employees shall abide by agency requirements in this matter.

b. The employee shall provide written notice of the intent to resign as of a specific date and the employer shall acknowledge the receipt of this notice in writing.

References

1. References shall be factually correct and include all pertinent data.
2. References shall state the relationship of the writer to the subject of the reference.
3. References shall be limited in content to material that has been made known to the subject of the reference during the course of his employment.
4. A copy of the letter of reference shall be made available to the subject of reference on his request.

NOTES

1. "NASW Procedures for Adjudication of Grievances" (rev. ed.; New York: National Association of Social Workers, 1970). (Multilithed.)
2. For more detailed suggestions about the conduct of financial aid programs, *see* "Establishing and Administering Financial Aid Programs in Social Work Education: A Guide to Standards and Practices" (New York: Council on Social Work Education, undated).

C. AFFIRMATIVE ACTION

35/AFFIRMATIVE ACTION AND JOB SECURITY: POLICY DILEMMAS

SHIRLEY M. BUTTRICK

A conflict among legitimate rights carries a corresponding obligation to search for remedies that are as equitable as possible. It is in this spirit that the thorny relationship between affirmative action, unionization, and seniority (tenure) is here examined. For while the struggle has been to achieve affrmative action in hiring and promotion that struggle has taken place within an economy of expanding opportunity. Given a situation of contraction or a nogrowth, the issues involved in layoff, as well as in hiring and promotion, surface. The resulting polarization and escalation of racial tension make incumbent the search for solutions.

Do the demands to equalize employment by increasing the percentage of minority and female employees on corporate and university payrolls mean that they are entitled to some special consideration when cutbacks are made? How can layoffs proceed without compromising either the equal employment opportunity obligation (EEO) or the obligation to organized labor? How can promotions be handled in the presence of an increasingly tenured faculty?

To put the discussion in proper perspective, the significant legislation should be noted. Three federal laws and one executive order are important: namely Title VII of the 1964 Civil Rights Act; the Equal Pay Act of 1963 as amended; Title IX of the educational amendments of 1972; and Executive Order 11246 as amended by 11375.

Title VII of the Civil Rights Act covers all employers with fifteen or more employees. It makes it unlawful to discriminate against an individual in hiring and firing, or with respect to compensation, terms, conditions, and privileges of employment because of race, color, religion, sex, or national origin. The most important guidelines pertain to hiring and promotion criteria. Criteria must be spelled out in objective terms. Also, criteria which may seem to be neutral but which adversely affect women or minorities are unlawful unless the employer can demonstrate that the skills measured by the criteria—bona fide occupational qualifications—are actually necessary in the performance of the job. The 1972 amendments expanded the jurisdiction of the Equal Employment Opportunity Commission to include all educational employers, major educational public elementary and primary school systems as well as public and private institutions of higher education. The Equal Pay Act of 1963 prohibits discrimination in regard to wages or fringe benefits based on sex, and in 1972 this act was amended to cover executive, administrative, and professional employees.

Executive Order 11246 has included coverage of sex discrimination since October, 1968, when it was amended by Executive Order 11375.[1] The requirements of the executive order are based on the contractual relationship between the federal government and employers holding contracts with the federal government. As a condition of doing business with the federal government, the employer is required to meet a higher standard than that imposed on employers in general by Title VII. Under the executive order, all employers with federal contracts in excess of $10,000 must agree to take affirmative action to:

1. Eliminate all discriminatory practices against women and minorities.

2. Eliminate, through the establishment of goals and timetables, any underutilization of women or minorities in their work force whether or not the underutilization is a result of prior discriminatory practices.[2]

Employers with contracts in excess of $50,000 must, in addition, develop and maintain an Affirmative Action Plan (AAP). Employers are evaluated on their good faith efforts to meet these goals. In addition, employers awarded contracts in excess of one million dollars must have their AAP's audited and approved prior to issuance of the contract.

Title IX has been in effect since July 1, 1972, and covers sex discrimination in student admissions, treatment of students, and employment of faculty for all educational institutions receiving federal monies from grants, contracts, loans, and so forth. Through this legislation almost every educational institution—elementary, secondary, and postsecondary—is explicitly prohibited from engaging in sex-discriminatory practices. Because the final Title IX regulations were not issued until August, 1975, it is still too soon to determine how the Office of Civil Rights will move.

The main import of the Civil Rights Act is that it permits the Department of Health, Education, and Welfare (HEW) to investigate discrimination and compel its elimination on the basis of the financial relationship between the federal government and the institution; it does not have to wait until a complaint has been filed.[3]

There are some who are still unclear about the concept of equal employment opportunity and affirmative action. EEO refers to the right of all persons to work and to advance on the basis of merit, ability, and potential. Affirmative action represents a way of achieving that goal. This is why there is recognition of the need to analyze the work force, to identify practices that serve to deny women and minorities equal pay, equal privileges, and equal opportunity for employment and promotion. It follows also that conditions of underutilization of women and minorities must be identified and steps taken to correct such underutilization as well as other inequities. What has been misunderstood is that it is "illegal" to have an institution or a department "reserve" a specific position for a female or a minority candidate and thereby exclude other potential candidates from consideration.

While there is much established civil rights law in the area of hiring and promotion, legal guidelines with regard to dismissal and layoffs are only now beginning to take shape. For example, the National Association for the Advancement of Colored People (NAACP) is currently involved in litigation against the policy of determining layoffs, furloughs, and dismissals by seniority.[4]

Case law is also developing around the variety of issues involved in sex discrimination in employment. The courts appear to be moving in the same forceful manner they showed in their decisions on racial discrimination. However, since the bulk of the sex discrimination cases has been filed only during the past few years, most of the key decisions so far have been made at the lower or appellate court levels. The situation is further complicated by the fact that case law has progressed along two different legal paths: under Title VII of the Civil Rights Act and under the 14th amendment to the Constitution. Thus, case law is more highly developed in relation to the specific issues of hiring, promotion, and testing qualifications than, for example, to layoffs.[5]

Take, for example, the case of *Griggs* v. *Duke Power Company*. In that case, Chief Justice Warren E. Burger of the Supreme Court wrote, for a unanimous court:

The objective of Congress in the enactment of Title VII was to achieve equality of employment opportunities and remove barriers that have operated in the past to favor an identifiable group of white employees over other employees. Under the act, practices, procedures or tests neutral on their face and even neutral in terms of intent cannot be allowed if they operate to "freeze" the status quo of prior discriminatory employment practices.[6]

In *Albermarle Paper Company* v. *Moody* the Supreme Court made back pay a right of victims of discrimination in all but exceptional circumstances.[7] It also tightened the standards an employer must meet in order to use an employment test that disqualifies minorities at a higher rate than it does nonminorities.

More recently, in *Watkins v. Local No. 2369*, Federal District Judge Fred J. Cassibry held that the Continental Can Company's plant in Harvey, Louisiana, should not be permitted to use a seniority approach that had the effect of laying off forty-eight out of fifty black employees, mostly because all but two of them had been hired since 1965.[8] Another view appears to reject Judge Cassibry's line of reasoning. The decision of the Court of Appeals in the Seventh Circuit stated that Title VII speaks only to the future and that an employment seniority system embodying the "last-hired, first-fired" principle does not of itself perpetuate past discrimination. "To hold otherwise would be tantamount to shackling white employees with a burden of past discrimination created not by them but by their employer."[9]

In industry there is seniority born of unionization; in universities, tenure born of academic freedom. The issue involves the relationship between tenure, seniority, and affirmative action and the critical effect of employment and layoffs upon these relationships. The conflicting and competing claims all have merit. One cannot erode the progress of the last five years, but the claims of seniority of service are indeed serious ones. It is somewhat encouraging to find organized labor searching for some compromise; that is, for a system of plant-wide seniority rather than seniority by job category or by department. In the meantime, the consistent logic of the courts continues to be that people should not be adversely affected as a result of race or sex.

ISSUES

Even if the issue of layoffs in an economic downturn had not arisen, a problem would still exist in any field or area that was neither actively expanding nor in flux. Thus, we have reached the point in universities, for example, where the tenure decisions of the 1960s may burden the entry of new people into the system. In such a case, the issue will be even more sharply drawn as to whether existing criteria for entry, promotion, and tenure may be at odds with affirmative action criteria. Chait and Ford lean heavily in this direction. They point out that the typical assistant professor has between three and seven years to demonstrate qualifications for tenure. These are years, beyond the doctorate, where women are disadvantaged by childbearing and other responsibilities. Further, they see the Griggs decision as lending support to their view that "credentials" as a criterion for tenure may also be at odds with affirmative action.[10] They lean on a lower federal court decision, namely, *Armstead v. Starkville Municipal School District*, as providing additional substance for their view. In that case, the court declared that a public school board had unlawfully discriminated against blacks by tying teachers' appointments and retention to the attainment of a master's degree and specified scores on graduate record examinations that had not been validated as accurate predictors of job performance.[11] The implications of such decisions are that the employers (colleges) have the burden of showing that any given requirement has a clear relationship to job performance.

By 1972, colleges and universities with tenure systems (85 percent of the total) had a median of 41 percent to 50 percent of their faculties on tenure.[12] Given present circumstances, vacancies need to arise from turnover rather than from expansion. The clear effect of tenure, however, is to limit turnover and thus to come into conflict with affirmative action. Unions also offer job security, which vies with tenure. Moreover, academic freedom can just as well be safeguarded through "conditions of employment" clauses. Unlike tenure systems, unions can protect everyone within the bargaining unit and so shift the burden of proof on to management to demonstrate incompetence.

Regardless of one's opinion of the feasibility and desirability of unionization for institutions of higher learning, the fact is that by the fall of 1973, 212 postsecondary institutions had collective bargaining agents. While affirmative action sets up a challenge to the criteria and procedures used to accord tenure, unions also pose a challenge by taking on the traditional goals of tenure, namely employment security and the protection of academic freedom. Does this mean that affirmative action and unionization are themselves compatible? Not at all. Teachers' unions have historically supported fixed pay scales. Such "lock-step" systems are based on length of service and specific credentials. They tend to bar an administrator from offering different salaries to equally qualified employees. Given the realities of the market place, this lock-step system conflicts with affirmative action recruitment. To the extent that retrenchment leads to layoffs, seniority as practiced by unions (unless new formulas are found) will adversely affect minorities and women.

In a January, 1973, directive, William Hodgson, then Secretary of Labor, ordered the Bethlehem Steel Plant at Sparrows Point, Maryland, "to correct a seniority system that has been found to perpetuate the effects of past discrimination in the assignment of blacks to jobs in departments with limited advancement opportunities." As authority to act, Hodgson cited Executive Order 11246, the same order that governs affirmative action for colleges and universities.[13] Chait and Ford maintain that affirmative action and unionization are likely to bring an end to current tenure systems. Where affirmative action conflicts with unionization, they believe federal and stage agencies will settle for affirmative action. Could be!

In the meantime, both unions and academic institutions have begun to search for ways to maintain the best of their tenure and seniority systems while permitting some innovation and flexibility.

DIRECTIONS

Universities have begun the process of rethinking and changing their traditional tenure commitments. The most pressing reason is financial. Some universities now require an extended probationary period, others have set tenure quotas, some offer only renewable contracts (which are usually renewed). The aim is to provide both financial and curricular flexibility, and in this respect, tenure guidelines and affirmative action plans have some elements of compatibility, at least in the short run. For that matter, unionization and affirmative action plans may be somewhat compatible in the long run. For as women and minorities become a more significant constituency, union policies which discriminate against them will have to undergo change.

As tenure has come under increasing attack, even its staunchest supporters have begun to consider the choices to be made in arriving at some reasonable guidelines. What are the choices and what shall the stated policy be? In a situation where there is little or no growth in the total number of faculty members, what are the limits to the tenuring-in process? What are the critical variables that must be considered?

The American Association of University Professors, justifiably uneasy with the setting of tenure limits, has identified several variables which must be considered, such as the annual attrition rate of those who have tenure, the annual promotion rate, and the fraction of tenured faculty lost by attrition who are replaced by nontenured appointments.[14] Each one of these variables represents a possible policy position which can affect the tenure ratio. For example, it is possible to achieve a tenure ratio of 0.67 by doing all replacements at the nontenured level, with a tenured attrition rate of 0.05 and an annual promotion rate of 0.10. It is also possible to keep the desired tenure ratio of 0.67 by replacing half of the tenured losses by tenure appointments if the attrition rate were 0.05. In that case, the promotion rate would have to drop to 0.05.[15]

All of this is intended to emphasize that there are choices to be made, that tradeoffs are possible between attrition, promotion, and replacement, and that it is useful to make such choices explicit. One way to decrease the tenuring-in problem is to raise standards. Or the annual promotion rate can be lowered, and a faculty member spend more time in a non-tenured rank. Greater turnover can be encouraged within the tenure ranks. The tenure ratio is itself a choice variable. But when an acceptable ratio has been chosen, a set of policies compatible with it should be stated. Such decisions involve knowing the tradeoffs that are involved and should be made with the full participation of faculty members.

The illustrations utilized for tenure decisions are also applicable to seniority decisions. New York City Human Rights Commissioner Eleanor

Holmes Norton has been asking employers to consider cost savings by means such as a reduced work week, shift changes, payless work days, and job cuts across categories and departments to spread the burden. Certainly business, caught between minority and feminist organizations, organized labor, and the civil rights enforcement machinery, wants some formula that will allow layoffs without jeopardizing either its EEO obligations or its obligations to organized labor. All are in agreement that the issue is prickly. Yet all are equally agreed that traditional methods are no longer workable and that modifications in the seniority system are in order. Had the recession gone much deeper, there would have been no way to avoid a solution, however faulty. The problem is not easily resolved to anyone's satisfaction, for the clash of interests is potentially explosive. Serious ideas must be brought forward and pat answers discarded. It is to be hoped that this discussion will make a small contribution in that direction.

NOTES

1. Roslyn Kane, *Sex Discrimination in Education*, Vol. I. This report was prepared under contract No. 300–75–0205, Education Division, National Center for Education Statistics, Department of Health, Education, and Welfare, 1976.
2. Regulations issued pursuant to Executive Order 11246, 41 C.F.R. 60–2.
3. Kane, *op. cit.*, p. x–7.
4. The NAACP argues for "racial ratios," that is, it asserts that an employer should have the same proportion of blacks after a layoff as it had before the layoff.
5. For an excellent summary of selected cases, see Kane, *op. cit.*, Section XI, pp. 1–19.
6. *Griggs* v. *Duke Power Co.*, U.S. Supreme Court, 1971, 401 U.S. 424 S. Ct. 849, 28 L. Ed., 158 (1971).
7. U.S. Supreme Court, 10 FEP 1181, June 25, 1975.
8. *New York Times*, January 29, 1975, p. 17.
9. *Ibid.*
10. Richard Chait and Andrew T. Ford, "Affirmative Action, Tenure, and Unionization," in Dyck Vermillye, editor, *Lifelong Learners: Issues in Higher Education* (San Francisco: Jossey Bass, 1975), p. 125.
11. *Armstead* v. *Starkville Municipal School District*, 325F. Supp. 560 (1971).
12. Chait and Ford, *op. cit.*, p. 126.
13. *Ibid.*, p. 129.
14. "Surviving the Seventies, report on the Economic Status of the Profession, 1972–1973. Part III: Tenuring-in." 59th Annual Meeting of the American Association of University Professors, AAUP *Bulletin*, LIX (1973), 198–203; Richard R. West, "Tenure Quotas and Financial Flexibility in Colleges and Universities," *Educational Record*, Spring, 1974, pp. 96–100.
15. See AAUP *Bulletin*, *op. cit.*, p. 20, for the formula which illustrates the limit to the Tenuring-in process where there is no growth in total faculty.

36/THREE KEY ISSUES IN AFFIRMATIVE ACTION

CATHERINE LOVELL

As we attempt to implement affirmative action policies, three key issues always arise. *First,* the distinction between affirmative action and "non-discrimination"; *second,* why preferential hiring and the setting of target quotas are necessary to the affirmative action process; and *third,* why traditional standards of "quality" must be reexamined.

Until these issues are resolved, successful affirmative action programs cannot be implemented and substantial progress toward eliminating job discrimination will not be made. Their resolution will require fundamental shifts in individual values as well as changes in some of our collective norms.

UNDERSTANDING THE DIFFERENCE BETWEEN AFFIRMATIVE ACTION AND NON-DISCRIMINATION

The distinction between affirmative action and non-discrimination is the difference between the *active* and the *passive* mode. It is illustrated by the difference between management by objectives and incrementalism. All of our public agencies have been "equal opportunity employers" operating under fair employment practices laws for nearly 30 years. What those laws require are policy statements against discrimination. The absence of overt discrimination has sufficed to meet this standard. Action is left to the individual applicant. Affirmative action, in contrast, requires more than passive non-discrimination by the organization—it demands active programs of broadly applied preferential hiring systems. It requires definition of objectives for redressing employment imbalances and implementation of plans for reaching those objectives.

Setting operational goals, and developing criteria for measurement of progress toward these goals, is much talked about these days in management theory. Administrators, however, still more often than not observe such decision rules more in theory than in the doing, particularly in situations of strongly conflicting objectives and values. Yet, goal setting, action programs, and evaluation are the *modus operandi* of affirmative action. Affirmative action demands more from organizational leaders than lack of prejudice and belief in equal opportunity; operationalizing affirmative action requires leaders to take action stances in which priorities are reordered and time and energy is allocated to affirmative action *above other goals.*

There are many reasons why such a shift is extremely difficult even if the administrator is basically unprejudiced. Many see affirmative action as a diversion from "real" organizational goals. How do we answer the director of a city public works department who says, "My job is to repair roads and keep the storm drains operating. I need the best engineers I can get for that. My job isn't to solve social problems"?

Questions of this variety must be satisfactorily answered if affirmative action is to go forward. Public managers must be convinced to broaden their perspectives and to redefine their standards of performance if the values inherent in affirmative action are to be upgraded to an operational level. This will require new standards for evaluating what is important in public organizations and strategic revisions of reward systems to support new standards.

WHY IS PREFERENTIAL HIRING AND THE SETTING OF TARGETS AND QUOTAS ABSOLUTELY NECESSARY TO THE PROCESS?

Affirmative action guidelines require specified objectives, usually translated into numerical quotas, as minimum goals for the employment of minority individuals and women. Numerical objectives have emerged for the present as the only feasible mechanism for defining with any clarity the targets of action and the criteria for evaluation of progress toward achieving them within a given period of time. Thus, the courts have upheld the validity of goals and quotas in civil rights enforcement efforts and have stated that color-consciousness and sex-consciousness are both appropriate and necessary remedial postures.[1]

Nevertheless, the issue of preferential hiring has assumed the proportions of a major national controversy. The issue is partly one of varying definitions of the situation. Preference and compensation can be seen as words of positive connotation or as words of condescension and disparagement. Preference can be defined as choosing the more highly valued candidate at a given point in time and circumstance, and compensation can be defined as redress for past failures to reach the actual market of human resources available to our organizations. From a very different perspective, these words in combination may be defined as "reverse discrimination."

The characterization of preferential hiring and quotas as reverse discrimination provides a crutch for those who would avoid the changes in organizational behavior required by management by objectives. Obviously, to the extent that quotas as targets for progress become job "slots" and maximums rather than minimums, they perpetuate race and sex discriminations. Otherwise, the argument is diversionary and should be treated as such.

Until we are ready to recognize that years of experience with passive non-discrimination in the public sector have not substantially changed its white, middleclass, male-dominated employment patterns and until we are ready to set objectives wherein results are what counts, it is unlikely that change will take place. Yet, when people with differing perspectives are asked to agree on concrete goals, and must attempt to reach collective agreement on priorities, conflict becomes inevitable.

However, we have learned to submerge conflict in organizations by avoiding explicit goal statements. We escape confrontations by letting statements of *intent* substitute for *action* plans in the most controversial areas. Conflict is also avoided by allowing sub-units to pursue their primary objectives with as little pressure as possible on them to agree on or produce on broader system goals. To the extent that affirmative action clashes with individual values or requires diversion of resources from each sub-unit's highly ranked goals it is met with avoidance or outright resistance. A serious affirmative action program, therefore, demands substantial departures from traditional policy-making practices and managerial styles.

WHY MUST OUR TRADITIONAL STANDARDS OF "QUALITY" BE REEXAMINED?

Most attacks on preferential hiring programs are grounded in the assumption that the quality of performance and work standards will be severely diminished as a result of the systematic employment of minorities and women. They are also grounded in the assumption that few "qualified" Blacks, Chicanos, other minority individuals, and women are available. Both assumptions stand on the third assumption that present criteria of merit and procedures for their application can be accepted uncritically and have yielded the excellence intended. We have not asked ourselves why the use of certain standards has resulted in the virtual exclusion of women and minorities from many professional positions and almost all high-level positions. To the extent that the use of our present standards has resulted in this exclusion (or inclusion in only token proportions), our organizations have been denied access to important sources of intellectual and physical vitality. Thus, the logic of affirmative action says that where a particular criterion of merit, even while not discriminatory on its face or in its intent, operates to the disproportionate elimination of women and minority group individuals, the burden on the organization to defend it as an appropriate criterion rises in direct proportion to its exclusionary effect.

The problems raised by the quality issue are probably the most difficult of those faced in affirmative action. Questioning our accepted standards of quality strikes at tradition and destroys some of the most important groups of our individual self-definitions. The less secure the institution, occupational group, or individual concerned, the more threatening such examination becomes. Degrees and other labels provide a much more comforting definition of quality than does a continuing evaluation of job performance. The more the occupational group is involved in processes of professionalizing itself or is striving for higher status, the greater the tension between those processes and inclusionary requirements. All of these changes increase exclusivity. Attempts at implementation of affirmative action in police departments, for example, are running head on into the federally financed drive to "professionalize" according to traditional measures—particularly degree attainment.[2]

The case of several state colleges in California which are undergoing a change of status from colleges to "universities" provides us with another example. In this instance one of the main criteria for change of status is the number of PhD degree holders on the faculty. Teachers with master's degrees who had been receiving excellent evaluations from deans, peers, and students are suddenly being reevaluated according to a more "professional" standard, i.e., the PhD. Job performance is the same, but some are now being dismissed or not advanced because external criteria have changed. Any attempt to implement affirmative action programs in this atmosphere of degree consciousness is difficult. Suggestions that alternative standards of faculty quality be considered (for example a bachelor's or master's degree plus experience, cultural knowledge, ability to relate to students, ability to serve as a minority role model, and warmth, energy, and decency) are met with fears about lowering standards and allusions to the importance of "quality." We see here two conflicting sets of standards about what is important and what quality means.

Organizational leaders dedicated to pursuing inclusionary policies must be prepared to meet the "quality" issue head on. The development of alternative measures of accomplishment is essential to the success of affirmative action programs at this period in time. A complex of social factors has combined to exclude minorities and women from the higher levels of formal educational attainment, and great numbers have pursued avenues of development other than that of formal education. Yet, their experience paths prepare them to bring new perspectives, different values, and perhaps even equal or higher capabilities to many public jobs. If, as we say, our objective is the best person for the job, we are *committed* to affirmative action.

Finally, in the broadest sense, a public employee group representative of the differing values and various perspectives in our total society is essential to public accountability. Any procedures which exclude multiple experience paths and disparate values from organizations *will* in these terms *lower standards* of public accountability as well as organizational effectiveness.

NOTES

1. For a summary of court decisions regarding quotas, see Herbert Hill, "Preferential Hiring, Correcting the Demerit System," *Social Policy*, July-August 1973, pp. 96–102.
2. For further discussion of this problem as it relates to an actively professionalizing sheriff's department, see Catherine Lovell, "Accountability Patterns of the Los Angeles County Sheriff's Department," *Institute on Law and Urban Studies*, manuscript, November 1973.

D. LABOR RELATIONS
IN SOCIAL AGENCIES

37/UNIONS AND VOLUNTARY
AGENCIES

MILTON TAMBOR

In recent years social workers in both public and private agencies have increasingly organized for the purpose of union representation. For example, a survey of the membership of the Metropolitan Detroit Chapter of the National Association of Social Workers (NASW) indicated that more than 50 percent of the respondents belonged to a union, and nearly 75 percent approved of social workers joining unions.[1]

Within the social work profession, standards of personnel practices have been formulated by NASW that relate to such factors as tenure, promotions, salaries, hours of work, leaves, layoffs, retirement, and various insurance benefits.[2] On labor-management relations, the association takes the following position:

NASW supports the collective bargaining process between organized labor and management as one means of providing a rational and coherent method of solving problems inherent in employee-employer relationships and thereby achieving conditions of employment conducive to optimum service to clients.

Professional values will guide the manner in which NASW members, whether as union members or part of management, participate in collective bargaining.[3]

Some social workers have argued that NASW should become a collective bargaining agent.[4]

Now that their colleagues in the teaching profession have entered the collective bargaining arena and thus have set the precedent, there is evidence that social workers no longer consider unionizing as unprofessional. Rather, they recognize that collective bargaining may produce many gains, such as reduced case loads, greater job security, improved procedures for dealing with grievances, and increased salaries and benefits. Such concerns are always important. They are especially relevant for social workers now, in view of inflation, a tight job market, and other current economic conditions. In fact, unionization of social workers is already moving ahead, especially in the public sector. One international union, the American Federation of State, County, and Municipal Employees (AFSCME), currently represents more than 50,000 employees in city, state, and county welfare departments and nearly 10,000 social service employees in private nonprofit agencies.

This article does not aim to analyze the concrete economic and noneconomic benefits that result from union organizing. Such a discussion would involve a comparison of union contracts in organized agencies with personnel practices of nonorganized agencies.

Rather, the focus is on the broader political impact of unionization: first, the effects on power relationships within the individual voluntary organization between direct service staff and policy-makers (that is, administrators and board members); second, the influence of collective bargaining on budgeting and planning practices that involve the funding organization and the individual agency. The case example utilized will be the volunteer agencies of Metropolitan Detroit. The union's role as an advocate of clients—a partisan supporting the struggles of oppressed groups within the community and an agent representing workers' interests for greater control in the planning and delivery of services within the voluntary agencies—will also be depicted.

BACKGROUND

Local 1640, Community and Social Agency Employees, AFSCME, Council 77, represents approximately 700 social service employees in 18 private agencies in the Metropolitan Detroit area. The five-year-old union represents social workers with master's or baccalaureate degrees, paraprofessional employees, clerical personnel, and maintenance workers. Most of the agencies involved receive the bulk of their budget allocation from United Community Services (UCS), which is the major budgeting and planning body for volunteer social services in the area. The fund-raising campaign is administered by United Foundation. UCS, through its budget committees, reviews and determines agency budgeting requests annually, provides for budgeting appeal procedures, and stipulates the mechanics of monthly fiscal reporting for each agency.

Under provisions of Michigan state law, public and private nonprofit employees have the right to select a labor organization as their exclusive bargaining representative.[5] Procedures include filing with the Michigan

Employment Relations Commission a petition that defines the bargaining unit and presents an expression of interest by 30 percent of its employees. The employer may extend voluntary recognition, but in most cases the commission authorizes and conducts a formal election.

ORGANIZING PROCESS

In the initial stages of organizing, a group of employees usually invites a union representative to discuss the benefits of union representation. Employees' grievances may be directed toward job classifications, work loads, inadequate salaries and benefits, or conditions for layoffs or discharge. Notwithstanding the existence of personnel practices, employees are generally aware of their lack of power in effecting improvements or correcting inequities, inasmuch as the final authority rests with the executive director and the agency board. The nonprofessional employee is in an especially vulnerable position regarding job security. Although clericals and paraprofessionals may have greater seniority or longevity than the professionals— thereby serving a vital function in the continuity of the agency's program— their status is low, their salaries and benefits are depressed, and they have minimal opportunities for mobility. On the other hand, the professionals, who are operating with a greater degree of security and higher marketability of skills, set greater expectations on personnel practices and are much less apt to tolerate inequities. Significantly, if professionals and nonprofessionals decide to unionize together, besides having increased strength as an employee unit, they then recognize their mutual concerns more clearly, thus improving rapport.

In this initial phase there is usually informal communication among employees, especially outside the agency. The administrators of the individual agency similarly engage in intensive communication—meeting with supervisory or middle-management staff, discussing with the agency board, consulting other agency directors or legal counsel.

With the filing for an election, the union's request for recognition becomes formalized. At this point the bargaining unit becomes defined, and some employees may be formally designated as supervisors and confidential employees and therefore ineligible to vote. In eligibility disputes, requests for formal hearings can be made or a separate supervisory bargaining unit may be formed. The significance of defining the unit is that the agency may need to clarify staff positions, modify some employee classifications, and possibly change its administrative structure.

POWER STRUGGLE

The hard campaigning usually begins after the setting of the date for the union election. The issues in the power struggle between agency and union are employee rights versus management prerogatives—which may be compared to the labor-management confrontations that occur in private industry. The union contends that collective bargaining results in job protection, improvement in salaries and benefits, elimination of favoritism, and greater employee participation in decision-making. The agency argues that the union is an outside party, may be responsible for strikes and picket lines, can adversely affect relationships between staff and administration, and may act against the best interests of employees.

Specific agency strategies include written communications and meetings with employees. In some cases, there may be direct or indirect harassment—for example, threat of layoffs or discharge, or perhaps promises of increased salaries. However, in rare situations, agencies may decide against any campaigning or even agree to union recognition without an election. Most frequently, the union's position is defensive, because meeting and communicating with employees occurs outside of work hours and off agency premises.

If the majority of the employees vote for union representation, then formal structures of representation for both employees and administrators are developed. For the employees, this process entails the election of officers, stewards, and a negotiating committee. Leadership and membership responsibilities are delineated, and contract proposals are drawn up. Similarly, the agency administrators designate their bargaining committee or legal counsel and plan their negotiating stance. In some instances, negotiations provide the initial opportunity for employees and board members to meet each other.

AN ACCOMMODATION

Despite the polarization arising from the organizing and the campaigning, the union and the agency usually arrive at an accommodation at the bargaining table with both parties making realistic compromises. A period of stabilization may be necessary to test the viability of the contract, including grievance procedures for handling disputes. However, when an impasse is reached at the bargaining table, when unresolved disputes accumulate, or when sudden administrative changes occur—such as layoffs or transfers—then the accommodation is likely to be disrupted.

Some agencies cannot accept the union's legitimacy, and no form of accommodation is possible. A "hard line" or punitive attitude toward employees is adopted. Administrators take strict disciplinary actions, adopt formal rules and regulations, and summarily reject union proposals. The employer may be trying to discourage other nonunion employees from organizing or may simply be intent on undermining or ousting the union. In turn, the union may counter by trying to develop leverage within the agency board, seeking support from other pressure groups or power blocs within the community, filing unfair labor practice charges, utilizing press and other media to publicize restrictive agency actions, or threatening or engaging in work stoppage.

Finally, a relationship of accommodation may be further expanded so that it approximates the European mode: of codetermination. In many agencies, negotiating wages, hours, and working conditions logically leads to the use of collective bargaining to effect changes in administrative policies and improve client services. This is more likely to occur when employees have been alienated from the agency's executive board and denied any voice in administrative decisions regarding policy. Most administrators resist these demands for changes, claiming that the union is encroaching on their authority and managerial rights, but some may be responsive to such a union-management partnership as being in the best interests of agency, clients, and workers. In one agency the executive reacted most favorably to union proposals for developing day care facilities and programs needed for black children. Besides the traditional provisions, a contract may therefore have provisions regarding union representation on agency boards and committees, and include procedures for effecting changes—such as special conferences offering opportunities for mutual discussion and decision-making on agency policies and client services.

AGENCY AUTONOMY

In the case example at Detroit, the early organizing and subsequent negotiations raised a serious question for the local union: the ability of individual agencies to bargain autonomously. In May 1969, after repeated efforts at mediation had failed, the union engaged in a strike of fourteen agencies. The union's position was that individual agency negotiations had reached an impasse and that meaningful negotiations could occur only if the funding and budgeting agencies, United Foundation and UCS, were involved in the collective bargaining process. The union specifically argued that budgeting controls exercised by UCS—including their past practices of establishing salary scales and ranges for agencies, as well as their planning and administering retirement and life insurance programs—significantly influenced individual agency bargaining. The union maintained that this involvement in labor-management relations should be legitimized within the framework of collective bargaining.

Five agencies fully supported the union position. They jointly became parties to an agreement with the union incorporating (1) the negotiation of a master contract that delineated bargaining items in which common agreement had been reached and that provided for supplementary agreements covering issues not specified in the master contract; (2) the endorsement of the formation of a study committee, made up of representatives of agencies, union, UCS, and United Foundation. This committee would recommend a collective bargaining mechanism that included job classifications, salary ranges, and a fringe benefit package to be applied to agencies.

In addition, the five agencies formulated a position paper pointing out that when UCS authorized agency upgrading of job classifications and established fiscal reporting procedures, it was applying centralized fiscal controls. The position paper summarized the problem as follows:

While these controls are necessary, and indeed desirable, the concept of agency autonomy becomes sometimes farfetched under the circumstances. During the past three years, UCS has always been the silent partner in the negotiating sessions. With limited funds and allocations our agencies would bargain up to a certain point, then we would be forced to admit that this was the final offer, since we cannot engage in deficit financing.[6]

On the other hand, UCS maintained that it was not the employer, but rather that each agency board assumed the full managerial functions regarding salaries and working conditions. Its basic contention was that direct or indirect participation would result in less freedom in allocating funds in response to community needs. Its primary obligation was toward contributors in the community and its secondary obligation was to agencies providing services. UCS explained its position thus:

The UCS Board has adhered to a policy which places full employer responsibility in the hands of the individual board and its executive. The voluntary system for a great many years has been decentralized in terms of philosophy and service. It seems illogical to move toward centralization in the voluntary system at a time when we are moving toward decentralization in education and other public services.[7]

Nine agencies argued against UCS involvement in bargaining for the following reasons: autonomy of agencies and boards, agency independence in determining employment policies and practices, and variations among agencies as to the nature of bargaining units, services, and funding arrangements. Administrators of nonorganized agencies expressed concern that UCS involvement in bargaining would mean a disproportionate gain in benefits and salaries for organized employees at the expense of those unorganized.

REVIEW COMMITTEE

The review committee appointed to study the issue received testimony from all interested parties. Its recommendations generally supported the position of agency autonomy in collective bargaining. However, the committee pointed out that a number of budgeting and planning procedures were linked explicitly to labor-management violations—for example (1) an agency's making an allocation in its budget for the employment of an agency attorney as the bargaining representative, and (2) an individual agency's sharing with UCS specific information that involved and affected collective bargaining agreements. The committee proposed that a communication channel be developed between UCS and the union for the discussion of mutual interests and concerns and that collective bargaining be coordinated with the budgeting timetable.[8] At the same time, the committee legitimized UCS participation in labor-management relations by suggesting that UCS make information available on "the prevailing rates and trends for comparable work among agencies."[9]

One immediate result was joint planning and coordination between agencies on labor-management issues. For example, unionized agencies exchanged information on existing contract salaries and benefits. Some agencies used the same legal counsel for bargaining, and they conducted joint training sessions for middle management in the administration of the union contract. Even in some nonorganized agencies personnel practices were revised in accordance with patterns developed in union contracts—frequently as a means of preventing any further organizing. For the union, negotiations were coordinated so that minimal agency standards for salaries and benefits could be established. Besides this upgrading, greater standardization and uniformity in both the organized and nonorganized agencies may result.

The author's position is that unionization has and will continue to influence the collective bargaining process in the private agencies. New communication links have developed, budgeting and planning procedures are being modified, and as organizing gains are realized—including the union representation of the employees of the funding agencies—it may be necessary for all parties concerned to create new forms of bargaining. The alternative is for agencies to reduce the number of staff positions to meet contract demands for higher salaries and benefits but this way they would lose future funding for those vacancies.

COMMUNITY ADVOCACY

Just as issues of advocacy and questions of policy may become important to the bargaining of the individual agency, so too can the relevance and adequacy of services in the voluntary field become concerns of the union as well as the community. Much criticism has been leveled at the voluntary system for its middle-class orientation and lack of service to the black, Chicano, and poor white communities. In practice, traditional agencies continue to be budgeted in increasing amounts, while inner-city, grassroots community groups are denied such funding. Boards of the funding and planning agencies and of the individual agencies are made up essentially of suburban whites and business executives. A recent survey of the voluntary field in the Metropolitan Detroit area documents these conditions.[10]

In 1971, UCS responded to such criticism by developing a plan for broadening citizen participation within its board. The union argued strongly against the proposed reorganization plan, contending that the same interests would be exercising power and controlling the decision-making process. Instead, as an alternative course of action, the union joined in a coalition with church and neighborhood groups, the Detroit Chapter of NASW, the Social Welfare Workers Movement, the Welfare Rights Organization, the Association of Black Social Workers, and the Student Organization of Wayne State University School of Social Work. The coalition, People United for Community Services, proposed a plan providing for community control and testified at public hearings conducted by UCS. More recently, the union supported funding policies relating to services rather than to the agency per se.

In the author's experience, employees' concerns for job security and improved working conditions can be combined in negotiations with changes in the structure and delivery of social services and expansion of the work force in the voluntary field. Many instances can be cited of social service employees supporting and being supported by welfare rights groups, whether in radical caucuses or in union negotiations, on issues of mutual concern. The fact is that the social service employee, in either the public or private sector, is defined and must act as both an employee and an agent on behalf of clients.

For boards and administrators of many volunteer agencies, union interest among staff represents a serious threat to existing relationships. Thus many executives react to unionization by personalizing—that is, bemoaning the ingratitude of staff and blaming the union as a troublemaker. Also, collective bargaining challenges the tradition in the voluntary agency that defined altruistic roles and service expectations for social workers and denied their self-interest as wage earners. Some staff, especially older workers, assume without question that the volunteer dollar is insufficient to provide equitable salaries and benefits.

It seems evident, however, that these attitudes are changing dramatically. In the past many employees accepted lower salaries and benefits in the voluntary field and tolerated the agency's paternalism toward clients and staff as preferable to the more bureaucratized and depersonalized work conditions that prevailed in public welfare institutions. Now, many social service employees identify with the needs and aspirations of the labor movement—that is, they are seeking salary increases to protect against inflation and rises in cost of living and are demanding job security to guarantee employment in a difficult job market. For such employees, volunteerism is not incompatible with unionism; rather, they have concluded that a restructuring of budgetary priorities for improved employee wages and benefits is necessary. For more radical workers, the climate of paternalism in the private agency may be definitely oppressive. For these workers, union representation not only provides protection against discharge when they engage in advocacy, but it can serve as a vehicle for transferring power from the middle-class agency and its board to the workers and to the poor and minority groups within the community. Some agency administrators may, in fact, share these objectives.

NOTES

1. *Metropolitan Detroit Chapter, NASW, Newsletter,* June, 1970.
2. *NASW Standards for Social Work Personnel Practices* (Washington, D.C.: National Association of Social Workers, 1971).
3. *Ibid.,* pp. 12–13.
4. *Metropolitan Detroit Chapter, NASW, Newsletter, op. cit.*
5. *See* State of Michigan, *Labor Relations and Mediation Act—Act 176 of the Public Acts of 1939 As Amended* and *Public Employment Relations Act—Act 336 of the Public Acts of 1947 As Amended.*
6. "Position Paper on UCS-Agency-Union Relationships" (Detroit, Mich.: Presented jointly by the Boards of Directors of Children's Aid and Family Service of Macomb County, Children's Aid Society, Franklin Wright Settlements, Inc., Neighborhood Service Organization, and UAW Retired Workers Centers, Inc., July 2, 1969). (Mimeographed.)
7. "Philosophy and Rationale for UCS Position on Agency Union" (Detroit, Mich.: Board of Directors, Unity Community Services, May 27, 1969). (Mimeographed.)
8. Malcolm Carron, S. J., Malcolm Denise, and Douglas Fraser, "UCS-Agency-Union Question," Report of Review Committee (Detroit, Michigan, November 10, 1969). (Mimeographed.)
9. *Ibid.*
10. *See* Greenleigh Associates, Inc., *Summary Study of United Community Services of Metropolitan Detroit* (Detroit, Mich.: Greenleigh Associates, Inc., 1968); and "United Foundation Priorities Report," submitted by Special Study Committee in report to United Foundation Board of Directors, January 1971.

38/UNIONIZATION AND THE PROFESSIONAL EMPLOYEE: THE SOCIAL SERVICE DIRECTOR'S VIEW

LAWRENCE C. SHULMAN

The question of unionization and the professional is one which generates much heat and limited light, much anger, frustration, confusion, and little analysis, evaluation, or understanding. Passions are abundantly in evidence, no matter which side of the question one supports. Thinking about issues, problems, and implications of unionization—particularly in relation to hospital social service departments—has become increasingly polarized. This is an unfortunate development. A stance which proclaims "I, or we, are on the side of the angels" is not productive in our current context. The professional social worker must always remain skeptical, questioning all facile assertions and easy solutions. Militant rhetoric (which, by the way is not equated with radicalism) in defense of one's interests or ideals may satisfy one's soul. In the organizational context, however, it can only inhibit legitimate debate, which has been and must remain a hallmark of our profession.

There are many of us who are opposed to the concept of unionization of professionals. It is also quite certain that there are many who are sympathetic to trade unionism. Indeed, many of us have been involved, as professional social workers, in trade union struggles in the past on behalf of clients, or nonprofessional fellow employees, or as employees of social agencies who were themselves unionized. The professional social worker, believing as he must in social justice, equality, economic opportunity, and human dignity, cannot help but have been sympathetic to many of the struggles of trade unionism over the past three or four decades. But while this may be true, many of us are now questioning what may be viewed as the increasingly narrow role of trade unionism. Most of us in socially responsible administrative roles find ourselves caught in the middle—between ideals and social reality. And so we need to raise the legitimate questions and anxieties of concerned professional human beings. Today, it is especially important for all vested interests, professional social workers among them, to be both responsive and responsible.

At the risk of being obvious, permit me a broad generalization: the pace and sweep of social, economic, political, and technological changes are transforming every aspect of our lives in fundamental and unpredictable ways. They are placing great strains on all social institutions, including hospitals. Unionization is one of these forces. Its impact on hospitals is becoming more evident and problematic.

This paper will look at the background for unionization of professional social workers and try to identify why this has come about, particularly in hospitals. Then it will explore some of what are seen as eight important issues for the profession of social work, and their impact on hospitals and management personnel. Finally, it will recommend some courses of action, identify some problems which will probably continue to frustrate us for years to come, and attempt some professional and organizational prophesy.

For many years, social workers (and agency administrators) debated the question: Are unionization and professionalization compatible or antithetical? This is Issue Number 1. While this might still be a good question for academic debate in graduate schools of social work, life and the realities of our society have answered that question. Social workers are unionized and the trend seems to be on the increase. In the New York City area, and in many other metropolitan areas, social workers in agencies, in antipoverty programs, in hospitals, have joined unions. District 37 (AFSCME–AFL–CIO) represents social workers in city hospitals. Local 1707 of that same union has represented social workers since the late 1950s in all the Federation of Jewish Philanthropies' affiliated agencies (with the exception of the Federation hospitals). Local 1199 of the National Hospital Union (RWDSW–AFL–CIO) has been extremely active in the voluntary hospital sector and now has 26 social service departments organized in New York City hospitals. Two other social service departments have elections pending.

The professional has internalized the controls of his profession—the skills, values, goals, and particularly its code of ethics. He has a strong service ideal in which personal profit is supposed to be subordinate to the client's interest when the two are in conflict.

But, the professional social worker is not an independent practitioner. He exists and functions within a social agency context. In the hospital, he works in a large, complex organization. The bureaucracy sets the conditions and benefits of employment, the standards, controls, policy, and volume, and affects the quality of his professional job. The professional social worker has viewed himself, and, regrettably, has been viewed by most hospital administrators, with certain notable exceptions, as a marginal professional in the hospital. He has felt himself to be powerless in the multipower systems of a hospital and, indeed, has been powerless, relative to the doctors, the administrators, even the nurses. He sees the hospital system as being basically in need of change, basically in conflict with some significant values he holds as a professional, and basically unresponsive.

While being marginal has its advantages, powerlessness creates numerous problems and provides great frustration to the professional, as employee or as director of a social service department. He has many important professional skills and areas of unique knowledge which can be beneficial to both his patients and to his organization, particularly at a time when the social determinants and components of health and illness are coming to be seen to be as vital, and perhaps even more important to the health of our citizenry than our technological and technical medical skills. If the challenge to our health care system in the seventies is our capacity to organize rationally and to deliver quality, comprehensive services to all in our nation, then the professional social worker has a vital contribution to make.

Yet, in all too many hospitals, the social worker is not part of the decision-making process, or the policy-making center. He develops a sense of "outsiderness," of being a stranger in his desired homeland. The hospital, as institution, becomes "they" and "The Doctors" and "The Administration," who do not share his values and goals, nor understand his role. This is Issue Number 2. Why does this occur? How does social work develop power in a medical setting?

The incompatibility of professional and administrative orientations has been indicated by several writers. Warren Bennis states that professionals derive their rewards from standards of excellence internalized and reinforced through professional identification. They are committed to the task, the service, not to the agency; to their standards, not to their boss. They are not good company men. They look to their colleagues and professional associations rather than to their place of employment for their values, their rewards, their status. Administrators, conversely, generally find satisfaction only within the organization. Thus a structured conflict is bound to exist.[1] This is Issue Number 3.

When one feels powerless in an organization, particularly if professional needs conflict with institutional needs, external controls are often sought to confront a perceived unresponsive bureaucracy. Professional staffs seem to be saying that they want greater bargaining power on bread-and-butter issues. Many have perceived unionization as a benefit. The union becomes a new ally of formidable strength, with greater powers than the social work director to raise salaries, improve personnel benefits, and alter conditions of employment. Indeed, social service employees are viewing the union as a vehicle for achieving a greater voice in the issues beyond bread-and-butter concerns—such issues as a policy and decision-making voice, program development, standards and criteria of work. They say, "If we have to carry out program and administrative decisions, we must have an input in formulating them."

This thrust toward participatory democracy is evident in all our social institutions—the schools, the government, among consumers. The demand is for a new way of looking at decision-making and power. Social work is, of course, not alone in this trend. Witness the increasingly militant actions of teachers, where professionally trained middle-class people are using unionization as a potent weapon for change—or, by contrast, for resistance to change when such is perceived as a threat to their own status, power, control, and values. The name of the game is power, as it always has been. But new players have entered the game, new coalitions which have rapidly altered the relationship of powers and shifted power to new institutional forces.

But if power is the goal, is the union the proper mechanism for the redistribution of it for professionals? How, we must ask, does one reconcile the Canon of Ethics of the social work profession with legitimate trade unionism? How do we reconcile the inevitable structured conflict between the professional norm of serving the patients' interests, and the union norm of serving the members' interests? Should a union have a say in professional matters, a voice in the determination of professional practice? This would be a change from the historic role of unions. This cluster of questions is Issue Number 4.

Might not the proper vehicle be the professional society? Perhaps. But our professional organization—NASW—has not become a guild concerned with wages and benefits as well as defining demonstrated skill and criteria for competency, as have the American Nurses Association and the American Physical Therapy Association!

Social work as a profession has identified strongly with the struggles of the black and Puerto Rican minorities for civil rights, justice, and equality of opportunity.* Social workers as individuals, particularly the younger, more recently graduated professionals, have been deeply and actively involved in these social movements which have roused the passions of our times. There will be little argument, I believe, with the observation that the unionization of the nonprofessional employees in hospitals, the majority of whom are black and Puerto Rican, was a concomitant of the civil rights struggles in the United States and gathered strength from the increasingly militant stances of the ethnic minorities in recent years. Was it not understandable, therefore, that professional social workers, who more often than not came from working-class and lower-middle-class backgrounds, and supported unionization efforts on behalf of minority groups as an effective means of social change and more equitable economic redistribution, should have considered unionization for themselves for similar, if not necessarily comparable, reasons?

Ethnicity has been the catalytic force for unionization. It has been sustained and nurtured by administrative and organizational insensitivity. Paradoxically, the trade union movement, itself, reflects these same resistances to change, to maintain the status quo. Witness the confrontations

* Editor's note: Social work also has identified itself with the struggles of other ethnic minority groups.

between the minority groups and the construction unions, or the teacher's union, in the 1968 New York City teacher's strike.

Anne Somers, a brilliant and incisive commentator on the health field, stated it quite clearly:

There is no question but that the problem of moving from initial organization to peaceful collective bargaining is far more difficult for both management and union leaders than it would be if it were not so intimately tied up with racial problems. But this is like saying that a sick man would be healthy if he wasn't sick. The problem is with us. The legacy of exploitation, hypocrisy and bitterness cannot be avoided and the hospital industry—a principal employer of minority group labor—will pay the price for years to come, which is to say that society will.[2]

This leads to a loaded question: Are the hospitals, particularly the nonprofit hospitals which developed out of the potent and progressive forces of voluntarism—of man's concern for his fellowman—are these institutions going to continue to abdicate to the unions the issues of concern for the health and welfare of minority group members as employees and as consumers in the health care system? How shall we respond to this social and moral imperative? This is not an easy question to answer.

This raises the question of what the social responsibility of a union, any union, is or has been in delivery of human services. We must get rid of the romantic notion of the social role of unions. They are in business to help and promote their members' interests. That is their reason for existence, plainly and simply stated. It is a powerful interest group, among many interest groups in the hospital.

Any interest group has areas of conflict, neutrality, and congruence with other interest groups. The interests of the employee often are not congruent with the interests of the hospital or of patients—just as, in a similar fashion, the interests of the AMA (which is a union, and a very effective one at that) have not always been in the best interests of patients and the effective organization and delivery of health care.

But unions are not monolithic. They are made up of many subgroups and interests. When a union includes both nonprofessional and professional members, internal conflict is inevitable. In this respect, the union leadership runs into the same problems as do administrators in hospitals, in trying to reconcile divergent groups toward a common goal. Thus, it has been submitted, and only somewhat facetiously, that administrators of hospitals and administrators of unions are more comfortable with each other than they are with professional constituents, who are seen as, at best, somewhat maverick but necessary, at worst as just too independent and a wee bit crazy.

Not only is it predicted that we will see increasing strains within individual trade unions themselves, but we shall also see more conflicts of jurisdiction between various trade unions. We already have seen evidence of this within some of our municipal hospitals which have affiliation contracts with various voluntary hospitals and university medical centers. In several of these hospitals which have made the headlines on a regular basis during the past year, jurisdictional disputes have arisen between District 37 and Local 1199. In one newly opened municipal hospital, the situation has had a serious effect on the ability of the Social Service Department to plan and carry out community-oriented programs to be staffed predominantly by indigenous workers in the area. The dispute has arisen because one part of the Social Service Department, on municipal hospital lines, belongs to one union, and the other section of the Social Service Department, on affiliation contract positions, belongs to the other union. The resultant jurisdictional and operational conflicts for power and balance have limited the capacity of the director of social service of that hospital from hiring the community personnel which he and his staff deem necessary effectively to operate this new health program. Add to that the fact that salary scales and personnel benefits under the two separate union contracts are markedly different, and you have an area of conflict which will affect the climate and operational effectiveness of a social service department.

What the union contract does is present a new structure and environment in which the social work administrator must function. And the use of structure is something with which we, as social workers, should be quite knowledgeable. But the basic, perhaps the most crucial problem for the social work director in a hospital department is that we, as middle-management personnel, basically do not know how to deal with unions. This is Issue Number 5. We tend to be caught in the middle between the union demands and the management needs of the organization. We are charged with the basic implementation of an agreement into which we ourselves have had little input, and union agreements, particularly as they relate to professional departments, do have a tremendous amount of ambiguity built into them. During negotiations with the unions, we have to try to maintain what we feel is the professional integrity of the department.

Most social work directors have had little experience in dealing with unions and therefore lack the administrative skill. We very often tend to feel insulted, defensive, squeezed. We do not know how to reach for the common ground that will enable us to begin working out a modus vivendi. Enormous strains are placed upon our administrative competency and on the traditional way social work directors have run their departments. This has been grounded on a combination of professional values, personal relationships, and all too often a "reward and punishment" concept of leadership.

A new concept of administrative leadership must begin to emerge. A basic part of this must be a viable concept of staff participation in the decision-making process. No longer is edict administration possible, nor personal leadership alone. The dilemma posed for us is how to give administrative leadership and involve our staff in a process of participation without giving up legitimate administrative authority.

This new concept of administrative leadership has no place in it for the old "reward and punishment" approach. The entire concept should be antithetical to professional practice. Our staffs are now very clearly telling us that if reward and punishment is where it's at, then they want constraints on capricious rewards and punishments of the bureaucracy. And social work directors are very clearly members of the bureaucracy.

Given the situation where professional goals, union goals, and management goals do not always coincide, the challenge to us is: How shall we develop a climate where planning and programming on common areas can take place? This is Issue Number 6. This will take much ability and courage on the part of middle-management personnel and hospital administrations. How can administrators involve constituent groups without giving up authority? Surely highly developed skills are needed in this area, skills which few of us have and which few of us have learned in our professional graduate education. Administration among constituent groups is a political process, a tension relationship in which mediating skills, intergroup skills, are absolutely necessary. While political trade-offs may constantly take place, social work directors have to learn how to represent their interests in a clear, honest, and strong manner. This will take a tremendous toll on many social work directors. Discomfort may become a way of life rather than a temporary state. Perhaps a question that administrators will need to ask before hiring social work directors will be "How do you deal with unions?"

Were such a question asked of many of us, we would be hard pressed to answer intelligently or comfortably. But competence in dealing with unionized staffs must become part of our new bag of skills.

Unionization will force upon us the necessity of learning new ways of operating and administering, just as unionization will surely force the hospital itself to look at its multipower systems and the way these affect the delivery of service. But if we can find selected areas of common ground, then conflicts can be approached differently. While conflicts may be inevitable, they can also present us with many opportunities. For example, there are a number of areas where union and hospital can find common ground and where the influence and impact of the social service department can be quite substantial.

One of the major concerns that management has always had is in retaining a stable work force. This is an area of concern for the union as well, for it is to their interests to maintain a stable membership. Would it be too presumptuous to suggest that the union and the hospital together set up day-care programs for staff to enable women who wish to stay in the work force to remain in the hospital? Surely we all are aware of the possibilities and opportunities offered to a social service department for an important role in such a program. Along the same lines, programs to upgrade and meet increasing manpower needs are an area of common ground for union and hospital.

But some conflicts transcend administrative skills. When the inevitable conflicts between union and management do arise, the end product may be confrontation and the use of that ultimate union weapon—strike. This raises one of the most vital of questions which were alluded to earlier, the one of social responsibility. The dilemma this poses to social workers is enormous. If the responsibility to the patient is a paramount professional value, how do people who provide vital human services justify removing of these services? Can social responsibility be maintained under trade union action? In our complex society, can groups continue to push only their own narrow interests, and say "To hell with the patient, the student, the consumer"? Where is the public interest? Just as in the New York City teacher strike and its aftermath, which left deep scars on New York City, a strike in the New York City hospitals would be viewed in the same way by the anxious, frustrated, discontented public, a large percentage of whom said to the teachers and to the Board of Education "A plague on both your houses." If unrestrained self-interest of the parties leads to a New York City hospital strike, it is inevitable that both union and management will have to be held accountable to the public. One might prophesy that the next group conflict will be between the unions and management on the one hand, and the public—the consumers—on the other.

Finally, there are two other very important issues to consider. The seventh issue is the recent trend that we see in hospitals (six so far) of social work supervisory personnel joining the union. This has serious implications for social work administrations. As union members, won't supervisors have conflicts of role and identity? Can supervisors have as many administrative responsibilities? Can they be asked to determine quantity or quality standards regarding such things as workloads, performance, etc.? Line staff could put pressure on a supervisor regarding average work standards or expectations. If a worker were to call a unionized supervisor unfair in his expectations of the worker, he might then ask the union to intercede. This places the supervisor in a position where he may have to choose between agency expectations and union loyalty. Therefore, one might postulate that the social work director will no longer be able to delegate certain responsibilities to his supervisors. Not all of us will welcome that necessity.

The last issue is that of the day-to-day effect of union contract on social work departments. How do we encourage the development of skills and professional growth, and the maintenance of standards of performance, under a union contract? Can or should skill and competence incentives be built into a contract? Will the contract become a sinecure for mediocrity, and indeed even incompetence, as has occurred in some parts of the Civil

Service system? If salaries continue to rise, as we all expect they will, will not hospitals demand of social work administrators more specific standards and criteria on input versus outcome? Will we not be subjected to increasing cost–benefit analysis, to come up with specific criteria of how many staff are needed in a specific hospital, to determine what the productivity output of a social worker really is?

Many difficult tasks lie ahead of us. What the future holds for hospital social work departments depends on whether the union and management view each other as inevitable and continual antagonists, or as potential allies in certain areas.

The union, as well as management, has a great stake in the financial stability of the hospital system, a system which has been chronically underfinanced. If the union is seen as a part of the hospital system instead of adversarily, hostilely outside of it, then it is logical that it be a significant part of the political, economic, and legislative struggle to improve and rationalize the financing, structure, and delivery of health care in New York City and the nation. The pros and cons of that debate is left for us all to consider.

NOTES

1. Warren Bennis, *Changing Organization* (New York: McGraw-Hill, 1968), p. 25.
2. Anne Somers, *Hospital Regulation: The Dilemma of Public Policy* (Princeton: Princeton University Press, 1969), p. 69.

39/COLLECTIVE BARGAINING IN
VOLUNTARY AGENCIES

HOWARD HUSH

The move toward trade unionism and collective bargaining by the professional employees of voluntary agencies in the social welfare field poses some harsh questions: Will unions destroy, or save, the voluntary agency? Will the contributors to united community funds support hard bargaining by professional employees or will they withdraw their support in protest?

Who is "management" in the collective bargaining process of a legally autonomous agency supported by a united fund?

For the uninitiated in such matters, the response to these questions may be explosive, violently prejudiced or partisan, or heavily flavored with the so-called puritan ethic—and perhaps only remotely related to reality. For many of us involved in the administration of large voluntary agencies in the Detroit area, where collective bargaining is in its third year, the response to these questions is likely to be one of studied restraint and evasion.[1]

Why are such questions, once they become a part of everyday reality, almost beyond approach? The fact that they are virtually unapproachable is, in itself, part of the problem. There is a communication blockage that is difficult to remove or circumvent. I should like to suggest some of the factors contributing to the difficulty of meaningful exchange.

1. Most professionals in the field of community and social service are sympathetic to organized labor and collective bargaining on philosophical grounds. Moreover, the profession of social work has been so throughout its history. Problems arise, however, when a philosophical, humanitarian view of workers' rights, which evolved from the needs of employees paid by the hour in an industrial, profit making enterprise, is applied to the collective bargaining process involving salaried personnel in a nonprofit community service enterprise in which "management" and "labor" are of the same educational and professional background and, presumably, have the same goals.

2. A collective bargaining relationship is by definition a conflict relationship between employer and employee. The conflict is out in the open; it is legally recognized; most of the ground rules for dealing with the issues are set by federal or state law or regulation. By legal definition, certain elements of an organization are "management" and certain other elements are "labor." Furthermore, the adversary relationship is not restricted to the bargaining table at a given season of the year. In varying degrees it pervades the whole organization. It may be minimal, it may peak at certain times of the year, or it may flare around certain issues. But it is never completely absent.

3. In a voluntary social welfare agency, there is likely to be lack of sophistication on both sides of the bargaining table. For example, when members of the staff believe, as too many still do, that a collective bargaining relationship is simply an orderly, businesslike way of employing someone to get more salary for them and that all other attitudes, relationships, and conditions of employment remain unchanged, they are naïve. They are overlooking the fact that an outside, third force—the union—is an entity in and of itself; it is part of the Establishment; it has its own thrust and its own political and survival pressures; and it has its well established techniques for protecting and promoting its own self-interest. Staff members are beginning to learn that a collective bargaining agreement is a two-way

instrument that defines in legal terminology what both administration and staff can and cannot do.

4. Finally, a collective bargaining relationship does not pose new questions so much as it puts into very sharp focus some old and very difficult questions: What are an employee's services worth in dollars? What values determine the worth? Who makes the judgment?

As if these questions were not troublesome enough, the problem of employee compensation is compounded by concepts of "charity," "dedication," and "sacrifice," which are now obsolete. Whether one likes it or not, these concepts are "out" as far as most urban employer-employee relationships are concerned, and one had best not try to use them to avoid paying decent salaries. At the same time, I believe that professional social workers must share with the general community and with boards of directors a substantial responsibility for their own compensation problems. Too many of them enjoy a kind of disengagement from the general community and do not get beyond the sterile complaint, " 'They' should pay 'us' more."

THE DILEMMAS AND THE ISSUES

For the Staff

The dilemma for the professional employee can easily become one of a conflict of loyalties. How much of his loyalty belongs to the union? How much to the agency? How much to the client? How much to the community? To what extent should he be guided by his own hard nosed, short term self-interest? Being faced with this dilemma provides a heyday for the person who lives by confusion and enjoys conflict for the sake of conflict. But it is a nightmare for the person who likes a quiet, diligent pursuit of his goals, an orderly arrangement of his loyalties, and a minimum of organizational commotion.

There is, too, a shift in the climate of relationships among staff, administration, and board. Relationships tend to become depersonalized, rigid, and legalistic. There is more sensitivity to the concept of "ultimate authority" in administration—not the particular decision or the basis for it, but who has the authority to make it.

Perhaps the greatest problem for professional employees is that so many of them are inexperienced and naïve about the ramifications of a collective bargaining agreement. For example, one member of an agency staff, who was an officer of the union and an especially active member of the bargaining team, requested a "merit" salary increase for himself after the contract had been signed for the current year. The agency administrator was dumbfounded by the simple innocence of the request and the lack of sensitivity to the broad implications of collective bargaining for the agency and for the financing of the program. The staff member, however, was even more dumbfounded to discover (1) that one purpose (and certainly the effect) of a collective bargaining relationship is to deny to administration discretion in individual salary adjustments based on merit, competence, or superior performance and (2) that the very contract he had just signed would not permit the agency to give him or anyone else in the bargaining unit the kind of individual salary adjustment he had requested.

For the Executive Director

The dilemma for the agency executive director is no less troublesome than it is for the staff. First, whether he likes it or not, he *is* management and he cannot avoid this role in relation to his staff and his board; he and the board sit on one side of the bargaining table and the members of the staff bargaining committee sit on the other side. Fundamentally, his role must be clear. It is true, however, that he also can retreat into isolation, a kind of legal sanctuary, if his survival is at stake.

Second, once a contract is signed, he is responsible for ensuring that it is fulfilled. The terms of the contract affecting salary, fringe benefits, insurance, working conditions, and so on cannot be modified by either the board of directors or the staff bargaining unit. The operating authority is the contract; it is not the board of directors, the personnel committee, or the agency's administrative staff.

Of greatest concern to some executive directors is the development of a kind of legally and morally justified disengagement among staff, administration, and governing board. Each of the three segments of agency operation tends to become legally defensive, more concerned with what it can and cannot do and less concerned with what it should or should not do. Particularly during the actual bargaining process, suspicion and conflict of interest among the segments are intensified. Long term common interests and goals, if indeed they exist, tend to become obscured by more immediate concern with short term goals and the struggle for power.

For the Board

The initial response of the governing board to the fact of a collective bargaining procedure may be one of surprise and disappointment. Very quickly, however, the attitude can become one of detached sophistication. Of necessity, the board has to take an official position on the issues; it must follow the rules of the collective bargaining process; it must eventually agree to a settlement.

It should not be surprising to executives (but it has been to many) to find that their boards relax quickly in the presence of a collective bargaining agreement, with some discomfort, to be sure, but almost with relief. Why? Because a collective bargaining agreement provides an orderly, legalistic resolution of issues involved in employer-employee relationships. The board becomes one step removed, more detached. It relies upon the collective bargaining machinery; it looks to the labor negotiator (usually an attorney, and a "must" for the employing agency) for advice and direction; and it depends upon the executive to administer the final contract. Just as the fact of a collective bargaining agreement influences the operation of the agency at the staff level, so it also has a pervasive effect on the relationship among board, administration, and staff.

HOPE FOR THE FUTURE

In this era of the "participation explosion," it is both fashionable and easy to play the game of confusion, of challenge for the sake of challenge, and of simple scapegoating. Nevertheless, with respect to salary issues and the collective bargaining process in voluntary agencies, the situation is not hopeless, unless we want to make it so. What are the sources of hope for the future?

We can hope for greater sophistication on the part of staff members in the adaptation of the collective bargaining process to the social agency setting. Specifically, we can hope that they will have conviction enough to challenge the outside union's "pros," many of whom know only the union contract model of the hourly rated employees in a profit making enterprise in the industrial community. They must evidence a high degree of sophistication even at the time they first consider the move toward a collective bargaining relationship. What are the issues, both short term and long term? What are the implications for staff, for agencies, and for the financial structure of voluntary agencies? What are the alternatives to collective bargaining?

These questions are not easily answered. And the answers are likely to reflect emotions, values, and moods much more than facts or rational judgments. But at least these questions should be asked before, not after, the decision is made to seek a collective bargaining relationship. I am persuaded that it is in part because such questions were never seriously considered that we have a much higher staff turnover rate in the Detroit agencies, particularly among union officers and members of bargaining teams, after contracts have been signed. Also there are a few bitter souls who now say that neither the professional association *nor* the union seems able to deal with the compensation problem. The staff's problem does not necessarily reflect, however, the failure of unions and collective bargaining. Rather it reflects the staff's initial lack of understanding, its unrealistic expectations, and the lack of a national model for collective bargaining for public service personnel—social workers, teachers, nurses, policemen, and so on.

We can also hope that once the staff makes the decision to engage in collective bargaining it will adopt a more critical attitude toward certain concepts very important to the union movement among hourly rated industrial employees. Take, for example, the concept of seniority and the traditional trade union position that seniority should be the primary factor in determining wages, promotions, demotions, dismissals, and so on. When rigidly applied to a professional service, the seniority concept has a disastrous effect; too many of the rewards are reserved for tenure, even though performance may be mediocre. Yet young professional social workers, with a proud disdain for the Establishment and for people over thirty years of age, can sit at the bargaining table and defend the traditional labor concept of seniority when matters of self-interest are at issue, apparently unconcerned with the inconsistency.

On the part of administration and board, we can hope for sharper, more realistic decisions in the over-all management of the agency's program. The decisions must be sharper, often hard nosed, simply because the pressures of collective bargaining put the issues and the conflicts into sharper focus. I should like to offer three illustrations.

1. The assessment of professional performance during a six-month probationary period assumes critical importance. During this period, the administration may have full discretion in keeping or not keeping a staff member, but it has very little discretion after the staff member's name has been placed on the seniority list. Administration must make a clear decision, one way or another, at the end of the probationary period; no evasion, no wait-and-see attitude, and no sentimental indulgence can be permitted.

2. The salary issue must be faced squarely in a collective bargaining agreement; there is little, if any, room for an appeal to "dedication" or "sacrifice" and the like. Each party at the bargaining table has a paid advocate to defend his position. The competitive spirit is dominant. Sentiment, if any, is likely to be rhetorical or theatrical; sheer self-interest takes on a vigor and frankness strange to some of us. It is not my intent to judge or to suggest what is "right" or what is "wrong." I want only to highlight the shift in climate and the compelling pressure to face issues openly and squarely.

3. Inevitably the pressures on the agency's budget will sharpen the issues with respect to program, priorities of service, and effectiveness of performance. We can hope that, as operating costs increase because of the improved benefits for the staff, the administration and the board will become increasingly critical of the traditional ways of delivering service—particularly if there has had to be a curtailment of service. In the automobile plants, for example, as labor costs went higher, there was a shift to more and more automation. Probing by administration and board will cause discomfort for many practitioners—usually a conservative force in agency operation—but collective bargaining is a two-way street. If used well, it can bring benefits to clients and to the community, but the benefits cannot be taken for granted.

THE CRUCIAL QUESTION

Will the outside union destroy, or save, the voluntary social agency? It will probably do neither. But it will provide a measure of the community's current commitment to the voluntary agency. It may force the community to decide how far it will go beyond token support. In the meantime, if the union is sensitive to the issues, it will have to decide how far it will go in a gamble with the future of the voluntary agency.

NOTE

1. In this article I am setting forth only my own observations and reflections on the implications of collective bargaining in one metropolitan area.

Part VII

SOCIAL SERVICE
INFORMATION SYSTEMS

Stimulated by pressure from funding, planning and monitoring agencies for accountability, and the developing availability at reasonable cost of technology and hardware, social agencies have sought increasingly to establish management information systems and procedures in their daily operations. Apart from such external demands, administrators are more and more aware of useful functions of a well-conceived system of data collection and dissemination as it serves the purposes of enhancing the quality of service delivery.

The following are among the *general* functions of social services information systems:

- planning and policy development
- decision-making
- coordination of client services

It is clear that these aspects of agency work require an adequate data base so that development can be rooted in objective reality rather than subjective judgment. In the absence of significant and accurate data, organizations move in a vacuum, unrelated to client need and community requirements.

There are other *specific* purposes to which systematic information can be directed—for institutional management, for service delivery, and for research, as follows:

Institutional Management
- budgeting
- program development
- program monitoring
- public relations
- evaluation
- cost analysis
- social and legislative action

Service Delivery
- referral and follow-up
- continuity of service

- service integration and coordination
- tracking clients (to keep clients from getting "lost")
- recording
- staff evaluation

Research
- knowledge building
- social problem analysis
- program evaluation
- practice testing

The accumulation of service statistics has always been part of the social agency's activities, and they are generally included in annual reports and as documentation for budget requests from funding agencies. What is required is a systematic and purposive rationale that makes it possible to achieve many of the objectives suggested above. An adequate information system encompasses a series of processes, including systematic classification, indexing and coding, and data collection, storage, processing, retrieval, and transmission. This can be done manually, or through automated or electronic data processing. The choice between these alternatives is a function of volume, complexity (number of variables required for classification and retrieval), and cost.

Experience suggests that the establishment of a competent information system is best achieved through a collaborative process between service professionals and information specialists. The former are in a position to indicate the "what," "who" and "why" of the system. Knowledge of the substance of the particular program, its goals and objectives, its relevant elements, the purposes to be pursued, and the significant relationships between variables, provides guides to the specialist in designing the appropriate technology, the "how" of the system. Data thus becomes information when it is put to significant use. Administrators need to know the potentials of an information system, and how to use the technician productively. They need to determine what information is needed, for what purposes, who needs to provide it, and where to use it. They are in the best position, in consultation with the staff, to define the three major types of data required—patient oriented, program oriented, and personnel oriented. Research requirements need to be defined by appropriate personnel designing both evaluative and experimental protocols.

Well-designed and technically competent plans for data use are necessary but hardly sufficient for the establishment of an agency information system. Professionals in the organization need to participate in the operation as well as the planning of the enterprise. Unless staff members accept and adhere to the requirements of the design, the system cannot work. "Staff involvement in the study design, and implementation stages [is] a necessary condition for success" (Nelson & Morgan, 1973). Many attempts at rational data use have failed, not so much because they are poorly designed, but because of resistance by the staff who had to provide the necessary data. Sometimes this resulted from lack of clarity about the information categories and coding system utilized. More generally, work overload and lack of conviction about the importance of the additional work requirements were at fault.

It cannot be stressed too much that acceptance of a new system must be carefully engineered. This is an important area of organizational change. A most significant role for the administrator lies precisely in this process of engendering compliance to the organizational requirements of a new information plan. A phased implementation process is clearly indicated, during which there should be continuous testing of steps in the technical design. Both professional and clerical feasibility are necessary, as is the step-by-step training of staff.

A good, comprehensive information system is often costly. It may take considerable time and effort to develop and adapt a system to tailor-made agency requirements. Start-up costs may be substantial in both financial and staff terms. Continuous operation of the system may similarly be expensive. These costs need to be considered carefully before an agency embarks on a full program. Pressure for accountability and auditing requirements by funding agencies, legislatures, and by governmental bodies purchasing services may suggest no alternative but to install a competent system. Professional considerations about quality of service and effective evaluation are also significant.

The selections in this section review several experiences in public and voluntary social agencies in developing social service information systems. Donahue and his associates record the experience of a public child welfare agency that instituted a reporting effort intended to relate service productivity to operating costs and so to provide a realistic picture of performance and resource allocation. Based on the conceptual framework developed by Robert A. Elkin, they worked out a distribution of direct-service time among service elements (e.g., homemaker services or family life education), and services (i.e., programs that incorporate service elements, for example, adoptions, or community services). Productivity measures were adopted and related to cost allocation. The ways in which the Social Service Information System (SSIS) was used are detailed, with special reference to the setting of agency goals and the ongoing process of program review and evaluation.

Catherwood reviews the process engaged in by a consulting firm in developing a management information system in a city–county welfare department. Starting with a delimited test area, and in coordination with a unit supervisor, a review was made of the existing information system, major weaknesses were identified, a case-and-goals classification developed, forms designed, and a strategy of implementation of the new system worked out. The article makes it clear that information selected for use and coding must pass the utility test—"What value is the information after it is produced?"

Young describes a computerized management information system developed for a voluntary child-serving agency, which was intended to make information quickly available and adapted to make possible the assessment of the quality of services provided. The key importance of training the service delivery staff in the use of the system is made clear. Young specifies the objectives of the system, identifies the specific elements of the data base growing out of these objectives, and reviews briefly the overall operation of the system. The article is useful as an indication of the potential use of computer technology in providing information to administrators, supervisors, and direct-service personnel in enhancing service to clients, and in evaluating both service and program achievements.

REFERENCE

Nelson, C., and Morgan, L. "The Information System of a Community Mental Health Center," *Administration in Mental Health* (Fall 1973):28.

40/THE SOCIAL SERVICE INFORMATION SYSTEM

JACK M. DONAHUE, ELIZABETH ANGELL,
ALOYSIUS J. BECKER, JUDITH CINGOLANI,
MARILYN NELSON, AND GEORGE E. ROSS

Many social service agencies need a reporting system that functions on an ongoing basis, is relatively simple in execution and takes into account staff time, caseloads, measurable staff accomplishments and operating costs. The Social Service Information System (SSIS) described in this article was developed in response to this need. The system was designed by the regional administrative staff of the East St. Louis Region of the Illinois Department of Children and Family Services. This is a public child welfare agency mandated to provide protective services to abused, neglected, exploited and dependent children; foster home and institutional care; adoptions and licensing services for day care homes and centers, local child welfare agencies and private child care institutions. The agency also provides family counseling, services to unmarried parents, homemaker services, purchase of day care, and community services such as family life education.

The East St. Louis Region consists of three district offices covering seven counties in southwest Illinois. Each local office offers a full range of services in its own area. The seven counties in the region contain a wide range of urban, suburban and rural socioeconomic groups. The agency employs 98 persons in the region.

The SSIS has been tested, assessed and developed to its present form during the last 4 years. It has proved adaptable to program change and expansion, and has been implemented statewide, with some revisions, by the Illinois Department of Children and Family Services.

DEVELOPMENT OF THE SYSTEM

The foundation of the SSIS is the utilization of time by direct service staff. It is a method of determining how direct service staff allocate their time in relation to defined productivity measures and operating costs.

From a conceptual framework developed by Elkin,[1] which defines the work of a social service agency in terms of services, elements and activities, came the method for gathering information on direct service workers' utilization of time. It was then fairly easy to determine a method for entering costs relative to direct service workers into the various services. As the system developed, a more sophisticated method was devised to convert this information into a formula that also distributes general operating costs and costs of nondirect service staff into services.

Elkin described three levels of agency operations—activities, service elements, and services. Activities are daily actions by staff in carrying out job responsibilities, such as interviewing and recording. Service elements are the aggregate of activities directed toward an objective and target group, such as homemaker services to the intact family or work toward making a child legally free for adoption. Services are identifiable programs consisting of service elements that constitute a clearly defined major objective of a social service agency. All three levels are event-oriented rather than process-oriented. They have clear beginning and ending points that provide the basis for time studies, cost analysis and management information systems.

As modified for use in the agency, the system uses only services and elements, with cost accounting integrated into it. Costs are distributed among the services according to percentages established by direct service time allocations. The exception to this percentage distribution are costs clearly identified as belonging to a specific area such as foster care payments, which obviously belong only in foster care service.

Consideration was given to reporting on all three aspects—activities, services and service elements—but since the objective was to develop a system that could be ongoing and would not consume an inordinate amount of staff time, this alternative was rejected. It was decided that the additional information provided by reporting activities within each element would not be sufficiently useful to justify the more complicated reporting system. The system is set up in such a way that activities could replace elements on the recording forms. This could be done on a periodic basis if this information would be useful; at this time there is no basis to show that this would be of value.

The system is designed to provide various cost figures on a monthly basis, such as the cost of an entire service area, the average monthly cost per opened case within a service, and costs for defined units of agency productivity, such as the cost for completing a home study for an adoptive applicant. The system is not designed to provide exact costs for individual cases.

CONCEPTUAL BASE

Using Elkin's criteria for service and elements, a method for coding and allocating direct service staff time was developed. This information is provided by direct service staff on a daily, ongoing basis. Seven major services that encompass the total range of objectives and operations of the agency in this region were identified and defined. They are: Services to Children in Their Own Homes; Adoptions; Substitute Care-Foster Home; Substitute Care-Institutional; Services to Unmarried Parents; Licensing of Community Facilities; and Community Services. Within each service, identification was made of elements that, together, cover every task performed by direct service staff in that service, and are distinguishable from each other.

Elements can be described as event-limited work units related to a secondary objective of the service in which they appear, such as "work toward making a child legally free for adoption." With few exceptions, they are defined in such a way that statistical units of cost can be determined for each element. At present, this agency is extracting costs for only a few of these elements.

The process of defining elements is determined by theoretical considerations, perceived needs for certain kinds of information, or a need to emphasize a particular aspect of a service. One example can be found in the Substitute Care-Foster Home Service. It was decided to separate "work with, or in behalf of, the foster child" into those activities directed toward establishing and maintaining a placement that would provide beneficial experiences for the child and those activities designed to implement a specific plan for moving the child into a permanent arrangement, such as return to his family or adoption.

During the 2 fiscal years preceding the development of the system, reporting was based on services and activities. Although this yielded some useful information, it did not facilitate determination of unit costs, which in some cases are directly related to a specific element. It was also believed that reporting by services and elements would provide more useful information for program monitoring by supervisory and administrative staff.

The use of Elkin's concepts was limited, since his framework could not be applied to the work of clerical and administrative personnel. Their services are supportive, rather than direct service to the client. Since the goal was a system that would encompass all costs and the functions of all staff, it was decided to distribute clerical and administrative costs according to the percentages established by the services and elements into which direct service workers code their time. The alternative would have been to define these as major services of the agency—which they are not—and define elements for the duties of administrative and clerical personnel. In addition to the fact that this was seen as irrelevant information, there would be no way to show the costs of these supportive services relative to the costs of a particular aspect of direct service. Administrative and clerical services are not a major objective of the agency and cannot be viewed as major services according to the criteria already described. The rationale for the indirect allocation of administrative and clerical time is that all of the agency's staff have as their *raison d'etre* the direct services provided to clients. The costs of providing these services must involve the cost of supportive services that enable the agency to function so that direct services can be provided. Obviously, although some clerical and administrative staff time can be identified with specific services, most of their time would be difficult, if not impossible, to allocate clearly into one or another. For this reason, indirect allocation was chosen.

It was also recognized that direct service staff do not spend all their working time providing direct services. Part of their job is to provide service to the organization in ways that enable that organization to continue to function. A major part of this is to provide input of information that ensures accountability and continuity of records. In addition, many of the staff are involved in administrative processes through participation in general staff meetings and committees for program review and evaluation. The aggregate of these activities is designated as "organizational maintenance."

The other major area of service in an agency is that of staff development, a service provided by the agency. Most of the time direct service workers spend in staff development and organizational maintenance relates to one of the service areas either directly or by the area in which the worker spends most of his direct service time. These two areas, organizational maintenance and staff development, are elements to be included in each service so that all working time can be recorded.

Thus, the four functions that enable an agency to fulfill its purpose are accounted for in the system. These functions are: direct services that the workers provide to the clients; services that the workers provide to the organization; supportive services that administrative and clerical staff provide to workers and to the organization; and staff development services that the agency provides to staff.

PRODUCTIVITY MEASUREMENTS

Measures of productivity were defined in two ways: by determining numbers of clients being served in the different services, and by defining certain units of production in each service. In some services, subunits that relate to a single element within a service are defined.

For each service unit, there was defined a cost to which all the costs of that service relate. The choice of units of production was made according to how useful this information would be administratively. Theoretically, a subunit could be defined and a cost figure attached to all elements from all services. The system is designed so that this could be done if circumstances demand; only a few subunits were selected for which costs would be extracted on an ongoing basis. For example, the major unit of cost for the adoption program is an adoptive placement, since all the time and costs of that service relate to making the placement and maintaining and legalizing it. The provision of 1 hour of homemaker service to a family is a subunit in Social Services to Children in Their Own Homes. This subunit is related to a specific element and includes not only the staff time involved in hiring, training, placing and supervising homemakers, but the costs of homemaker salaries and a prorated share of overall agency costs according to the percentages previously mentioned.

It was recognized that in counting open cases, the system did not account for the fact that not all clients receive the same amount of service and in some cases a client will receive no services in a particular month. It does, however, provide an average cost per month for keeping a case open for service in a particular service area.

An examination of the quality of each service, the frequency of contact or the intensity of involvement is not the province of this system. This aspect of agency operations is dealt with later in the discussion of the relationship between this system and ongoing program review. Program review is oriented toward qualitative evaluation of services.

STEPS IN THE SYSTEM

The primary source of information for the SSIS is the day sheet kept by each direct service worker to record his daily activities (see accompanying chart). The sheet is used for other purposes as well. Workers record mileage for travel and other reimbursable expenses; names and dates of contacts recorded are used as an aid in later case recording. In addition, the records are used to keep track of how many service contacts are made with clients for whom cost of service is reimbursable through federal funds.

The major use of the day sheet, however, is as a source document for the SSIS. Time is allocated in blocks of at least quarter hours and designated as to what service and under which element it should be counted. Each week, direct service hours in each element are totaled on the day sheets and submitted to unit supervisors, who compile monthly totals of hours in each service and element. At this stage, case counts and production figures for each supervisory unit are added. These monthly unit statistics are then reported on intermediate documents—a series consisting of one sheet for each service area. These reports are used to compile a monthly report from each district office in the region.

Administrative and clerical time is not figured directly into the hours of service under each element, since the major consideration for the system is the relative percentages of the elements within each service; the addition of this prorated time would not alter these percentages. For each office within the region, the direct service hours in each service are added and percentages are computed for each service; the percentages for the seven services total 100.

This set of percentages is used to distribute monthly operating expenses among the services not specifically identified as belonging to only one serv-printing. The same percentage is used to determine the average number of ice. Operating expenses include such costs as rent, equipment, utilities and staff working in each service. This is necessary because many of the direct

DAILY SERVICE SHEET

PLACE	ARR.	DEP.	MI.	ACTUAL CASE NAME	/	CONTACT	SERV. ELEM. CODE	HOURS	G	CLIENT I.D.
					/					
					/					
					/					
					/					
					/					
					/					
					/					
					/					
					/					
					/					
					/					

				OTHER EXPENSES (SPECIFY)			WORKER	
BREAKFAST	$				$		WKR. S.S. NO.	$
LUNCH	$						SUPERVISOR	$
DINNER	$						DATE	$
PER DIEM	$						OFFICE	$
LODGING	$							

CFS 863-1 (1/'74)

SERVICE I SOCIAL SERVICES TO CHILDREN IN THEIR OWN HOME

1.00	INTAKE/INFORMATION/REFER.
1.01	ABUSE INVESTIGATION
1.30	HOMEMAKER SERVICES
1.31	DAY CARE SERVICE
1.32	FAMILY PLANNING
1.40	MAINTAIN FAMILY
1.41	PREPARE FOR PLACEMENT
1.43	WORK - WITH COURT
1.48	AGENCY MANAGEMENT
1.49	ORGANIZATIONAL MAINT.
1.50	STAFF DEVELOPMENT
1.51	WORK WITH VOLUNTEERS
1.52	WORK WITH ADVOCATES

SERVICE II ADOPTION

2.00	INTAKE/INFORMATION/REFER.
2.01	ABUSE INVESTIGATION
2.10	STUDY/LICENS, PROCESS
2.30	HOMEMAKER SERVICE
2.40	PREPARE - FAMILY/CHILD
2.42	PLACEMENT SUPERVISION
2.46	LEGALLY FREE CHILD
2.47	SUBSIDY RE-EVALUATION
2.48	AGENCY MANAGEMENT
2.49	ORGANIZATIONAL MAINT.
2.50	STAFF DEVELOPMENT
2.51	WORK WITH VOLUNTEERS
2.52	WORK WITH ADVOCATES

SERVICE III SUBSTITUTE CARE FOSTER HOME

3.00	INTAKE/INFORMATION/REFER.
3.01	ABUSE INVESTIGATION
3.10	STUDY/LICENS, PROCESS
3.20	WORK - FOSTER HOME
3.30	HOMEMAKER SERVICE
3.31	DAY CARE SERVICE
3.32	FAMILY PLANNING
3.40	WORK - NATURAL FAMILY
3.42	WORK - PERMANENT PLCMT.
3.43	WORK - WITH COURT
3.44	WORK - PLACED CHILD
3.48	AGENCY MANAGEMENT
3.49	ORGANIZATIONAL MAINT.
3.50	STAFF DEVELOPMENT
3.51	WORK WITH VOLUNTEERS
3.52	WORK WITH ADVOCATES

SERVICE IV SUBSTITUTE CARE INSTITUTIONAL

4.00	INTAKE/INFORMATION/REFER.
4.01	ABUSE INVESTIGATION
4.30	HOMEMAKER SERVICE
4.32	FAMILY PLANNING
4.40	WORK - NATURAL FAMILY
4.42	WORK - PERMANENT PLCMT.
4.43	WORK - WITH COURT
4.45	LIAISON - CHILD/FACILITY
4.48	AGENCY MANAGEMENT
4.49	ORGANIZATIONAL MAINT.
4.50	STAFF DEVELOPMENT
4.51	WORK WITH VOLUNTEERS
4.52	WORK WITH ADVOCATES

SERVICE V SUBSTITUTE CARE GROUP CARE FACILITY

5.00	INTAKE/INFORMATION/REFER.
5.01	ABUSE INVESTIGATION
5.30	HOMEMAKER SERVICE
5.32	FAMILY PLANNING
5.40	WORK - NATURAL FAMILY
5.42	WORK - PERMANENT PLCMT.
5.43	WORK - WITH COURT
5.44	WORK - PLACED CHILD
5.45	LIAISON - CHILD/FACILITY
5.48	AGENCY MANAGEMENT
5.49	ORGANIZATIONAL MAINT.
5.50	STAFF DEVELOPMENT
5.51	WORK WITH VOLUNTEERS
5.52	WORK WITH ADVOCATES

SERVICE VI SUBSTITUTE CARE INDEPENDENT LIVING

6.00	INTAKE/INFORMATION/REFER.
6.01	ABUSE INVESTIGATION
6.30	HOMEMAKER SERVICE
6.31	DAY CARE SERVICE
6.32	FAMILY PLANNING
6.40	WORK - NATURAL FAMILY
6.42	WORK - PERMANENT PLCMT.
6.43	WORK - WITH COURT
6.44	WORK - CHILD IN I.L.
6.48	AGENCY MANAGEMENT
6.49	ORGANIZATIONAL MAINT.
6.50	STAFF DEVELOPMENT
6.51	WORK WITH VOLUNTEERS
6.52	WORK WITH ADVOCATES

SERVICE VII UNMARRIED PARENT SERVICE

7.00	INTAKE/INFORMATION/REFER.
7.01	ABUSE INVESTIGATION
7.30	HOMEMAKER SERVICE
7.32	FAMILY PLANNING
7.40	WORK - UNMARRIED PARENT
7.42	WORK - PERMANENT PLCMT.
7.43	WORK - WITH COURT
7.48	AGENCY MANAGEMENT
7.49	ORGANIZATIONAL MAINT.
7.50	STAFF DEVELOPMENT
7.51	WORK WITH VOLUNTEERS
7.52	WORK WITH ADVOCATES

SERVICE VIII LICENSING AND REGULATION OF COMM, FACILITIES

8.00	INFO TO COMMUNITY/REFERRAL
8.10	STUDY/LICENS, PROC - DC HOMES
8.11	STUDY/LICENS, PROC - DC CENTERS
8.12	STUDY/LICENS, PROC - INSTITUTIONS
8.13	STUDY/LICENS, PROC - AGENCIES
8.14	STUDY/LICENS, PROC - GR HOMES
8.20	DEVELOPMENT - DC HOMES
8.21	DEVELOPMENT - DC CENTERS
8.22	DEVELOPMENT - INSTITUTIONS
8.23	DEVELOPMENT - AGENCIES
8.24	DEVELOPMENT - GR HOMES
8.48	AGENCY MANAGEMENT
8.49	ORGANIZATIONAL MAINT.
8.50	STAFF DEVELOPMENT
8.51	WORK WITH VOLUNTEERS
8.52	WORK WITH ADVOCATES

SERVICE IX COMMUNITY SERVICES

9.00	PUBLIC INFORMATION/REFER.
9.20	RESOURCE DEVELOPMENT
9.30	HOMEMAKER SERVICE
9.32	FAMILY PLANNING
9.45	LIAISON WORK - COMMUN.
9.48	AGENCY MANAGEMENT
9.49	ORGANIZATIONAL MAINT.
9.50	STAFF DEVELOPMENT
9.51	WORK WITH VOLUNTEERS
9.52	WORK WITH ADVOCATES

service staff work in more than one service, as services are defined in the system. The same procedure is used for clerical and administrative staff. Salaries of direct service workers, supervisors, clerical and administrative staff are distributed among the services in the same manner. Finally, those costs directly attributable to a specific service are entered under that service.

This part of the district's monthly report, which is contained on a single sheet of paper, includes the number of direct service hours in the services and elements and a breakdown of staff, salaries and operating costs into services. The format of this report allows for vertical tabulation of cost items and gives the total cost of each of the seven services that have been defined.

Regional costs are handled in a similar manner. Monthly reports from the district offices are combined. When direct service hours from all offices are totaled, a new set of regional percentages for the services is computed. This new set of percentages is used to distribute regional staff salaries and regional office operating expenses among the services. As in the districts, costs clearly attributable to a specific service are added to only that service, rather than being distributed by percentage.

Case counts and production figures are also reported monthly. These are related to the combined costs for the entire region in the preparation of the regional report. The system can accommodate these computations being performed at the district level, as well as at the regional level.

Case movement for the month is shown in terms of cases opened during the month, cases closed, total cases served, and an end-of-the-month balance of opened cases. A subsystem had to be developed to provide for accurate and consistent case counts. This subsystem is usually maintained by a unit secretary or other clerical person.

Specific measures of productivity were defined and are reported monthly; these, too, are combined into the regional totals. In the regional summary, costs, production figures and case counts are brought together.

For each service, there is a total cost that takes into account that service's share of the total expenses of the region, as well as costs directly attributable to that service. An average cost per open case for the month and the average number of cases carried per month by a worker in each service is also computed. In the regional summary, elements within services are broken down by percentages showing what percentage of the total time in that service was spent by direct service staff performing that element. The final step is the determination of unit costs in each service. As previously mentioned, a major unit of cost is defined for each service to which all costs of that service relate. A major unit of cost for Substitute Care-Foster Home Service is one 24-hour period of foster home care for a child. By definition, this is the payment to the faster homes and the costs of services rendered to or in behalf of the children. The number of individual days of foster care provided during the month is divided into the total expenditure of the service to arrive at the cost of this unit.

Subunits are always related to a specific element within a service; this adds an extra step to these computations. One of the subunits in Social Services to Children in Their Own Homes is the cost of 1 hour of homemaker service to a family. The definition of this element is "all activities in planning and arranging for homemaker services, including work with the homemaker to ensure effective delivery of services." The subtotal cost of the entire service, which includes the prorated share of general expenses but not costs directly attributable to the service, such as homemakers' salaries, is multiplied by the element percentage. The salaries paid to homemakers during the month are then added to this figure and the total amount is divided by the total number of individual hours of homemaker service provided during the month to arrive at the subunit cost.

Although cost figures are done on a monthly basis, it is obvious that in many instances one monthly figure seen by itself will have little meaning. For example, one of the agency's responsibilities is the licensing of child-caring institutions in the region. Most months will show no production in that item although hours may have been devoted and so recorded. Adoptive placements, although a less extreme example, often fluctuate in numbers from month to month. In such situations, average unit costs can also be computed on an annual or semiannual basis for a more meaningful indication of cost. However, the fluctuations in unit costs from month to month can be a valuable administrative monitoring tool.

HOW SYSTEM INFORMATION CAN BE USED

The cost information described in the preceding section is the most basic and obvious data supplied by the SSIS. Detailed and consistent reporting of the costs of services and costs of units of production is a primary objective of the system. The SSIS provides a wealth of other information.

Accurate case counts in the various services are obtained in such a way that the rate of case turnover can be shown. In a public agency where there are great demands on a limited number of staff, quick and effective provision of services becomes vital.

The relative amounts of direct service time in each service, and an examination of those elements into which time is concentrated, are useful in program monitoring for unit supervisors, as well as other administrative staff. A foster care supervisor who sees most of his unit's time devoted to maintenance work with the child or the foster parent and very little to work toward moving the child into permanent placement can more effectively query the causes.

Since cost items are listed in a manner compatible with previously established bookkeeping systems, spending within various line items can be monitored to prevent excessive surplus or deficit during the fiscal year. Budget construction and defense are also facilitated by this type of record keeping. After the system has been in operation long enough to establish valid unit costs, this information can serve as a base for determining how much funding is necessary to achieve a certain production level.

The SSIS provides information useful for determining trends in clientele, shifts in service demands and priorities. This information can be used to adjust resource allocations and staffing patterns to allow the agency to be more responsive to changing circumstances. Trends in element percentages, caseloads and unit costs can be examined monthly by staff; this can serve to help staff quickly identify—and intervene in—problems in program functioning.

Potentially, one of the most useful aspects of the SSIS for an agency is in the negotiation of contractual arrangements between public and voluntary agencies for the provision of specific services. If, for example, agencies are negotiating an agreement with a voluntary agency to provide homemaker services for a public agency, a realistic price can be more easily determined if the public agency has some indication of how much it costs to provide the service internally. This is equally applicable to the voluntary agency in this kind of negotiation.

The particular value of the SSIS is that it brings most of this information into one reporting system.

RELATIONSHIP OF SYSTEM TO GOAL SETTING AND TO REVIEW AND EVALUATION

There are two major aspects of the East St. Louis Regional operations to which the SSIS is related—the setting of goals consistent with the "management-by-objectives" approach to administration, and an ongoing process of program review and evaluation. A basic principle of goal setting is that the goals be feasible. Goals that are too low or too high make the entire procedure irrelevant and can have adverse effect on staff morale and productivity.

Information obtained through the SSIS is of great assistance in setting realistic goals in accordance with the resources allocated by the Illinois Department of Children and Family Services at the state level. If the system were also implemented at the state level, the same would apply to the resources allocated to the department by the Illinois Legislature.

Program review and evaluation, like the goal-setting process, was not developed specifically in conjunction with the SSIS. Once the system was developed, however, it became obvious that the system and the review and evaluation process complemented each other. The SSIS is primarily concerned with the quantitative and financial aspects of agency operations, while review and evaluation are focused on qualitative considerations.

The SSIS was not intended to provide qualitative review, although much of the information it provides is useful for this purpose. The implication of total reliance on the SSIS for monitoring purposes is that efficiency and cost may be overemphasized to the detriment of the maintenance of quality services. An ongoing review and evaluation process has been operating in the East St. Louis Region since the initial implementation of the SSIS.

REVIEW AND EVALUATION

Although the general area of program review and evaluation is extensive enough to merit separate treatment, following is a brief description of its purpose and function.

Although program functioning is monitored for quality on an ongoing basis, a full review and evaluation of a program (or part of a program) provides an opportunity for staff to step back periodically from their day-to-day involvement and examine the program intensively. The clue for review areas is often found in the monthly SSIS reports completed for the region. In most instances a member of the regional staff has primary responsibility for conducting the evaluation, working with a group of direct service workers and other staff involved in the program. Some of the questions addressed by the review committee might be:

How effectively is the program functioning in terms of accomplishing service objectives and meeting the needs of clients?

Are there identifiable trends in client populations and their service needs, and if so, how can the agency most effectively respond to these changes?

Are there trends in service delivery, and if so, are they a result of planning for meeting clients' needs or are they a result of external or internal stresses that might threaten the provision of quality service?

What are the current or anticipated problems in the functioning of the program, what causes these problems and what alternatives are available for correcting them?

What are current or anticipated staff development needs?

Are the information systems related to the program efficient and functional? Can they be streamlined to release more staff time for provision of service?

In some instances a review might focus on a specific question of current concern, such as the effectiveness with which the agency is using paraprofessional staff, or the effects of the adoption of a formal intake policy.

The final report contains recommendations for improving or maintaining service delivery, based on the information gathered by the review committee. After approval by the regional director, those changes that can be implemented locally are put into effect. Recommendations that require changes in department policies or procedures are submitted to the state office for consideration.

We have found that, in addition to providing a base for program development, program review and evaluation provide an opportunity for all staff working in a program to have meaningful input into its functioning, as well as providing them with a valuable learning experience.

CONCLUSIONS

The SSIS was developed to provide ongoing information about the functioning of a public child welfare agency, covering all aspects of operations in a way that relates productivity to operating costs. It is based on the distribution of direct service time among services and service elements using a framework developed by Elkin.

Since full implementation of the system in the East St. Louis Region took place July 1, 1972, and statewide July 1, 1973, it is still in an evaluative stage. However, parts of the system were in use during the 2 preceding years and their usefulness has been established. Direct service workers state that the daily reporting does not consume an inordinate amount of working time. Staff resistance to the system has been alleviated by their recognition that reporting of elements is more relevant to service delivery than other methods of reporting. It is recognized that the SSIS is in an early stage of development and that problems may still arise. The initial months of operation have revealed minor problems of implementation and interpretation, but no obvious flaws in the basic structure have been discovered. The definitions of services and elements were tailored for local operations, and it is likely that implementation by other agencies would necessitate the identification of other major service areas.

Consultation with data-processing personnel during the construction of the SSIS has indicated that the system can easily be adapted to computerized operations. In the programming of the SSIS for statewide use, it is possible that the only information necessary will be the workers' daily reports. Other necessary information is already being supplied to data processing by current reporting systems. It is also expected that the SSIS can be used to meet the more comprehensive reporting standards to be issued by the Department of Health, Education and Welfare.

REFERENCE

1. Elkin, Robert. A *Conceptual Base for Defining Health and Welfare Services.* New York: Child Welfare League of America, Family Service Association of America, Travelers Aid Association of America, 1967.

41/A MANAGEMENT
INFORMATION SYSTEM
FOR SOCIAL SERVICES

H. R. CATHERWOOD

ORIGINS OF THE SYSTEM

The state executive director was polite but firm. "I'm sorry," he said, "but we really have no problems for an outside consultant. No need at all. Please leave me . . ." and then he interrupted himself. "Say, there is one area. If you could develop something it would be the greatest boon to all welfare people that I can imagine."

He went on to tell a story. "I go to see the chairman of the appropriations committee," he began, "and say to him 'Joe, next year we have to have more caseworkers. Our services delivery staff is helping more people, their caseloads are up 50 percent, we just can't get the job done with present staff.' Joe then asks me a few questions. 'What do you mean by services? What kind of services? Who do you help? What kind of people? Why do they need help? How many of them get jobs after you help them? How many of them are really hopeless cases? How many are alcoholics? How many people can one worker handle at one time?'"

The executive director smiled. "I can't answer any of these questions," he said. "We can give Joe a lot of statistics on categories, intake, terminations and that, but we can't really tell him what service workers do or for what kinds of people. Now that eligibility work has been split off, those social services staffs in my county offices stand out in my budget like sore thumbs. If you find an answer to that one, every department in the country could use it."

INITIATION OF THIS STUDY

After many days of library research, talks with officials of HEW Region VIII, discussions with state and county welfare directors, and some hard thinking, my firm prepared a proposal (jointly with management services division of Touche Ross & Co.) to the Denver, Colorado, city-county welfare department. The proposal was for the design of a management information system for the adult and medical services section of the department and it set out the need for such a system as follows:

We believe that the need for better management information regarding social services is greater today than ever before. In January 1969, new regulations were issued by HEW (Part 220, Chapter II, Title 45, Code of Federal Regulations) relating to "service programs for families and children." These require that the staff for services be full time and that the determination of eligibility and the provision of financial assistance be done by others. As these staffs are isolated from other duties, as their size and importance within the organization increases, and as their salaries and other expenses become more clearly identifiable and increase in absolute amounts, budget authorities and appropriating bodies will increasingly be asking the question—what services?—as well as questions about the kind, scope, extent, and effectiveness of these services. Welfare departments will need to have established information systems to provide at least some of the answers to these questions.[1]

As to the identification of the needs for services, the reporting of services rendered, etc., and the use of this information for planning and control, only rudimentary systems usually exist in a welfare office. New cases are assigned to social workers either in rotation or on the basis of the personal knowledge of the line supervisors. The social workers prepare descriptive statements identifying the needs of their clients, plan the services to be given, and the services are rendered in the field under the direction of the supervisor. Higher authority is usually informed about these activities in terms of the numbers of social workers and supervisors assigned to each category, the number of cases receiving services in the respective categories, the number of cases per worker, and the number of "contacts" or "service calls."

Usually the reporting of even these data is done in such a way as to throw a substantial clerical burden on the caseworkers. Furthermore, a lack of management information often requires that special searches be made, sometimes involving reading of case files, when it is necessary to locate certain kinds of cases or obtain data as to the services being rendered.

The management information system that we propose will, to the extent practical, be designed to answer the following questions:

1. Based on the present caseload, how many cases need social welfare services?

2. What services, by kinds, do they need, and for how long?

3. What is the prognosis for the several cases? How many are probably hopeless and likely to remain permanent charges of the state? How many would benefit from intensive services and of what kind? How many of the cases should be expected not to need assistance after some interval, say a year?

4. What does a review of the cases after a period (such as six months) show as to progress? Have their service needs decreased, remained the same, or increased? What, in short, has been done for them?

5. Are the cases assigned properly to workers? Do the assignments bear any relation to the services needed and the special interests and skills of the workers? After taking into account the kind and extent of services needed

by the caseload, do the assignments fairly balance the work loads of the caseworkers?

6. What is the level of productivity of the workers or of the supervisory units, after making allowances for the services being rendered? What are reasonable work standards for service cases?

7. What are the costs of the services being rendered? Is it possible that an economic benefit (including a direct saving in appropriated monies) could be obtained by rendering one kind of intensive service for a short time rather than another on a permanent basis? Should there, in other words, be a concentration of money and service resources on certain cases and certain kinds of services? If so, which cases and which services?

8. What cases were recently discharged from the rolls and why? What services had they been receiving? Can these services correctly be identified as having produced some degree of rehabilitation?

The proposed system was planned to be a manual one—certainly until its usefulness had been fully demonstrated. It was designed, however, so that it might be converted to EDP with a minimum of trouble. The proposal to design such a system was accepted by the Denver department and was presented to the Colorado State Board of Social Services in April, 1970. The comments made during the discussion are interesting:

The chairman said that it is rather shattering when he looks at some of these statements, such as "What cases were recently discharged from the rolls and why?" If these county people have been administering the department for the past seven years and do not know why they are discharging people from the rolls, then we are in a bad situation. The state director answered that it is a matter of determining the kinds of social services an adult person could use and should have when he comes in and applies for AND (AD) or OAP or AB. . . . There has to be some way of recording what the caseworker did for this person. . . . Did it solve the problem? These are the kinds of questions we are getting now from legislators, getting from Congress, and that is why HEW is interested in this. The department has been spending a lot of money for what we call casework social services, and what are the results, how do we measure it? . . . The federal auditors were here the other day and they were critical that our case records did not note the social service applied. . . . We do not have a system for . . . recording the service as it is rendered. . . . We have for a long time been worrying about assistance payments and money. Now, we are talking about giving services to people to help them. . . .

COLLECTING THE FACTS

In November, 1970, we went to work. Six units (which comprise a supervisor and five workers) were selected as the test area. One of the supervisors was detailed to work with the consultants later in the project, when the case classification plan was to be prepared.

We first reviewed all of the principal forms and records kept by the adult services caseworkers, finding—as everyone expected—a number of overlapping clerical chores done by caseworkers, some records that were of dubious value, and several areas where state-required forms demanded a great deal of office time. Although we reported these matters to management, we took the general position that there is no use fighting City Hall and went on about developing the MIS.

We found a management information system already in operation, based on a monthly transportation and contact report. In addition to being a claim for reimbursement for the use of the worker's automobile on official business, caseworkers were required to post to this form each contact with a client or on behalf of a client (the collateral contact), including the date, name of the person contacted, his address, the assistance category involved, whether the contact was in the office or field, and the mileage involved in the contact. The forms submitted each month contained from thirty to sixty entries (one to a line) and obviously made substantial demands on caseworkers' time.

The reports (after being used to pay mileage) were routed to a research and statistics unit, where they were used to prepare a Monthly Worker Report. This report showed, for each worker and each supervisor unit, the days worked during the month, the numbers of field and office visits, and a calculated contact rate expressed as a percentage (based on the assumption that a field visit requires one hour and an office visit half an hour). We recommended that the contact reporting system be abolished, for three principal reasons:

1. The contact is not in itself a particularly significant unit of performance. Some contacts are long, others short, some cases require numerous contacts, others can be well-handled with few contacts, and in some cases multiple contacts merely mean that the worker did not do the work right the first time. It is by no means true that a worker who makes four contacts a day is twice as productive as one who makes two contacts.

2. Both supervisors and workers say that the contact statistics mean little to them and several supervisors state that the contact rate is meaningless.

3. The posting of contacts on the monthly transportation and contact report takes up worker time that could better be spent otherwise.

We further found that the workers were using a desk card as a ready reference to save referring to case files whenever routine information was needed. These cards were also used as ticklers for the next visit to the client—the annual visit in the case of nonservice clients. The cards also contained space to record visits to clients, including a soon-to-be-obsolete classification of the services delivered on such visits. The posting of visits and services rendered, if faithfully done, require appreciable amounts of worker time.

Having thus cleared away the underbrush—or at least mapped the location of the worst thickets—we proceeded to the design of the proposed system.

CASE CLASSIFICATION

We first addressed ourselves to the problem of classifying cases. We decided that there should be two taxonomic systems, one classifying cases by the services they need, and the second classifying them according to goals. The first classification plan would answer the question: What help do these people need? The second would answer the question: What kind of person, taking him all in all, is this client? We met, of course, the objection that "You can't classify people"—to which we replied that hospitals classify patients by diseases, the Army classifies people by skills, and the census classifies them by economic criteria. We are not, we said, really "classifying people"—we are merely classifying certain objectively defined characteristics of the people whom we serve.

Because of the existence of a state services classification, we decided to adopt the state codes applicable to the adult categories, as follows.*

B. Information and referal services
C. Protective services
D. Services to enable persons to remain or return to their homes or communities
E. Employment services
F. Health needs services
G. Money management services
H. Homemaking and housing services
I. Education services
K. Self-support services for the handicapped

To these nine classes of services we added another for annual visits to clients not otherwise requiring (or wanting) service.

We then developed the goals classification. The introduction to the plan reads as follows:

The goals classification plan set out in this memorandum is intended to provide social workers and their supervisors with an orderly, logical, and structured plan for describing and categorizing adult clients according to the goals appropriate to each case. Whereas the services classification plan relates to objectives (better housing, combating despair), the goals classification relates to the kind of person the client—taken as a whole—is believed to be. The plan is a taxonomic system by which a social worker experienced with the kinds of adults who

---

* Code A is not relevant.

receive public assistance can answer the question of another experienced worker: What kind of case is this?

The seven goals classes that have been identified have been arranged in descending order of intensity of need for service, ranging from those needing most attention and casework time to those needing service only rarely (the last class includes clients who decline service). Four of the classes have, for convenience, been grouped as "intensive," two as "maintenance level," and one as "basic."[2]

The goals classification plan is as follows:

Intensive
1. Short-term rehabilitation
2. Crisis control
3. Long-term rehabilitation
4. Protection

Maintenance Level
5. Chronically ill
6. Unresponsive

Basic
7. Adequate marginal adjustment or independent

It should be noted that a given client at a given time can be assigned to only one class—unlike the case of the services classification where a client may need help toward several objectives. It should also be noted that temporary changes in the status of a client would not require reclassification. Thus a client in any of the other seven classes might temporarily need crisis intervention but no reclassification would be necessary—provided that the worker expected the client to return to his normal level of functioning.

It should further be noted that the priorities given to the several goals represent a statement of agency policy, in that higher priority cases are expected to be given more attention and time than those of lower level.[3]

The goals classification plan then gives, in considerable detail, a definition of each goal and, under the heading of "typical characteristics," a number of examples of that goals class.

The proposed MIS contemplates that each client will be classified at the time the worker receives the case for service (the classification could be done at intake). One or more service needs would be identified in the course of working up the case and preparing the case plan, and the client would be assigned to a goals class. These decisions would appropriately be reviewed with the unit supervisor.

These decisions would be recorded on the back of a desk card designed

EXHIBIT A
Desk Card

Age:		Sex:			CASE CLASSIFICATION					
Date										
Worker										
Goal										
S E R V I C E	B									
	C						ˌ			
	D									
	E									
	F									
	G									
N E E D S	H									
	I									
	K									
	A V									
	Misc									

for the purpose (see Exhibit A). The front of the card shows the usual data about the client—name, etc.

The left-hand column of this form would, of course, be used the first time the case was classified. The date of classification, worker identification, and the number identification of the goals class would be entered. Checks would be made opposite the appropriate letter code for the services needed by the client. At regular intervals thereafter, or when the status of the client changed, the next column would be used to reclassify the case. It should be noted that case movement—progress or retrogression—would be clearly visible by looking at a succession of classifications.

The front of the desk card would continue to be used for ready reference including the tickler for date of next visit and provision for recording the dates of successive client contacts. Age and sex data are duplicated between the front and back of the form for convenience in use.

SERVICES DELIVERY

Having covered the matter of case classification, we were confronted with the other face of the coin—what system should be established to produce information about caseworker activity?

Our previous research showed that the problem had been met in other agencies in various ways. Some made intensive pilot runs—during a week or a month, every employee reported exactly how much time he spent in various activities. In at least one case, increments of five minutes were used and coffee breaks and restroom visits were seriously required to be reported. We felt that such pilot studies—even if employees would take them seriously—were biased by the fact that everyone wanted to make a good showing during the test period. The results during, say, a two-week test could not with any accuracy be extrapolated to a year. Furthermore, such extrapolations conceal changes in work loads and priorities of working time that are vitally important for management to know.

Another method, of course, was to ask the caseworkers to report on only the service delivery part of their activities. They might, at the least, report on what services they had delivered during a stated time period. They might be asked to report time spent on service delivery, according to a standard classification of services or of activities necessary to render such services. They might be asked to classify their time according to the goals toward which they were assisting their clients—so much time on rehabilitation cases, so much on the health problems cases, so much on the nonresponsive. We rejected these simply because they did not give a full and rounded presentation of what workers are really doing—such reports were at best fractional and incomplete.

We faced, however, solid opposition to the only other alternative—the preparation on a regular, recurring basis of time reports covering all working time, reports balancing out to forty hours a week. The opposition centered on the implication that the report would be used as a surveillance tool—that the supervisor would examine every entry and ask questions such as "Why did you take two hours talking to the doctor?" "How could you spend an hour going three blocks away, only to find the client not at home?" We found that this quite understandable resistance centered on the assumption that the time report would contain a descriptive statement as to how each increment of time was spent—such as "home visit to Mrs. Brown." We therefore wholly eliminated any such requirement and merely asked the worker to classify his own time, hopefully at the end of each day, in his own way, using the same code for services that he used for reporting to the state and in our proposed classification of services. In addition, he would put down time spent in nonservice matters, such as overhead (paperwork), professional development, and special projects (of which a number occurred during our study). The form that we suggested is shown in Exhibit B.

Although this form identifies the work done by classes of services and other activities, it does not contain enough detail to be used (except perhaps by the most ill-willed supervisor) as a surveillance tool and of course is not so intended. Increments of time would be recorded in units of an hour, estimated by the worker himself. Space is provided for comments if the worker desires to use it. Space is also provided for reporting total contacts made during the day, for the benefit of those who cling to the reporting of such artifacts. We estimate that the form would require, at a maximum, ten minutes time a day. At the end of the week, it would be totaled and cross-totaled and be given to the supervisor.

EXHIBIT B
Report of Professional Activity

REPORT OF PROFESSIONAL ACTIVITY							Employee:						Week:		
Cont.	Spec.	Ohd.	P D	B	C	D	E	F	G	H	I	K	AV	Misc.	T
M O N D A Y	Comments:														
Cont.	Spec.	Ohd.	P D	B	C	D	E	F	G	H	I	K	AV	Misc.	T
F R I D A Y	Comments:														
						Weekly Totals									
Cont.	Spec.	Ohd.	P D	B	C	D	E	F	G	H	I	K	AV	Misc.	T

The simplification of the form, together with the argument that lawyers, doctors and—yes—even management consultants use such a "swindle sheet" appeared to be convincing to the rank and file of workers. They may have been influenced, too, by the statement that some such report of professional activity is essential to telling their story to the public—and the appropriation committee.

INFORMATION DERIVED FROM THE SYSTEM

At this point in the description of the proposed system, we have described the input of information using the desk card and the report of professional activity. Let us now describe the output of the management information system.

Information about the active service case loads would be compiled at intervals of perhaps three months. A report would be prepared for each worker, showing the number of cases by category and by goals, as well as the total number of services required by the caseload (which might total two or three times as many as the case count). The reports for the several workers in a unit would be consolidated for the unit and, presumably, for groups of units under a common senior supervisor.

Information about the professional activities of workers would be compiled at least once every four weeks and it might be desirable to compile it every two weeks. The two or four reports from each worker and the supervisor would simply be added and the totals would be entered under the name or number of the caseworker on a report showing the time expended on various classes of service (or overhead activities) by each worker and

EXHIBIT C
Analysis of Caseloads

ANALYSIS OF CASELOADS	Social Worker or Unit								
Period:									Totals
Total Case Counts									
AND									
AB									
OAB- A									
OAB- B									
TB									
Total caseload									
Goals Classification of Service Cases									
Short-term rehabilitation									
Crisis control									
Long-term rehabilitation									
Protection									
Chronically ill									
Unresponsive									
Adequate or independent									
Total service caseload									
Service Needs of Service Cases									
Information & referral									
Protective									
Remain or return									
Employment									
Health									
Money management									
Homemaking & housing									
Education									
Self-support handicapped									
Annual visit									
Miscellaneous									
Total service needs									

the unit. This report would follow a routine similar to that of the report on the caseload. The proposed form is shown in Exhibit C and the format of the analysis of professional activities is shown in Exhibit D.

VALUE OF THE INFORMATION PRODUCED

Any proposed management information system must be tested as to the usefulness of the information output and must be subjected to the question, "What value is the information after it is produced?"

In regard to the present proposal, we would answer the question at two levels in the hierarchy—from the points of view of supervisors and of middle management. The advantages of the system from the point of view of supervisors, we believe, are as follows:

1. The classification of the case load by goals gives the supervisor better control—when you have a large number of disparate entities the problems

EXHIBIT D
Analysis of Professional Activities

ANALYSIS OF PROFESSIONAL ACTIVITIES	Social Worker or Unit							
Period:								Totals
Special project								
Overhead								
Professional development								
Total nonservice								
Information and referral								
Protective								
Remain or return								
Employment								
Health								
Money management								
Homemaking & housing								
Education								
Self-support handicapped								
Annual visit								
Other								
Total service								
Total time								
Contacts								
Comments:								

are hard to identify and grasp and a system of classification is a great help. A plan for organizing the case load under a goals classification gives peace of mind.

2. The goals classification makes it possible for workers to allocate their time to those goals that need primary attention—the first four. If they must, they can give scant attention to the goals 5–7 cases. The supervisor can help his workers direct their efforts accordingly.

3. The goals classification makes it possible to make treatment plans for various kinds of cases, by providing a classification of cases. The goals indicate what kind of person the client is and hence what may be the appropriate treatment. The supervisor can then better direct the efforts of his workers and the techniques they use with specific groups of cases.

4. The classification of a given case according to the goal for that case and the services needed by the client, taken in conjunction with his age, provides a profile description of the case. The worker and the supervisor have a common language (or a set of handles) by which a case can be defined and identified. This should be especially useful in dealing with cases transferred from other units using the same system of classification—the worker would not have to start from scratch.

5. The services classification provides an orderly way of identifying the problem areas for each client. The supervisor can then explore with the worker the specific problems under each service need.

6. The service needs statistics for each worker's caseload gives the supervisor information as to the quality of the load—whether it is predominantly of certain kinds of service needs and what they are.

7. In time and on a gradual basis, the more sophisticated data provided

by the system as to the composition of caseloads may make it possible to shift some cases from one worker to another, to equalize caseloads and recognize special aptitudes and interests among the several workers.

8. The professional activity report makes it possible to ask questions of workers at the weekly supervisor-worker conferences as to why so much time was spent on a particular matter—such as overhead or a particular kind of service.

9. The activity report gives the supervisor a sense of awareness as to how each worker is spending his time—what is going on in the unit. This is particularly useful if the supervisor is absent for one or several days. In the case of the occasional malingerer, the report would help the supervisor check his subjective judgement that the worker is not using his time properly—to pinpoint malingering. This need occurs mainly in the case of new workers during the probation period.

10. Reporting time instead of contacts is much more significant both for the supervisor and for the workers—who agree in this opinion.

11. The "special" column on the activity report should be useful from time to time for a variety of special checks—such as determining the amount of time devoted by workers during a given trial period to testing proposed forms, time devoted to communications with eligibility technicians, or the time devoted to crisis intervention on behalf of clients prematurely discharged from state institutions. Once the time data for such activities are established, it would be easy to extrapolate the time figures on an annual basis and express them as dollar costs.

12. The data available to a supervisor as to the composition of case loads and the time devoted to various activities by workers should give him objective data to use in making the annual ratings of workers. To an extent, they should permit the supervisor to set up normal productivity standards.

Middle management (by which we mean section and division heads) would profit from several of the foregoing advantages, especially in dealing with individual supervisors and caseworkers. The system output would come to the three middle managers principally, however, in the form of the analysis of professional activities (every two or four weeks) and the quarterly analysis of caseloads. Their reports would, of course, be in summary form—that is, they would show totals by units rather than by individual workers.

We believe our management information system has great potential as an administrative tool in the field of public welfare. It allows a greater degree of control and flexibility at the supervisory and middle management level; frees the line worker to use his time in the most productive manner; and, perhaps most important, facilitates accurate diagnosis and clarity of thought regarding the individual client.

NOTES

1. Kansas-Denver Associates and Touche Ross and Co., "Proposal for Development and Installation of a Social Services Management Installation System for the Denver Department of Welfare," (unpublished report, January 28, 1970).
2. *Ibid.*
3. *Ibid.*

42/MANAGEMENT INFORMATION SYSTEMS IN CHILD CARE: AN AGENCY EXPERIENCE

DAVID W. YOUNG

As child care agencies become increasingly accountable to their funding sources, their communities and others, they are being called upon more and more to provide to third parties and to their boards of directors adequate information on the effectiveness of their programs. Additionally, many agencies continue to encounter administrative dilemmas that result from a growing complexity of service delivery patterns and from a continuing concern for the unmet needs of a constantly changing client population.

In part, these problems stem from the traditional manner in which data are collected and presented. Statistical information in the child care field and in many social service fields is usually presented in a highly summarized manner, and often with a considerable lag between the time of an event and the time it is reported statistically. However, administrators of social agencies require both detailed and timely information. To be useful, this information must be presented in a format that a) permits a quick review, b) facilitates the pinpointing of problem areas, c) assists in the determination of responsibility for action, and d) contains a capacity for followup and evaluation.

For example, in many child care agencies administrators receive a monthly or quarterly report summarizing the number of admissions, transfers and discharges. Although this information may be helpful for maintaining control over such factors as maximum population levels, it is only marginally useful for assessing the quality of service being delivered. More useful information would consist of reports that list the children involved, the appropriateness of the admission, the reason for the transfer, and whether the discharge was timely and as planned. This information would be even more useful if it were presented in a form that could be quickly scanned so that potentially inappropriate admissions, transfers or discharges were indicated. These instances could then be followed up and corrected if necessary.

THE TIME FACTORS

Manual preparation of reports that call for collection of a broad range of data, plus selection and presentation of portions of these data for administrative review and analysis, could be extremely time-consuming. Further, the development of special administrative reports presenting information concerning new agency emphases or new problem areas could be difficult. For example, an agency wishing to place increased emphasis on adoption might require a special list of all children who were under the age of 3 from families with an abusive parent, and in need of legal action to free them for adoption. In most agencies, manual preparation of such a list would require considerable effort from both casework and clerical staffs.

In an attempt to resolve this dilemma of the increasing need for detailed management information and the problem of delay in obtaining it by traditional manual methods, the Edwin Gould Services for Children agency of New York City has developed a computerized management information system. The system, called the Child Record System, contains a broad base of data on each child in care with the agency, and facilitates a wide variety of both regular and special analyses and comparisons. The latter characteristic allows the agency's administrators to determine more accurately the child's overall needs and the appropriate program to meet those needs, to evaluate more thoroughly the progress toward state child objectives, and to review more objectively the agency's ongoing programs.

The Child Record System was developed over a period of about 2 years,[1] and has been in operation for about 2 years. During these 4 years a great deal was learned about the application of management information system technology to the child care field. This paper presents some of that knowledge for professionals and others interested in the application of management information systems technology to the child care field.

The paper begins by reviewing the historical development and objectives of the system, discussing the basic decisions made by the agency in defining the scope and capabilities of the system. It then describes the overall operation of the system. Next the content of the data base and the process of report design are examined. Finally, the paper considers the potentials of the system and new directions being taken by the agency as a result of using the system.

HISTORY OF DEVELOPMENT

Conceptually, the Child Record System grew out of a variety of administrative problems confronting the management of Edwin Gould Services for Children. Specifically:

• As the agency's population expanded, the quantity of data to be maintained and tabulated was growing to unmanageable proportions.

• As service emphasis shifted from custodial foster care to adoption, aftercare and prevention, the information necessary for effective management of the new programs and services increased and changed in nature.

• As the size and turnover rate of the agency's population increased due to the new emphases, it became increasingly difficult for supervisors and program directors to be personally acquainted with each client and his or her needs and problems.

• As the quantity of information in each child's case record grew, due both to increased city and state reporting requirements and to new information being collected on biological parents and other involved persons, the effort required to summarize case information increased as well; the preparation of statistical analyses covering children with special characteristics or needs became an almost impossible task, thereby complicating program planning for these children.

Because of these problems and an administrative emphasis on full accountability for day-to-day decisions affecting clients, the decision was made to develop a computerized management information system.[2]

OBJECTIVES OF SYSTEM

At the outset, the agency's principal goal was to develop an information system that would retain and display when necessary the full range of objective case information on each child or on groups of children with similar characteristics. The hope was that such a system would facilitate program planning and eventually substitute for all but the narrative portions of each child's case record.

As the system developed, the agency's program directors began to focus on more explicit objectives. Among these were:

• to develop a variety of case management reports pinpointing problem areas and indicating situations requiring administrative attention or casework action.

508 DAVID W. YOUNG

- to give casework and supervisory staff useful and up-to-date reference information on each case in their caseloads.
- to summarize, tabulate and compare any given items in the case records at any given time, in order to prepare or assist in the preparation of special reports or population summaries.
- to prepare monthly control or "tickler" reports informing caseworkers and clerical staff of specific action required of them by the city or state on behalf of a client.
- to facilitate the access and summary presentation of data concerning specific areas of interest for certain categories of the client population, in order to assist in evaluating agency performance.

Early in the development process, the agency made three key decisions that had a major impact on the scope and usefulness of the system. The first was to accumulate a large data base on each child, covering a wide variety of potentially useful areas. This posed possible problems in terms of keeping the information current and accurate; however, it was believed that the advantage of having complete data available outweighed potential problems. Additionally, the large data base allowed the agency to make full use of a computer-based information system's capability to store and maintain large quantities of data without sacrificing the ability to "retrieve" and analyze any portion of the data base with speed and accuracy.

The second decision was to avoid use of standard report formats. It was felt that such formats would require the agency to analyze specific predetermined data elements that could become outmoded as agency objectives and client needs changed. Instead, the agency decided to develop a system providing complete flexibility of report formats and report design.

The third decision was to give the system an "end-result" as well as a "service-input" focus.[3] That is, caseworkers would be asked to designate a planned goal for each child and estimate a date for achieving it. This decision reemphasized the agency's concern with evaluation and overall program accountability.[4] Further, service needs of both children and biological parents became an integral part of the system.

In the 1½ years following these decisions, considerable effort went into a) the development of the specific elements of the data base, b) the construction of computer-readable codes, c) the preparation of data entry forms, d) the writing of computer programs, and e) the instruction of caseworkers in the use of the system.

TRAINING THE CASEWORKERS

Caseworker instruction was perhaps the most important of these tasks, since the agency had placed a high priority both on giving the system a casework orientation and on involving caseworkers in the use as well as submission of information. Casework staff participated in many decisions concerning the nature and scope of the information system, and explanations of the data entry forms and coding structures were given at agencywide meetings. Several other steps were taken to assist caseworkers:

• A special uncoded report—the Verbal Child Record Printout—was prepared to facilitate case reference and updating by caseworkers.

• An instruction manual was written, giving detailed information on the use of the system by caseworkers.

• The system is used to help caseworkers prepare city and state reports.

• Many of the regular summary reports prepared from the system are distributed to the caseworkers, so that they are aware of the kind of information being utilized by the administrative staff.

The training of caseworkers to complete comprehensive information forms and to update data regularly began early in the design stage and is still in progress.[5] The agency believes this process has been aided by the emphasis placed on caseworker participation, particularly on "information feedback." Caseworkers either receive or have access to information supplied to supervisors and program directors.

The system was put into use in early 1971, and has been fully operational since. Because of the flexibility in both data base components and report formats, the system has also been an evolving one. New information has been added to the data base and new types of reports are regularly designed and prepared to meet agency and staff needs.

OVERALL OPERATION OF THE SYSTEM

Original Data Collection

Data collection for the Child Record System begins when a child is admitted to the agency. At that point the caseworker responsible for evaluating the child completes three data entry forms: an *Intake* form, a *Natural Parents* form and a *Foster Parents* form.

Following a staffing of each case and the transfer of casework responsibility from the intake to the undercare division, an *Undercare* data entry form is completed by the caseworker assigned to the child.

Report Preparation

Once each month a series of computer listings is prepared, giving detailed clerical information. These listings help clerical personnel and caseworkers to comply with city, state, and other reporting requirements. For example, clerical personnel receive listings of all children admitted, transferred within the agency, and discharged during each month. Caseworkers also receive listings of children in their caseloads for whom certain city or state reports are required.

Once each quarter a variety of case-management or other computer reports is prepared. One is the Verbal Child Record Printout, prepared for

CHILD RECORD SYSTEM -- SYSTEMS FLOW CHART

From: Caseworkers
(for new cases
only --
monthly)

From: Clerical
Staff
(monthly)

Foster
Parents

Natural
Parents

Undercare

Intake
Form

Other
Clerical
Information

Notices of
Admissions
Discharges
Transfers

Verbal Child
Record Print-
outs WITH
CHANGES
MARKED

Keypunch
and
Check

Additions
Changes
Deletions

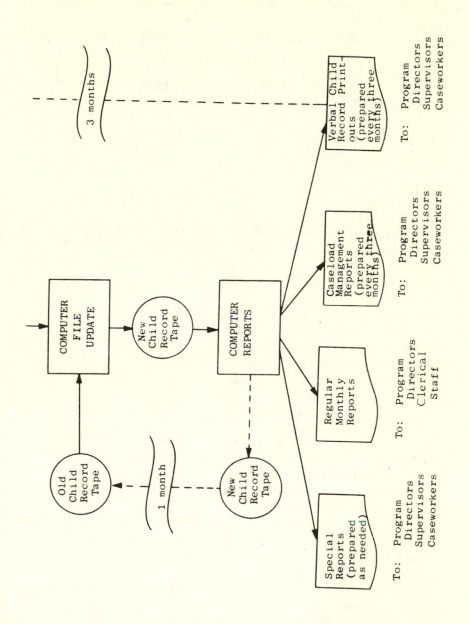

each child in care and sent to the caseworker in a binder containing the printouts for his or her complete caseload. Other reports such as an Analysis of Discharges, an Analysis of Plans To Be Completed in the Following Quarter, and an Analysis of Plans Not Completed on Schedule are also prepared at this time.

During each quarter, the system is used on an as-needed basis to prepare listings and reports in response to special requests, which may come from the administrative, casework or clerical staffs, or from the city or state. In some instances, information from the Child Record System itself is adequate to respond fully to the request. In others, Child Record information is distributed to caseworkers and clerical staff to assist them in preparing the reports.

Updating

Objective case information, such as caseworker changes, foster home changes, and status change, is updated monthly by the clerical staff. Updating of more subjective case information, such as problem appraisal, plan for the child, and service needs, is done quarterly by the caseworker. The caseworker reports any changes in or additions to a child's record by writing directly onto the corresponding Verbal Printout. The printouts are returned by caseworkers shortly before the end of each quarter; changes and additions are keypunched, and updated printouts are returned to caseworkers the first week of the next quarter (see the accompanying Systems Flow Chart).

DATA BASE CONTENT AND REPORT DESIGN

As mentioned earlier, two of the key decisions made in the development of the Child Record System were to accumulate a large data base, and to maintain flexibility in report design. To allow latitude in the creation of the data base, each child's record was designed to consist of about 2000 coded data positions.[6] Currently 1200 of those positions are in use, covering information in each of the following areas: basic identifying characteristics; service needs; recreation; IQ; remediation programs; vocational interests and needs; physical and mental health; adolescent sexual behavior; natural parents; and foster parents.

Additionally, the data base consists of a permanent record and a changeable record. Data known when a child first entered the agency is entered into both records. Thereafter, the changeable record is updated monthly and quarterly, as discussed previously, while the permanent record is left unchanged. This procedure was developed to facilitate computer-based comparisons between a child's characteristics at the point of admittance and at various points in the future.

Flexibility in report design is achieved by means of a computer program called the Report Generator.[7] The Report Generator is activated by three sets of control cards:

• *The scan and select control cards,* which specify the characteristics a child's record must possess in order to be selected for a report;

• *The sort control cards,* which specify the order into which the selected records are to be sorted and the "hierarchy" of the sorted cards; and

• *The verbal control cards,* which specify what information from each selected record is to be printed on the report, the location in which it is to be printed, and if it is to be printed in coded form or not. If an uncoded form is desired, the verbal control cards specify what kinds of verbal designations are to replace the codes. The verbal control cards also determine the report headings to be used.

The flexibility thus created allows administrative and professional staff to develop reports without extensive assistance from computer experts. When interest is expressed in a particular problem or a particular category of child, a clerical person responsible for the operation of the system works with the child care professional to determine the specific information needed. A report format is designed, control cards are keypunched, and the report is prepared.

POTENTIAL OF THE SYSTEM; NEW DIRECTIONS

Owing to the built-in flexibility of the Child Record System, both in terms of report preparation and data base content, the system is constantly changing. Changes are usually in response to an expressed need from the casework or supervisory staff, but occasionally result from modifications in city or state reporting requirements. Additionally, the system has been modified on occasion to accommodate agency accounting functions. Finally, the agency intends to implement a full-scale planning, reporting, and evaluation system.

In sum, the Child Record System has been a useful tool to program directors, supervisors and caseworkers at Edwin Gould Services for Children. It has assisted them in meeting more effectively the needs of their clients, and in evaluating the overall results of their efforts, thereby adding a valuable dimension to the agency's program and service accountability.

NOTES

1. Development funding for this and several other child care information system efforts in New York City was provided by the Edwin Gould Foundation for Children. Potential users of such systems may be interested in two monographs published by the Gould Foundation: *Child Welfare and the Computer: A Projection of Potential,* by Brandt R. Allen and Alexander B. Horniman, 1969; and *Child Welfare and the Computer: Four Years Later,* by Brandt R. Allen and David W. Young, 1973.

2. For a discussion of the system's beginnings, see "Case Costing in Child Care: A Critical Step Toward Increased Accountability in Social Services," by David W. Young, *Child Welfare*, LII, 5 (May 1973).
3. Emphasis on end results is generally lacking in the New York City child care system. This is in no small way a result of the city's system of reimbursement to voluntary child care agencies for services delivered. The reimbursement system financially penalizes an agency that discharges a child from care. See *Examination of New York City Child Care Reimbursement System*, by Brandt R. Allen et al., the 1971–1972 Prize Cases, Public Policy Program, John F. Kennedy School of Government, Harvard University, February 1972.
4. Work is under way in the agency to develop a more sophisticated evaluation system focusing on the relationship among goals, subgoals and service needs.
5. Caseworkers point out that time spent on forms cannot be spent with clients. An agency must recognize this "trade off."
6. Each record consists of 26 data cards with 80 columns per card, for a total of 2080 data positions. Card input is utilized so that system maintenance and operation does not require a computer professional. Once the cards have been read by the computer (the agency rents time—about 2 hours per month—on an IBM 360 Model 30), they are processed by a combination of magnetic tape and disk.
7. The early conceptual and design work for this computer system was performed by Thomas T. Goldsmith and James E. Hirst, management consultants to Edwin Gould Services.

Part VIII

ORGANIZATIONAL CONFLICT AND CHANGE

Social service organizations, like all organizations, are dynamic, evolving social systems, composed of interrelated units concerned chiefly with the attainment of specific goals. Organizational life tends to be characterized in part by pervasive processes of conflict and change, some planned, some unplanned. Among the major functions of administrators is their role in the management of these processes.

Change in organizations is endemic, propelled by both internal and external pressures. Social agencies inevitably respond to the impact of changing social circumstances which define new social needs and new client potentials growing out of the new or elaborated social problems to which their goals are directed. Such factors as demographic shifts, technological developments, developing social pathologies, and structural inequities, among others, create an agenda for social response that calls for organizational adaptation and innovation. Since the sociocultural, political, and technological environment of social practice constantly undergoes modification, both social planning and intervention are pressed to respond in novel ways. They create an ethos and ambience for social development, and determine the ebb and flow of policy, resource allocation, and program development.

As social agencies respond to new social tasks and incorporate new technologies, they move from one steady state to another, and in the process tend to upset an established equilibrium. Any disruption of the reward system, organizational "turf," status, or power tends to lead to resistance and frequently to conflict. The interdependence of change and conflict has often been noted in the literature, and this interrelation is reciprocal—change leads to conflict, and conflict often powers the change process.

The many and diverse constituencies of the social agency project a multiplicity of interests and needs that are sometimes contradictory and sometimes antagonistic. Conflict between and among these interest groups creates a force field within which administrators function. It is their responsibility so to manage these conflicts that the service goals will not be compromised, and the organization's strength will not be impaired. Administrators are well advised to anticipate conflicts within the staff, between staff and trustees, within the board, and between their organizations and others upon which they depend and with which they interact.

The literature on planned organizational change and the conception of social practitioners as change agents is substantial.[1] The rhetoric of change is even more pervasive. Experience suggests, however, that engineering change in organizations is extremely difficult. Constraints even on executive authority need to be recognized. Change and conflict require political insight, that is to say, they must be viewed in terms of the dynamics of power and influence. Perhaps the appropriate metaphor would suggest the "power steering" function of the administrator.

The selections which follow analyze relevant concepts that inhere in these processes of conflict and change, providing clues for the development of strategies for their management. Slavin reviews the potential values and functions served by conflict, identifies a series of key concepts essential for its understanding, and catalogues four sets of strategies available to practitioners in responding to conflict situations. He develops a typology which suggests the essential conditions under which one or another response is appropriate. The key here is the relationship between goals and strategies. Varying degrees of goal congruence between conflicting parties are paired with specific action models to provide a good "fit."

Patti focuses attention on the efforts of lower participants in organizations to initiate and sustain change where resistance is likely to come from organization members located in higher positions in the hierarchy. This is the obverse of the problem where those invested with organizational authority find resistance from below to their initiatives for innovation and change. While not specifically dealing with the question, Patti implies that varying obstacles stand in the way of planned change depending on the point of entry of change-directed activities. Change action can originate externally to the organization, say, from funding sources or public interest groups, or internally, from lower, middle, or higher participants. In each instance, tactics and strategies for effective implementation differ. Patti makes the point that where lower participants engage in change efforts, a set of variables determines the nature of the resistance they can expect from above. These analytical elements provide clues to the identification of various response patterns likely to be effective. Organizational resistance to change may be a universal institutional characteristic. The extent of that resistance and its organizational location will, however, tend to vary depending upon the specific relation of forces in time and space. Intervention strategy depends on such an assessment if it is to be appropriately responsive to the specific tasks at hand.

Brager puts the spotlight on political considerations in organizational change. He contrasts the social practitioner's role in helping clients and in attempting to influence organizations to humanize their services. In pursuing the latter objectives, activities need to be directed at such processes as coalition building, political trading, identifying and dealing with resistance, resource mobilization, establishing goal and value linkages, interest tending, and management of stress. Brager sees these organizational behaviors as an essential part of professional skill, entailing both method and substance. They involve both diagnostic understanding of organizational dynamics and problem-solving technology directed to organizational innovation and change.

NOTE

1. For a recent compilation, see Thomas, John M., and Bennis, Warren G., eds., *Management of Change and Conflict* (Baltimore, Md.: Penguin Books, 1972).

43/CONCEPTS OF SOCIAL CONFLICT: USE IN SOCIAL WORK CURRICULUM

SIMON SLAVIN

The current social turbulence in the nation, affecting, as it does, some of its most central institutions, and not least of all the universities, underscores the significance of conflict processes for the development of social practice and social policies. Few aspects of social work practice unfold without evidence of conflict, competition, or rivalry between individuals, groups, organizations, and/or institutions. Such conflict is pervasive in community life. Its very universality suggests that conflict is a property of social organization.[1] Quincy Wright, a careful student of the subject, suggests that "conflict in some form . . . is probably an essential and desirable element of human society." A society cannot exist without competition and conflict."[2]

While little empirical evidence is recorded on the subject, one has the impression that social workers frequently find themselves involved in interpersonal and intraorganizational disputes, that social agencies are frequently in competition and conflict with one another, and that social agency participants and adherents are frequently pitted against other institutions in the community, competing for scarce resources and attempting, through a variety of patterns of organization and action, to affect changes in their modes of operation and service delivery. One might have expected that this general circumstance would have led the profession to a careful study of the processes of social conflict and, consequently, to the development of insight and skill in dealing with them. In fact, little has been done in this field. This paper is a modest contribution to this lacuna in professional development. It will suggest a number of concepts central to an understanding of social conflict and to its management, and will review briefly a suggested typology of conflict strategy. The underlying assumption here is that some range of conflict concepts is essential for a well-designed social work curriculum, and, while most of these ideas seem especially relevant for community organizing work, its very pervasiveness in organizations suggests similar relevance for all aspects of social work practice.

The current study of conflict is advanced by the realization that "all conflicts have common elements and general patterns."[3] Considerable effort has recently gone into conflict analysis as a consequence of the imperative need to deal with problems growing out of the international threat of nuclear war. The conjunction in time of the civil rights revolution and the weaponry revolution has raised the interest in conflict and conflict control or management to a new high level.

SOCIAL CHANGE AND CONFLICT

Perhaps no relationship is more central to conflict than that of change. According to LaPiere, "Any change always involves considerable stress both individual and collective . . . in the process of being accomplished, the change produces its own stress and strains—discontents, frustrations, discussions and disappointments."[4] The extent to which change touches deeply felt values or interests is the extent to which it is likely to lead to overt conflict. The rate of change also has its consequences for conflict. The more rapid the rate of change, the more likely it is to upset existing social relationships and the more likely it is that conflict will result.

Social change implies a movement away from the *status quo*, a shift in the norms and relationships that compose the social equilibrium at any specific point in time. Such an equilibrium in a social system satisfies certain interest groups and, conversely, has a negative impact on other groups and individuals. Those who benefit from the existing arrangements resent change and tend to resist its manifestations. Thus, change tends to breed conflict between interest groups because it challenges the conventional basis of reward distribution. Under certain conditions, these strivings lead to organized conflict. The greater the disparity, the greater the likelihood that individual dissatisfaction and perception of inequality will assume collective forms.

Conflict and change have a reciprocal relationship—each is both source and product of the other. Change leads to conflict and conflict to change. These are natural processes characteristic of social systems.[5] Within certain limits, some aspects of these processes can be moulded and directed through deliberate social action.

The central purpose for focusing on conflict is to develop diagnostic insight into conflict elements and processes and to provide principles that can serve as a guide to change agent activities. These should make it possible to plan ways of maximizing the creative and productive function of conflict.

THE NATURE OF CONFLICT

Kurt Singer has defined conflict as "a critical state of tension occasioned by the presence of mutually incompatible tendencies within an organismic whole, the functional continuity or structural integrity of which is thereby threatened."[6] In a similar vein, Boulding suggests that "conflict may be defined as a situation of competition in which the parties are aware of the in-compatibility of the potential future positions and in which each party wishes to occupy a position that is incompatible with the wishes of the other."[7] It is the perception of the existence of the incompatible prefer-ences, the mutual desire to achieve these preferences, and the behavior ex-pended in the direction of gaining such positions that essentially charac-terize a state of conflict. The sheer existence of contradictory positions and preferences may constitute competition, rivalry, or hostility, but not neces-sarily conflict. Competition is a concurrent striving by social entities for scarce objects, while conflict implies antagonistic struggle directed against one another. The chief objective in competition is the scarce object. In conflict it is injury, destruction, or defeat of an opponent.[8]

THE POSITIVE FUNCTIONS OF CONFLICT

That conflict can be destructive is part of conventional wisdom and com-mon sense. It is increasingly recognized, however, that conflict can also be functional for individual, group, and societal welfare. A fairly substantial literature has now appeared that points to the ways in which conflict has integrative and beneficent consequences for group and community life.[9]

Perhaps the most thoroughgoing significance of conflict grows out of the ways in which it places issues and problems on the community's agenda, calling attention in dramatic and often irresistible ways to social circum-stances that require change action. When the normal procedures of com-munity decision-making are nonresponsive to imperative social need, con-flict forces a facing of social issues and, in so doing, makes possible their attempted resolution. The absence of conflict under conditions of social disadvantage is often expressive of inertia, complacency, or deliberate in-action that permits the continuation of exploitative social relations in the community. Even the threat of conflict often results in responsive action.

Once conflict has broken out, the very process whereby parties contend with one another has the effect of sharpening interest and compelling thought about the issues at stake, of advancing and defending alterna-tives,[10] of distinguishing divergent points of view,[11] and of deepening analy-sis. Mutual challenge requires probing into the implications of opposing viewpoints. What appears simple and uncomplicated may, in fact, assume multiple and complex dimensions calling for further examination and clarification. Implicit in social conflict behavior is a form of reality testing not unlike that which takes place in therapy groups where, according to Frank, "the occasion of conflict is seen as a means of evoking and clarifying the distortions and neurotic attitudes which are highlighted by the strug-gle, whether it is resolved or not."[12]

Conflict is essentially an expression of a relationship between social en-tities that often mirrors unequal access to scarce objects that are socially valued. Such relationships often represent differential status positions. Conflict can have the effect of restructuring relations between groups,[13] without conflict, group accommodation can result in subordination.[14] Intergroup struggle compels recognition of group interest and group integrity, and, if pursued with strength and persistence, of group demands. Minorities find a place in the arena of competing interests and decision-making when they assert their collective will in opposition to those they perceive as responsible for maintaining the *status quo*. In this process, the locus of power is laid bare, making possible a real confrontation between true contenders. Much community power is latent and camouflaged and operates through intermediary agents, formal and informal. When conflict is sufficiently intense, the real wielders of power are likely to be revealed. Negotiation can then take place with people in a position to make real commitments.

Neighborhood residents perceived as alienated and apathetic move into action whenever there is a threat of displacement as a result of urban renewal, highway construction, slum clearance, and the like. Their engagement in the conflict to keep their homes mobilizes energies and creates group identity and collective awareness that effectively dispels isolation and anomie. Negroes involved in the civil rights movement and in struggles for local control give evidence of community participation and involvement that defy stereotypes of apathy and detachment.

The role of conflict in moving organizations to creative effort has been frequently noted. Thus Katz suggests that "organizations without internal conflict are on their way to dissolution. A system with differentiated substructures has conflict built into it by virtue of its differentiated subsystems. If it moves toward complete harmony, it moves toward homogeneity and random distribution of all its elements. Entropy takes over."[15] Conflict, on the other hand, both "within and between bureaucratic structures provides means for avoiding the ossification and ritualism which threaten their form of organization."[16] Challenge engenders response and stimulates the search for new and better ways of doing things. Its absence tends to lead to complacency and acceptance of inbred habits of thought and action.

Finally, there is some recognition that conflict leading to violence may also be functional for society. While violence, with its destructive potentials, is generally considered to be antithetical to democratic processes, under certain conditions it serves to mobilize indifferent or callous authority in the direction of positive social change that modifies oppressive or exploitative social practices. Thus, prison riots often lead to institutional reforms; violent racial conflicts can lead to legislative reform and social policy development. There is, of course, always the possibility that violence may bring more repressive counter-violence. The context and environment of violence, the nature of predisposing issues and events, the strength, political and otherwise, of the parties involved, the degree, nature, and intensity of the violence behavior, all define whether one or another consequence is likely to be forthcoming. A clue to the diagnostic value of violence is suggested by Nieburg: "Demonstrations of domestic violence serve to establish the intensity of commitment of members of the political system."[17] Low commitments either in scope or intensity have less meaning for challenge to the *status quo*. High commitments may be ultimately irrepressible. Violence tends to point to weaknesses in a social or organizational system, and hence suggests modifications that may help establish new equilibria. "The risk of violence," Nieburg states, "is necessary and useful in preserving natural societies."[18]

KEY CONCEPTS IN CONFLICT

There are a number of elements that inhere in any conflict situation and that provide a conceptual basis for conflict analysis. They include parties, issues, power, goals, boundaries, alliances, equity, and strategies of conflict management. Each is reviewed briefly in the next section.

Parties

Conflict, which depends upon incompatible preferences, implies at least two polar aggregates, each seeking to achieve its preferences in the face of a challenge by the other. Parties to a conflict can be individuals, groups, and/or organizations, theoretically suggesting nine possible types of conflict. At one end there are conflicts between individuals and at the other, between organizations.

Conflicts between individuals may have their sources in incompatible personality needs, in differing reference group identity, or in contrasting ideological beliefs and sentiments. Planned actions to deal with individual conflict will inevitably be influenced by diagnostic judgments thus made. Individual conflict is often expressive of group or organizational conflict, and may become an important source of collective conflict as others rally to an individual's cause in controversy and as existing organizations recognize their inherent interest in the fate of individuals mobilized by such interest.

Conflicts that grow out of group differences, such as are characterized by ethnic minorities, labor, religious adherents, and the like, tend to heighten group consciousness and to assume organizational forms.[19]

Perhaps the most significant conflicts in community life are those in which organizations are the parties involved. Such conflicts take place both within and between organizations. The larger an organization, the greater the likelihood of differing sentiments and values among its members. Lines of communication and control tend to be more tenuous as distance increases between rank-and-file participants and successive levels of authority, making organizational compliance more difficult. Subgroups, cliques, and friendship clusters tend to form and become potential sources of organizational deviance. When sub-group sentiments are perceived to be violated by the organization's policies and practices, intra-organizational conflict tends to occur.

Another source of internal conflict grows out of the organizational structure that differentiates member roles. Such differentiation tends to establish conflicting interests on the part of members who occupy diverse organizational roles. Higher participants who constitute the organization's leadership do not necessarily have the same structural interests as lower participants, even if they share the same ideals, goals, sentiments, and values. For example, rank-and-file trade union members are chiefly concerned with the benefits they derive from union membership, such as wages, hours, fringe benefits, and the like. Union leaders may be more interested in considerations of union security and stability, as well as *their* benefits, which take the form of salaries, perquisites, and power. Higher salaries for union executives may require higher dues payments from members. In this connection, one might note that unions frequently discourage, and even actively oppose, unionizing efforts among their own employees.

The more successful an organization becomes, the more it tends to establish a system of vested interests among its higher participants. Organizations tend to be preoccupied with their own maintenance needs as they deal with the problem of organizational survival and growth. For members of an organization's secretariat, such maintenance concerns tend to have a direct personal reference. For them, the organization may mean employment, status, and power, in addition to ideology or sentiment. The possibility of organization becoming an end in itself for such role incumbents potentially places them in opposition to other role participants. Thus, organizations frequently are the arenas for disaffection and revolt of members against leaders, stockholders against corporation executives, young Turks against entrenched bureaucrats.

Conflicts between organizations grow out of competition for like or scarce resources. These may be finances, leadership, friends, adherents, public attention, etc. Such conflicts are greatest where resources are relatively fixed, so that competing moves take on the character of a zero-sum-game—what one organization gets diminishes the "take" of the other. For example, welfare organizations frequently tend to appeal to the same set of voluntary foundations for funds, to the pool of community leaders for their attachments, and to the same central source of distribution of centrally gathered funds.

Interorganizational conflicts often take on intraorganizational forms simultaneously. This is a consequence of either differing values or divergent interests between higher and lower participants. The goals promulgated by constituent parts of an organization may not only differ, but may also find points of linkage with similar segments of competing organizations. Thus, the common structural characteristics of the leadership core of two organizations in conflict may lead to common aims that override their differences. Collective bargaining negotiations between the union officialdom and the employer representatives frequently lead to implicit understandings that take precedence over the common strivings of union members and their official representatives. At a certain point, particularly where stalemate appears, in achieving a settlement the interests of the higher participants of one party (union officials) frequently are more congruent with the interests of their counterparts of the second party (employer representatives) than with those of their lower participants (union members). Situations such as these lead to charges by lower participants of "selling out" to the enemy or of "betraying the members." They tend characteristically to lead to the employment of secret negotiations prior to or at the same time that official talks are being held.

Such secret dealings frequently involve third or fourth parties who are free to reformulate positions taken by the competing organizations or to develop entirely new lines of inquiry. Secret dealings tend also to lead to the use of "spies" to ferret out secrecy moves, to the public issuance of rumors concerning parallel moves made by the parties, or reports of secret "deals" made.

Issues

Parties are generally joined in conflict with respect to some substantive matter that has significance and meaning to the contestants. The degree to which there is a potential investment of feeling or an attachment of significance to these issues has an important bearing on how intense a particular conflict is likely to be and the ways in which it can be effectively handled. Conflict issues involve events that have divergent consequences for people affected by them. These frequently arise out of divergent interests among social units located in a competitive or conflict field. Interests are goals and objects that have salience for individuals, groups, or organizations and, when perceived and understood, tend to provide direction to their actions. Such interests may be material (they have economic or political value), psychological (they confer status or grant control and power), or structural (they grow out of different locations in social structures or organizations). Assessing the interests that motivate members of opposing parties can be a difficult task, since actions that promote interests are not always expressive of them on the surface. Much of the rhetoric of conflict is carefully designed to hide the underlying motivations and to demonstrate ways in which stated positions accord with conventional and idealistic sentiments. The task of the practitioner often is to help reveal the latent content of observed behavior of opponents and, at the same time, make manifest the actual, if unperceived, interest of members of his own system.

Among the most difficult and intractable conflicts are those that grow out of differing and conflicting values and beliefs. Groups with strong ideological roots tend to develop attachments of intensity on the part of their adherents. They tend also to be uncompromising as a way of insuring their purity, continuity, or growth. Maintenance of rigid group boundaries and the administration of more or less rigid criteria of belief commitments tend to characterize such groups. Most, if not all, social conflict contains an element of value incompatibility. The extent to which such differences lie at the base of a particular conflict depends in part on value ordering. Strong value orderings inhere in organizations whose goals are defined by strong ideological or religious commitments. Political organizations that are ideologically rooted similarly have strong value orderings and tend to be involved in sharp conflicts with opposing groups professing contradictory or competing values.

Whether an organization with strong value orderings will tend to be more or less uncompromising in a conflict situation will depend on: (1) the degree of internal cohesion, (2) the degree of centralization of internal organizational control, and (3) the degree and exclusiveness of commitments to group or organizational values.[20] Where these elements are positive and extensive, organizations will be ready for conflict that is intense and of substantial duration. They will respond to challenge quickly and will tend to initiate conflict where they perceive possible invasion of their rights or preserves.

The social work practitioner works in a complex value field where the values of his profession, his employing agency, his client system, the community at large, and his own value preferences frequently diverge, even if they do not assume outright conflict forms. In his contact with other professionals and other agencies, he frequently comes up against the same value barriers.

It is highly likely that some aspect of value or interest divergence can be identified in all conflict situations.[21] The more strong value elements conflicts have, the greater the difficulty one can expect in dealing with them. Similarly, the greater the vested interest at stake, the more tenacious and uncompromising parties tend to be.

Power Relations

There is general consensus in the literature that power and its distribution is a concept that is central to an understanding of conflict. To some it is *the* core concept that helps explain both the genesis and course of conflict, and it plays a crucial role in defining strategies to be used in its management. Thus North *et al.* state: "It is evident . . . that a conflict is always concerned with a distribution of power. Indeed, an exertion of power is prerequisite to the retention of a share in the determination of future relations—as well as for the acquiring or retaining of other benefits perceived as the 'reasons' for conflict."[22]

In what is perhaps the most ambitious attempt to develop a theory of social conflict, Dahrendorf places central emphasis on the relationship of dominance and subordination that characterizes the structure of authority in associations such as industry, the state, and the church.[23] Authority is defined as legitimate power. For him, the distribution of authority in associations is the ultimate "cause" of the formation of conflict groups.

The power dimension is a variable quantity in conflict relationships. The more fundamental the issue at stake, the more significant power becomes and the higher one reaches into the power hierarchy in the course of struggle. The relative distribution of power not only has an impact on the course of conflict, but becomes itself a value and an interest. In this sense, it is both an instrument and a cause of conflict. The exclusion of some segments of the population from the structure of power creates conditions for collective redress. Their bid to play a part in the processes of community decision-making that affect their circumstances of living serves as a rallying point in the contest that attempts to effect a redistribution of power. The values they assert are democratic insofar as a broader sharing of power advances democratic goals. A restructuring of power is also an interest in the sense that enhanced power, on the part of those who have little, leads to a greater capacity to achieve both latent and manifest interests.

The uses of power in the course of conflict is largely determined by the extent to which contending parties have access to power resources. While power is a property of social systems, it is manifested through persons located in certain segments of the social structure. Where access to such persons and, through them, to organizations in which they wield influence is open, conflict strategy is based in part on reaching them and attempting to attach them to the cause at hand, a phenomenon I call power steering. Differentiation within any strata of power frequently leads to competitive bidding for such support by the parties in conflict. Where, however, access is closed or limited, conflict parties tend to build their own bases of power. This they do through the recruitment of large numbers to the cause and the imaginative use of tactics that mobilize support and release social energy.

Goals

Parties are drawn into conflict with one another because they compete for a limited supply of goods, objects, values, or positions. It is the scarcity of these resources that creates conditions of conflict.

In each conflict there is a potential payoff to the parties. These constitute the conflict goals that bring the parties into contact with one another. It is the very commonality of interest that defines the nature of the conflict. It is important to identify specifically what the conflict goals are and how realistic and salient they are to the involved party. Planned conflict is goal-directed. The goals have an important bearing on the significance of the conflict and the ways in which it is conducted.

There is a significant relationship between intensity and scope on the one hand, and the expected pay-off in planned conflict on the other. Practitioners and participants need to make judgments as to whether there is enough to be gained to warrant the amount of social energy expended in any particular conflict campaign. Small effort for major gains may be totally unrealistic and result in a waste of collective energy. Major effort expenditure that yields little in desired directions can, similarly, have a negative effect on group morale. In general, the more substantial the goals and the greater the stakes, the more intensive must be the planning that goes into developing a conflict effort.

Boundaries

Conflict takes place within a particular field where moves of one party can be made that result in its aggrandizement at the same time that another party is diminished. Thus, there is an "area" occupied by conflict that has a quasi-spacial dimension. The parameters of this conflict space can be determined by the specific resources possession of which is at issue, by the physical area occupied by the parties, by the extent of organizational membership, by claimed jurisdiction, or by the kinds and number of issues that engage the contending parties. Where the boundaries defining the claims, interests, or values of different parties are in dispute, conflict may result. Those who claim rights and responsibilities within their perceived boundaries tend to resist invasion.

The boundary concept is important to the practitioner in helping him match organizational resources to organizational goals in planned conflict. Conflict can become dysfunctional when too much "ground" is covered or when the organizational effort attempts to accomplish too much. To a considerable extent, the intensity of conflict may determine its utility. The absence of conflict or too little conflict may be indicative of the strength of the mechanisms that maintain the equilibrium of the *status quo*. On the other hand, a conflict can go beyond the boundaries of maximum intensity to the disadvantage of the concerned party. This is as true of intraorganizational conflict as it is of interorganizational or community conflict. While conflict within an organization helps maintain its viability and creativity, too much internal conflict can lead to its dismemberment. The stronger an organization and the greater the attachments of its members, the more conflict it can tolerate. There are, however, limits beyond which no organization can contain conflicting elements and survive. Much the same is true of conflict in the community. Conflict tends to create a reactive response. The extent of the response is determined by the nature of the challenge and by the strength and will of the opposing parties. Too much planned conflict can stimulate overwhelming counter-reaction and result in negative rather than positive consequences. One of the persistent problems in planned conflict grows out of the unplanned and often undisciplined attachment of segments of the community that can result in unanticipated mass behavior.

Alliances

Social conflicts frequently involve more than two prime parties. Other individuals, groups, or organizations may feel a stake in the issues under contention. There is a tendency for multiple party conflicts to polarize around one or the other of the major contenders. This is clearly seen in politics and in wars. Political alliances and coalitions are traditionally a part of the political process. This is true in the two-party system as well as in those countries where multiple parties exist. The latter tend to join together several political organizations that are more or less stable and that shift with circumstances. In the former, single parties are themselves composed of coalitions of formal or informal interest groups. There may, in actuality, be a wider range of interests and beliefs *within* each of two opposing political parties than between them. Wars bring together different national states which share some common interests or values in two opposing camps. Effectiveness in conflict in both war and politics often depends on the nature and strength of the alliances formed to do battle.

Conflict groups in the community have a similar interest in knowing and cultivating potential allies and friends. In some instances, they strive to establish formal coalitions. Informal alliances without organizational ties play, perhaps, an even more important role. The ability to sustain a conflict position and to resist attack frequently depends on the extent to which allies are recruited and their support maintained. However, the greater the reliance on coalition members, the more the pressure develops to release part of the objectives of the conflict.

Coalitions and alliances are, in the long run, frequently unstable. Their capacity to sustain cooperative effort depends largely on the degree of perceived congruence of goals. Where goal linkage has short-run dimensions, alliances fall apart when the proximate goals are achieved, or when defeat is apparent. Victory brings into focus the long-range intra-group differences, and sets a new stage for conflict in which new and divisive interests or values appear. Thus the united effort in World War II produced an effective coalition until the point of surrender. Having achieved the immediate common goal—defeat of the Axis powers—the longer-run differences in national aims, interests, and philosophies asserted themselves in new national policies that pitted former enemies against former allies. Victory seems to sow the seeds of its own destruction.

After defeat, coalitions tend also to splinter, each group blaming the other, while frustration and disillusionment tend to reduce group cohesion and the attachments of members to the cause.

Equity

Social conflicts have their own dynamics, form, and structure, irrespective of the nature of the issues that brought them about. They do, however, also deal with substantive matters that have greater or lesser significance for people they involve or affect. Except for unrealistic conflicts that deal with sheer ventilation, there is often an underlying ethical and humanistic base that motivates the constituents of the parties opposing one another. In wars as in social life, a small determined nucleus of high morale and dedication often oppose even seemingly overwhelming forces with considerable effectiveness.

Part of the task of the practitioner is his assessment of where equity lies in the conflict between parties. Most indigenous social movements engage in conflict with forces of superior power and resources. The collective action directed toward constructive social change in the community often takes the form of conflict between power and equity.

Strategies of Conflict Management

Once conflicts have gotten underway they have their own life cycle—beginning, middle, and end. Even the most acrimonious and heated conflict comes to an end with some new circumstance and relationship between the parties. Wars end in treaties, strikes in settlements, unhappy marriages in separation or divorce. The task of the social practitioner—union organizer, civil rights leader, or community organizer—is to help conduct his side of the battle in such a way that positive consequences are maximized and costs minimized.

There are a variety of ways in which conflicts are conducted and brought to some more or less stabilized conclusion. Such modes of resolution bear a relationship to the nature, sources, types, and intensity of specific conflicts. Some lend themselves to certain approaches that would be totally inappropriate in other situations. The use of an inappropriate strategy may well lead to an intensification of hostility and prolonged conflict or to early defeat of one of the parties. A needed area of research lies in the empirical study of conflict types and the strategies of conflict management that are useful and productive in each type. Even the best intention and motivation can lead to a sequence of negative and unanticipated events because the "wrong" strategy was applied, or because it was planned poorly.

Where the dominant element in conflict concerns the struggle for power and control, the use of persuasion and dissemination of information in the hope of developing better human relations can hardly be expected to lead to effective settlement. On the other hand, where the differences between parties are narrow and the common interest readily perceived, severe forms of action—such as attempted suppression of one party by the other—will more likely result in exacerbating the conflict and a disruption of settlement rather than in speedy resolution.

A simplified classification of conflict strategies suggests itself. There are at least four major groupings of approaches to conflict management, within each of which there are a variety of adaptations. At one extreme are orientations that are intended to prevent the outbreak of overt intergroup hostility or to remove the negative consequences of interparty conflict. They attempt to apply rational methods of a problem-solving character to a situation that might otherwise deteriorate. At the other end of the spectrum lie orientations based on the avowed opposition and hostility of the parties that lead to "declarations of war." Here parties lack a common perception of goals, and at least one of the parties thinks it can compel the other to concede or disappear. The situation is one of win-lose confrontation. A middle range of conflict approaches aims at some accommodation or blunting of the demands or positions of the parties. There is no likelihood that the issues can be ignored and no proximate wish to destroy the opposing side. Differences are negotiated and bargaining processes organized. These strategies are based on some minimal degree of common goal perception or community of interests. Here, both parties "win," in a sense, in contrast to the circumstance where one party wins and the other loses.

The general strategies and their adaptations are shown in the following chart:[24]

STRATEGIES OF CONFLICT MANAGEMENT

Integrative	Utilitarian	Negotiative	Coercive
Super-ordinate Solution	Fait Accompli	Direct bargaining	Suppression
	Cooptation	Third party	Radical protest
	Persuasion and	negotiation	Non-violent protest
	dissemination	Conciliation	Violent protest
	of information	Mediation	
	Early containment	Arbitration	

Integrative Strategies. The classic demonstration of integrative problem-solving is found in the intergroup experiments of Sherif and his associates. After creating intense hostility between two groups of boys in a camp setting, Sherif set about the task of dispelling the hostility and antagonistic behavior. The key was found in introducing *superordinate goals* into the relationship between the parties—"goals that are compelling for the groups involved, but cannot be achieved by a single group through its own efforts and resources."[25] This strategy is contingent on the possibility of locating potentialities for such goal linkages and of finding creative ways of directing action toward common ends.

Utilitarian Strategies. A variety of approaches are included in the strategies that I have labeled utilitarian. The *fait accompli*, as described by Gordon Allport, suggests that unpopular or highly controversial changes should be initiated directly, firmly, and without equivocation. "Official policies once established are hard to revoke. They set models that, once accepted, create habits and conditions favorable to their maintenance. . . . Clear cut administrative decisions that brook no further argument are accepted when such decisions are in keeping with the voice of conscience."[26] Where feelings run deep and issues indicate sharp controversy, the *fait accompli* attempts to set action in a potential conflict field before opposing forces have time to mobilize their resources and develop momentum for counterattack.

Much has been written about cooptation as a mechanism for dealing with external threat and securing organizational survival. Selznick, who developed the concept out of his analysis of the TVA, concluded that the "absorption of nucleuses of power into the administrative structure of an organization makes possible the elimination or appeasement of potential sources of opposition."[27] There may, however, be unintended and unanticipated consequences that follow upon the introduction of opposing elements into an organization's decision-making structure. Goals may be muted or modified, as in the case of the TVA, or, if the opposition is powerful enough, it may lead to organizational takeover, resulting in a form of counter-cooptation.

The utility of a stratagem of *early containment* of conflict grows out of Coleman's study of a wide variety of community conflicts. "Social controversy," he concluded, "sets in motion its own dynamics."[28] Once begun, conflicts become elaborated, moving from specific to general issues, then to new and different issues, and, finally, from disagreement to antagonism and personal vilification. Dealing with potential differences at relatively early stages can have the effect of limiting hostile escalation.

In the American ethos of consensus, a natural approach to the management of conflict lies in the attempt to deal with differences through *persuasion and dissemination of information.* Where differences reflect deep attachments to values or interests, persuasion may, however, have little impact. It works best where the level of conflict intensity is low, and where the basis of difference is faulty or blocked communication, or misunderstanding. Persuasive and educational devices can correct misperceptions and distortions, but rarely can they deal effectively with realistic and deeply felt differences.

Negotiative Strategies. The strategic approaches to conflict discussed so far all involve circumstances in which an overall common goal and identity of interest can be built into the conflict field, or where some pattern of action can be organized that has the effect of "sidetracking" or freezing potentially explosive hostility while maintaining the viability of the system in which divergence appears. Another set of procedures lend themselves to situations where these potentials are absent but where some degree of commonality as well as difference can be brought into the perceptual field of the parties to the conflict.

Situations calling for negotiation through bargaining are characterized by a mixture of conflict and mutual dependence that bind parties to one another, yet compel each to contend for a division of resources in accordance with their differing interests. Most "ultimately involve some range of possible outcomes within which each party would rather make a concession than fail to reach agreement at all."[29] In the bargaining process, each party's actions are guided not only by what they think will advance their own position or maximize their payoff, but by what they divine the opposing party's choices and action to be. Party A's behavior depends in substantial part on his expectations of what Party B will do if Party A moves in direction X. But these are reciprocal expectations, where "one must try to guess what the second guesses, the first will guess the second to guess and so on."[30]

Negotiation and bargaining tend to be appropriate stratagems when power relations are relatively equal. In the words of Kirsh: "If collective bargaining is to be a process of private decision-making by the parties, free choice would necessarily presuppose equal power on each side of the bargaining table."[31]

Bargaining works best when it takes place between organized and solidary groups whose leaders reflect the views of their constituents,[32] when a minimum of covert intent can be read into moves made by opposing parties, when parties perceive the importance of coexistence "and act without threatening the survival of the other."[33] The essential mechanism at work is the perception that continued disagreement, antagonism, and overt conflict is more costly to both parties than an agreement that provides for some gain for each.[34]

Coercive Strategies. The final set of strategies in our typology of conflict management deals with situations in which coercion tends to be functionally appropriate. Up to this point we have discussed conflict patterns where a variety of procedures could be employed that relied in some way on a sharing or mutuality of goals even in the face of certain divergent or incompatible expectations. Where parties lack a degree of common reference and goals are mutually exclusive, the resolution of difference depends on an assertion of force or compulsion to gain ends not otherwise achievable. Coercive strategies come into play when other mechanisms have little hope of achieving change. The greater the disparity between projected group images and aspiration and the prevailing state of affairs, the more likely that force will enter the conflict arena. Coercion challenges the *status quo* and threatens interests enhanced by the existing social arrangements. It invariably calls forth counter-action and pressure to destroy or modify protest effectiveness. Thus, coercive approaches are characterized by open confrontation between parties, by more or less intense emotional or ideological investment in group goals, by strong group identity, and by sharp cleavage between organized entities.

A crucial consideration in analyzing such conflicts concerns the extent to which parties are either invested with power, have access to power resources, or are able to locate channels that permit maneuvering within relevant power systems. The presence or absence of accepted and legitimatized power resources predispose parties to the use of variants of coercive strategies. Consideration of the use of coercion in collective action turns on the relationships of conflict parties to goals, power, and commitment.

Coercive action, from one point of view, has as its purpose the creation of a new circumstance in the conflict where other, less drastic approaches become feasible. Aside from suppression and surrender, it serves to bring parties together as a consequence of contestual pressure where they formerly failed to find common cause for settlement. When coercion is effective, it leads to some pattern of accommodation or negotiated agreement, or to some indicated action, such as legislative or administrative enactment, that is responsive to the question at issue. Coercion does not necessarily solve problems, but it can create the conditions under which competing parties can develop shared goals that supercede, in part, the basis for pre-existing hostility. Thus strikes lead to the collective bargaining table, demonstrations to intercommunication and legislative action, school boycotts to new forms of intergroup decision-making, and rent strikes to conferences that propose remedies.

While there are many ways of identifying coercive approaches in community organization and social action, it may be useful to think of the following four types of activity: suppression, radical protest, non-violent protest, and violent protest. These are not necessarily mutually exclusive categories, but are suggestive, and represent differing traditions on the American scene.

A TYPOLOGY OF MODES OF CONFLICT MANAGEMENT

The selection of appropriate strategies in any specific conflict situation is largely based on the degree to which the goals or objectives of the parties are linked. Such goal relationships vary from total convergence to total divergence. The location of goals in this spectrum determines the aptness of particular strategies. Four sets of goal relationships parallel the four strategies suggested above.

When there is mutual identity of goals, they are said to be *superordinate*. Such goal identity can either be implicit in the relationship between the parties, awaiting only a new perception or consciousness, or it can be invented or created through deliberate manipulation of the situation that calls forth creative effort at restructuring the relationship.[35] Where goal differences can be submerged so that the discordant influences of goal conflict can be deflected, inhibited, or suppressed, at least overtly, one can speak of goal *sublimation*. There are many situations in which goal differences and sub-goal mutuality are both operative simultaneously. Parties may seek differing objectives, yet find a common need for identifying shared outcomes so that normative relationships can be established or re-established. Such a mixed goal circumstance indicates some degree of goal *convergence*. Finally, when parties are motivated by clearly opposed goals and seek the imposition of one for the other, we have goal *divergence*.

The combination of four strategies and four sets of goal relationships yields 16 possible relationships between goals and strategies, and can be charted as follows:

STRATEGIES OF CONFLICT MANAGEMENT

Goal Relationships	Integrative	Utilitarian	Negotiative	Coercive
Identity	1	2	3	4
Sublimation	5	6	7	8
Convergence	9	10	11	12
Divergence	13	14	15	16

In practice, the utility of a particular strategy will generally depend on the degree to which it is congruent with the goal circumstance that inheres in the conflict. In the table above, these tend to be located in boxes 1, 6, 11, and 16.

Because the power phenomenon is so central to conflict, it may be useful to speculate about its relationship to the four congruent conflict modes suggested above. In type 1, power may be a negligible ingredient. The identity of ends and the rationality implicit in the methodology of conflict management can override power differences. Problem-solving is likely to be less destructive and to require less energy expenditure than other approaches. In the case of type 6, it is likely that power differences will be modest. Unequal power will tend to seek more assertive methods and be unprepared to pursue anything other than the full fruits of combat. Overwhelming power will tend to lead to coercive strategies and will characterize type 16. When winner can take all, why settle for anything less than total victory? Power weakness on the other hand, which tends to be met by non-recognition or suppression on the part of those in authority, may present few alternatives to coercive action in circumstances where divergent goals have strong salience. Type 11 is best indicated when there is a relative parity of power. Negotiation proceeds most productively when the power of the parties is roughly equal. Parties with superior power tend to ignore or overwhelm the weaker foe rather than cohabit the conference table.

CONCLUSION

This discussion has underscored the importance of social conflict processes for an understanding of planned action for social change. It stressed the positive and creative functions of conflict and suggested a set of concepts that are useful for analyzing conflict situations and in planning conflict action. A proposed typology of conflict management strategies suggests routes for subsequent research that can shed further light on appropriate practitioner and client system response to potential or actual threat or disruption growing out of conflict potential inherent in social and organizational relationships.

NOTES

1. Raymond W. Mack, "The Components of Social Conflict," *Social Problems* Vol. 12, No. 4 (Spring, 1965). "Wherever human beings are found (1) social organization exists, (2) social conflict ensues, and (3) social conflict is, at least to some extent, deprecated" (p. 388). *See also* Ralf Dahrendorf, *Class and Class Conflict in Industrial Society* (Stanford, Calif.: Stanford University Press, 1959), p. 208; and E. E. Schattschneider, *The Semi-Sovereign People* (New York: Rinehart and Winston, 1960), p. 71, "All politics, all leadership and all organization involves the management of conflict."
2. Quincy Wright, "The Nature of Conflict," *The Western Political Quarterly*, Vol. IV (June, 1951), pp. 197–198, 200.
3. Kenneth E. Boulding, *Conflict and Defense* (New York: Harper and Row, 1962), p. 189.
4. Richard T. LaPiere, *Social Change* (New York: McGraw-Hill Book Co., 1965), p. 478.
5. Alvin L. Bertrand, "The Stress Strain Element of Social Systems: A Micro Theory of Conflict and Change," *Social Forces*, Vol. 42, No. 2 (October, 1963).
6. Kurt Singer, "The Resolution of Conflict," *Social Research*, Vol. XVI (1949), p. 230.
7. Boulding, *op. cit.*, p. 5.
8. Raymond W. Mack and Richard C. Snyder, "The Analysis of Social Conflict— Toward an Overview and Synthesis," *The Journal of Conflict Resolution*, Vol. I (June, 1957), p. 218.
9. George Simmel, *Conflict and the Web of Group-Affiliation* (Glencoe, Ill.: The Free Press of Glencoe, 1955); Lewis A. Coser, *The Functions of Social Conflict* (Glencoe, Ill.: The Free Press of Glencoe, 1956); Robert C. North, Howard E. Koch, Jr., and Dina A. Zinnes, "The Integrative Functions of Conflict," *The Journal of Conflict Resolution*, Vol. IV, No. 3 (September, 1969); H. L. Nieburg, "The Uses of Violence," *The Journal of Conflict Resolution*, Vol. VII, No. 1 (March, 1963); Joseph S. Himes, "The Functions of Racial Conflict," *Social Forces*, Vol. 45, No. 1 (September, 1966).
10. Gary W. King, Walter E. Freeman, and Christopher Sower, *Conflict over Schools*

(East Lansing, Mich.: Institute for Community Development, Michigan State University, 1963), p. 35.

11. Lyle E. Schaller, *Community Organization: Conflict and Reconciliation* (New York: Abingdon Press, 1966), p. 77.

12. Jerome D. Frank, "Training and Therapy," in *T-Group Theory and Laboratory Method: Innovation in Re-Education,* Leland P. Bradford, J. R. Gibb, and Kenneth D. Benne, eds. (New York: Wiley and Sons, 1964), p. 450.

13. Dan W. Doddson, "The Creative Role of Conflict in Intergroup Relations," Mimeo, undated, p. 4.

14. Robert C. Sorensen, "The Concept of Conflict in Industrial Sociology," *Social Forces,* Vol. 29, No. 7 (March, 1951), p. 266.

15. Daniel Katz, "Approaches to Managing Conflict," in Robert L. Kahn and Elise Boulding, *Power and Conflict in Organizations* (New York: Basic Books, 1964), p. 114.

16. Lewis A. Coser, "Social Conflict and the Theory of Social Change," *The British Journal of Sociology,* Vol. VIII (September, 1957), p. 200.

17. Nieburg, *op. cit.,* p. 54.

18. *Ibid.,* p. 43.

19. Dahrendorf, *op. cit.,* distinguishes between *"quasi-groups,"* which are "aggregates of incumbents of positions with identical role interests," and interest groups, which have "common modes of behavior" (p. 180). Thus, quasi-groups are the recruiting ground for interest groups. Industrial workers constitute a quasi-group; trade unions, an interest group.

20. Mack and Snyder, *op. cit.,* p. 234.

21. Vilhelm Aubert, "Competition and Dissensus: Two Types of Conflict and Conflict Resolution," *The Journal of Conflict Resolution,* Vol. VII, No. 1 (March, 1963), p. 29.

22. North *et al., op. cit.,* p. 370.

23. Ralf Dahrendorf, "Toward a Theory of Social Conflict," *The Journal of Conflict Resolution,* Vol. II, No. 2 (June, 1958), pp. 177–178.

24. For a somewhat similar general classification, see Herbert A. Shepard, "Responses to Situations of Competition and Conflict," in Robert L. Kahn and Elise Boulding, eds., *Power and Conflict in Organizations* (New York: Basic Books, 1964), p. 33. See also Robert C. North, *et al.,* p. 368; and J. David Singer, "The Political Science of Human Conflict," in Elton B. McNeil, ed., *The Nature of Human Conflict* (Englewood Cliffs, N.J.: Prentice-Hall, 1965), p. 141.

25. Muzafer Sherif, *In Common Predicament* (New York: Houghton Mifflin Co., 1966), p. 88. See also Muzafer Sherif, O. J. Harvey, B. Jack White, William R. Hood, and Carolyn W. Sherif, *Intergroup Conflict and Cooperation: The Robbers Cave Experiment* (Norman, Oklahoma: University of Oklahoma Book Exchange, 1961); Muzafer Sherif, "Superordinate Goals in the Reduction of Intergroup Conflict," *American Journal of Sociology,* Vol. 63 (1958); Muzafer Sherif and Carolyn W. Sherif, *Groups in Harmony and Tension* (New York: Harper and Bros., 1953).

26. Gordon W. Allport, *The Nature of Prejudice* (New York: Doubleday and Co., Anchor Edition, 1958), p. 471.

27. Philip Selznick, *The TVA and the Grass Roots* (New York: Harper and Row, 1966). Cooptation is defined as "the process of absorbing new elements into the leadership or policy-determining structure of an organization as a means of averting threats to its stability or existence" (p. 13).

28. James S. Coleman, *Community Conflict* (Glencoe, Ill.: The Free Press of Glencoe, 1957), p. 17.

29. Thomas C. Shelling, *The Strategy of Conflict* (Cambridge, Mass.: Harvard University Press, 1960), p. 70.

30. *Ibid.*, p. 87.
31. Benjamin S. Kirsh, *Automation and Collective Bargaining* (New York Central Book Co., 1964), p. xi.
32. John A. Fitch, *Social Responsibilities of Organized Labor* (New York: Harper and Row, 1957), p. 40.
33. Herman Lazarus and Joseph P. Goldberg, *The Role of Collective Bargaining in a Democracy* (Washington, D.C.: The Public Affairs Institute, 1949), p. 21.
34. Robert P. Blake, Herbert A. Shepard, and Jane S. Mouton, *Managing Intergroup Conflict in Industry* (Houston, Texas: Gulf Publishing Co., 1964), pp. 76–77.
35. Richard E. Walton, "Two Strategies of Social Change and Their Dilemmas," *The Journal of Applied Behavioral Change*, Vol. 1, No. 2 (April-May-June, 1965), p. 171.

This paper was originally presented at the CSWE Seventeenth Annual Program Meeting held in Cleveland, Ohio, January 21–24, 1969.

44/ORGANIZATIONAL RESISTANCE AND CHANGE: THE VIEW FROM BELOW

RINO J. PATTI

INTRODUCTION

Bureaucratic organizations have come to occupy a position of almost unique disfavor among human service professionals. Recognized by most as a necessary evil, such organizations tend in general to be characterized as sluggish, uncreative, and mired in rules and procedures which prevent the professional from offering the service he would otherwise be able to provide unfettered by these constraints. Bureaucracies are further criticized as being inherently preoccupied with maintenance and self-perpetuation, often to the extent that consumer welfare is sacrificed.[1] It is not my intent to elaborate on this critique except to point out that it has tended to obscure the necessity of analyzing each organization in terms of its receptivity or resistance to innovation. In too many instances, conventional wisdom about "the bureaucracy" has served as a substitute for careful differential assessments of organizations and their varying capacities for change.

In this paper I direct attention to four variables which can provide the internal change agent[2] with a partial framework for analyzing the magnitude and nature of the resistance he will likely encounter in efforts to effect organizational change. The four variables to be discussed are (1) the nature of the change proposal; (2) the value orientation and decision-making style of the decision maker; (3) the administrative distance between the practitioner and the decision maker; and (4) "sunk costs," that is, the investment an organization, or some part thereof, has made in the arrangement the initiator of change intends to alter. In presenting this analytic framework my intent is to provide a practitioner with a tool that may enable him to make a differential assessment of resistance. Such an assessment, as I suggest later in the paper, is crucial to making an informed choice of change objectives and interventional strategies.

In what follows, organizational resistance will be viewed from the perspective of the administrative subordinate who, in a given instance, must obtain the approval of his superior for changes he is proposing. Thus, in this context, the subordinate is any employee, be he administrator, supervisor, direct-service worker, researcher, or program analyst, who is actively attempting to influence decision makers at some point further up in the administrative hierarchy to adopt his plan of action.

For the most part, discussions of organizational resistance tend to view the agency from the top down or, more specifically, from the vantage point of high-level administrators who generally have the authority to institute changes they consider desirable.[3] This is to be expected since these actors carry a major responsibility for initiating and managing change. At the same time this perspective has, at best, limited value for the low-power practitioner because his interest, his information, his experience, and, most certainly, his authority are likely to be distinctly different from those of his counterpart in higher administrative circles.

DEFINITIONS AND ASSUMPTIONS

Before proceeding with an analysis of those variables which have some bearing on resistance to change, it is first necessary to define some terms and state the major assumptions that will be central to the following discussion.

Change will refer to the formal acceptance of a proposed addition, modification, or deletion in administrative policy, program, or procedure by a person, or persons, with authorization to do so. I will not be concerned here with other kinds of changes, often just as important, that occur in the informal system (e.g., interpersonal relationships, communication, distribution of power) and for which no formal decision is required. Nor will I be concerned with modifications in policy, program, or procedure that fall within the authority domain of the practitioner himself. For example, if a caseworker decides to initiate group treatment for certain of his clients, or to modify his own record-keeping system, and has the authority to do so without gaining the formal approval of someone in the hierarchy, we will not consider this a change for our purposes.

Resistance refers to those forces or conditions within the organization that tend to decrease the likelihood that decision makers will accept or act favorably upon a proposal for change initiated by an administrative subordinate. No effort will be made to address the resistance that may arise from a decision maker's judgment that a proposed innovation is not sound or beneficial to the agency or the clientele it serves. Innovations are not inherently desirable, and in any given instance a supervisor may simply reject a new course of action out of a conviction that it will not add to, or may detract from, an agency's service capability. Resistance arising from this source will not be dealt with here.

In what follows, it will be assumed that the practitioner is attempting in good faith to effect change in the organization's policies, programs, or procedures in order that it may be a more effective instrument for the delivery of social services. I will further assume that the change agent is competent and responsible in the performance of his professional role and that his involvement in the change effort is not intended to divert attention from or displace responsibility for his own personal or professional inadequacies. Finally, I will proceed on the assumption that he has conscientiously attempted to formulate his proposal on the basis of the best and most complete information available to him. It is necessary at this point to observe that unless these conditions have been met, the resistance the administrative subordinate encounters may be attributable more to him than to the organization he seeks to change.

THE CHANGE PROPOSAL

Since the range of change proposals made by practitioners may be as diverse as the activities that occur in the field of social welfare, I will attempt to focus this discussion by conceptualizing such efforts in terms of two dimensions: *generality* and *depth*. These dimensions are selected because on the face of it they seem to be critically related to organizational resistance.

Generality refers to the scope or pervasiveness of the proposal; in simple terms, the size of the organizational unit that will be affected by the changes sought. Three levels of generality are proposed here:

1. *Component*—those change efforts that seek modifications in organizational arrangements or operations which have relevance primarily for the change agent or for a small group with whom he interacts on a day-to-day basis (e.g., supervisory unit).

2. *Subsystem*—those change efforts that seek to alter the arrangements

or operations of an entire unit or class of organizational participants (e.g., a department, district office, all caseworkers).

3. *System*—those efforts aimed at changing some aspect of the organization that will have operational implications for its entire membership.

In reality, changes at either of the first two levels of generality are likely to affect the third, but our concern here is not with the eventual ramifications of the change but with its intended, first-order consequences.

The second dimension concerns the *depth* of change that is sought.[4] Again, three levels are suggested:

1. *Procedural*—those proposed changes that seek to alter the rules and procedures guiding the day-to-day behavior of employees who are carrying out the policies or programs of the agency. The goal here is to facilitate the flow of work activities or to utilize resources more efficiently, not to alter the substance or purpose of the services provided. Examples might be improved methods of interdepartmental referral, the development of mechanisms for increased communication and coordination among staff (e.g., interdisciplinary team conferences), or the introduction of new statistical forms to enable an agency to monitor its workload better.

2. *Programmatic*—those innovations aimed at modifying the operating policies or programs carried out by an organization in order to implement its basic purposes and objectives. The focal concern is to substantively alter the services that an agency provides so that it can more effectively accomplish its mission. Changes at this level may take the form of new treatment modalities (e.g., family therapy, behavior modification) or the addition of programs such as day care, job placement, or homemaker services.

3. *Basic*—those efforts that are aimed at changing the core objectives of an agency. The intent is to effect a fundamental shift in the organization's mission so that it will address itself to a different set of problems and outcomes. Examples here might be transforming a character-building agency into one that seeks to correct emotional disturbances in children, or changing a custodial institution into one that is committed to rehabilitation.

When these variables of generality and depth are related to one another a ninefold classification of change proposals emerges. It is my premise that as either the generality or the depth of a proposal increases, the resistance to be expected from organizational decision makers is, all other things being equal, also likely to increase. This is to be anticipated since the more fundamental and far-reaching the proposal, the greater the costs of innovation and the potential for instability are likely to be. Not only must the agency devote a greater than usual share of its resources to establishing new arrangements and behavior patterns, but the period of transition is almost certain to be accompanied by a lessening of the decision maker's ability to predict and control employee behavior and the reactions of external support groups.

VALUE ORIENTATIONS OF DECISION MAKERS

Practitioners in the lower reaches of social welfare bureaucracies may often assume that organizational decision makers will be resistant to proposals emanating from below. Unfortunately, this assumption often serves to deter administrative subordinates who would otherwise promote their ideas for change. A more useful perspective would be to proceed on the premise that superiors vary considerably in their receptivity to innovation, and thus in how they react to proposals for change.[5]

One approach to making such a differential assessment involves an analysis of a decision maker's value orientations. *Values* are defined here as the personal goals held by an official that serve to guide his organizational behavior, especially how he decides issues. They are a reflection of those conditions he believes will produce a sense of self-fulfillment, satisfaction, or accomplishment. The assumption here is that, notwithstanding limits to rationality,[6] a decision maker consciously attempts to choose those courses of action for the organization which are most likely to maximize the prospect of attaining the goals he holds most important. Personal goals are not necessarily self-aggrandizing or selfish in the conventional sense. They may include values that the decision maker perceives as altruistic or in the public good.

The following list of personal goals[7] indicates something of the range of values that may influence decision-making behavior. While all of these goals may be perceived as important, the decision maker is likely to arrange them in a hierarchy so that some are more important in influencing his behavior than others. Thus the attention of the practitioner should be directed not toward the presence or absence of certain values but toward their relative position in the decision maker's goal hierarchy. In other words, while all goals may be operative in some degree, it is likely that some are more consistently salient than others. The goals include:

1. *Power*—authority and control over organizational behavior
2. *Money*—increases in income or income substitutes
3. *Prestige*—respect and approval from those who are responsible for funding the agency, determining promotions, hiring and firing, etc.
4. *Convenience*—avoidance of conditions that will require additional personal efforts
5. *Security*—protection against losses of personal power, prestige, or income
6. *Professional competence*—respect from peers for knowledge, technical proficiency, or professionally ethical behavior
7. *Client service*—achieving maximum program effectiveness and efficiency in the interest of better service to clientele
8. *Ideological commitment*—maintenance of the agency as an instrument of an ideology or philosophical stance[8]

This scheme does not exhaust the range of values that may motivate decision-making behavior, nor does it account for the fact that each proposed innovation may well call into play a somewhat different constellation of personal values from a superior. For example, under ordinary circumstances, if a decision maker places high value on the retention of power but a particular proposal has no implications for his ability to achieve this goal, then another value (e.g., convenience) may become a dominant factor in his consideration. Nevertheless, despite its limitations, the scheme provides the change agent with a point of departure for assessing those goals that are likely to influence the superior's decision on his proposal at a given point in time.

An analysis of literature further suggests that these personal goals are not randomly distributed among decision makers but rather tend to cluster characteristically in certain organizational role types. Brief profiles of each of three modal types—the conserver, the climber, and the professional advocate—are presented to illustrate the relationship between goals and decision-making behavior.[9]

The *conserver* is, as the name implies, largely concerned with maintaining his place and routine in the organization. His primary preoccupation is with security and convenience, that is, with maintaining whatever power, prestige, privilege, and income he now possesses. As one might expect, decision makers who are conservers tend to consider any significant change in the status quo, especially if it affects their domain, anathema. Such officials are often fearful, cautious, and lacking in self-confidence. They are likely to be alienated from the organization and its mission and secretly somewhat pessimistic about the effects of its programs. Cynicism about new efforts or ideas tends to be expressed in terms of failures associated with past similar ventures. Conservers frequently divorce job and social life, concentrating most of their creative energies in the latter arena. Although some administrators may be conservers by personality predisposition, such an orientation tends more often to be a product of longevity in the organization, advanced age, lack of promotional opportunities, and a declining sense of personal efficacy produced by years of frustration and disappointment while fighting the good fight.[10] This is not meant to imply that all officials approaching retirement are conservers but merely that there is a considerable tendency for those who have been in the bureaucracy a long time to develop this orientation.

The decision-making behavior of the conserver, as the preceding profile suggests, will tend to approximate what Gawthrop refers to as a "consolidative" orientation. He defines consolidation as "a deliberate and conscious effort to resolve demands for change regardless of source solely in the context of existing organizational structures, if at all possible."[11]

In contrast to consolidation, innovation (at the other end of the decision-making continuum) represents "a deliberate effort on the part of executive officials to search for improved performance programs, to diagnose organizational weaknesses in advance, and to predict as accurately as possible the consequences of innovative change."[12]

The consolidative bias of the conserver does not mean that such decision makers indiscriminately reject all proposals for change, because to do so would obviously be to court disaster. Rather, consolidative behavior is more likely to be manifested by a failure to seach for, or identify, emergent problems and issues. The conserver tends to be relatively impervious to informational inputs regarding program gaps or deficiencies until such information, through the sheer weight of repetition or wide popular acceptance, takes on the nature of conventional knowledge. Finally, when conditions requiring change are upon the organization and some response is imperative, the change implemented is likely to be incremental and modest.

The *climber*, the second modal type of decision maker, is primarily concerned with acquiring power, position, and prestige.[13] He does this in a number of ways, including assiduously cultivating those in authority who have the power to affect his personal fortunes, taking on responsibilities or functions not previously associated with his job in order to increase the scope of his office, and moving opportunistically from one job to the next in search of more money and status. The climber's apparent commitment to the goals and programs of an organization is, in fact, likely to be an allegiance to the regime in power, whether this regime be the board, legislature, or chief executive. He thus systematically avoids dissenting from or criticizing organizational policies as well as interpersonal conflicts with superiors or important constituents. The climber is not excessively burdened with moral ambiguity or ethical conflicts and tends to resolve such matters as they arise, quickly and decisively. He values action, efficiency, and "getting things done." In short, his concern is with the "how" rather than the "why." It goes without saying that the climber is ambitious, but it is also true that he tends to be energetic and hardworking. The boundaries between work and personal life are extremely permeable, and frequently these dimensions become undifferentiated parts of his existence. The climber tends to become involved in a variety of community activities that bring him high visibility and contact with elites. It is these involvements that frequently provide opportunities for upward mobility.

It is probably most difficult to anticipate the decision-making style of the climber and thus his reaction to a specific proposal for change. In terms of Gawthrop's consolidative-innovative continuum, the climber's decision-making behavior would probably be characterized mainly by its inconsistency. That is, since he relates to his job opportunistically, one would expect him to act similarly regarding change. Accordingly, changes in public sentiment, funding patterns, or the views of important constituents are likely to be reflected in his decision-making behavior almost immediately. The climber's goal hierarchy makes him no more inherently disposed toward one style of decision making than another. If stability and continuity are the currency of the time, then he is most likely to take a consolidative approach. If experimentation is fashionable, then he is likely to encourage and support proposals for change.

There are, however, two factors which over time would seem to constrain the climber's decision-making inconsistency. The first is that the climber, concerned as he is with upward mobility, must establish some kind of track record, a history of accomplishments. Since this is more likely to occur if he is *doing* rather than *not doing* something, we would expect him to be inclined to innovation. It is also probably true that the climber cannot afford an extreme image. He can afford to be tagged neither as timid or unimaginative on the one hand nor as brash and revolutionary on the other. This being the case, one might expect the climber to operate in the middle ranges of the consolidative-innovative continuum but seldom, if ever, and certainly not for long, at one end or the other.

The *professional advocate*[14] does not deny the goals that are characteristic of the climber, particularly with regard to power and prestige. The distinction lies in what each considers instrumental as apart from ultimate values. The climber considers the acquisition of power and prestige of paramount importance; the substance of what he is engaged in, the social goals of the enterprise, are his vehicle. The professional advocate, on the other hand, may acquire prestige, status, and power and may indeed actively seek such resources; their acquisition, however, is likely either to follow from or be used in the service of achieving some organizational objective.

The professional advocate is committed to his organization as an instrument of service. This commitment is more often to an image of what the organization can be and do rather than to what it is and is doing. He is likely to be identified with its goals and policies not because, as is true with conservers and climbers, this protects or advances some personal interest, but rather because it most closely approximates his professional ideals. The word "approximates" is crucial here because the advocate is seldom satisfied with what his organization is accomplishing and is likely to be its most severe critic. However, his displeasure does not ordinarily take the form of cynicism but is rather more likely to be expressed as a continual search for new approaches, personnel with fresh ideas, additional funds, enlarged jurisdiction, etc. His dissatisfaction with what is leads him to experiment. Critical, ambitious, and sometimes even imperialistic, the advocate often finds himself in conflict not only with members of his own staff but with executives of other agencies and even, on occasion, his own board. His relations with those in authority stand in sharp contrast to the climber's. While the latter is likely to celebrate authority figures and defer to them on substantive issues, the advocate sees them as resources to be persuaded and enlisted in the cause of enhancing his organization's effectiveness.

Given this portrait of the professional advocate, one would expect his decision-making behavior to be strongly oriented toward innovation. This is likely to be reflected in a relatively high investment in searching the environment (both internal and external) for incipient or emerging trends, issues and problems, feedback regarding current program operations, and proposals for change. Since the professional advocate places considerable emphasis on informational input, his capacity to receive unorthodox or unpopular recommendations will probably be somewhat greater than that of either the conserver or the climber, as will be his ability to tolerate the uncertainty and tension involved in receiving and processing such a wide range of stimuli. Concerned as he is with problem solving and goal attainment, the advocate tends not to avoid rather considerable departures from existing policy and program directions, when such departures are in the interest of increased effectiveness. He is prepared, in short, to adopt fundamental and far-reaching changes and to bear the costs of instability and conflict that frequently accrue, if these changes promise an improved capacity for goal attainment.

While the professional advocate has a bias toward innovation, he can also be a staunch defender of the status quo if the changes suggested are contrary to the ideological or philosophical stance he espouses.

In summary, I have suggested in this section that administrative superiors, indeed all organizational actors, tend to behave in ways that will maximize certain personal goals that they consider most important. I have further suggested that a superior's goal hierarchy tends to be reflected in certain modal role orientations, most particularly in approaches to decision making when change is called for. These modal types are seldom observed in their pure form, but my contention is that the practitioner who is attempting to promote an innovation can utilize this typology as a point of departure for analyzing the resistance that he is likely to encounter from decision makers.

ORGANIZATIONAL DISTANCE

Another variable which appears to be crucial in assessing the potential resistance that may be encountered in efforts to change is what might be called *organizational distance*. In this context, organizational distance refers to the number of administrative levels between a subordinate who is making a proposal and the administrative superior who must ultimately decide upon it. All other things being equal, it is suggested that the greater the distance a proposal must traverse, the greater the likelihood that it will meet with resistance at the point of decision. Thus, if this premise is correct, one would expect to have greater success in gaining approval from an immediate superior than from, for instance, an agency executive who is three or four levels higher in the administrative hierarchy.

At the outset it is important to note that my concern is with those processes (forces and conditions) that are natural concomitants of organizational distance. These processes can be augmented or neutralized by the actors in a change scenario, that is, they can be consciously manipulated by subordinates and decision makers to affect the outcome of the change proposal. In the discussion that follows, however, I will focus only on ways in which distance itself can generate resistance to changes initiated by subordinates. Two major aspects are considered here: the processes that affect the substance and relevance of a proposal as it is communicated through one or more intermediaries; and the conditions under which the proposal is considered and decided upon.

The greater the number of intermediaries through which a proposal for change must be communicated, the more vulnerable it becomes to information loss, distortion, and delay.[15] One or more of these may have the effect of altering a proposal's substance or diminishing its timeliness.

First, it is in the nature of multilevel organizations that every subordinate must condense the information he conveys to his superior. Were this not the case, the sheer bulk of information emanating from below would soon grow to unmanageable proportions. The caseworker communicates only a portion (indeed, a small portion) of what he considers relevant information to his superior, who in turn further collapses the information for presentation to his superior. This "winnowing process"[16] occurs at each level and inevitably entails a certain amount of information loss. While proposals (suggestions, recommendations) are less subject to condensation than information bits, here too the pressures of time frequently require that they be simplified or abbreviated in the course of passing through the communication network. As a consequence, it is not at all unusual for a proposal initiated several levels down to be only a skeleton of itself when presented to the decision maker. That this occurs is evidenced by the frequency with which change agents can be heard to complain that their proposal was oversimplified or inadequately represented in the decision-making forum.

In addition to information loss, a proposal for change often becomes distorted as each intermediary inevitably filters it through his own perceptual screen. Values, vested interests, past experiences, feelings toward the practitioner—all these influence the intermediary's perception of what will be favorably or unfavorably received in the upper echelon. A proposal that may incur disfavor from superiors, for example, is often presented with somewhat less enthusiasm and vigor.

There is finally the matter of time. Since the timeliness of the proposal is often as crucial as its substance, delays that occur in the process of communicating across several administrative levels can have a determinate influence on the outcome. Such delays need not be motivated by opposition, although the popularity of phrases like "pigeonholing" and "sitting on" is testimony to the fact that they often are. More pertinent here is that intermediaries often delay transmitting a proposal because their superiors are preoccupied with other matters or overloaded.

Singly or in combination, these processes can have the effect of making a proposal for change less acceptable to decision makers. This need not occur inevitably, but it seems fair to conclude that the greater the number of intermediaries, the greater the likelihood that information loss, distortion, or delay will take its toll on a proposal for change.

Organizational distance would also seem to be important to an assessment of potential resistance insofar as it is related to the conditions under which change proposals are considered and decided upon. First, the further removed a practitioner is from the ultimate decision maker, the more likely it is that their respective organizational perspectives and criteria for decision will differ. The needs, interests, and priorities of incumbents in various echelons do differ, and these differences tend to become more sharply delineated as organizational distance grows. While these varying perspectives need not be in conflict, it frequently happens that they are.

Second, and not unrelated to the point just made, the more distance there is between the change agent and the decision maker, the less opportunity there will be for sustained face-to-face interaction between them. In very practical terms this means less opportunity for the change agent to elaborate, argue, persuade, and compromise. This is perhaps best illustrated by the not unusual experience of being given fifteen minutes on the crowded agenda of an executive staff or board meeting to present a proposal. The constraints of time, unfamiliarity, and differences in language become formidable barriers to a persuasive presentation. Under these circumstances, it is not unusual for the subordinate to feel that he has not adequately represented his recommendations. Contrast this with a proposal made to an immediate supervisor with whom the practitioner has day-to-day interaction: this context permits the actors to explore their respective points of view, probe motivations, develop common referents, and negotiate differences. The obvious point is that the context in which a proposal is made and a decision arrived at is itself an important determinant of the outcome.

Finally, the higher a change agent must go in the administrative hierarchy for decision, the more likely his proposal is to come into competition with the interests of other groups. At each successive level in the administrative hierarchy, the decision maker is confronted with an increasingly complex array of contending interests that must somehow be mediated. For the practitioner, this fact has important ramifications because it means, in effect, that as the array of competing interests becomes more varied and complex, his proposal will be weighed against a set of criteria that go beyond the merits of his proposal. The further removed the initiator of change is from the decision maker, the less likely he is to have the information needed to anticipate or counteract these competing interests.

In summary, then, I am suggesting that the distance between the initiator of change and the decision maker can itself be a crucial determinant of the amount of resistance that a proposal will encounter. There are, of course, ways to counteract or neutralize the consequences of distance, but before these can be developed, the change agent must be aware of their potential for generating resistance.

SUNK COSTS

The variable of *sunk costs*[17] may also constitute the source of resistance to change efforts initiated by administrative subordinates. Sunk costs refer to the investments that have been made by an organization (or its members) to develop and sustain any institutional arrangement or pattern of behavior that is currently in force. Investments are here defined broadly as inputs of money, time, energy, or personal commitment. They might include, for example, the staff time and energy that have been devoted to recruiting, developing, and maintaining foster homes over a period of time, or the funds that have been expended to train workers in a new mode of treatment (e.g., behavior modification). More specifically, sunk costs might be represented in the money that has been spent to remodel and furnish a building so that it can accommodate program activity. An equally important, if more subjective, element of sunk costs is the personal commitments made by members of an organization to an existing arrangement. It might be difficult, for instance, to attach a dollar figure to a social worker's effort to establish interdisciplinary team conferences on a surgical ward, but the worker will surely be able to attest to the energy costs that have been incurred in the process.

This latter aspect of sunk costs is frequently associated with length of employment in an organization.[18] That is, the longer a person has worked in an agency, the more likely he is to have a personal stake in its existent programs, procedures, and objectives. Since this dimension of sunk costs is subjective and often difficult to elicit (who would admit that he is opposed to change?), length of employment can sometimes be used to make an assessment of potential resistance. One way to gain an indication of resistance to innovation in a bureaucracy might be to sum the total number of years of employment for all persons in the department or unit that will be affected by the proposed change, and divide it by the number of employees. The dividend, when compared to those of other departments, may provide one measure of the relative opposition to be expected.[19]

Generally, it would appear that the greater the magnitude of an organization's investment in some arrangement or pattern of behavior, the more likely it is that a change in that arrangement will be resisted. Sunk costs, in other words, generate an organizational bias toward continuity. There are, of course, conditions that serve to counterbalance this bias. If, for example, the benefits gained from an investment have been less than anticipated, or existing arrangements have produced dysfunctional consequences (e.g., unfavorable community reaction, client dissatisfaction, loss of funding), an organization may be willing to write these costs off as a bad investment and strike out on a new course of action. External inducements that promise rewards greater than those currently received can also make it worthwhile for an agency to sacrifice its investments. Nevertheless, where sunk costs are large, organizations are not likely to make such judgments quickly. They are rather more likely to opt for continuity than for change.

IMPLICATIONS FOR CHANGE AGENTS

Assessing potential resistance to a proposal for change does not of necessity predict the fate of that proposal. Indeed, the purpose of being able to anticipate resistance is precisely that the change agent can mobilize resources and conduct interventions in a way that will decrease or neutralize opposition. Thus, it is my position that this kind of analysis is crucial preparation for a low-power subordinate who, with limited resources, wishes to maximize the effect of his efforts.

The action implications which flow from an analysis of resistance are manifold and cannot be fully explored here.[20] For illustrative purposes, however, I will suggest several ways in which the kind of analysis previously developed can inform a practitioner's interventions.

Feasibility
A change agent's ability to achieve a goal is very likely to depend upon whether he chooses a feasible goal in the first place. But how is feasibility assessed? Following Morris and Binstock, we would contend that "if the proposed innovations are resisted by the target organization, the *feasibility* [emphasis added] of the planner's goals is determined by his capacity for overcoming that resistance."[21] An analysis of organizational resistance can be useful in determining feasibility by putting into sharper perspective the resources the change agent will need to achieve approval and implementation of his goals. If the practitioner finds that one or more of the sources of resistance are likely to be operative in the change situation, he is then in a position to appraise whether it is possible to mobilize the resources that will be needed to overcome that opposition. Is it likely, for example, that he will be able to generate sufficient pressure to convince a "conserver" decision maker to adopt a change that requires a major redirection of organizational focus? Can he reasonably expect to convince such a decision maker that his interests (goals) are better served by anticipating change

than by waiting until it is foisted upon the agency? If the conserver approves a proposal, can a staff that is heavily committed to the status quo be expected to implement it?

Answers to questions like these, even when one allows for the vagaries of prediction, can assist the change agent in deciding whether the resources he has, or can likely mobilize, are sufficient to the task at hand. If they are not, he may find it preferable to redefine his goals in terms that are more consistent with the resources he can muster.

Focus of Intervention

An assessment of resistance can also aid the practitioner in determining where to focus his interventions. If he finds, for instance, that the decision maker with a professional-advocate orientation is favorably disposed to a proposed change but declines to give approval because of anticipated adverse effects on the morale or efficiency of staff, then it may be a better use of the subordinate's time and energy to focus his attention on the staff. Efforts to persuade or influence them to accept a proposal may not only free the decision maker to give his approval but insure that the change, once authorized, will be effectively implemented.

In another situation, the change agent may find that the major obstacle to gaining approval for his recommendations is simply his failure to represent his ideas adequately to the decision maker. Here again, he may decide that it is not pressure upon the superior which is indicated so much as efforts to increase the likelihood that his proposal will be given a full hearing. This might be accomplished by cultivating the support of intermediaries in the communication network, dramatizing the proposal to draw the attention of the decision maker, going around the administrative hierarchy directly to the superior, etc. Finally, in those cases where the administrative superior's role orientation and decision-making style resemble those of the "climber," the practitioner may find that a most effective point of leverage is to achieve the support of some community influential who has access to the superior.

Type of Intervention

An assessment of resistance may also enable the practitioner to make a more informed choice of strategy. Let us assume for the moment that an administrative subordinate is proposing a change that is both high in generality and basic in character. Let us further assume that the worst possible combination of resistive forces is at work, that is, a conserver decision maker at some distant point high up in the hierarchy and a staff that has for many years worked at developing and maintaining the agency's programs. Under these circumstances, the change agent who would pursue a consensually oriented strategy, based solely on information giving and rational persuasion, is very probably doomed to fail. A more suitable strategy in this scenario is likely to be one that makes it costly for the organization to pursue its present course, one that assumes fundamental differences between the subordinate and the decision maker, in short, a strategy characterized by aggressiveness, stridency, and coercion. The practitioner may not be inclined to pay or impose the costs that are associated with this approach, but he should not assume that the kind of change he is seeking can be accomplished without this magnitude of commitment.

On the other hand, one who is seeking approval for a modest program or procedural change in a relatively new agency with a professional-advocate executive and a shallow hierarchy is equally misled if he adopts a conflictually oriented strategy. To do so under such circumstances may not only elicit spurious resistance to his proposal but use up personal credit the change agent might wish to call on in future endeavors.

CONCLUSION

This paper has been an effort to translate selected aspects of organizational theory into analytic concepts that can have some practical utility for administrative subordinates who are attempting to promote change in their agencies. The four variables discussed—the nature of the change proposal, the decision maker, organizational distance, and sunk costs—are suggested as analytic focal points for the practitioner who wishes to assess the resistance he is likely to encounter in seeking change. While a certain degree of resistance is to be expected in virtually any proposal for change, the contention of this paper is that it will vary significantly from one situation to another depending upon the particular configuration of variables that obtains. It is further argued that an assessment of the quality and quantity of resistance is crucial if the change agent is to make an informed choice of intervention strategy.

It is important to note that the four variables discussed in this paper are only some of those that will determine an organization's resistance to change. Others that could not be dealt with here, but which require attention, are the nature of an organization's external environment (including its sources of legitimation and funding), its stage of development, and its technology. All of these appear to have some bearing on resistance and should eventually be part of an analytic scheme employed by change agents.

It is my hope that this paper serves simultaneously to provide lowpower change agents with a beginning framework for organizational analysis and to stimulate further inquiry into this crucial aspect of change methodology.

NOTES

1. See, e.g., Robert Presthus, *The Organizational Society* (New York: Random House, Vintage Books, 1962); and Warren G. Bennis, "Beyond Bureaucracy," in *American*

Bureaucracy, ed. Warren G. Bennis (Chicago: Aldine Publishing Co., 1970), pp. 3–16. Critiques more specific to social welfare can be found in Irving Piliaven, "Restructuring the Provision of Social Services," *Social Work* 13 (1968):34–41; and Robert Pruger, "The Good Bureaucrat," *Social Work* 18 (1973):26–32.

2. Hereafter the terms "practitioner" and "administrative subordinate" are used interchangeably with "change agent."

3. See, e.g., Alvin Zander, "Resistance to Change: Its Analysis and Prevention," in *Social Work Administration*, ed. Harry Schatz (New York: Council on Social Work Education, 1970), pp. 253–57; and Paul Lawrence, "How to Deal with Resistance to Change," *Harvard Business Review* 47 (1969):4–13, 166–76.

4. This scheme for classifying depth of change is adopted from Anthony Downs, *Inside Bureaucracy* (Boston: Little, Brown & Co., 1967), pp. 167–68.

5. The empirical evidence on this point is scanty and somewhat inconsistent. Weinberger's analysis of agency executive behavior led him to the conclusion that administrators tend to resist making decisions that involve the reordering of goals or the reallocation of resources (Paul E. Weinberger, "Executive Inertia and the Absence of Program Modification," in *Perspectives on Social Welfare*, ed. Paul E. Weinberger [New York: Macmillan Co., 1969], pp. 387–94). Tangential but apparently supportive evidence is reported by both Epstein and Heffernan, who found agency executives to be conservative in their attitudes toward social change strategies that are likely to have a disequilibrating effect on agency behavior (Irwin Epstein, "Organizational Careers, Professionalization and Social Worker Radicalism," *Social Service Review* 44 [1970]:123–31; Joseph Heffernan, "Political Activity and Social Work Executives," *Social Work* 9 [1964]:18–23). A somewhat different profile of executives' reactions to change emerges from Hanlan's partial replication of Epstein's study. He concludes, e.g., "On the basis of these limited findings, these executives cannot be characterized as a group within the profession who are most resistant to social action strategies," and later, "The study findings reported here, while limited to a small selected sample, provide some challenge to the assumption that these social work executives are co-opted into conservative and non-social action directions by nature of their occupancy of hierarchical positions" (Archie Hanlan, "Social Work Executives. Recent Graduates, and Social Action Strategies," unpublished paper [n.d.], pp. 11, 13). One source of the inconsistency reported in these studies may be the fact that executives, as I suggest here, fall into subgroupings with distinctly different value orientations.

6. In the context of a single decision-making episode, insufficient information, emotional stress, inability to foresee consequences, etc., may prevent the decision maker from rationally choosing, from among the available courses of action, those that will maximize the potential for goal attainment.

7. This is a modification of a list suggested by Downs, pp. 84–85. Goals 6, 7, and 8 are different from those suggested by Downs. The modification is necessary to reflect some of the distinct features of the culture of social work.

8. This goal category refers to those decision makers whose primary goal is to preserve or maintain an agency because of their commitment to some broad principle like the maintenance of ethnic identity or the value of private or volunteer philanthropy. The preservation of the agency becomes a vehicle for promulgating a particular ideology which, in the administrator's view, serves the public interest.

9. This typology was constructed from an analysis of several classification schemes that attempt to relate goals and role orientation to the behavior of organizational officials. While these schemes conceptualize organizational behavior in rather different ways, there are notable areas of agreement and overlap among them (Downs, pp. 88–111; Presthus [n. 1 above], pp. 164–268; Alvin Gouldner, "Cosmopolitans and Locals: Toward an Analysis of Latent Social Roles," *Administrative Science Quarterly* 2

[1957]: 281–306, 444–80; and Leonard Reissman, "A Study of Role Conceptions in Bureaucracy," *Social Forces* 27 [1949]: 305–10). The designations "conserver" and "climber" are borrowed from Downs.

10. See Downs, pp. 96–99.
11. Louis C. Gawthrop, *Bureaucratic Behavior in the Executive Branch: An Analysis of Organizational Change* (New York: Free Press, 1969), p. 181.
12. *Ibid.*, p. 182.
13. Presthus (pp. 164–204) refers to these officials as upward mobiles.
14. The professional advocate shows characteristics of Presthus's "ambivalent" and Gouldner's "cosmopolitan," but differs from both because of his high commitment to the agency.
15. An elaboration of impediments to upward communication in bureaucracies can be found in Daniel Katz and Robert L. Kahn, *The Social Psychology of Organizations* (New York: John Wiley & Sons, 1966), pp. 245–47; and Gordon Tullock, *The Politics of Bureaucracy* (Washington, D.C.: Public Affairs Press, 1965), pp. 137–41.
16. Downs, p. 117.
17. See James G. March and Herbert A. Simon, *Organizations* (New York: John Wiley & Sons, 1966), p. 173; and Downs, pp. 195–96.
18. Jerald Hage and Michael Aiken, *Social Change in Complex Organizations* (New York: Random House, 1970), p. 97. Some functional aspects of personal commitment to organizational arrangements are discussed in Donald Klein, "Some Notes on the Dynamics of Resistance to Change: The Defender Role," in *Concepts for Social Change*, ed. Goodwin Watson (Washington, D.C.: National Training Laboratories, 1967), pp. 26–36.
19. Victor Thompson, *Bureaucracy and Innovation* (University: University of Alabama Press, 1969), pp. 61–88. See this source for suggested approaches to measuring resistance to innovation in complex organizations.
20. A further discussion of factors that should be considered in choosing and planning change strategies can be found in Rino Patti and Herman Resnick, "Changing the Agency from Within," *Social Work* 17 (1972):48–57.
21. Robert Morris and Robert H. Binstock, *Feasible Planning for Social Change* (New York: Columbia University Press, 1966), p. 94.

45/HELPING VS. INFLUENCING:
SOME POLITICAL ELEMENTS
OF ORGANIZATIONAL CHANGE

GEORGE BRAGER

The dehumanization of clients by social welfare organizations is a commonly observed phenomenon.[1] Differences may exist among professionals about how pervasive or limited, how direct or subtle, how crippling or cruel it may be, but that dehumanization occurs, frequently in some service organizations and at times in all of them, is no longer contestable. Nor are there significant disagreements regarding the social work response. Minimally, we are counseled that "the professional's commitment to the social well-being of persons demands the continuous examination of existing policies, programs, and services of institutions."[2] More militantly, it is suggested that the worker is "a partisan in a social conflict and his expertise is available exclusively to serve client (as opposed to agency) interests."[3] But although we have been exhorted regarding the need to humanize the organizations within which most of us work, and have sometimes ourselves led the chorus, little has been written that would directly guide us in practice.[4]

To paraphrase a former presidential nominee, exhortation in the pursuit of a good cause is a virtue, and this paper will not violate the social work "norm of exhortation." It follows in that tradition, for it implicitly urges social workers at whatever level of hierarchy to seek to expand their autonomy and change agency procedures and policies which violate client interests. What is urgently required, however, is a practice technology of organizational innovation,[5] and although we have no pretension that this paper will fulfill that need, it is intended to suggest some considerations and actions which might be useful in gaining autonomy and seeking change. In what follows we note a generally overlooked distinction between the social worker as "helper" and as "influencer," and then focus on three elements in the change process: choosing a problem and its solution, assessing and mobilizing pro-change forces; and finally, assessing and neutralizing the opposition. Essentially, our interest is in the political aspects of the process; that is, those steps required to gain sufficient influence to achieve the desired values or ends.[6]

If practitioners are to avoid either frustration or fantasy, we first need to comment briefly on the constraints in attempting change from within. Whatever truth there is in the accusation by which social workers downgrade one another (i.e., the profession's lack of commitment to social change or its ineptness in the pursuit), the reproaches do tend to overlook inherent limitations. Power derives in large measure from how a society or an organization defines the essentiality of the function of a particular occupational group. By this standard, it is not lack of commitment or ineptitude which limits the influence of social workers, but rather the norms of the society (e.g., to blame the victim for his ills) and the functions of organizations (e.g., when social work is intended to "regulate the victim," or when it is noncritical to organizational purpose). Some measures to counteract these limitations, such as disengagement from the disadvantaged, are not in conscience available to use, and others, such as education or public relations, provide a less easy solution than critics have tended to credit.

Nevertheless, change often occurs in incremental steps, and we believe, with Naomi Gottlieb, that "workers can create oases of independent behavior even within the limitations of a controlling hierarchical institution, permitting somewhat more creative possibilities for themselves."[7] Even if an influence attempt is as small as winning some measure of autonomy for the worker or revising a procedure to aid a single client, it is worthy of professional attention and, therefore, of professional skill.

But this aspect of skill has tended to be neglected or confused in our overriding interest in clinical method. One condition of effectiveness, for example, is to discriminate between the techniques and values which are appropriate to providing personal services from those appropriate to promoting agency responsiveness to clients. Although the principle that different cases require different remedies has wide acceptance, its practice implication in this instance has not often been recognized.

"HELPING" VS. "INFLUENCING"

When we fail to distinguish between methods of "helping" clients and "influencing" agencies, we risk the use of "principles" which may be effective in individualized service but which are ineffective in humanizing bureaucratic structures.[8] There are at least three major differences between "helping" people and "influencing" organizations; they concern: (1) the uses of power; (2) commitment to goals; and (3) worker-"client" relationships.

In providing personal services, the worker is likely to be in a commanding and authoritative position. Thus, one text urges that he increase "his appreciation of how the recipient of his service feels in the less powerful, one-down, and unreciprocating role."[9] Typically, he strives to reduce the inherent inequality between the giver and the receiver of a service. In attempting organizational change, on the other hand, the case is reversed, and the worker may well understand the "one-down" role through experiencing it. His task is not the reduction of his power, but its increase. There is scant organizational impact without the uses of power, and how one may generate and maximize resources for influence is a critical methodological task.

It is generally agreed that "helping" a recipient of service entails a commitment to a process rather than to a specific end, that worker and client jointly engage in problem-solving, and the client is final arbiter of the goal to be sought. (This is appropriate because of the power imbalance mentioned previously, among other reasons.) Although there are ambiguities in the way these principles are applied, they at the least provide guidance for the worker. Conversely, almost by definition, an organizational change attempt entails a commitment to a particularized objective. Furthermore, change pursued by middle and lower hierarchical levels in an organization is ordinarily so difficult, the cards usually stacked so largely against them, and the need for circumspection in the attempt so frequently great, that commitment to a goal—and indeed, zeal in its pursuit—is a necessary if insufficient condition for a successful outcome.

Finally, in "helping," the importance of the relationship between the receiver and the giver of service is central. Concomitant with this emphasis is the worker's obligation to be authentic, to present himself openly and honestly.

The empathetic worker is advantaged in either "helping" or "influencing," and nothing that we will say is intended to minimize the importance of relationship skills in gaining organizational influence. Whether the method of influence is consensual or conflictual, interpersonal ability will be called for, and may at times mark the difference between success and failure. Nevertheless, relationship is not the primary motive force in most organizational change attempts. More important are the resources which can be mustered to mobilize support for the chosen objective. Two resources, to be sure, are personal attractiveness and solidary relations, but these are two among many. Furthermore, other organizational actors may be adversaries, in which case an honest and open presentation of self is only sometimes appropriate. Finally, the primary emphasis in "influencing" is exchange relations. Workers must assume that persons respond in large part from their self- and organizational interest, stemming from their role, function, location in the hierarchy, professional or other reference groups, and the like, and that a salient question is "What's in it for him to do what I want?" Influencing organizational change often entails trading; each party gives something to get something. The worker must thus consider what he has (or has access to) which the other wants (or wants to avoid) badly enough to pay the worker's price. This mode of thinking, which is essentially political, is a requirement of "influencing," and must be cultivated by those who would encourage the humanization of organizations.

In sum, to "influence" organizations rather than to "help" individuals requires committing oneself to a specific objective and action without the aid or corrective of client interaction, much less the sanction of an employing organization. It necessitates that the worker seek to enhance his power, thereby impelling a far different set of techniques, some of which we indicate in the remainder of this paper. And it demands a professionally conscious involvement in the implicit and explicit trading which oils the gears of organizational engines.

CHOOSING THE PROBLEM AND ITS SOLUTION

As with most social processes, initiating organizational change contains both substantive and methodological elements. Some or all of the following steps are likely to be included in the process: the identification and definition of a problem, the formulation of goals, the review of alternative solutions or actions, the assessment and mobilization of resources (that is, the marshalling of pro-change forces and/or neutralizing those opposed), the choice of a feasible alternative which "satisfices" the desired end, and its implementation. These phases are often implicit; they may be interdependent; and while some are primarily substantive and some primarily political, all of them contain a measure of both. For present purposes, we shall restrict ourselves to three political aspects of the process: (1) choosing the problem, goal, and problem solution; (2) assessing and mobilizing the pro-change forces; and (3) assessing and neutralizing the opposition.

It is a truism that some problems are easier to solve, some goals more subject to specification, and some solutions simpler to implement.[10] Thus, the characteristics of proposed innovations make them more or less amenable to adoption.[11] The more obvious the advantage of a problem solution is over current practice, for example, the easier it will be to win support. Similarly, the more likely a solution can be tested on a limited basis, such as in a demonstration program, or the more likely it can be reversed if necessary, the greater its chances of adoption. Chances are also enhanced if the implementation of an innovation requires a lesser use of scarce resources. Conversely, the more radical a problem solution, the more difficult it will be to gain acceptance. Acceptance will also be more difficult when innovations are particularly complex, have a widespread effect on other organizational actors, or require the approval of a number of levels or functional subgroups. The practice implications of these points are apparent. When the worker is able to shape the innovation in the direction predisposing acceptance, he will maximize the possibility of a successful outcome.

The most significant determinant of a successful or failed outcome, however, is whether the innovation is perceived to be consistent with the values, interests, and prior experiences of those who must approve the action, or whether they perceive the problem or solution to be threatening to them. The more consistent with their values, interests, and past experiences, the more acceptable the innovation. The more threatening, the more resistance it will induce. And the greater the resistance, the more power, or resources for influence, which must be brought to bear by those promoting the change.

The point has extensive practice implications. Three will be cited. First, there is the requirement that the worker explore, infer, or know how the problem impinges on the interests of potential decision-makers before he proceeds. There is a risk inherent in this exploration that the worker will reveal his change interests before he has sufficiently prepared for the effort; that is, before he has thought through how the change might best be introduced, by whom, and with what initial support.

A second practice ramification stems from the operative word "perceived"; that is, whether the proposed solution is *perceived* to be consistent with or threatening to the interests of those who must approve the change. Whatever the reality, the views of parties regarding what an action means for them is the crucial determinant of their response. It is their definition of the situation that matters, and definitions are manipulable. One way is to revise the content of a proposal to fit the other's perspective. Another is through the argument used in the proposal's support. A problem may be defined in its most benign and nonthreatening manifestation. For example, the desirability of citizen involvement in agency affairs can legitimately be argued as a self-help mechanism, which is nonthreatening, rather than as a means of increasing consumer influence on policy, which is threatening. Another technique is to refer to the change effort itself as no change or hardly one at all. Organizations avoid new measures in part because of the risk and uncertainty which they generate; this is one of the reasons why, in addition to fashion, pointing to the experience of other agencies in adopting a similar innovation is so often used in promoting a new idea.[12] Thus, if change is viewed as no change, the threat of change is minimized. An example is provided by Henry Street Settlement which, in radically altering its program, developed a policy statement which read in part as follows: "The statement is fully in accord with the history of Henry Street. It selects from that history a particular emphasis and highlights it as a central purpose. . . ."[13] Another means, beyond the mere assertion of the fact of no-change, is to allow a new idea to percolate without pressing for action until the idea hardly seems innovative at all. Thus, leaders of organizations in which vote-taking is required sometimes introduce agenda items for discussion only. After a number of such discussions, the item is presented for a decision. If the participants are not already talked out, they at least cannot maintain that their views did not receive a hearing, and are more likely to accept the inevitability of the item's adoption. The item has, in short, ceased to be an innovation and has become a position to be formally ratified.[14]

There is a final and important practice ramification to be noted. We have suggested that when the perception of a problem is consistent with a target's interests, less power is necessary to effectuate a change; and that when interests are perceived as threatened, the worker's resources for influence must be greater. Since these two factors vary in tandem, effecting change demands minimally that they be brought into balance. Thus, if the worker's resources are insufficiently potent for the problem he seeks to solve, he is faced with one of two alternatives, short of relinquishing the effort entirely. One is to revise his problem, goal, or solution to reduce its threat. This may be done by limiting its scope, "settling for less," or through other techniques such as offering a solution which is more in conformance with the position of important others than he had originally planned.

A second alternative, in attempting to balance power resources and problem solutions, is to seek additional resources through such methods as eliciting support from members of the organization's elite or by mobilizing a coalition of forces. In bringing power and problem into conformance, the worker must thus not only know how his innovation impinges on those whose approval he needs, but also what his own current or potential resources for influence are, the scope and locus of pro-change forces, and the source and basis of potential opposition. It is with this information that he implements his plans for walking the methodological tightrope among the field of conflicting forces which characterize organizations.

ASSESSING AND MOBILIZING PRO-CHANGE FORCES

Lewin's force field analysis has been used by behavioral scientists as a conceptual framework for the study of organizational development and change. Systems, according to Lewin, operate in a given pattern and retain equilibrium as long as a relative balance of forces is maintained.[15] Driving forces (i.e., those that push in a particular direction) are at any single moment offset by restraining forces (i.e., those which retard movement in that direction).[16] For change to occur, there must initially be stress or tension which "unfreezes the system," at which time the forces driving in one direction may be strengthened or added to, or the restraining forces may be reduced or removed, thus establishing a new equilibrium.

Dalton, reviewing a series of empirical studies regarding administratively directed change, notes that initial stress or tension was associated in almost every instance with a successful outcome.[17] Social workers will find little to surprise them in this result. One practice technique, crisis intervention, is based on the understanding that the stress of crisis opens (or in Lewin's words, "unfreezes") a system to new influences. Thus, before initiating change, there must be stress or tension within an organizational system which can be put to the uses of the innovative attempt. Short of that, the worker must create and focus stress from the latent dissatisfactions to which all complex systems are subject. Creating a receptive climate for change through using, highlighting, or focusing stress is thus ordinarily a first step in a change process.

Furthermore, the location of organizational stress will serve as a pointer directing to potential pro-change advocates. The coalitions, or factions, which compose a large organization are more fluid than is generally credited. The finely attuned practitioner will have communication lines into varied factions in order to locate those stresses which signal support (or opposition).

In using Lewin's conception, one theorist refers to levels of knowledge, values, attitudes, and feelings as primary motive forces driving toward or restraining change.[18] The intensity of these attitudes influence their potency as forces to move or resist change, since how or whether people will act in particular circumstances depends on how intensely they feel about the circumstances. Curiously enough, however, willingness to take action is perhaps no more related to strength of feeling about an event than it is to the person's belief that he can effect the outcome of the event. Thus, Mohr, in a study of 29 health organizations, found that motivation to innovate by health officers was four and a half times greater when their resources were high than when they were low.[19]

The attitudes and feelings which impel driving and restraining forces are not separable from the people who hold them. It is the power of the proponents and opponents of an issue which, in our judgment, constitutes the singlemost determinant of the force for and against change. Ultimately, successful innovating depends on the cards the worker and his pro-change allies hold (and how skillfully they play the game) as against the resources (and skills) of those who would resist the change.

There is an extensive literature on the sources of power such as wealth, the backing of solidary groups, etc.,[20] and we will not detail them here. Briefly, however, we note three which are generally available to middle and lower ranking staff. The first is expertise. Expertise is a more or less compelling resource depending on the organization's need for it and its availability in the marketplace. Wax notes, for example, that in a multifunctional setting "the more (important) social service becomes to the people with the greatest power . . . the more power social service commands by virtue of its control of a scarce . . . resource."[21] A second resource for influence is access to information, and a closely related attribute, control of communication. When staff possesses the information needed on which to base a wide variety of policy issues, it is in a position to influence the direction of those decisions. Furthermore, as the link between administration and service users, staff may indirectly affect agency program and policy by how it interprets agency authority to the consumers of service or selects client communications to report to upper level staff. And if upper level ranks *need* the information of staff to perform their tasks creditably, this may contribute to their dependence on the lower ranking information-

holders, which in turn subjects them to the others' influence. A third resource is personal attractiveness. As persons are seen as attractive, the social
rewards which they have to dispense, such as gratitude, approval, and recognition, become more valued currency. Not only may upper-ranking members trade policy concessions for social rewards, but personal attractiveness
is useful in gaining peer participation in developing coalitions to promote
issues of mutual interest. Thus, personal attraction, or informal leadership,
or access to it, provides a potentially important contribution to the coming
together of a pro-change alliance.[22] Indeed, it is the forging of such an alliance, either informally (e.g., in a caucus or through a grapevine) or formally structured (e.g., in a duly constituted committee) that pro-change
conception is mobilized into a pro-change process.

ASSESSING AND NEUTRALIZING
THE ANTI-CHANGE FORCES

How the innovator handles potential opposition is a critical element in attempting change. For one thing, a problem solution which does not create
significant resistance obviously requires fewer resources and lesser influence-
mobilization than one which does. Even latent opposition which can be
kept quiescent or unorganized is hardly opposition at all. Sometimes workers, in their zeal to stir potential supporters to action, overlook the fact
that activism can also arouse a dormant but stronger opposition force. Second, people tend to communicate with others of similar interest and persuasion, and are thus less in touch with opposition positions and persons.
Studies indicate that outside groups are undervalued in comparison to
one's own and that in competitive situations they are undervalued even
more.[23] Thus, there is the danger that the potential opposition may be unknown, ignored, or, what may be worse, underestimated.

There are four factors regarding anti-change forces which are directly
pertinent to practitioner intervention. They are: (1) the bases or grounds
on which change may be resisted; (2) the organizational actors who might
oppose the efforts and with what resources for influence; (3) the countervailing interests of the anti-change advocates; and (4) the intensity of the
opposition.

We have mentioned that organizations—and more importantly for our
purpose, subunits of organizations—strive to limit uncertainty. This is a
major reason for what appears to be organizational imperialism, i.e., the
encroachment on the goals, functions, and tasks of other groups. In broadening the boundaries of its domain the organization seeks to limit dependence on its environment, particularly in areas of undependability or unpredictability.[24] By incorporating tasks subsidiary to its core practice but which
contribute to its mission, the organization wins greater control over its
process and overall operations. This helps to explain why family agencies,

for example, would generally prefer to operate their own homemaker service rather than call on a centralized homemaker program available similarly to all of the agencies in a community.

Subunits within organizations are responsible for different goals and task accomplishments as well.[25] They too strive to reduce uncertainty, though their encroachment is likely to be internally directed against other subunits. This, we would argue, is an inevitable dynamic of the structure of complex organizations. So too is the competition between subunits in relation to resource allocation whether, as in a university, it is over the finite number of student-customers or course offerings, or, as in a social agency, over the funds or personnel for one particular service as opposed to another. It is this dynamic which is responsible for many attempts to change organizations. And for the resistance to change as well.

We are suggesting, in other words, that potent anti-change forces are generated by proposals which challenge or appear to challenge a subunit's current share of organizational autonomy or scarce resource. Just as subunits struggle to expand or protect their "turf" from incursion, so too do individuals within subunits—and on much the same grounds. Individuals guard the privileges and satisfactions accruing from their roles and statuses. Innovations which, even inferentially, dispute their expertise, expose their actions to question or criticism, create ambiguities in what is expected of them, deprive them of authority, or reduce their esteem in their own or other eyes are likely to call forth strong anti-change reactions.

There are of course other grounds for resistance, although we believe that the above set constitutes the most potent one. Innovations which violate subunit norms or professional and personal values are next in significance, though in good measure organizational norms and values are the outgrowth of organizational interests; that is, they serve to invest one's interests with moral justification.[26] Other anti-change forces stem from inertia, psychological investments in things-as-they-are, lack of information regarding the problem or the consequences of current policy, fear or uncertainty regarding the outcome of a proposed change, as well as such structural impediments as rules and the law. With the exception of the latter, all of these may constitute relatively tractable anti-change forces. It is a serious diagnostic mistake to assume without sufficient evidence that a proposed change threatens organizational interests since success is almost as endangered by overestimating the opposition as by underestimating it. The appropriate intervention depends of course on the basis of the anti-change position. If it is inertia, the proposed change must be made to appear worth the effort; if it is lack of information, knowledge can be a corrective; if it is fear of the future, time and reassurance may be sufficient. And rules may as often be used to legitimize a worker's position as to oppose it.

For diagnostic and interventive purposes, *who* might oppose a change is as important as *why* it might be resisted. The locus of potential anti-change forces may be inferred by reference to the interests and values of subunits or individuals on which the proposal impinges. Confirmation of the worker's inferences must be done unobtrusively, but is important because it informs him what power resources he may be up against, and therefore the feasability of his proposal, the extent to which he must mobilize counter resources, and what might be his tactic of choice. In efforts of clearly unequal contest, for example, the more the worker will have to accommodate his conceptions to the interests of potential opponents, and the more he will use collaborative tactics such as education and persuasion.[27] Or as put by Wax, the worker will then have to "maintain contact ideologically with the basic values of significant others, or he becomes a psychological outsider or a social deviant, and neither of these roles is conducive to social influence."[28]

Identifying potential anti-change advocates is important on two other practice grounds. First, it will suggest who might be the best initiator of the change idea, for who initiates or argues a proposal has significance for who will oppose or support it. Obviously, for example, a competitive subunit or an untrustworthy source as initiator will hardly endear an idea to those whom one would hope to sway. Second, identifying potential opposition has considerable relevance for the sequence of the process. Apolitical workers believe that their task is to develop a persuasive case and bring it to the closest authority. Those who are more adept will first consider whether there is a need to build support by seeking out natural allies on a particular issue, and if so, will ensure that this support is made evident, however indirectly, as the change idea is considered. In other words, if the worker goes prematurely to a potential anti-change advocate, particularly someone with decision-making responsibility, he may be prevented from going any further by a flat "no." In thus courting instant defeat, he forgoes his chance of developing support, and also relinquishes his opportunity of introducing his idea to other decision-makers or subunits where the climate for its adoption is more auspicious.

Assessing the other interests and values of potential opponents, apart from those directly related to the proposed innovation, is also useful. In conflict situations, overt or covert, an understanding of a target's countervailing interests suggests where pressure may be applied most tellingly. And in collaborative actions, it may indicate the something-of-interest to potential opponents which, in being anticipated, may be included in the change package. Or an exchange may be effected (e.g., "I'll support you on that issue if you support me on this one"). The worker who would influence organizations will have already proferred support or favors to others, knowing that reciprocity is the expected norm.[29] The favors granted yesterday are the credits which can be redeemed tomorrow. Politically speaking, it is better to give than to receive.

One caution needs mention. Although reciprocity is an expected norm, it cannot be invoked in crass commercial terms, for that violates another norm, namely that we act on issues on the basis of merit and put aside extraneous considerations. Thus, if the worker will support a potential opponent on an issue important to the latter in return for his support on some other matter, the "contract" has to be negotiated with indirection, or what in other circumstances is sometimes called "tact."

Finally, the intensity of the anti-change force will determine what resources it will commit to obstruct the change, and therefore what the worker has to contend with.

Although it is difficult to assess anti-change intensity until one is into the process, one means of both exploring and meliorating it is to talk initially only about problems and to avoid any reference to remedies. If there is no common ground on problem definition, the discussion might best be terminated. If common ground is found, however, solutions might then be sounded out, and the worker could elaborate on those suggestions of the other which are compatible with his own projected plans. Or as the worker proffers his own notions, he may revise them if they meet with objection, if accommodation is not unduly costly and he requires the other's support. Finally, if a common solution has evolved from the interaction, the worker can generously give credit where credit may not be due. In other words, he he has to grant the approbation which comes from initiating a good idea to the potential-adversary-turned-sympathetic-supporter. In practice, of course, the process is not as simple as the above makes it sound, but in skeletal form it represents a not uncommon method of persuasion.

We note, in conclusion, that the complexities of increasing worker autonomy and influencing agency procedures and policies have only been suggested in this paper. We have examined three of a number of possible elements in the process, those relating to problem solutions, pro-change forces, and potential opposition. Hopefully though, it has become clear that if social workers are to develop the skill to influence their agencies, if only as minimally as to define their own activity on behalf of clients, they will have to add political consciousness to their clinical outlook.

However halting the worker's first steps may be, they are likely to be steps well-taken. We learn through trial and error and contribute to theory by accumulating experience. Even the awareness of the need for innovation and how it might be accomplished inhibits the ready assumption that things-as-they-are prescribe how things-will-always-be. It is perhaps too much to hope for the "controlled explosion" referred to by one sociologist;[30] that is, that the demand in one sphere of innovation can encourage more general reorganization. But some theorists have observed that the major reason for programs' continuing without change is because the participants do not search for or consider alternate courses.[31]

We conclude with the hope (and it may be a pious one) that social workers will one day come so far that they will have to deal with the new problems and devise the new solutions which will result from their having engaged and solved the old ones, for the process of change is circular.

NOTES

1. For just one example, see Naomi Gottlieb, *The Welfare Bind* (New York: Columbia University Press, 1974). Gottlieb, in her study of the interaction between public welfare staff and welfare rights groups describes some of the ways in which the welfare system dehumanizes both clients *and* staff (pp. 115–22).
2. Harold Goldstein, *Social Work Practice: A Unitary Approach* (Columbia South Carolina: University of South Carolina Press, 1973), p. 88.
3. Charles Grosser, "Community Development Programs Serving the Urban Poor," in Ralph Kramer and Harry Specht, *Readings in Community Organization Practice* (Englewood Cliffs, N.J.: Prentice-Hall, Inc., 1969), p. 297.
4. For two notable exceptions, see Rino J. Patti and Herman Resnick, "Changing the Agency from Within," *Social Work* 17, no. 4 (July 1972); and John Wax, "Power Theory and Institutional Change," *Social Service Review* 45, no. 3 (September 1971).
5. There is a considerable body of useful theory in organizational development, but its major focus is change from the top down.
6. Wamsley and Zald refer to a political system as a structure of rule which has two major components: ethos or values and power. Gary L. Wamsley and Mayer N. Zald, *The Political Economy of Public Organizations* (Lexington, Mass.: Lexington Books, 1973), p. 17.
7. Gottlieb, *Welfare Bind*, p. 130.
8. For an eloquent example of this confusion, see William Schwartz, "Private Troubles and Public Issues: One Job or Two?" *Social Welfare Forum* (New York: Columbia University Press, 1969).
9. Goldstein, *Social Work Practice*, p. 87.
10. We group problem, goal, and solution together for the sake of convenience, largely because the tactical considerations of each are often similar. In reality, however, each recognition of a problem which is acted on generates feedback which amends the problem. This, in turn, influences the goal and how it gets specified, generating further feedback. The new information then tends to further alter the process and may revise the substance of the solution.
11. Some of these are detailed in Gerald Zaltman et al., *Innovations and Organizations* (New York: John Wiley & Sons, 1973), chapter 1.
12. *Ibid.*, p. 36.
14. National Federation of Settlements and Neighborhood Centers, *Making Democracy Work* (New York: NFSNC, 1968), p. 14.
14. The importance of objective reality in shaping perception ought not be underestimated, however, nor should the targets of a change effort, since people ordinarily understand where their short-term interests lie. "Creative" definitions of a problem are unlikely to influence perceptions unless there is ambiguity or ambivalence in the target's position, and transparently guileful arguments adversely affect a worker's credibility.
15. Kurt Lewin, "Group Decision and Social Change," in T. M. Newcomb and E. L. Hartley, eds., *Readings in Social Psychology* (New York: Holt, Rinehart & Winston, 1958).
16. David H. Jenkins, "Force Field Analysis Applied to a School Situation," in Warren G. Bennis et al., eds., *The Planning of Change* (New York: Holt, Rinehart & Winston, 1962), p. 238.

17. Gene W. Dalton, "Influence and Organizational Change," in Gene W. Dalton et al., eds., *Organizational Change and Development* (Homewood, Ill.: Richard D. Irwin and the Dorsey Press, 1970), pp. 234–37.
18. Jenkins, "Force Field Analysis," p. 238.
19. Lawrence Mohr, "Determinants of Innovation in Organizations," *American Political Science Review* 63 (1969).
20. For some examples, see Robert A. Dahl, "The Analysis of Influence in Local Communities," in Charles R. Adrian, ed., *Social Science and Community Action* (East Lansing: Michigan State University Press, 1960), p. 32; and Terry N. Clark, ed., *Community Structure and Decision-Making* (San Francisco: Chandler, 1968).
21. Wax, "Power Theory," p. 278.
22. For a more complete examination of lower ranking resources for influence, see George Brager and Harry Specht, *Community Organizing* (New York: Columbia University Press, 1973), chapters 10 and 11.
23. Bernard M. Bass and George Dunteman, "Biases in the Evaluation of One's Own Group, Its Allies and Opponents," *The Journal of Conflict Resolution* 7, no. 1 (March 1963).
24. Thompson makes this point in *Organizations in Action*.
25. Wamsley and Zald, *Political Economy*, p. 66.
26. Lazarsfeld and Thielens posit that ideology results from self-interest, selective perception, and processes of mutual reinforcement. Paul Lazarsfeld and Walter Thielens, *The Academic Mind* (New York: Free Press, 1958).
27. The range of tactics available to the worker extends from collaborative (problem-solving, education, persuasion), to campaign (political maneuvering, bargaining, mild coercion), to contest or disruptive tactics. Part IV of Brager and Specht, detail these.
28. Wax, "Power Theory," p. 277.
29. Alvin Gouldner, "The Norm of Reciprocity," *American Sociological Review* 25, (1960): 161–78.
30. Cyril Sofer, *Organizations in Theory and Practice* (New York: Basic Books, 1972), p. 302.
31. James March and Herbert Simon, *Organizations* (New York: John Wiley & Sons, 1958), p. 174.

INDEX